W9-APP-026

SALEM HEALTH
CANCER

SALEM HEALTH
CANCER

Second Edition

Volume IV
Procedures
Appendixes

Editors

Michael A. Buratovich, Ph.D.
Spring Arbor University

Laurie Jackson-Grusby, Ph.D.
Children's Hospital Boston, Harvard Medical School

Editor, first edition

Jeffrey A. Knight
Mount Holyoke College

SALEM PRESS
A Division of EBSCO Information Services, Inc.
Ipswich, Massachusetts

GREY HOUSE PUBLISHING

∞ The paper used in these volumes conforms to the American National Standard for Permanence of Paper for Printed Library Materials, Z39.48-1992 (R2009).

Note to Readers

The material presented in *Salem Health: Cancer* is intended for broad informational and educational purposes. Readers who suspect that they or someone whom they know or provide caregiving for suffers from cancer or any other physical or psychological disorder, disease, or condition described in this set should contact a physician without delay; this work should not be used as a substitute for professional medical diagnosis or staging. Readers who are undergoing or about to undergo any treatment or procedure described in this set should refer to their physicians and other health care team members for guidance concerning preparation and possible effects. This set is not to be considered definitive on the covered topics, and readers should remember that the field of health care is characterized by a diversity of medical opinions and constant expansion in knowledge and understanding.

Library of Congress Cataloging-in-Publication Data

Publisher's Cataloging-In-Publication Data
(Prepared by The Donohue Group, Inc.)

Names: Buratovich, Michael A., editor. | Jackson-Grusby, Laurie, editor.
Title: Cancer / editors, Michael A. Buratovich, Ph.D., Spring Arbor University, Laurie Jackson-Grusby, Ph.D., Children's Hospital Boston, Harvard Medical School.
Other Titles: Salem health (Pasadena, Calif.)
Description: Second edition. | Ipswich, Massachusetts: Salem Press, a division of EBSCO Information Services, Inc.; Amenia, NY: Grey House Publishing, [2016] | Editor, first edition, Jeffrey A. Knight, Mount Holyoke College. | Includes bibliographical references and index. | Volume I. Diseases, Symptoms and Conditions: Achlorhydria – Ovarian epithelial cancer – Volume II. Diseases, Symptoms and Conditions: Paget disease of bone – Zollinger-Ellison syndrome, Medical Specialties, Organizations, Social and Personal Issues – Volume III. Cancer Biology, Carcinogens and Suspected Carcinogens, Chemotherapy and Other Drugs, Complementary and Alternative Therapies, Lifestyle and Prevention – Volume IV. Procedures.
Identifiers: ISBN 978-1-61925-950-8 (set) | ISBN 978-1-68217-230-8 (vol. 1) | ISBN 978-1-68217-231-5 (vol. 2) | ISBN 978-1-68217-232-2 (vol. 3) | ISBN 978-1-68217-233-9 (vol. 4)
Subjects: LCSH: Cancer.
Classification: LCC RC265 .C336 2016 | DDC 616.99/4–dc23

First Printing

PRINTED IN THE UNITED STATES OF AMERICA

▶ Contents

Appendixes

▶ Complete List of Contents

Volume 1

Volume 2

Diseases, Symptoms, and Conditions

Medical Specialties

Organizations

Social and Personal Issues

Volume 3

Cancer Biology

Carcinogens and Suspected Carcinogens

Chemotherapy and Other Drugs

Complementary and Alternative Therapies

Lifestyle and Prevention

Volume 4

Procedures

Appendixes

▶ ABCD

Category: Procedures
Also known as: Jewett staging system or the Whitmore-Jewett staging system (for prostate cancer)

Definition: There are two distinct ABCD rating systems for cancer. The first uses the symbols *A*, *B*, *C*, and *D* to define the stages of prostate cancer. The second uses these designations to describe the early warning signs of melanoma, the most serious type of skin cancer.

Cancers monitored: Prostate cancer and melanoma (each with its own distinct ABCD rating)

Why performed: After detecting prostate cancer, the physician will evaluate the stage of the tumor according to its size, its location, and the extent to which it may have spread to other parts of the body. This information is important for choosing the best treatment plan. Staging of prostate cancer is based on the findings of clinical tests, mainly a digital rectal examination, a test to measure the level of prostate-specific antigen (PSA) in the blood, and transrectal ultrasonography.

For melanoma prevention, the American Cancer Society recommends monthly skin self-examinations. The ABCD guideline serves as a reference when looking for any suspicious changes in the appearance of spots or sores that do not heal. Usually, this means monitoring any variation in the size, shape, or color of a mole. Any suspicious mole should be checked by a physician, who may decide to resect an abnormal-looking lesion and send the tissue for pathological review.

Results: The ABCD rating for prostate cancer is used to classify the disease into four basic stages.

- Stage A: Localized disease in which the cancer is very small, confined to the prostate gland, not palpable during a rectal examination, and identified by high PSA levels and biopsy.
- Stage B: Localized disease in which the cancer is larger and confined to the prostate gland, but a lump is palpable during a rectal examination.
- Stage C: Regional disease in which the cancer has grown through the prostate capsule and into surrounding tissues, perhaps into the seminal vesicles.
- Stage D: Metastatic disease in which the cancer has grown into the pelvic area or has spread to the lymph nodes, bones, or other parts of the body.

The ABCD rule for melanoma detection lists the four usual warning signs of the disease for most types of melanoma.

- A (asymmetry): The two halves of the skin lesion are dissimilar.
- B (border irregularity): The lesion has ragged or poorly defined edges.
- C (color): The color of the lesion is uneven with different shades of brown or black.
- D (diameter): The lesion is usually greater than 6 millimeters or 0.25 inch.

Anna Binda, Ph.D.

See also: Melanomas; Moles; Premalignancies; Prostate cancer

▶ Abdominoperineal Resection (APR)

Category: Procedures
Also known as: Abdominoperineal excision, anorectal excision, anoproctectomy

Definition: Abdominoperineal resection (APR) is the surgical removal of the anus, rectum, and surrounding membrane called the mesentery, as well as the lower part of the colon supported by that mesentery. The upper part of the colon is rerouted through a new opening (ostomy) in the lower abdomen, forming an opening called a stoma.

Cancers treated: Low rectal cancer, advanced anal cancer, metastatic pelvic disease

Why performed: APR is performed to remove cancerous tissue, thereby curing or controlling the cancer or relieving symptoms of advanced disease. APR is the preferred procedure for large rectal tumors and tumors near the anal sphincter, but other tumor characteristics and patient-specific factors are also considered.

Patient preparation: A series of medical tests are completed to plan effective treatment and to evaluate the patient's fitness for major surgery. A specialist counsels the patient and helps choose the location for the stoma required by an APR. Radiation therapy, chemotherapy, or both may be recommended before the procedure. Certain patient medications may need to be stopped, the patient's bowel must be cleaned, and the patient's stomach must be empty.

Steps of the procedure: APR is scheduled in a hospital. Sensors are placed to monitor the patient's condition. An intravenous line is started, and an antibiotic is infused.

General anesthetic is administered, and a breathing tube is placed. The patient is positioned, a urinary catheter is inserted, and the incision sites are prepared.

APR is a complex operation requiring incisions first on the abdomen (abdominal resection) and then on the perineum (perineal resection), which may be performed by one or two surgeons. Abdominal resection prepares the lower colon and rectum for removal during the perineal resection and forms the stoma. Perineal resection frees the anus and removes all the diseased tissue. In some instances, the abdominal resection may be performed laparoscopically; however, this approach will remain controversial until long-term studies prove its safety and efficacy for APR.

To begin, the surgeon makes an midline incision in the abdomen large enough to see the tumor and to examine lymph nodes and other organs for metastases. If the tumor is removable, then the procedure continues.

Within the abdomen, rectal blood vessels are tied, and the mesentery is clamped. The lower colon is freed from attachments. The peritoneum is divided, enabling the surgeon to free the rectum. The tied blood vessels and clamped mesentery are divided and sealed. Then, the ostomy opening is made in the abdomen. The colon is divided. The lower end of the colon is covered and tucked below the peritoneum for removal during the perineal resection, and the peritoneum is closed. The upper end of the colon is passed through the ostomy opening, the colon segment is sized to an appropriate length, and the edge of the cut end is folded back and stitched to the abdomen, forming a stoma. Next, other organs are examined for cancer; if other lesions or metastases are found, then they may also be removed. Finally, the abdominal cavity is inspected and cleaned, and the abdominal incision is closed.

On the perineum, the surgeon makes an elliptical incision around the anus. Blood vessels are clamped, then tied as needed. The anus is freed from attachments, including as much surrounding tissue as possible without disturbing major blood vessels, nerves, and healthy organs; however, if the cancer has spread into these structures, then part or all of these structures may be included. The anus is pulled out, as well as the rectum and lower colon freed during the abdominal resection. All tissues are taken to the laboratory for histopathologic evaluation. Finally, the pelvic cavity is inspected and cleaned, and the perineal incision is closed, with a small tube inserted to drain excess fluid.

After the procedure: Anesthetic is stopped, and the breathing tube is removed. The urinary catheter and the intravenous line are kept. A clear collection pouch (ostomy appliance) is fitted over the stoma. The patient is transferred to the recovery room, then to a hospital room. Medications are given to control pain and infection. The patient slowly progresses to a normal diet. The ostomy is monitored; once it starts functioning, the patient learns how to care for the stoma, empty and change pouches, and manage bowel function. At home, the patient follows the physician's instructions about medications, activities, and diet. Further treatment with radiation therapy, chemotherapy, or both may be recommended.

Risks: APR is moderately safe, with low mortality. Risks relate to anesthesia, infection, and inadvertent damage to other structures. Side effects are common because of the complex anatomy and the difficulty of operating within the bony pelvis. The most frequent side effects are urinary dysfunction and infection, perineal infections or bleeding, and ostomy-related problems. Less frequent side effects are male impotence and infertility, abdominal wound infection, and intestinal obstruction.

Results: The long-term outcome varies considerably with patient-specific factors (such as disease stage, overall health, and body characteristics), among medical institutions (as a result of surgical protocol and specialized experience), and with therapeutic combinations. The five-year survival rate has increased as the recurrence rate has decreased because of more complete removal of diseased tissue and more effective therapeutic combinations. Survival is improved significantly by the removal of metastases.

Patricia Boone, Ph.D.

For Further Information

American Cancer Society. *Detailed Guide: Colon and Rectum Cancer Surgery*. Available online at http://www.cancer.org.

American Cancer Society and National Comprehensive Cancer Network. *Colon and Rectal Cancer: Treatment Guidelines for Patients*. Version IV. Atlanta: American Cancer Society, 2005. Available online at http://www.nccn.org.

Levin, Bernard, et al., eds. *American Cancer Society's Complete Guide to Colorectal Cancer*. Atlanta: American Cancer Society, 2006.

See also: Anal cancer; Anoscopy; Appendix cancer; Colectomy; Coloanal anastomosis; Colorectal cancer; Colostomy; Crohn disease; Enterostomal therapy; Ileostomy; Laparoscopy and laparoscopic surgery; Rectal cancer; Sexuality and cancer

▶ Accelerated Partial Breast Irradiation (APBI)

Category: Procedures

Definition: Accelerated partial breast irradiation (APBI) is an alternative to traditional radiation therapy after lumpectomy that can reduce the time of treatment from weeks to days. It is considered an experimental procedure by many doctors.

Cancers treated: Breast cancer

Why performed: Radiation therapy is given after a lumpectomy to kill any cancer cells that remain in the breast. Accelerated partial breast irradiation is an alternative therapy that delivers radiation in a way that reduces the time and number of treatments required. Radiation therapy usually requires visits to the outpatient center or clinic five days a week for six or seven weeks. APBI reduces the amount of time required for treatment to about five days in total.

Patient preparation: Patients who are undergoing accelerated partial breast irradiation treatment are generally enrolled in a clinical trial, because the procedure is still considered experimental. A clinical trial is a carefully controlled study, supervised by doctors who are also researchers, that is designed to investigate the risks or benefits of a new or experimental procedure. Different types of APBIs are being investigated in clinical trials, using different methods and techniques. As a result, the patient preparation for APBI will differ depending on the specifics of the therapy. In general, the preparation for APBI is the same as for any other radiation therapy treatment.

Steps of the procedure: Just as with traditional radiation therapy, the actual time elapsed during a treatment of accelerated partial breast irradiation is usually very short. The time that it takes to get the equipment and patient set up, however, may be significant. First, the patient and the patient's breast are positioned appropriately for the machine. During traditional radiation therapy, the entire breast receives radiation. During APBI, however, the only part of the breast that receives radiation is the area around the lumpectomy site. Therefore, the breast must be positioned very exactly so that the right area receives the radiation. To place the breast in the correct position, the cancer care team may label the breast with marker or tattooing. The patient should check with her cancer care team to see if these marks are temporary.

Once the breast and equipment are correctly positioned, a dose of radiation is given to the breast. Radiation machines deliver beams of high-energy particles to the tissue that destroy cancer cells. Accelerated partial breast irradiation uses amounts of radiation during treatment that are higher than those used by traditional radiation therapy. This is part of the reason that the treatment time of APBI is so short.

After the procedure: After the procedure, the patient may experience fatigue, as well as pain or swelling in the breast. Aftercare depends on the procedure that is used. Patients should discuss aftercare with their cancer care team before the day of the first procedure so that anything needed, such as transportation home after the procedure, can be arranged in advance.

Risks: Some risks are associated with any procedure involving radiation. With an experimental therapy such as APBI, ongoing clinical trials are trying to determine any long-term side effects that may result from the procedure. Most studies, however, have found the risks associated with APBI to be relatively mild, not greater than risks associated with traditional radiation therapy, and decreasing over time.

The most common side effects of APBI are believed to be fatigue, skin changes similar to sunburn in the treated area, swelling in the breast, breast heaviness, and breast discoloration. The creation of small, hard nodes in the breast is also possible. These nodes are not dangerous, but they can occasionally be mistaken for a return of the breast cancer when felt or seen on a mammogram. A very rare but extremely serious possible complication of any radiation to the breast is the development of angiosarcoma, an aggressive form of cancer.

Results: Studies done comparing women who received APBI and those who received traditional radiation therapy after lumpectomy have generally found comparable rates of recurrence, even after many years. Researchers, however, are still conducting more studies and clinical trials. Most studies have been conducted only on very specific groups of women, and more research is being done to study the larger population of women with breast cancer to help determine whether APBI is a technique that could be beneficial to all women, and should be integrated into standard breast cancer treatment practices. The results that any individual woman experiences after APBI will depend on many different factors, including genetics, the type of original cancer, and the size of the original cancer.

Helen Davidson, B.A.

For Further Information

Pasqualini, Jorge R., ed. *Breast Cancer: Prognosis, Treatment, and Prevention.* 2d ed. New York: Informa Healthcare, 2008.

Smith, Terry L. *Breast Cancer: Current and Emerging Trends in Detection and Treatment.* New York: Rosen, 2006.

Torosian, Michael H., ed. *Breast Cancer: A Guide to Detection and Multidisciplinary Therapy.* Totowa, N.J.: Humana Press, 2002.

Winchester, David J., et al. *Breast Cancer.* 2d ed. Hamilton, Ont.: BC Decker, 2006.

See also: Afterloading radiation therapy; Breast cancer in children and adolescents; Breast cancer in men; Breast cancer in pregnant women; Breast cancers; Cutaneous breast cancer; Ductal Carcinoma In Situ (DCIS); Invasive ductal carcinomas; Invasive lobular carcinomas; Lobular Carcinoma In Situ (LCIS); Lumpectomy; Lumps; Mastectomy; Medullary carcinoma of the breast; Radiation therapies; Radiofrequency ablation

▶ Acupuncture and acupressure for cancer patients

Category: Procedures

Also known as: Traditional Chinese medicine (TCM), complementary and alternative medicine (CAM), Oriental medicine (OM)

Definition: Acupuncture is a technique in which hair-thin, sterile, disposable needles of varying lengths are inserted into the skin and muscles at specific anatomical points (called acupoints) in order to treat ailments, including pain and certain diseases. It is one branch of traditional Chinese medicine (TCM) that originated in China around four thousand years ago to prevent, diagnose, and treat diseases in both humans and animals.

Acupressure is a variation of acupuncture, in which therapists or patients press on acupoints with their fingers instead of inserting needles. Only specifically trained, licensed professionals can treat patients using acupuncture needles, but patients can be taught (preferably by a licensed professional) to perform acupressure on themselves. In 1996, the Food and Drug Administration (FDA) approved the acupuncture needle as a medical device. In 1997, the National Institutes of Health (NIH) began evaluating the safety and effectiveness of acupuncture as a complementary and alternative treatment.

According to TCM principles, fourteen meridians are theorized to course invisibly along the body surface, including six paired and two unpaired channels. These meridians correspond to and connect with certain internal organs and physiological systems as understood in both traditional Chinese and Western medicine. Every acupoint is named and numbered according to its location on a specific meridian (for example, P6, or pericardium 6).

Upon needling, the acupuncturist attempts to unblock, move, or alter what TCM refers to as the qi or chi (pronounced "chee") of the body. This qi is a vital force that is thought to flow along the meridians and throughout the body and organ systems. TCM posits that qi is formed from a merging of yin and yang, which are opposite energy states that permeate the universe. An imbalance of yin and yang in the body is thought to lead to a disruption of qi, leading to disharmony in physical and psychic well-being and thus to certain ailments or diseases. The acupuncturist (or acupressure practitioner) tries to restore a healthier balance of yin and yang in the patient. Many Western and Eastern acupuncturists currently blend TCM theory with modern understanding of neuroanatomy and the immune and other physiological systems.

Cancers diagnosed or treated: In Western cancer management, acupuncture and acupressure are primarily used to mitigate the side effects related to conventional cancer treatments such as chemotherapy, radiation treatment, and surgery, or side effects of the disease itself. These side effects include chemotherapy-related nausea and vomiting, dyspnea (shortness of breath in advanced cancer cases), pain (either from a conventional treatment or the cancer itself), fatigue, depression, vasomotor symptoms (hot flashes), and treatment- or cancer-related immunosuppression. In most instances, the acupuncture or acupressure interventions are used in addition to state-of-the-art pharmaceutical treatments, such as antiemetic therapy (such as Odansetron) for nausea and vomiting.

Why performed: Cancer patients and their clinicians often resort to acupuncture and acupressure (and other alternative medical treatment modalities) for symptoms that are not amenable or are unresponsive to traditional therapies. Sometimes they are used to augment the effectiveness of conventional medicines, as in the case of antiemetic therapies for nausea and vomiting, which can lead to weight loss and depression.

Some patients (and their clinicians) are seeking a more holistic approach to healing, viewing acupuncture and acupressure as methods that restore harmony to the body, treating the whole person instead of just the disease. Often patients take solace in the "mysterious" mechanisms underlying alternative treatments. Many acupuncturists are intrigued by the TCM philosophies and theories, at the same time applying current Western knowledge of anatomy and neurophysiology to their techniques. Most acupoints correspond to specific nerve pathways or receptors and/or highly vascular areas. There is strong evidence that acupuncture modulates neurotransmitters, leading to the release of endogenous opioids (endorphins and enkephalins) for analgesia (pain relief). Manipulation of certain acupoints stimulates the autonomic nervous system, leading to changes in blood circulation and engaging components of the immune and endocrine systems (proteins called cytokines or the release of endogenous corticosteroids and other hormones). These procedures can also alter blood pressure, heart rhythms, and body temperature. Not all the mechanisms involved in successful acupuncture and acupressure treatment are understood, and they remain a subject of scientific investigation. Some skeptics still believe that they work primarily via the placebo effect.

Patient preparation: Very little patient preparation is required for these procedures. The patient disrobes to the extent required for examination and the placement of acupuncture needles or accessibility to acupressure points. Some acupuncturists will take a patient's medical history and ask questions about diet and exercise. Some will also look at the patient's tongue and feel his or her pulse in order to make a TCM diagnosis and appropriate acupoint prescription tailored to the patient's needs. A more Westernized approach would be to apply a standard point prescription for a particular malady, omitting such TCM elements as tongue and pulse exams.

Steps of the procedure: The acupuncturist will feel for the appropriate acupoints, often massaging the area prior to needle insertion. The skin is then cleaned with an alcohol wipe and the needle is inserted until the practitioner feels some resistance and/or the patient feels a tingling or cramping sensation. This is referred to as "obtaining the qi," or *De Qi*. Many practitioners then manipulate the needle, using hand technique (*shou fa*) to move, supplement or drain the qi and/or yin and yang. The needles are then usually left in place for ten to twenty minutes.

In acupressure, the patient or practitioner applies pressure to the acupoints for a few minutes, repeating this action at intermittent intervals over a specified period of time. Sometimes a band with an attached stud is applied over an acupoint and the patient is instructed to press the stud into the point at prescribed intervals in an effort to obtain a *De Qi* response during point stimulation.

Sometimes an acupuncturist will apply a small electric current to the needles in a technique called electroacupuncture. This is another method of stimulating the acupoints. Various other methods of stimulation are employed as well. Moxibustion applies heat to the acupoints using burning mugwort herb (*Artemisia vulgaris*). Aquapuncture is a technique in which acupoints are injected with drugs, vitamins, flower essences, herbal extracts, or other fluids for longer-term stimulation of acupoints.

After the procedure: A properly treated patient should experience relaxation, deeper respiration, and increased vitality following acupuncture, since energetic balance has supposedly been restored. For treatment of specific cancer-related symptoms, some immediate relief is expected, followed by delayed improvement, especially after multiple acupuncture or acupressure sessions.

Risks: Acupuncture should be avoided in patients with thromobocytopenia or aplasia or in those treated with

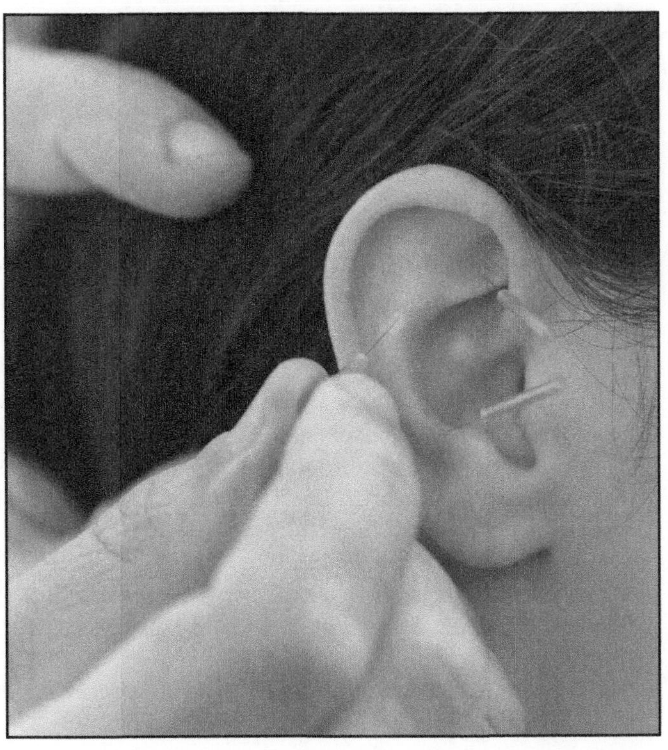

A patient receives an acupuncture treatment. (iStock)

anticoagulants. Some common side effects are bruising, local bleeding, and mild pain in the treated areas. The risk of infection is small if sterile, disposable needles are used. There is a very small risk that the lungs or other internal organs can be punctured if a needle is placed too deep.

Results: The results of many random, controlled clinical trials have demonstrated that acupuncture is effective for reducing episodes of acute vomiting following chemotherapy for breast and other cancers. The same and other studies have shown that acupressure at certain acupoints is effective for reducing episodes of acute nausea following chemotherapy. Both acupuncture and acupressure have been more effective for prophylactic treatment of vomiting and nausea following conventional cancer treatment rather than stopping these symptoms once they have started. One study indicated that the effectiveness of acupuncture for reducing vomiting episodes following chemotherapy was increased for up to twenty-four hours when acupressure followed needling therapy.

One review of acupuncture for the relief of cancer-related pain found that ear acupuncture (stimulation of acupoints corresponding to different body areas on the ear) was effective for reducing cancer-related pain. Other clinical trials have shown that acupuncture helps reduce the number of hot flashes in men being treated with hormones or surgery for prostate cancer and women being treated with tamoxifen or related hormone therapies for breast cancer. Investigators, however, have noted a dearth of random, double-blind, controlled clinical trials for proving the effectiveness of these alternative therapies. The development of a sham acupuncture needle (the needle withdraws into the shaft upon "insertion" at true acupoints) is expected to improve the rigorousness of these trials and to provide substantive evidence for or against acupuncture-related therapies.

Lisa J. Shientag, V.M.D.

For Further Information

Ezzo, J. M., M. A. Richardson, and A. Vickers. "Acupuncture Point Stimulation for Chemotherapy-Induced Nausea or Vomiting." *The Cochrane Database of Systematic Reviews* 2 (2007).

Hyangsook, L., K. Schmidt, and E. Ernst. "Acupuncture for the Relief of Cancer-Related Pain: A Systematic Review." *European Journal of Pain* 9, no. 4 (August, 2005): 437-444.

Sagar, Stephen M. *Restored Harmony: An Evidence Based Approach for Integrating Traditional Chinese Medicine into Complementary Cancer Care.* Hamilton, Ont.: Dreaming DragonFly Communications, 2001.

See also: Bone cancers; Bone pain; Complementary and alternative therapies; Home health services; Integrative oncology; Living with cancer; Pneumonia; Side effects; Smoking cessation

▶ Adjuvant therapy

Category: Procedures

Definition: An adjuvant therapy is any treatment given after the primary treatment to increase the likelihood of killing all cancer cells.

Cancers treated: Many types, including cancers of the breast, colon, kidney, ovary, and testicle

Why performed: After the primary treatment removes or kills a detected primary tumor, additional cancerous cells or microtumors may still be present in the body. Adjuvant therapy may be administered to help prevent the recurrence of cancer after the primary tumor is removed. Generally, the larger the primary tumor size at detection, the larger is the probability that residual cancer cells may be left behind following surgery. Cancer cells can break away from the primary tumor and metastasize even when the disease is in an early stage, and they exist in a form too small to detect by radiological or laboratory testing.

Patient preparation: In the decision regarding whether to undergo adjuvant therapy, a number of prognostic factors enter into the determination, such as patient age, size of primary tumor, spread to lymph nodes, and microscopic appearance of the cancer cells. Doctors consider these factors and others in order to estimate the likelihood of recurrence. The higher the risk for recurrence, the greater is the motivation to pursue adjuvant therapy options. Local adjuvant radiation treatment typically commences about three to six weeks following the primary treatment. If a combination of chemotherapy and radiotherapy as adjuvant therapy is chosen, then usually chemotherapy is received first followed by radiation, although they may be administered simultaneously in some cases. It is not known how effective adjuvant therapy may be if started later than six weeks following primary therapy.

Steps of the procedure: The term "adjuvant therapy" actually encompasses many different treatment forms, including chemotherapy, radiation, hormonal therapy, targeted therapy, or some combination thereof. Adjuvant therapy can be either systemic or local. Chemotherapy, for instance, is given by mouth or injected into the bloodstream. Adjuvant chemotherapy is administered in cycles of treatment followed by recovery and typically lasts for three to six months. Side effects from adjuvant therapy such as chemotherapy or radiation may be experienced. For example, the effects of adjuvant chemotherapy may include loss of hair, loss of appetite, vomiting, diarrhea, mouth sores, psychological distress, and some loss of cognitive brain function. Medications are available to help control vomiting and nausea induced by chemotherapy. Researchers at the University of Rochester have reported that treatment with modafinil (Provigil) can alleviate the cognitive symptoms of so-called chemo brain experienced in certain cancer treatment regimens. Longer-term side effects may include infertility.

Another example of adjuvant therapy is hormone adjuvant therapy to treat breast cancer. Hormone adjuvant therapy is used on breast cancer cells that have been found to be estrogen or progesterone receptor positive. Some standard hormone therapies include the synthetic hormone tamoxifen and aromatase inhibitors. Tamoxifen as an adjuvant therapy has been found to decrease the chance of recurrence in women with early-stage hormone receptor positive breast cancer. It is also used to treat women who are at risk of one day developing breast cancer. Aromatase inhibitors are used as adjuvants to reduce the levels of estrogen in postmenopausal women; they include anastrozole (Arimidex), exemestane (Aromasin), and letrozole (Femara). These drugs are not to be used by premenopausal women. Combination adjuvant therapies comprising hormone treatment together with chemotherapy are also available for some patients.

After the procedure: It is advised that patients undergo regular checkups following adjuvant therapy in order to monitor any cancer recurrence. Hormone adjuvant therapy, such as used to treat some forms of breast cancer, involves longer-term procedures, with five-year regimens recommended.

Risks: The risks associated with different forms of adjuvant therapy are similar to the risks of corresponding primary treatments with chemotherapy, radiotherapy, or hormone therapy. The main risk of declining to participate in adjuvant therapy is the possibility of cancer cells spreading undetected to other parts of the body. While patients with invasive cancers are often urged to consider undergoing adjuvant therapy, other options are available. Patients who turn down the option of adjuvant therapy are advised to participate in regular follow-up clinical examinations to facilitate the detection of new tumors. This alternative is often referred to as "watchful waiting." Some of the side effects of hormone adjuvant therapy mimick the symptoms of menopause, such as hot flashes and an increased risk for the development of osteoporosis.

Results: The goal of adjuvant therapy is to make primary treatment more effective and result in years of disease-free survival. Successful adjuvant therapy is marked by a lack of detectable tumor recurrence or metastasis formation in the months and years following primary therapy.

Michael R. King, Ph.D.

For Further Information

Henderson, I. Craig, ed. *Adjuvant Therapy of Breast Cancer*. Boston: Kluwer Academic, 1992.

Kirkwood, John M., ed. *Strategies in Adjuvant Therapy*. Malden, Mass.: Blackwell, 2000.

Murphy, Kevin. *Adjuvant Chemotherapy Guide*. Available online at http://www.cancerguide.org.

Salmon, Charles G. *Adjuvant Therapy of Cancer*. Philadelphia: Lippincott Williams & Wilkins, 1993.

Other Resources

Mayo Clinic

Adjuvant Therapy for Breast Cancer Guide
http://www.MayoClinic.com

National Cancer Institute

http://www.cancer.gov

See also: Biological therapy; Chemotherapy; Hormonal therapies; Pain management medications; Radiation therapies; Watchful waiting

▶ Afterloading radiation therapy

Category: Procedures

Also known as: High dose rate remote afterloading (HDR)

Definition: Afterloading radiation therapy is a form of high dose rate brachytherapy that uses a computer-controlled machine called an afterloader to deliver radiation from iridium 192 directly to a tumor. Iridium 192 is a radioactive source that emits high-energy gamma rays, a type of radiation that is used to kill cancer cells. The radioactive source is contained in the lead-shielded machine and welded to a stainless steel cable that is inserted into the tumor through catheters, needles, or balloons placed in the tumor or tumor bed. Afterloading radiation therapy is considered a temporary implant because the radioactive source does not remain in the patient, and the patient is not radioactive.

Cancers treated: Lung cancer, breast cancer, prostate cancer, head and neck cancers, uterine cancer, cervical cancer, esophageal and bile duct cancers, soft-tissue sarcoma, rectal cancer, others under study

Why performed: The use of a high-dose remote afterloader provides more targeted therapy to the tumor, or to the tumor bed after the bulk of the tumor is removed in surgery. The afterloader provides more accurate dose delivery to the target site while better protecting normal tissue. Its use also provides a shorter course of therapy of approximately one week, as compared to external beam radiation therapy, which takes place over four to six weeks. The dose distribution is more even, and there are fewer hot (overdose) spots or cold (underdose) spots. Side effects occur less often with HDR therapy.

Patient preparation: Planning for the use of afterloading radiation therapy often begins before an initial surgery, depending on the type of cancer and its site. The surgeon and the radiation oncologist will confer, as the catheters used in administering the radiation may be placed at the time of the initial surgery for the cancer. Catheters or needles may also be placed in an outpatient setting under local anesthesia or other sedation.

Imaging or radiology studies may be used to assist in treatment planning for the optimal radiation dose delivery to the tumor site and to verify the location of the catheters, especially if it has been a few weeks since their placement. A simulation is done to visualize the tumor or tumor site in comparison to adjacent organs and tissues using a computed tomography (CT) scan or X ray. This procedure assists the radiation oncologist in planning the amount of dose that the afterloader will deliver. The simulation data are then loaded into a treatment-planning computer, which calculates the dose needed.

Steps of the procedure: The patient arrives in the radiation oncology center and may change into a gown prior to receiving treatment. For some prostate treatments, needles may be placed prior to the treatment under local anesthesia. Upon entering the treatment room, the patient is assisted to a comfortable position that also allows access to the ends of the catheters or needles. The treatment catheters or needles from the patient are attached to the transfer tubes from the afterloader. The treatment personnel leave the room but can observe the patient using closed-circuit television and an intercom for communication. The treatment data loaded into the HDR unit control the movement of the source into the patient and the time that the source remains at various stops along the catheters or needles in order to achieve the distribution of dose planned. The source is placed in the patient for approximately ten to fifteen minutes, but a single treatment may take up to one hour or more.

The complexity of the treatment, the site being treated, and the strength of the radioactive source will dictate the time involved. The radiation oncologist will discuss the number of treatments needed based on the disease, but treatment times vary from a few days to slightly more than a week.

After the procedure: Depending on the site being treated, the patient may need to stay in the hospital or may be allowed to go home between treatments. A bandage may be placed over the catheters. After all treatments are complete, the catheters are removed by clipping the sutures holding the catheters, and they are withdrawn. A small amount of bleeding may occur, but it is quickly controlled with direct pressure, and a bandage is applied over the site.

Risks: Risks are related to catheter movement out of the site being treated. It is important for patients to tell the radiation staff if a catheter seems to have moved, or if it gets snagged on clothing or the bandage at any time. A misplaced catheter or needle may deliver radiation to normal tissues or organs, causing radiation burns. There is a risk that cancer cells may be missed by the radiation.

Results: Outcomes vary by the disease being treated, but success rates for HDR treatments are comparable to other forms of treatment in most instances.

Patricia Stanfill Edens, R.N., Ph.D., FACHE

For Further Information

Hoskin, P. J., and P. Bownes. "Innovative Technologies in Radiation Therapy: Brachytherapy." *Seminars in Radiation Oncology* 16, no. 4 (October, 2006): 209-217.

Hoskin, P. J., K. Motohashi, P. Bownes, L. Bryant, and P. Ostler. "High Dose Rate Brachytherapy in Combination with External Beam Radiotherapy in the Radical Treatment of Prostate Cancer: Initial Results of a Randomized Phase Three Trial." *Radiotherapy & Oncology* 84, no. 2 (August, 2007): 114-120.

National Cancer Institute. *Radiotherapy and You: Support for People with Cancer*. Available online at http://www.cancer.gov/cancertopics/radiation-therapy-and-you.

Other Resources

American Cancer Society
http://www.cancer.org

American Society for Therapeutic Radiology and Oncology
Patient Web Site
http://www.rtanswers.org

See also: Brachytherapy; Cobalt 60 radiation; External Beam Radiation Therapy (EBRT); Intensity-Modulated Radiation Therapy (IMRT); Iridium seeds; Proton beam therapy; Radiation therapies; Radiofrequency ablation; Stereotactic Radiosurgery (SRS)

▶ Alkaline Phosphatase Test (ALP)

Category: Procedures
Also known as: ALKP, alk phos, alkaline phosphatase total

Definition: Alkaline phosphatase (ALP) is an enzyme that helps in the process of digestion and bone development. All tissues contain ALP. Higher concentrations are found in the liver, bone, kidney, and intestines. Various processes within the tissues release ALP into the blood. By measuring ALP blood levels, doctors can determine the presence of liver and bone disease, including cancer. ALP levels are determined by testing serum or plasma on an automated chemistry analyzer.

Cancers diagnosed: Cancers of the bone, renal cells, liver, gallbladder, and bile ducts

Why performed: The test is done as a part of a chemistry or liver panel to detect liver or bone disease. Once a diagnosis has been made and treatment started, the test may be done to determine if treatment is effective or if disease has progressed or returned.

Patient preparation: The patient may be asked not to eat or drink or take certain medications for six to twelve hours prior to the test.

Steps of the procedure: A small sample of blood is collected from a vein and placed in a tube. In children, blood may be obtained from a capillary in the heel or finger.

After the procedure: A small gauze or cotton ball is applied at the site of needle insertion. The patient is asked to apply pressure. The person collecting the blood observes the site for bleeding and may apply a bandage. The bandage may usually be removed in thirty to sixty minutes.

Risks: Risks from the procedure include bleeding, bruising, hematoma (bleeding under the skin), fainting, light-headedness, or the need for multiple needle sticks to obtain a sample.

Results: Normal ALP levels vary by the patient's sex and age and by the analyzer used. Each laboratory establishes a set of normal ranges based on this information. The physician receives a report of the test results with the normal values established by the testing laboratory.

Elevated levels indicate the possibility of liver or bone disease, including the presence of a tumor. The test does not distinguish from which tissue the increased amount of alkaline phosphatase comes. The physician may order other blood tests, including an alkaline phosphatase isoenzyme test that determines if the increased ALP comes from bone, liver, or intestine. Other procedures such as X rays may also be ordered. Following cancer treatment, ALP levels are expected to decrease. If levels remain high or increase, then some cancer may remain or has returned.

Wanda E. Clark, M.T. (ASCP)

See also: Immunocytochemistry and immunohistochemistry; Paget disease of bone; Placental alkaline phosphatase (PALP)

▶ Alpha-Fetoprotein (AFP) levels

Category: Procedures
Also known as: Total AFP, AFP-13 percent, alpha-fetoglobulin, αFP, AFP tumor marker

Definition: Alpha fetoprotein (AFP) is a protein produced by fetal tissue and by tumors. There are several forms of AFP. The test for AFP generally measures total AFP. The test is performed on serum or plasma on an automated chemistry analyzer.

Cancers diagnosed: Cancers of the liver, testes, and ovaries

Why performed: The AFP test is done to detect and monitor cancers of the liver, testes, and ovaries. Physicians may order the test for patients with chronic liver disease because of the high risk of developing liver cancer. Because AFP is also produced by a fetus, AFP levels are generally higher in pregnant women. A test for AFP done on pregnant women is not done to detect a tumor but is used with other data to detect possible abnormalities in the developing fetus.

Patient preparation: No special preparation is necessary.

Steps of the procedure: A small sample of blood is collected from a vein and placed in a tube. In children, blood may be obtained from a capillary in the heel or finger.

After the procedure: A small gauze or cotton ball is applied at the site of needle insertion. The patient is asked to apply pressure. The person collecting the blood observes the site for bleeding and may apply a bandage. The bandage may usually be removed in thirty to sixty minutes.

Risks: Risks include bleeding, bruising, hematoma (bleeding under the skin), fainting, light-headedness, or the need for multiple needle sticks to obtain a sample.

Results: Normal AFP levels vary by the patient's sex and age and by the analyzer used. Each laboratory establishes normal ranges based on this information. The physician receives a report of the test results with the normal values established by the testing laboratory.

AFP decreases at birth, and adult levels are normally low. Elevated levels are present in liver cancer and in some cancers of the testes and ovaries. Generally, higher levels of AFP indicate a larger tumor. The test is not considered specific for diagnosis, but it is an indicator that a tumor may be present. Physicians may order imaging studies and additional laboratory tests to determine the presence of a tumor. Some physicians order a test called AFP-13 percent, as 13 is one of the forms of AFP that make up the total. An increased percentage of AFP-13 to total AFP indicates an increased risk of developing liver cancer or a poorer prognosis. AFP levels usually return to normal within a month of treatment.

Wanda E. Clark, M.T. (ASCP)

See also: Ataxia Telangiectasia (AT); Beckwith-Wiedemann Syndrome (BWS); Germ-cell tumors; Pathology; Placental alkaline phosphatase (PALP); Proteomics and cancer research; Testicular cancer; Yolk sac carcinomas

▶ Amputation

Category: Procedures

Definition: Surgical removal of all or part of a limb as a result of peripheral vascular disease, trauma, tumor, infection, or congenital anomaly.

Cancers treated: Soft-issue neoplasias (malignant fibrous histiocytoma, fibrosarcoma, rhabdomyosarcoma, synovial sarcoma); bone malignancies (osteosarcoma, chondrosarcoma, adamantinoma, Ewing sarcoma)

Why performed: Amputations are performed to remove extremities that are severely diseased, injured, or no longer functional. Amputation has five goals: removal of all diseased tissue; relief of pain; proper wound healing; prevention of metastatic spread of tumor cells; and construction of a stump that will permit useful function. Amputation as a musculoskeletal procedure is often accomplished as an alternative to limb salvage and should be considered a reconstructive maneuver. Because of the psychological implications and the alteration of body self-image with amputation, a multidisciplinary team approach should be taken to return the patient to a maximum level of independent function. The process should be considered the first step in the rehabilitation of the patient rather than a failure of treatment.

Epidemiologic data on the incidence of amputation in the United States from 1993 to 2003 show that the number of lower-extremity amputations increased 14 percent, from 99,522 to 123,379 cases. Average hospital charge for this procedure increased 40 percent, from $24,332 to $34,046. Nearly two-thirds of amputations are performed in individuals with diabetes, even though these individuals represent only 6 percent of the entire population.

Patient preparation: Amputation and subsequent healing depend on several factors, including vascular inflow, nutrition, and an adequate immune system. Prior to surgery, patients should be evaluated regarding these parameters. Patients with malnutrition or immune deficiency have a high rate of wound breakdown or infection. A serum albumin level below 3.5 grams per deciliter (g/dl) indicates a malnourished patient. An absolute lymphocyte count below 1,500 cubic millimeters is a sign of immune deficiency. If possible, amputation should be delayed in patients until these values can be improved by nutritional support. In severely affected patients, nasogastric or percutaneous gastric feeding tubes are necessary.

Oxygenated blood is a prerequisite for wound healing. A hemoglobin level of more than 10 g/dl is required.

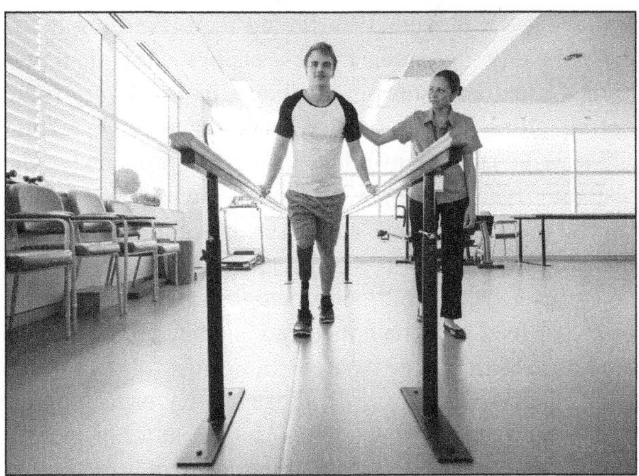

Treatment of some cancers involves amputation, which requires the patient to learn new living skills. (iStock)

Doppler ultrasonography has been used to measure vascular inflow and to predict the success of wound healing. An absolute Doppler pressure of 70 millimeters of mercury (mm Hg) and an ischemic index of 0.5 or greater are necessary at the surgical site. The transcutaneous partial pressure of oxygen (Tcp02) is now regarded as the gold standard in the measurement of vascular inflow. Values greater than 40 mm Hg correlate with acceptable healing rates.

Steps of the procedure: With regard to tumor stage and desired functional outcome, there are a variety of surgical procedures pertaining to upper-limb, lower-extremity, or axial skeletal amputation. Patients with musculoskeletal neoplasms face new choices in treatment with the development of limb salvage techniques and adjuvant chemotherapy and radiation therapy. If an amputation is chosen, then the incision must be planned carefully to achieve the appropriate surgical margin. These surgical margins are characterized by the relationship of the surgical incision to the lesion, to the inflammatory zone surrounding the lesion, and to the anatomic compartment in which the lesion is located. The four types of surgical margins include the following:

- intralesional: the surgical incision enters the lesion
- marginal: the surgical incision enters the inflammatory zone but not the lesion
- wide margin: the incision enters the same anatomic compartment of the lesion but is outside the inflammatory zone
- radical: the incision remains outside the anatomic compartment

After the procedure: A variety of wound care methods are used after amputation, including rigid dressings, soft dressings, controlled environment chambers, air splints, and skin traction. The use of an immediate postoperative prosthesis (IPOP) has been shown to be effective in decreasing the time to limb maturation and definitive prosthetic fitting. Rehabilitation and prosthetic fitting remain the primary postoperative goals.

Risks: The amputee is at risk for deep vein thrombosis (15 percent) and pulmonary embolism (2 percent). Prolonged postoperative immobilization, stagnation of blood due to ligation of large veins, delayed prosthetic fitting, and inactivity increase the overall risk of thromboembolism (clot). Approximately 80 to 90 percent of amputees experience some episodes of phantom limb pain, which are often severe but infrequent. Other major complications include failure of wound healing, infection, postoperative edema, joint contractures, and dermatological problems such as skin irritation as a result of improper prosthetic fit, breakdown over stump margins, and episodes of contact dermatitis.

Results: There is an ongoing controversy when comparing limb salvage to amputation with regard to energy expenditure to ambulate, quality-of-life measures, and the performance of activities of daily living. Studies suggest that functional outcomes are comparable with either limb salvage or amputation. Overall survival remains comparable with either treatment.

With some tumors, amputation may achieve better local disease control. Both treatment groups report quality-of-life problems involving employment, health insurance, social isolation, and poor self-esteem.

John L. Zeller, M.D., Ph.D.

For Further Information

Bone, M., P. Critchley, and D. Buggy. "Gabapentin in Postamputation Phantom Limb Pain: A Randomized, Double-Blind Placebo-Controlled, Cross-Over Study." *Regional Anesthesia and Pain Medicine* 27, no. 5 (2002): 481.

Doherty, Gerard M., and Lawrence W. Way, eds. *Current Surgical Diagnosis and Treatment*. 12th ed. New York: Lange Medical Books/McGraw-Hill, 2006.

Menendez, L. R., ed. *Orthopaedic Knowledge Update: Musculoskeletal Tumors*. Rosemont, Ill.: American Academy of Orthopedic Surgeons, 2002.

Peabody, T. D., et al. "Evaluation and Staging of Musculoskeletal Neoplasms." *The Journal of Bone and Joint Surgery: American Volume* 80, no. 8 (1998): 1204.

Skinner, Harry B., ed. *Current Diagnosis and Treatment in Orthopedics*. 4th ed. New York: Lange Medical Books/McGraw-Hill, 2006.

Other Resources

American Academy of Orthopedic Surgeons
http://www.aaos.org

American College of Surgeons
http://www.acs.org

See also: Bone cancers; Fibrosarcomas, soft-tissue; Hyperthermic perfusion; Juvenile polyposis syndrome; Limb salvage; Liposarcomas; Lymphangiosarcomas; Mastectomy; Neuroectodermal tumors; Occupational therapy; Orthopedic surgery; Sarcomas, soft-tissue; Surgical oncology; Synovial sarcomas; Veterinary oncology

▶ Angiography

Category: Procedures
Also known as: Arteriography, angiogram, arteriogram

Definition: Angiography is a general term for a minimally invasive imaging technique that uses real-time X rays and a special dye to see inside blood vessels, lymph nodes, and certain glands deep inside the body. The dye, known as a contrast medium, is injected into the body to highlight the vessels, lymph nodes, glands—and cancerous tumors—and make them easier to see. The contrast medium is a low-dose radioactive compound known as a radioisotope. The image created by the X ray is called an angiogram.

Cancers diagnosed or treated: Cancers of the lymphatic system, the digestive system, the lungs, the brain, and certain glands

Why performed: Doctors use angiography to detect and directly examine cancerous tumors and to show the blood flow to a tumor. A direct real-time view of a tumor and blood flow helps doctors diagnose and treat the cancer. With angiography, doctors can determine a tumor's size, appearance, and relationship to nearby organs and tissues; whether the tumor is growing or extending into nearby parts of the body; and whether cancer cells are spreading to other parts of the body. In some cases, doctors use the procedure to deliver medicine to a tumor.

Patient preparation: Patient preparation varies slightly depending on the part of the body to be examined and whether the patient is already in the hospital (inpatient) or having the procedure done and then returning home the same day (outpatient). Nurses help the inpatient prepare. Outpatients stay several hours in a recovery room before going home. Most outpatients receive a mild sedative to help them relax during the procedure. The test may take up to several hours. Generally, patients should not eat or drink anything for eight hours before the procedure.

Patients should tell their doctors if they are pregnant or breast-feeding; which medications they are taking, including aspirin; if they have any bleeding problems or are taking blood-thinning medications; if they have allergies to any substances or medications; if they suffer from asthma; if they have a history of kidney problems or diabetes; if they have blockage of the blood vessels caused by atherosclerosis (hardening of the arteries), high blood pressure, or aging; and if they think they will find it difficult to lie still during the procedure.

Steps of the procedure: A team of technicians and nurses led by a radiologist (a doctor who diagnoses diseases by studying X rays and other images) conducts the procedure. The procedure takes place in the radiology laboratory of a medical center. The patient wears a hospital gown and receives a mild sedative but remains awake. The patient lies supine on a table much like an operating table.

The surgeon makes a small incision near a blood vessel in the neck, chest, groin, or arm. Using real-time X rays displayed on a video screen for guidance, the surgeon then inserts a thin, flexible tube called a catheter into the vessel. The surgeon guides the catheter through the blood vessels until the tip reaches the area to be studied. Once the catheter is placed in the exact spot, the radiologist injects the dye. The dye travels through the catheter and to the blood vessels, making the target easier to see in the X ray. A round cylinder or rectangular box, known as a fluoroscope, takes the pictures. It moves both above and beneath the patient.

After the procedure: After the test, a nurse applies a pressure bandage at the site where the catheter was inserted. Some patients feel tenderness or soreness at the site. Depending on where the catheter was inserted, the patient may have to remain in bed—in the hospital or at home—from several hours up to a day. The patient receives pain medicine if needed.

Some people experience a headache, flushing of the face, or a salty or metallic taste in the mouth after the dye is inserted, but these feelings disappear quickly. Doctors generally recommend that patients drink extra fluids to help pass the dye from the body.

Risks: Angiography is a very common test. Both the X ray and the dye are safe. The exposure to radiation is low. There are, nevertheless, some small risks. There is a remote chance that a person may react to the contrast agent, or dye. Common contrast agents are iodine, barium, and gadolinium. In addition, patients may feel a slight burning sensation when the doctor injects the dye or some discomfort at the site where the catheter is inserted. Patients do not feel the catheter inside the body. There is a small risk of bleeding, pain, or infection at the site where the catheter is inserted.

Results: The angiogram shows that there are no problems if the dye flows smoothly through the blood vessels and no tumors appear in the lymph nodes or glands studied. If the angiogram reveals that blood vessels are not in their normal position or the blood is flowing in an abnormal pattern, then a tumor may be present. Doctors will then conduct additional tests.

Wendell Anderson, B.A.

For Further Information

Icon Health. *Angiogram: A Medical Dictionary, Bibliography, and Annotated Research Guide to Internet References.* San Diego, Calif.: Author, 2004.

Pagana, Kathleen Deska, and Timothy J. Pagana. *Mosby's Manual of Diagnostic and Laboratory Tests.* 3d ed. St. Louis: Mosby Elsevier, 2006.

Welch, H. G. *Should I Be Tested for Cancer? Maybe Not and Here's Why.* Berkeley: University of California Press, 2004.

See also: Bile duct cancer; Chemoembolization; Embolization; Endocrinology oncology; Exenteration; Eye cancers; Gallbladder cancer; Hemangioblastomas; Hematemesis; Hemoptysis; Imaging tests; Lymphadenectomy; Lymphangiography; Pancreatic cancers; Percutaneous Transhepatic Cholangiography (PTHC); Testicular cancer; X-ray tests

▶ Anoscopy

Category: Procedures

Definition: Anoscopy is the examination of the anus, anal canal, and lower end of the rectum with an endoscope.

Cancers diagnosed: Anal cancer, rectal cancer, cancer of an unknown primary site

Why performed: Anoscopy is a diagnostic procedure to evaluate the presence of hemorrhoids, anal fissures, abscess, inflammation, tumors (malignant and benign), foreign bodies, infection such as condyloma or warts caused by human papillomaviruses (HPV), and anal squamous skin lesions associated with the human immunodeficiency virus (HIV).

Patient preparation: The patient is instructed to clear stool from the rectal vault. A laxative, enema, or other preparation may be necessary for complete emptying of the rectum. For pediatric patients, their parents should be counseled on proper preparations for the procedure so that the patients' anxiety may be reduced. In emergency cases, preparation for the procedure may not be possible.

Steps of the procedure: The patient is asked to use a medical examination gown and to remove underwear. The position during the examination is either bending forward over the examining table or lying on the examination table on the patient's left or right side with both lower limbs drawn up to the chest. The doctor performs a digital rectal examination wherein a gloved, lubricated index finger is inserted into the rectum to check for abnormalities and structures that can block visualization; the prostate is also examined in male patients. The external area of the anus is examined prior to the anoscope insertion. The doctor then uses the anoscope, a tubular instrument with a light source, to view the anus, anal canal, and lower rectum. The anoscope is lubricated prior to its insertion into the anus and anal canal; the patient may be asked to "bear down" during the insertion, as during a bowel movement. During the procedure, the patient may feel some pressure and the urge to defecate. A biopsy may be obtained during the procedure, as needed. The doctor slowly withdraws the anoscope as the anal canal is viewed carefully.

After the procedure: Patients can return to normal activities. If a biopsy was taken, then the patient may be instructed to have a sitz bath daily to relieve mild pain.

Risks: No significant risk is associated with anoscopy. A small amount of bleeding and mild pain may occur if the patient has hemorrhoids or if a biopsy was obtained.

Results: Normal results will show no structural or color abnormalities. Abnormal findings include hemorrhoids, fissures, infections, abscess, inflammation, or tumors.

Miriam E. Schwartz, M.D., M.A., Ph.D., and Colm A. Ó'Moráin, M.A., M.D., M.Sc., D.Sc.

See also: Anal cancer; Hemorrhoids

▶ *APC* gene testing

Category: Procedures
Also known as: Adenomatosis polyposis coli gene testing

Definition: The *APC* gene is a tumor-suppressor gene that is often mutated in colorectal and other cancers. Most mutations leading to colorectal cancer occur spontaneously in the digestive tracts of affected individuals, but approximately 5 percent of cases result from inherited mutations in *APC*. Testing for mutations in *APC* usually involves determining the deoxyribonucleic acid (DNA) sequence of a patient's *APC* gene, but other screens are sometimes used.

Cancers diagnosed: Familial adenomatous polyposis, familial colon cancer

Why performed: Testing for mutations in the *APC* gene is performed to diagnose familial adenomatous polyposis (FAP), an inherited condition in which precancerous polyps form in the colon. Although these polyps are initially benign, they may develop into cancer if untreated. The DNA of patients exhibiting symptoms of FAP is sequenced to confirm diagnosis and to characterize the mutation in *APC*. Because FAP is an inherited disorder, genetic testing is often done in relatives of those afflicted with FAP in order to determine whether prophylactic treatment is required.

Patient preparation: Patients considering genetic testing may meet with a genetic counselor to discuss the benefits and risks of the test and the significance of negative, positive, and inconclusive tests. The material required for genetic testing is obtained from a blood sample.

Steps of the procedure: Blood samples are sent to a clinical laboratory that offers *APC* screening. DNA is purified from the blood sample, and the DNA that encodes for *APC* is amplified by polymerase chain reaction (PCR) and sequenced using standard, automated methods.

After the procedure: The patient may consult with a physician or genetic counselor to discuss the implications of the test results.

Risks: Complications from drawing blood are rare but may include pain, bleeding, hematoma, or infection. Because the information obtained from *APC* screening may have dramatic psychological effects, it is essential that patients be offered genetic counseling.

Results: Sequence analysis allows clinicians to identify the specific DNA mutation(s) present in a FAP patient. Once the mutation has been identified, close relatives can be screened to determine if they share the FAP-causing mutation. Patients who do not carry the mutation are at no greater risk for colon cancer than the general population. Colectomy (surgical resection of the colon) and other prophylactic treatment are recommended for individuals who carry cancer-causing mutations in the *APC* gene.

Kyle J. McQuade, Ph.D.

See also: Adenomatous polyps; Colorectal cancer; Desmoid tumors; Gardner syndrome; Genetic counseling; Genetic testing; Hereditary cancer syndromes; Hereditary polyposis syndromes; Tumor markers; Turcot syndrome

▶ Arterial embolization

Category: Procedures
Also known as: Transarterial bland embolization, transarterial chemotherapy, transarterial chemo embolization (TACE)

Definition: Arterial embolization is the intentional blockage of an artery, thus depriving a tumor of a blood supply, oxygen, and nutrients. In some cases, embolization is used to deliver drugs or other chemotherapeutic agents via blood vessels to induce the cytotoxicity of tumors.

Cancers treated: Hepatocellular carcinoma, tongue carcinoma

Why performed: In patients whose cancer is significantly advanced and for whom surgical options cannot be considered, or in conditions of metastasis outside the liver and inadequate hepatic reserves, arterial embolization is preferred as a viable alternative. This option is generally chosen when the tumor is greater than 4 centimeters in size and there are multiple lesions. Arterial embolization takes advantage of the fact that the liver receives its blood supply from two main sources, the hepatic artery and hepatic portal vein, and that the major supplier of blood to liver is the hepatic artery. During the embolization procedure, the hepatic artery is blocked. Embolization may be combined with chemotherapy or radiotherapy to enhance the effects of treatments.

Patient preparation: Patients are briefed on all the steps and options involved in the procedure. A hospital stay is generally required. Patients receive intravenous sedation to cause numbness and to mitigate pain.

Steps of the procedure: During the procedure, an angiographic catheter is introduced in the branches of the hepatic artery. Usually a dye is injected for contrast and to acquire images. The hepatic artery is then blocked with occluding agents such as polyvinyl alcohol beads, which are transported to terminal hepatic arteries and occlude the vessels. The liver can still be healthy and functional using a blood supply derived from the alternative route of portal veins. In cases where arterial embolization is combined with chemotherapy (as in transarterial chemo embolization, or TACE), an anticancer drug (such as doxorubicin) is injected through the catheter and then the artery is blocked. Pressure is applied to prevent bleeding after the procedure is performed. Sometimes radiotherapy is combined with arterial embolization.

After the procedure: An overnight stay in the hospital may be required. Generally, patients are advised to take adequate rest and avoid strenuous activities for at least twenty-four hours. The procedure may be repeated every six to eight weeks.

Risks: Total liver failure, although not common, is a risk associated with this procedure. Side effects termed "embolization syndrome," including nausea, abdominal pain, and mild fever, may ensue.

Results: Increasing evidence shows that this procedure increases the rates of survival in liver cancer patients. In cases where it is combined with chemotherapy, recovery is expedited as a result of the presence of increased and prolonged concentrations of drugs around tumors.

Geetha Yadav, Ph.D.

See also: Carcinoid tumors and carcinoid syndrome; Chemoembolization; Embolization; Hereditary Leiomyomatosis and Renal Cell Cancer (HLRCC); Hereditary non-VHL clear cell renal cell carcinomas; Hereditary papillary renal cell carcinomas; Kidney cancer; Leiomyomas; Living will; Urinary system cancers; Virus-related cancers

▶ Autologous blood transfusion

Category: Procedures
Also known as: Preoperative autologous blood donation (PABD), intraoperative blood salvage, postoperative blood salvage, acute normovolemic hemodilution (ANH)

Definition: Autologous blood transfusion is the collecting and reinfusing of a patient's own blood. Collection is done before surgery and/or during or after the surgical procedure.

Cancers treated: All types of cancer, based on the physician's decision

Why performed: Autologous blood transfusion is performed to replace blood lost as a result of surgery.

Patient preparation: A physician evaluates the patient to determine whether autologous transfusion is appropriate. The decision is based on established standards. The criteria that the physician uses include the likelihood of the patient needing blood during or after surgery, the type of cancer, and other medical conditions that the patient has. There must also be an autologous donor/transfusion program available to the patient, adequate time to collect blood prior to surgery, and equipment available for the collection and reinfusion of blood during surgery.

Steps of the procedure: The physician writes an order for autologous transfusion. For preoperative autologous blood donation (PABD), the patient donates one or more units of blood at a blood donor center. The donor center staff attaches special labels to the unit of blood indicating it is for a specific patient. Blood collected prior to surgery is stored for up to forty-two days, separately from other blood.

Two systems are available for the collection and reinfusion of blood during surgery. One system is semi-automated: Blood is collected, washed, and transfused to the patient. The other system is a suction system that collects the blood and returns it to the patient without washing. The patient is constantly monitored by anesthesia staff.

In acute normovolemic hemodilution, blood is removed, and, at the same time, a solution to maintain fluid volume is infused. The blood is collected into blood bags and may be stored for up to twenty-four hours if properly refrigerated. The patient is monitored by anesthesia staff during surgery and by nursing staff after surgery.

Postoperative blood salvage is not usually used for cancer patients.

After the procedure: Following the donation of blood prior to surgery, the donor center staff gives the patient refreshments and observes the patient for any signs of an adverse reaction. During and following the transfusion of autologous blood, anesthesia staff or a nurse monitors the patient for any signs of an adverse reaction.

Risks: The risks of PABD are infusion of the wrong unit of blood, which is very low. The risks of intraoperative blood salvage include reinfusing cancer cells and the reduction of platelets and other clotting factors. The risks of acute normovolemic hemodilution include a reduction of hemoglobin and oxygen-carrying capacity and the dilution of clotting factors.

Results: Ideally, autologous blood transfusion results in a decrease in blood loss and a better surgical outcome.

Wanda E. Clark, M.T. (ASCP)

See also: Transfusion therapy

▶ Axillary dissection

Category: Procedures
Also known as: Axillary lymph node dissection

Definition: Axillary dissection is a surgical procedure carried out to remove and examine underarm lymph nodes through an incision in the armpit region (axilla).

Cancers treated: Carcinoma of the breast, melanoma

Why performed: For persons with operable breast cancer or melanoma, axillary dissection is used to determine whether cancer has spread beyond the primary tumor. Because these primary tumor cells usually infiltrate axillary lymph nodes before invading distant organs, physicians recommend that nodes be removed and examined histologically for the absence or presence of malignant cells. The results will guide the treatment course.

Patient preparation: A few days before surgery, the patient undergoes a blood test, chest X ray, and electrocardiogram in order to assess general health. To avoid excessive bleeding, any blood-thinning medications are usually suspended at this time. Patients are cautioned not to eat or drink in the eight hours before surgery and, on admission to the hospital, are asked to sign an informed consent form.

Steps of the procedure: The operation, performed under general anesthesia, lasts up to two hours. The surgeon makes an incision under the arm and removes a section of fat that contains a cluster of lymph nodes. The incision is sutured, and a drain is generally inserted to remove excess fluid.

After the procedure: Most patients remain in the hospital overnight, longer if complications develop. Nurses monitor the patient until the anesthetic wears off and vital signs stabilize. The drain may be left in place until the first follow-up visit. Postoperative measures include medication to relieve pain, preventive care to avoid infection at the incision site, the use of compression bandages to reduce fluid retention, and stretching exercises to rehabilitate arm movement. No heavy lifting is allowed during the recovery period of up to six weeks.

Risks: The most common complications of axillary dissection are numbness under the arm, swelling of the arm (lymphedema) with feelings of tightness and reduced range of motion, and infection at the incision site.

Results: Before proceeding with an axillary dissection, the surgeon may decide to biopsy the sentinel lymph node (the very first node that drains fluid from the tumor). If no cancer cells are found, then no other nodes or only a few adjacent key nodes are removed. If tumor cells are detected, however, then a more extensive axillary dissection is performed to excise six to ten nodes or more. The greater the number of cancerous nodes, the less favorable is the prognosis for survival.

Anna Binda, Ph.D.

See also: Breast cancers; Cutaneous breast cancer; Lobular Carcinoma In Situ (LCIS); Lumpectomy; Lymphedema; Mastectomy; Melanomas; Mucinous carcinomas; Sentinel Lymph Node (SLN) biopsy and mapping

▶ Barium enema

Category: Procedures
Also known as: Lower gastrointestinal (GI) series, single-contrast barium enema, double-contrast barium enema, air contrast barium enema

Definition: A barium enema involves the insertion of barium sulfate, a radiopaque contrast medium, into the colon, the first section of the large intestine. This procedure is used with X rays as a diagnostic and screening test for colon cancer, colorectal cancer, and colon polyps, growths that are sometimes a precursor to colon cancer.

Cancers diagnosed: Colon cancer, colorectal cancer, colon polyps

Why performed: A barium enema with X rays is used to screen for and help diagnose colon cancer, colorectal cancer, and colon polyps. The American Cancer Society recommends screening beginning at the age of fifty, earlier for people with risk factors.

Barium sulfate shows up on X rays and highlights the shape of the colon better than X rays alone. A single-contrast barium enema uses barium sulfate that is inserted into the colon. A double-contrast barium enema involves inserting barium into the colon, emptying the colon, and then expanding the colon with air. The barium remains on the lining of the colon, and the air expands the folds of the colon to allow a better view.

Patient preparation: Patients consume a clear liquid diet for one to three days before the test. Patients are instructed to consume large amounts of water and to use laxatives and enemas on the day before the test. An enema may be repeated on the day of the test to make sure the bowel is clear of stool and gas. For women, a pregnancy test may be used to ensure that the patient is not pregnant. Patients should tell their doctor if they have a latex allergy.

A barium enema is an outpatient procedure that is performed at a hospital radiology department or an outpatient radiology center. A barium enema does not require anesthesia, and patients are awake. A single-contrast barium enema takes about forty-five minutes, and a double-contrast study takes about an hour to complete. Patients disrobe and wear an examination gown for the procedure.

Steps of the procedure: Patients lie on an X-ray table. An X ray is taken before the barium is inserted. Patients lie on their side for the barium insertion process. A well-lubricated plastic tube is gently inserted through the anus and into the rectum. Barium is slowly poured through the tube to fill the colon. The barium is monitored on a barium fluoroscope monitor. A balloon at the end of the enema tube is inflated to keep the barium in the colon. Patients may receive medication to relieve cramping.

X rays are taken from a variety of angles. Patients are asked to change positions, and the X-ray table may be tilted. Pressure may be applied to the patient's abdomen to help move the barium through the colon.

At the end of the procedure, the enema tube is gently removed. Patients empty the barium from the colon by using a bedpan or going to the bathroom. After the barium is removed, a few final X rays are taken.

For a double-contrast barium enema, the colon is drained of barium. The colon is then filled with air, and X rays are taken. When the procedure is complete, the enema tube is removed, and patients empty the colon of barium. A few final X rays are taken.

After the procedure: Patients should drink plenty of fluids to help remove the barium from their bodies. Bowel movements will contain barium for one to two days following the tests. The barium may make bowel movements appear pink or white in color.

Risks: A barium enema is a low-risk procedure. Occasionally, the barium may harden, resulting in constipation. Drinking extra fluids and using a laxative may relieve constipation. In rare cases, the bowel may become inflamed or perforated. Patients should contact their doctor if they experience bleeding, severe pain, fever, or no bowel movements within two days of the procedure.

Results: The X-ray films are read by a radiologist. The ordering doctor may review the films as well. A healthy colon and rectum are free of abnormal growths or polyps. Any abnormalities, such as cancer or precancerous tissues, are visible on the films. Abnormal results are followed with colonoscopy.

Mary Car-Blanchard, O.T.D., B.S.O.T.

For Further Information

Etzioni, D. A., et al. "Measuring the Quality of Colorectal Cancer Screening: The Importance of Follow-Up." *Diseases of the Colon and Rectum* 49, no. 7 (July, 2006): 1002-1010.

Fenton, J. J., et al. "Delivery of Cancer Screening: How Important Is the Preventive Health Examination?" *Archives of Internal Medicine* 167, no. 6 (March 26, 2007): 580-585.

Jimbo, M., et al. "Effectiveness of Complete Diagnostic Examination in Clinical Practice Settings." *Cancer Detection and Prevention* 30, no. 6 (2006): 545-551.

Pickhardt, P. J. "The Natural History of Colorectal Polyps and Masses: Rediscovered Truths from the Barium Enema Era." *American Journal of Roentgenology* 188, no. 3 (March, 2007): 619-621.

Rollandi, G. A., E. Biscaldi, and E. DeCicco. "Double Contrast Barium Enema: Technique, Indications, Results, and Limitations of a Conventional Imaging Methodology in the MDCT Virtual Endoscopy Era." *European Journal of Radiology* 61, no. 3 (March, 2007): 382-387.

Rosman, A. S., and M. A. Korsten. "Meta-analysis Comparing CT Colonography, Air Contrast Barium Enema, and Colonoscopy." *American Journal of Medicine* 120, no. 3 (March, 2007): 203-210.

See also: Adenomatous polyps; Barium swallow; Colon polyps; Colonoscopy and virtual colonoscopy; Colorectal cancer screening; Crohn disease; Diverticulosis and diverticulitis; Gallium scan; Imaging tests; Medicare and cancer; Ovarian cancers; Pancolitis; Premalignancies; Small intestine cancer; X-ray tests

▶ Barium swallow

Category: Procedures

Also known as: Barium swallow X ray, barium swallow exam, barium swallow test, barium meal, double-contrast barium swallow, upper gastrointestinal (GI) series, esophagraphy, esophagogram, esophagram

Definition: A barium swallow is a diagnostic test in which the patient ingests barium sulfate, a radiopaque contrast medium. It is used with X rays to detect mouth, throat, vocal cords, esophagus, stomach, and small intestine cancers.

Cancers diagnosed: Oral cavity (mouth) cancer; oropharyngeal (throat) cancer; vocal cord cancer, including laryngeal and hypopharyngeal cancer, glottic cancer, supraglottic cancer, subglottic cancer; esophageal cancer; stomach cancer; stomach polyps, which may precede stomach cancer; small intestine cancer, including carcinoid tumors, gastrointestinal stromal tumors, lymphomas, and adenocarcinoma

Why performed: A barium swallow with X rays is performed to help diagnose cancer of the mouth, throat, vocal cords, esophagus, stomach, and small intestine. When swallowed, barium sulfate shows up on X rays and highlights the linings of the above-mentioned structures. A double-contrast barium swallow involves swallowing substances that create air in the stomach to expand it, allowing a better view.

Patient preparation: Patients may be placed on a restricted diet a few days before the test. Patients should not eat, drink, chew gum, or smoke after midnight before the test. Patients receive instructions from their doctors about swallowing medications. The stomach needs to be empty for the procedure. In some cases, the stomach contents are removed through a tube placed in the nose. For women, a pregnancy test may be performed to ensure that the patient is not pregnant.

A barium swallow is an outpatient procedure that is performed at a hospital radiology department, outpatient radiology center, or doctor's office. The test does not require anesthesia, and patients are awake. A barium swallow usually takes from thirty to sixty minutes, depending on the extent of the procedure. Patients disrobe and wear a gown for the test. Patients need to remove metal objects that may interfere with the X rays, including glasses, dentures, and jewelry.

Steps of the procedure: The patient's vital signs are taken before the test and monitored during the test. Patients may sit, stand, or lie on an X-ray table for the procedure. Patients may be secured to the X-ray table if it is tilted to allow images to be taken from various angles.

X rays of the patient's heart, lungs, and abdomen are taken. Then, patients drink sixteen to twenty ounces of barium sulfate. The barium sulfate is mixed in a thick drink that may have flavor added to it; otherwise, the drink is described as tasting chalky. The examination table may be tilted or pressure may be applied to the patient's abdomen to help spread the barium. The barium is viewed on a barium fluoroscope monitor as it travels through the upper digestive tract. Still X-ray images can be taken at any time. Patients may need to drink more barium sulfate as the test progresses.

For a double-contrast barium swallow, the patient swallows baking soda crystals. The baking soda creates gas, and the air expands the stomach. Additional images are taken, and the patient is repositioned or the examination table is tilted as necessary.

After the procedure: Patients should drink plenty of fluids to help remove the barium from their bodies. Patients can eat a regular diet unless instructed otherwise. Bowel movements will contain barium for one to two days following the tests. The barium may make bowel movements appear white, gray, or pink in color.

Risks: A barium swallow is considered a low-risk procedure. The radiation exposure is low, but it carries a small risk of cancer. Patients may be allergic to the flavorings that are mixed with the barium drink. Occasionally, the barium may harden, resulting in intestinal blockage or constipation. Patients should contact their doctor if they have not had a bowel movement within one to two days of the procedure.

Results: The X-ray films are read by a radiologist. The ordering doctor may review the films as well. The linings of healthy structures are free of abnormal growths or polyps. Any abnormalities, such as cancer or precancerous tissues, appear as growths or polyps.

Mary Car-Blanchard, O.T.D., B.S.O.T.

For Further Information

Drop, A., et al. "The Modern Methods of Gastric Imaging." *Annales Universitatis Mariae Curie-Skuodowska* 59, no. 1 (2004): 373-381.

Gore, R. M., et al. "Upper Gastrointestinal Tumours: Diagnosis and Staging." *Cancer Imaging* 29, no. 6 (December, 2006): 213-217.

Hosaka, K. "Radiological Investigation of the Mucosae Around Early Gastric Cancers." *Journal of Gastroenterology* 41, no. 10 (October, 2006): 943-953.

Kunisaki, C., et al. "Outcomes of Mass Screening for Gastric Carcinoma." *Annuals Surgical Oncology* 13, no. 2 (February, 2006): 221-228.

Levine, M. S., and S. E. Rubesin. "Diseases of the Esophagus: Diagnosis with Esophagography." *Radiology* 237, no. 2 (November, 2005): 414-427.

Pasuawski, M., J. Zuomaniec, E. Ruci½ska, and W. Koutyk. "Synchronous Primary Esophageal and Gastric Cancers." *Annales Universitatis Mariae Curie-Skuodowska* 59, no. 1 (2004): 406-410.

Summers, D. S., M. D. Roger, P. L. Allan, and J. T. Murchison. "Accelerating the Transit Time of Barium Sulphate Suspensions in Small Bowel Examinations." *European Journal of Radiology* 62, no. 1 (April, 2007): 122-125.

See also: Diarrhea; Esophageal cancer; Gastrointestinal cancers; Gastrointestinal complications of cancer treatment; Imaging tests; Laryngeal cancer; Laryngectomy; Small intestine cancer; Stomach cancers; Throat cancer; Upper Gastrointestinal (GI) series; X-ray tests

▶ Bethesda criteria

Category: Procedures

Definition: Bethesda criteria are a standardized set of criteria that are used to identify potential cases of hereditary nonpolyposis colorectal cancer (HNPCC), or Lynch syndrome.

Hereditary nonpolyposis colorectal cancer: HNPCC is an autosomal dominant disease that is characterized by early age of onset (average is before the age of forty-five), tumor formation in a variety of tissues (endometrial, gastric, renal, ovarian, and skin), and microsatellite instability. HNPCC accounts for only about 3 to 5 percent of the cases of colorectal cancer, and the molecular and genetic testing that is required to diagnose this form of cancer can be quite time-consuming and costly. Therefore, it became important to set down a standardized set of criteria for identifying potential cases of HNPCC and to separate them from sporadic, noninherited forms of colorectal cancer.

History: In 1997, a group of experts met at the National Institutes of Health to discuss the state of research on HNPCC. They came up with a set of criteria, the Bethesda criteria, which expanded the previous Amsterdam criteria to include extracolonic tumor formation as well as more specific histological characterization. In 2002, the criteria were further revised to define tumors that should be tested for microsatellite instability (MSI), which is the frequent mutation of repetitive deoxyribonucleic acid (DNA) sequences due to defects in the mismatch repair machinery in the cell.

Criteria: Currently, the criteria for identifying a potential case of HNPCC are as follows:

- Colorectal cancer diagnosed prior to age fifty
- Presence of synchronous or metachronous HNPCC-associated tumors
- High microsatellite instability (MSI-H) histology diagnosed prior to age sixty
- One or more first-degree relatives diagnosed with an HNPCC-related tumor prior to age fifty
- Colorectal cancer diagnosed in two or more first- or second-degree relatives

Testing: If a patient meets the Bethesda criteria, a number of molecular and genetic tests are recommended. The ideal set of tests would include evaluation of microsatellite instability status as well as immunohistochemical analysis of tumors. In patients who show high levels of microsatellite instability and loss of expression of one or more of the DNA mismatch repair proteins, DNA sequencing of *MSH2* and *MLH1*, the two genes most commonly mutated in HNPCC, should be performed. Patients who have mutations in either of these genes show an increased risk of developing cancer, and they should therefore undergo frequent screening.

Lindsay Lewellyn, B.S.

See also: Ashkenazi Jews and cancer; Endometrial cancer; Ethnicity and cancer; Family history and risk assessment; *MLH1* gene; *MSH* genes; Pancreatic cancers; *PMS* genes; Turcot syndrome

▶ Bilobectomy

Category: Procedures
Also known as: Lobectomy, thoracotomy

Definition: A bilobectomy is a surgical procedure to remove two lobes of the lung.

Cancers treated: Various types of lung cancer

Why performed: A bilobectomy is performed to remove diseased lung tissue.

Patient preparation: Bilobectomy is performed under general anesthesia in a hospital with the usual preoperative preparation, such as physical examination, blood testing, and consultation with an anesthesiologist. In addition, an examination and additional lung tests will be done by a pulmonologist (a lung specialist).

Steps of the procedure: The surgical procedure is performed by a thoracic surgeon making a cut in the side; the rib cage is separated or cut away to allow the lungs to be seen, and the pleura (a membrane around the lungs) is also cut away. The lung being operated on may be deflated, and the other lung continues to work with the help of a breathing tube. The lobes of the lung are pulled apart and separated, and the diseased lobes are cut free and removed. Arteries and veins that have been cut are sealed or reconnected. A drainage tube is left in the chest wall to drain or suction out fluid and air. The procedure may take from two to five hours.

After the procedure: Pain medication will be used to make the patient more comfortable after the surgery. A hospital stay of about one week is to be expected; during hospitalization, breathing exercises as well as exercises for movement (range of motion) will be taught. Recovery at home can take several weeks, during which time pain medications may be used, the surgical incision site needs to be kept clean, and a gradual return to physical activity is recommended.

Risks: The risks of a bilobectomy procedure are a narrowing of the bronchi (the large air passages leading from the windpipe to the lungs), scar formation, injury to nerves during surgery that may cause numbness and tingling in the chest area, and leakage of air from the surgical site with partial or complete collapse of the lung.

Results: Surgery, including bilobectomy, is most effective for Stage I and Stage II non-small-cell lung cancer. Smoking cessation is of utmost importance to maximize surgical treatment as it improves wound healing and allows for the best outcome when additional therapies, such as radiation and chemotherapy, are used.

Vicki Miskovsky, B.S., R.D.

See also: Bronchoalveolar lung cancer; Esophagectomy; Lobectomy; Lung cancers; Mesothelioma; Pleural effusion; Pleurodesis; Pneumonectomy; Surgical biopsies; Thoracoscopy; Thoracotomy

▶ Biopsy

Category: Procedures
Also known as: Tissue sampling, fine needle aspiration, needle biopsy, percutaneous biopsy, core biopsy, incisional biopsy, excisional biopsy, endoscopic or laparoscopic biopsy, surgical biopsy, open biopsy, transvenous biopsy

Definition: A biopsy is the removal of a tissue sample for laboratory analysis to detect the presence of cancer cells.

There are several types of biopsy procedures. The type of biopsy procedure performed is dependent on the type of cancer suspected and the area of the body being examined.

In fine needle aspiration (also called needle biopsy or percutaneous biopsy), a very fine needle is inserted into the area and a sample of fluid or tissue is withdrawn through the needle into an attached syringe. This type of biopsy procedure may be used to remove tissue from an organ that is otherwise accessible only via surgery, such as the liver, pancreas, or lung. The advantage of fine needle aspiration is that it does not require a surgical incision. To place the needle accurately, ultrasound or computed tomography (CT) guidance may be used.

Similar to fine needle aspiration, core biopsy uses a larger needle to withdraw a greater sample of fluid or tissue. Ultrasound or CT guidance may be used.

In incisional biopsy, a scalpel or similar instrument is used to remove a portion of the suspected cancerous tissue via an incision made in the skin. Incisional biopsies are most commonly used to remove soft tissue, such as skin, connective tissue, muscle, and fat. For skin lesions, an incisional biopsy may be performed with a hollow, circular-shaped instrument (punch biopsy), or a razor may be used (shave biopsy). Depending on the type of procedure, the patient may be under general or local anesthesia.

In excisional biopsy (sometimes called open biopsy or surgical biopsy), a whole lump, tumor, or organ and a margin of normal tissue around it are removed. An excisional biopsy may be used to remove some types of tumors or suspected cancers that need to be removed entirely for an accurate diagnosis, such as the removal of lymph nodes to diagnose lymphoma accurately. General anesthesia is usually used for excisional biopsies.

In endoscopic or laparoscopic biopsy, an endoscope (small camera on a thin tube) is used to view an internal area and to identify the tissue for removal. The endoscope transmits magnified images of the area onto a video monitor to guide the physician during the procedure. The endoscope can be inserted through a natural body opening, such as the throat to remove esophageal tissue, or it can be inserted through a small incision. Surgical instruments attached to the endoscope or inserted through other small incisions can be used to remove the tissue. Endoscopic biopsy procedures are the most common type of biopsies. A laparoscopic biopsy procedure may be used when a tissue sample is needed from more than one area or when a larger tissue sample is needed. General or local anesthesia may be used, depending on the biopsy site.

A capsule biopsy is a type of laparoscopic technique in which a patient swallows a capsule that is connected to a thin tube. X rays confirm the proper positioning of the capsule, and a syringe attached to the end of the tube is used to withdraw a tissue sample into the capsule. The capsule and tube are gently removed, and the tissue sample is taken to the laboratory for analysis. This type of biopsy procedure may be used to remove a sample of tissue from the lower gastrointestinal tract.

Other biopsy procedures include colposcopic biopsies to identify and remove abnormal tissue from the cervix, transvenous biopsy to remove tissue via a catheter inserted into a vein in the neck, and bone marrow biopsy to remove a bone marrow sample through a needle inserted into the hip and withdrawn through a syringe.

Cancers diagnosed: Various, including breast, bone, gynecological, liver, lung, lymph node, skin, thyroid, urological, and gastrointestional cancers

Why performed: A biopsy is performed to diagnose and stage cancer when an abnormality is found during diagnostic tests. It also may be performed to determine the cause of unexplained symptoms or to match organ tissue before a transplant.

Patient preparation: Tests before the procedure may include blood tests, urine tests, a chest X ray, an electrocardiogram, CT scanning, magnetic resonance imaging (MRI), and other imaging tests. The patient preparation for a biopsy procedure varies depending on the type of procedure and biopsy location. In some cases, no special preparation is required. In other cases, the patient must not eat or drink for eight hours beforehand and is required to stop taking anticoagulant medications for several days before the procedure. The patient will receive specific preparation instructions from the health care team.

Steps of the procedure: Local or general anesthesia may be used, depending on the type of biopsy procedure and biopsy location. The biopsy site is cleansed, and a local anesthetic is injected into the area. In some cases, such as with sentinal node biopsy, a radioactive substance or dye is injected into the tumor and a scanner is used to locate the lymph node or tissue containing the radioactive substance or stained with the dye. The tissue sample or fluid is removed via one of the biopsy techniques.

The sample is sent to a laboratory for microscopic analysis by a pathologist. There are a variety of methods for processing tissue samples. Histologic sections involve preparing stained, thin slices of tissue mounted on slides, a process that may take up to forty-eight hours. With the histologic method, the tissue sample is placed in a machine that replaces all water in the sample with paraffin wax. The sample is embedded into a larger block of paraffin, sliced into very thin sections, and stained with dye to aid microscopic analysis. Frozen tissue analysis involves freezing the tissue, slicing it into thin sections, and staining the sections to aid analysis. Smears are tissue samples that are spread onto a slide for examination. The results of smears can usually be obtained very quickly.

After the procedure: The length of a patient's recovery and the steps for recovery vary depending on the type of biopsy procedure and biopsy location. The patient may stay in a recovery room for a certain amount of time after the procedure. The biopsy site is usually covered with a bandage or dressing. Medication is prescribed as needed for relief of pain, which may include discomfort at the biopsy site or muscle pain. An overnight hospital stay may be required for some fine needle aspiration, laparoscopic, and surgical biopsy procedures.

Specific instructions for driving, activity, incision care, medications, nutrition, and follow-up care are provided to the patient, as applicable. In some cases, the patient is not permitted to drive home after the procedure. Depending on the physician's instructions, the patient may be

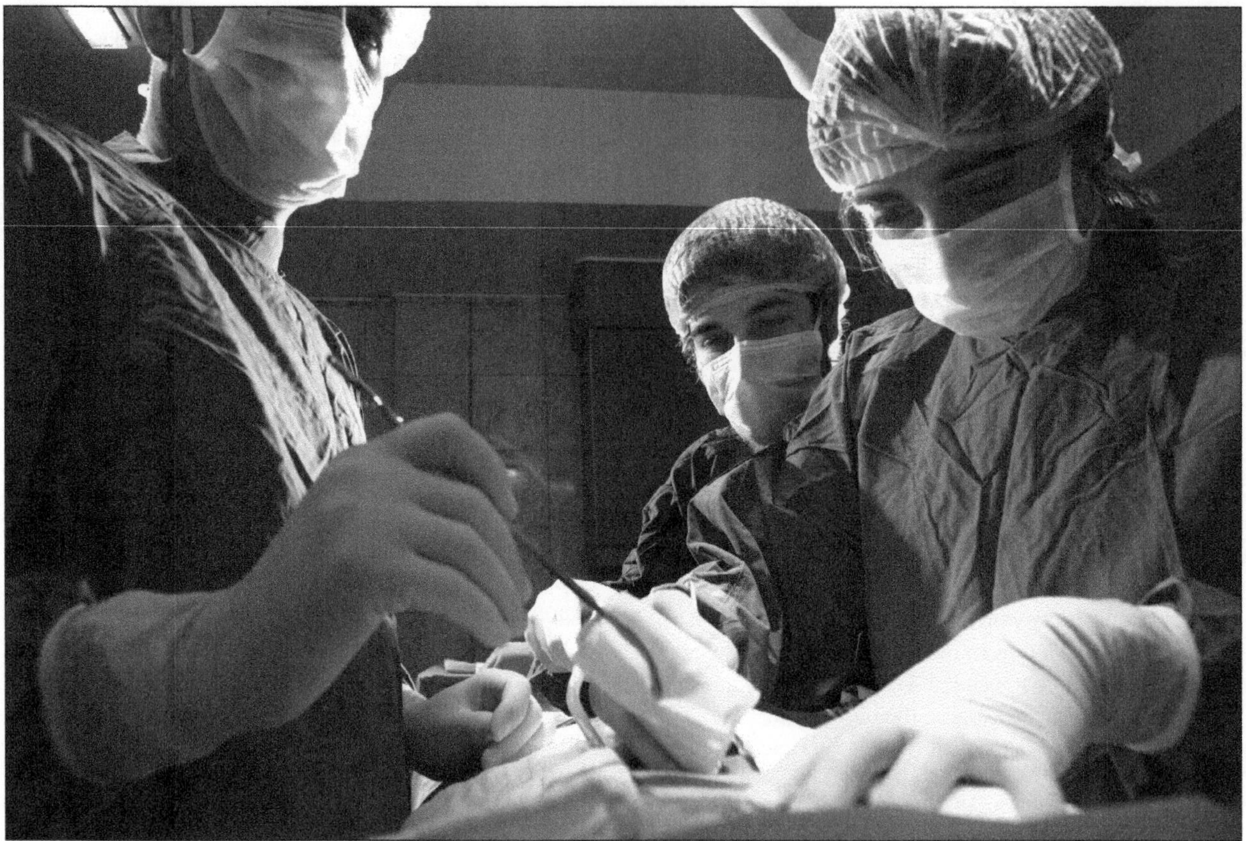

In incisional biopsy, a scalpel is used to remove a sample of the suspected cancerous tissue through an incision made in the skin. (iStock)

required to stay on bed rest at home for a certain amount of time after the procedure.

Risks: The risks of biopsy procedures are dependent on the type of procedure performed and the biopsy location. Possible risks of all biopsy procedures include bleeding and infection. The risk of death associated with biopsy procedures is generally very low. The physician may discuss specific mortality rates and risks with the patient, depending on the type of procedure performed.

Results: The tissue sample removed during the procedure is either normal, which means it is benign or noncancerous, or abnormal, which means it has unusual characteristics and may be malignant or cancerous. In some cases, the tissue that was obtained during the biopsy is not adequate to make a diagnosis, and a repeat biopsy procedure or a different type of biopsy procedure may be performed. The type of cancerous cells and extent of disease will help guide the patient's treatment.

Angela M. Costello, B.S.

For Further Information

DeVita, Vincent, Jr., Samuel Hellman, Steven A. Rosenberg, et al., eds. *Cancer: Principles and Practice of Oncology*. 7th ed. Philadelphia: Lippincott Williams & Wilkins, 2005.

McPhee, Stephen J. Maxine A. Papadakis, and Lawrence M. Tierney, eds. *Current Medical Diagnosis and Treatment 2008*. New York: McGraw-Hill Medical, 2007.

Ota, D. M. "What's New in General Surgery: Surgical Oncology." *Journal of the American College of Surgeons* 196, no. 6 (2003): 926-932.

Other Resources

American Cancer Society
http://www.cancer.org

National Cancer Institute
http://www.cancer.gov

RadiologyInfo
http://www.radiologyinfo.org

Society of Interventional Radiology
http://www.sirweb.org

See also: Anoscopy; Axillary dissection; Bone marrow aspiration and biopsy; Breslow's staging; Bronchoscopy; Colonoscopy and virtual colonoscopy; Colorectal cancer screening; Colposcopy; Computed Tomography (CT)-guided biopsy; Conization; Core needle biopsy; Culdoscopy; Cystoscopy; Cytology; Dilation and Curettage (D&C); Dukes' classification; Endoscopic Retrograde Cholangiopancreatography (ERCP); Endoscopy; Flow cytometry; Gastric polyps; Gleason grading system; Grading of tumors; Hormone receptor tests; Hysteroscopy; Immunocytochemistry and immunohistochemistry; Ki67 test; Laparoscopy and laparoscopic surgery; Laryngoscopy; Liver biopsy; Loop Electrosurgical Excisional Procedure (LEEP); Lumpectomy; Lymphadenectomy; Mediastinoscopy; Needle biopsies; Needle localization; Pap test; Paracentesis; Pathology; Pleural biopsy; Polypectomy; Premalignancies; Progesterone receptor assay; Prostate-Specific Antigen (PSA) test; Receptor analysis; Screening for cancer; Sentinel Lymph Node (SLN) biopsy and mapping; Sigmoidoscopy; Staging of cancer; Stereotactic needle biopsy; Surgical biopsies; Thoracoscopy; Thoracotomy; TNM staging; Upper Gastrointestinal (GI) endoscopy; Wire localization

▶ Bone marrow aspiration and biopsy

Category: Procedures

Definition: Bone marrow aspiration involves the removal of a bone marrow sample for laboratory examination. The bone marrow is where all blood cells are created. It is the job of the bone marrow to replace dead and dying red blood cells, white blood cells, and platelets. At times, cancer or other disease may cause this bone marrow production to stop or decrease. Sites for bone marrow aspiration and biopsy are typically the pelvic bone (ilium) or the sternum, larger bones that provide the best samples. A bone marrow biopsy can be performed by a hematologist, medical oncologist, internist, pathologist, or specially trained technologist. The patient can have a bone marrow biopsy at the bedside, in interventional radiology, and even in the operating room.

Cancers diagnosed: Leukemia, multiple myeloma, or polycythemia vera, cancers referred to as hematological malignancies; metastatic cancer

Why performed: A bone marrow biopsy is done to evaluate the functioning of the bone marrow and to determine the presence or absence of cancer.

Patient preparation: The patient will have the procedure explained and provide consent. A numbing medication is injected at the site; it may burn or sting a bit when first used. Once the numbing medication is injected, patients usually feel considerable pressure at the site but not necessarily pain during the procedure. When the biopsy is done in the hip, patients occasionally complain of a quick shooting pain down the leg, but it usually stops once the sample has been taken. A patient with a low platelet count may receive a platelet transfusion immediately before the procedure.

Steps of the procedure: The patient will be positioned for the procedure and needs to remain still until its completion. A patient who is having the pelvic bone biopsied will be placed on one side with pillows or blankets used to maintain positioning. A patient who is having the sternum biopsied will lie flat in the bed or on the table. The patient may be given medication for pain and relaxation. The site is scrubbed and cleaned, and then the patient is given medication to numb the site. A small cut is made into the skin. The procedure is done with a device that consists of a large hollow needle with an inner attachment (cannula) that allows for the bone to be accessed. The needle is used to make a hole into the bone. Once it is inside the bone, the middle of the needle is removed, and the large hollow needle is then resting in the center of the bone. A large syringe is used to extract a sample of the marrow (aspirate). The section of bone taken when the inner cannula was removed from the needle is also kept for pathology testing. The patient may have this procedure done on both hip bones or at multiple sites in order to establish staging of disease. The samples are placed on slides or in a liquid to preserve them until testing can be completed.

After the procedure: Pressure may need to be applied to prevent bleeding. The patient may be asked to lie on that hip to provide extra pressure immediately after the biopsy for ten to fifteen minutes. The cut is typically small enough that a bandage and a little pressure is all that is needed. Some patients may not be able to stop bleeding after the biopsy, usually because their platelet counts are too low. These patients may require a stitch or two at the bone marrow site to stop the bleeding. Patients may remain sore at the site for two to three days after the procedure. If this procedure was performed on an outpatient,

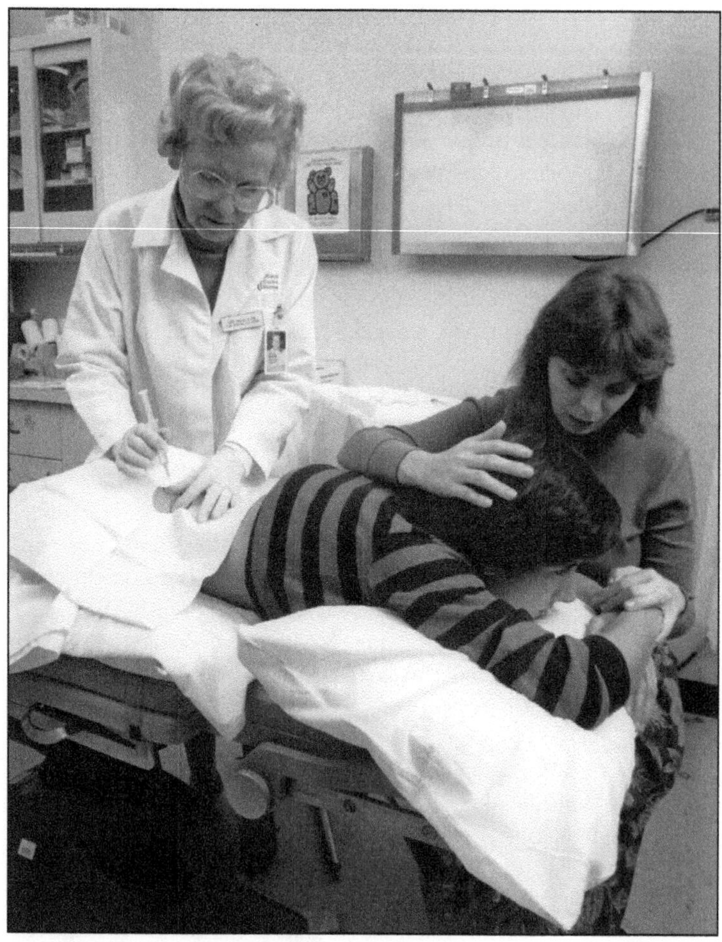

A young patient is undergoing bone marrow aspiration. (National Cancer Institute)

then the patient will not be able to drive home and will need a family member or friend to help.

Risks: The risks from performing a bone marrow aspiration and biopsy are minimal. As with any invasive procedure, there is a risk for infection. There is also a risk for bleeding and bruising with this procedure. If the sample is taken from the sternum (breast bone), then there is a risk of injury to the heart, lungs, and major blood vessels.

Results: Findings from the bone marrow aspiration and biopsy show what types of cells are in the bone marrow. The hematologist or pathologist will examine the samples with a microscope to determine what types of cells are present. The physicians are able to determine if these cells are normal, misshapen, or cancerous, as well as the stage of the cancer that may be present.

Bone marrow biopsies are also done to evaluate therapy. This is typically seen in leukemia patients. They will have a bone marrow biopsy completed prior to therapy and then a biopsy done at or around day fourteen to determine if the chemotherapy has destroyed the cells in the bone marrow.

Katrina Green, R.N., B.S.N., O.C.N.

For Further Information

Carrier, Ewa, and Gracy Ledinham. *One Hundred Questions and Answers About Bone Marrow and Stem Cell Transplantation*. Sudbury, Mass.: Jones and Bartlett, 2003.

Klag, Michael J., et al., eds. *Johns Hopkins Family Health Book*. New York: HarperCollins, 1999.

Weisbrot, Deborah M., and Alan B. Ettinger. *The Essential Patient Handbook: Getting the Health Care You Need—from Doctors Who Know*. New York: Demos Medical, 2004.

See also: Acute Lymphocytic Leukemia (ALL); Acute myelocytic leukemia (AML); Aplastic anemia; Blood cancers; Childhood cancers; Chronic Lymphocytic Leukemia (CLL); Chronic Myeloid Leukemia (CML); Eosinophilic leukemia; Fanconi anemia; 5Q minus syndrome; Flow cytometry; Hairy cell leukemia; Hematologic oncology; Hemolytic anemia; Histiocytosis X; Hodgkin disease; Immunocytochemistry and immunohistochemistry; Medulloblastomas; Multiple myeloma; Myelofibrosis; Myeloma; Myeloproliferative disorders; Neuroblastomas; Non-Hodgkin lymphoma; Polycythemia vera; Retinoblastomas; Rhabdomyosarcomas; Stem cell transplantation; Thrombocytopenia; Veterinary oncology; Waldenström macroglobulinemia (WM)

▶ Bone Marrow Transplantation (BMT)

Category: Procedures

Also known as: Peripheral blood stem cell transplantation (PBSCT)

Definition: Bone marrow transplantation (BMT) and peripheral blood stem cell transplantation (PBSCT) Peripheral blood stem cell transplantation (PBSCT) Stem cell transplantation are procedures used in cancer therapy to provide stem cells to a patient to replace those lost to disease, chemotherapy, and radiation. Stem cells may be obtained from patients themselves, a related or unrelated donor, or umbilical cord blood taken after the birth of a baby. Autologous transplants use the patient's own stem cells. Allogeneic transplants use stem cells from a related person; the donor is most often a parent or sibling, but an unrelated but matched donor or umbilical cord blood may be used. A syngeneic transplant is done with stem cells from an identical twin.

Cancers treated: Leukemia, lymphoma, multiple myeloma, and neuroblastoma; additional cancers eligible for transplant are being evaluated in clinical trials

Why performed: Cancer patients are often treated by high doses of chemotherapy and radiation to rid the body of cancer cells. Chemotherapy and radiation therapy target rapidly dividing cells in the body. Because cancer cells and stem cells divide rapidly, they both may be killed by the therapy. BMT and PBSCT are used to rescue patients after high-dose chemotherapy and radiation by replacing destroyed stem cells with healthy stem cells. Transplanted stem cells allow the bone marrow to begin producing blood cells needed by the body. Additionally, white blood cells from the donor may identify any remaining cancer cells in the patient's body and attack them as foreign, thus providing additional cancer cell killing. This phenomenon – the graft-versus-tumor (GVT) effect – is important in some kinds of leukemia treated with allogeneic transplants, since the GVT enhances the effectiveness of the transplant.

To understand bone marrow transplantation, it is important to understand the role of stem cells. Stem cells are found in the bone marrow and can develop into different types of cells in the body, such as blood cells. Blood cells originally begin as immature cells, called hematopoietic stem cells, which are constantly and rapidly dividing. Stem cells used in transplantation are not embryonic stem cells. Hematopoietic stem cells are located in the bone marrow, but some stem cells circulate in the bloodstream and are called peripheral blood stem cells. The role of hematopoietic stem cells is to produce cells that fight infection (white blood cells), carry oxygen (red blood cells), and prevent bleeding (platelets).

Patient preparation: The first step in the transplant procedure is determining the type of transplant that will be used by determining if the patient has a potential donor. Doctors try to minimize side effects by using stem cells that match as closely as possible the patient's own stem cells. There are different proteins on the cell surface, called human leukocyte antigens (HLAs), which are identified by a blood test. The success of the transplant depends on how close a match can be made between the donor stem cells and the patient's stem cells. Close relatives are the most likely sources of matching stem cells, but less than one-third of patients will have a matched sibling. Finding an unrelated, matched donor is possible in about one-half of cases, and the chance of a match increases if the donor and patient are of the same ethnic and racial background. If a potential donor is identified, then blood work will be used to determine the level of the match. A donor registry may also be used to identify donors who have offered to provide stem cells for transplantation if they match a patient in need.

If no donor match can be found, then the patient's own stem cells could possibly be used in an autologous transplant. Stem cells are obtained from the patient and then treated to remove any cancer cells. Extra stem cells are removed from the patient, as some healthy cells may be damaged when the cancer cells are removed.

Once the type of transplant is determined, the stem cells are obtained, or harvested. The liquid center of the bone is the source for stem cells used in BMT. The donor is given anesthesia to make the harvest procedure pain-free. General anesthesia or regional anesthesia, which numbs the area below the waist, is used. Large needles are inserted into the back of the hip (pelvic) bone or, rarely, the breastbone (sternum), and marrow is drawn out. The harvest procedure takes approximately one hour. The bone marrow is then treated to remove blood and bone fragments, and, if not to be used immediately, frozen with a preservative and stored until it is time to administer the stem cells to the patient. Stem cells that are frozen (cryopreserved) can be stored for many years.

If the doctor determines that a peripheral blood stem cell transplant is the best choice for the patient, then stem cells are harvested from the bloodstream rather than from the bone marrow. Autologous transplants often use peripheral blood stem cells (PBSCs). Apheresis is used to remove PBSCs with a machine that removes the stem cells and then returns the remainder of the blood, minus the stem cells, to the donor. Medicine that stimulates the growth of stem cells in the body may be given to the donor for several days before the harvest. Apheresis may take up to six hours. The cells are processed and frozen for future use.

Umbilical cord blood may also be a source of stem cells for transplantation. The mother requests that cells be harvested when the birth occurs. Cord blood banks

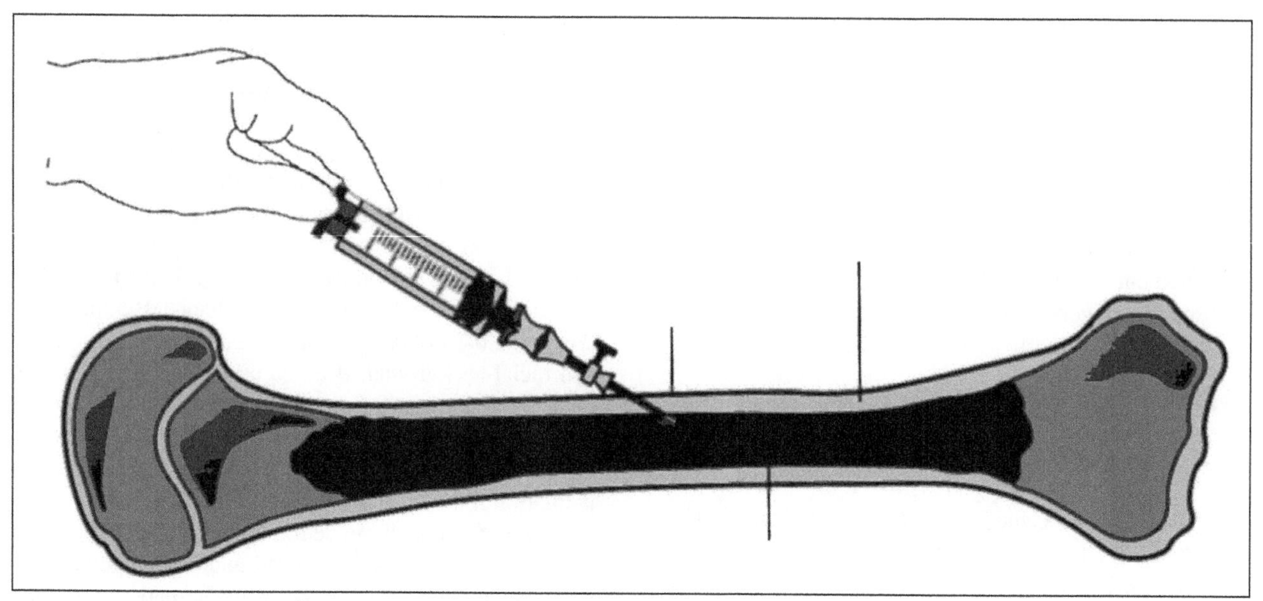

Bone marrow transplantation is used to treat several types of lymphoma.

may store the cells for potential use by the family at a later date or may be given to a public cord blood bank for use by any matching patient. Blood is taken from the umbilical cord and placenta and then frozen for storage. Since only a small amount of blood may be available, cord blood transplants are usually most effective in children or small adults.

Steps of the procedure: The patient usually receives high-dose chemotherapy (anticancer drugs) and radiation to rid the body of as many cancer cells as possible. Depending on the hospital program, the patient may be admitted to the hospital or may undergo the preoperative regimen as an outpatient. Once the regimen before the transplant is complete, the patient is ready to have the procedure. The stem cells are thawed and given through an intravenous line, as in a blood transfusion. The infusion of the stem cells may take from one to five hours.

After the procedure: Once the infusion of the stem cells is complete, the wait begins for the cells to graft (or take) and produce new blood cells for the patient. During this time, the patient may be in a room with special air filters and strict infection control guidelines because the patient has very few stem cells until the graft occurs, and the body is unable to fight infection or control bleeding. The wait for engraftment ranges from two to four weeks. High fevers, chills, shortness of breath, coughing, low blood pressure, and weakness may occur during and after the transplant. Following the transplant the patient is also at risk for infection, bleeding, and anemia until the new stem cells begin to produce new blood cells. With allogeneic transplants, the most significant complication that occurs is graft-versus-host disease, in which the donor's white blood cells recognize the recipient's cells as foreign and attack them as if they were a pathogen.

Once discharged from the hospital, the patient may face a variety of problems. Fatigue, physical problems lingering after the transplant, and psychological problems may occur. Frequent visits to the physician to follow progress after the transplantation and to manage symptoms are expected. The recovery period may be a year in length.

Risks: There is minimal risk involved with donating bone marrow or undergoing apheresis. If the match between donor and patient is not complete, then graft rejection may occur in rare instances. The most significant risks are infection, bleeding, anemia, and graft-versus-host disease. Patients may be unable to have children after a transplant due to the chemotherapy and radiation, and this topic should be discussed with the physician prior to the transplant.

Results: Survival rates after transplantation vary by disease, type of transplant, and the age of the patient. In related donor patient transplants, survival rates are 55 to 70 percent and 25 to 50 percent if the donor is unrelated. Bone marrow transplantation (BMT)

Patricia Stanfill Edens, R.N., Ph.D., FACHE
Updated by: Michelle Herdman

For Further Information

Jenks Kettmann, J. D., & Altmaier, E. M. (2008). Social support and depression among bone marrow transplant patients. *Journal of Health Psychology*, 13, 39-46.

Nadir, Y., & Brenner, B. (2007). Hemorrhagic and thrombotic complications in bone marrow transplant recipients. *Thrombosis Research*, 120(suppl. 2), 92-98.

Arora, M., Cutler, C.S., Jagasia, M.H., Pidala, J., Chai, X., Martin, P.J., ... Lee, S.J. (2016). Late acute and chronic graft-versus-host disease after allogeneic hematopoietic cell transplantation. *Biology of Blood and Marrow Transplantation*, 22, 449-455.

Other Resources

American Cancer Society
www.cancer.org/

National Cancer Institute
Bone Marrow Transplantation
http://www.cancer.gov

National Marrow Donor Program
https://bethematch.org/

See also: Blood cancers; Graft-Versus-Host Disease (GVHD); Immunocytochemistry and immunohistochemistry; Leukemias; Lymphomas; Organ transplantation and cancer; Pheresis; Stem cell transplantation; Umbilical cord blood transplantation

▶ Bone scan

Category: Procedures
Also known as: Bone scintigraphy

Definition: A bone scan is a procedure that can detect abnormalities in the skeleton. A radioactive substance (known as a tracer) is injected into the body and taken up by the bone. The tracer emits radiation in the form of gamma rays, which can be detected by a special scanning camera. More tracer will accumulate in areas of the bone that are actively rebuilding or breaking down (such as that in the presence of cancer) compared to the inactive areas.

Cancers diagnosed: Cancers that have spread to the bone (metastatic cancers), primarily breast, prostate, and lung cancers, and kidney and thyroid cancers to a lesser degree

Why performed: Cancer cells can spread from their primary location to the bone in a multistep process known as metastasis. Metastatic bone disease can result in bone pain and an overall decrease in the quality of life. Tumor cells residing in the bone can also cause bone destruction (known as resorption) as a result of both direct effects of the tumor and the activation of osteoclasts (a type of bone cell responsible for resorption). This process may result in weakened bones and a greater risk of bone fractures. Furthermore, calcium may be released from the bone as it breaks down, and elevated levels of calcium in the blood can cause loss of appetite, nausea, and exhaustion and can affect the heart and kidneys.

A bone scan is one method to detect if cancer has spread to the bone and to identify where the cancer is located. Bone scans can also be used to determine the stage of disease, as well as to examine how much bone damage is present. Additionally, bone scans may be performed to monitor the response to treatment, as some cases of bone cancers are treated with drugs such as bisphosphonates in order to reduce bone resorption.

Patient preparation: Very little prior preparation is required, and patients do not need to fast. At the time of the scan, patients must remove all metal objects (such as jewelry, zippers, and metal buttons), as they may interfere with the scan. In some cases, the clothes should be removed and the patients will wear a hospital gown.

Steps of the procedure: A bone scan will usually be performed in a hospital. The two stages of this procedure are the tracer injection and the scan.

A radioactive tracer will be injected into a vein in the patient's arm. Patients will then wait one to four hours to allow the tracer to be incorporated into the bone tissue. Drinking several glasses of water (at least four) will help to eliminate excess tracer through the urine. Patients will be instructed to empty the bladder before the scan begins.

For the scan, patients must lie still on a table while the scanning camera moves overhead and scans the body. The camera will detect the gamma rays emitted by the tracer that has concentrated in the bone. Sometimes the scans will be conducted when patients are in different positions in order to view the bones from various angles. On average, the bone scan lasts about thirty to sixty minutes.

After the procedure: Care should be taken when sitting up at the completion of the scan, as dizziness or lightheadedness may result from the extended period of lying down. Patients will be instructed to drink plenty of fluids for at least forty-eight hours after the bone scan to help eliminate the remaining radioactive tracer. Patients who are breastfeeding should also discard their breast milk for the first two days after the procedure.

Risks: Common risks include redness, soreness, or swelling at the injection site. In rare cases, patients have allergic reactions to the tracer.

Results: If the radioactive tracer is distributed equally throughout the bones, then the result will be considered normal. An abnormal result will occur when the tracer concentrates in distinct sites of the bone, resulting in "hot spots." Hot spots indicate that there is a lot of activity in the bone, both building and resorption, which may be a sign of tumor cells within the bone. Hot spots, however, may also be caused by a fracture or bone infection. Therefore, if hot spots are detected, the doctor will often suggest blood tests, biopsies, or other imaging tests in order to confirm the presence of cancer.

Elizabeth A. Manning, Ph.D.

For Further Information

Coleman, R. E. "Clinical Features of Metastatic Bone Disease and Risk of Skeletal Morbidity." *Clinical Cancer Research* 12, no. 20, pt. 2 (2006): 6243s-6249s.

Even-Sapir, E. "Imaging of Malignant Bone Involvement by Morphologic, Scintigraphic, and Hybrid Modalities." *Journal of Nuclear Medicine* 46, no. 8 (2005): 1356-1367.

Hamaoka, T., et al. "Bone Imaging in Metastatic Breast Cancer." *Journal of Clinical Oncology* 22, no. 14 (2004): 2942-2953.

Rosenthal, D. I. "Radiologic Diagnosis of Bone Metastases." *Cancer* 80, suppl. 8 (1997): 1595-1607.

Yoneda, T., and T. Hiraga. "Crosstalk Between Cancer Cells and Bone Microenvironment in Bone Metastasis." *Biochem Biophys Res Commun* 328, no. 3 (2005): 679-687.

Other Resources

American Cancer Society

How Is Bone Cancer Diagnosed?
http://www.cancer.org/docroot/CRI/content/CRI_2_4_3X_How_is_bone_cancer_diagnosed_2.asp?sitearea=

What Is Bone Metastasis?
http://www.cancer.org/docroot/CRI/content/CRI_2_4_1X_What_Is_bone_metastasis_66.asp

Mayo Clinic

Bone Scan: Using Nuclear Medicine to Find Bone Abnormalities
http://www.mayoclinic.com/health/bone-scan/CA00020

See also: Alveolar soft-part sarcomas; Beckwith-Wiedemann Syndrome (BWS); Bone cancers; Childhood cancers; Ewing sarcoma; Exenteration; Gallium scan; Glomus tumors; Imaging tests; Lacrimal gland tumors; Mantle Cell Lymphoma (MCL); Medulloblastomas; Myeloma; Nuclear medicine scan; Paget disease of bone; Pineoblastomas; Pneumonectomy; Radionuclide scan; Rhabdomyosarcomas; Richter syndrome; Spinal axis tumors

▶ Boron Neutron Capture Therapy (BNCT)

Category: Procedures

Definition: Boron Neutron Capture Therapy (BNCT) is a form of radiation therapy that brings together a stable isotope of boron (boron 10) and a beam of low-energy neutrons to target and destroy tumor cells while leaving adjacent tissue undamaged.

Cancers treated: Glioblastoma multiforme (GBM); perhaps other brain tumors and skin melanomas

Why performed: Treatments for high-grade gliomas are supportive but not curative. Patients with GBM die within three months when left untreated. Standard approaches using surgical resection, radiation therapy, and chemotherapy increase the median survival time to twelve months, with few patients surviving beyond five years. This is the case because tumor cells infiltrate into surrounding brain tissue and are not readily available to the surgeon, and because glioma cells tend to resist radiation and chemotherapy. Moreover, older patients respond poorly to all current therapies, and there has been no significant new approach to GBM treatment since the early 1980's. Researchers hope that BNCT will offer some improvement.

Patient preparation: Patient preparation is standard for radiation therapy. The size and location of the patient's tumor are determined using imaging studies such as magnetic resonance imaging (MRI) or computed tomography (CT) scans. Prior to neutron targeting, the patient's skin is marked to position the head correctly.

Steps of the procedure: The patient first receives an intravenous injection of boron 10 that has been chemically tagged to bind with the tumor cells. Neutrons created in a nuclear reactor and modified for BNCT treatment are beamed into the targeted tissue. Neutron activity slows during the ensuing collisions, resulting in a transformation into low-energy thermal neutrons. The boron atoms are then able to capture the thermal neutrons, resulting in boron disintegration into energetic lithium 7 and alpha particles. These cancer-destroying particles react in a very small area, thus confining the ensuing tissue destruction to the tumor.

After the procedure: There are no special procedures following BNCT.

Risks: The risks are minimal because the path length of the boron elements produced during the procedure is small, limiting the destructive properties to the size of a single cell and leaving nontargeted tissue unharmed.

Results: Although work on boron neutron capture therapy continues to hold promise, in general it has proved no more successful than standard therapies and so is not now a routine approach to treatment.

Richard S. Spira, D.V.M.

See also: Radiation oncology; Radiation therapies

▶ Brachytherapy

Category: Procedures
Also known as: Sealed source radiotherapy, endocurietherapy

Definition: Brachytherapy is a form of radiation treatment in which the radioactive source consists of small pellets or seeds, ribbons, or wire, each about the size of a grain of rice, that are placed into or next to the area being treated. Brachytherapy is from a Greek word meaning "short," so literally brachytherapy means "short distance treatment." It is unlike radiation from an external source, such as a machine, in which the radioactive beam is directed at the tumor from outside the body.

There are three types of brachytherapy delivery. Intracavity treatment involves radioactive implants that are placed inside a body cavity, such as the uterus. In interstitial treatment, radiation implants are placed directly in the tumor. They are often permanent and used in prostate cancer treatment. In unsealed internal radiation therapy, radioactive materials are injected into a vein or body cavity.

Brachytherapy can be either permanent or temporary. Permanent brachytherapy, or low dose rate (LDR) brachytherapy, is often called seed implantation and involves placing small radioactive seeds at or near the tumor and leaving them there permanently. This is typically used in the treatment of prostate cancer. The radioactivity of the seeds decreases over time, and the seeds left inside the patient cause no discomfort or harm. Temporary brachytherapy, or high dose rate (HDR) brachytherapy, involves radioactive seeds that are left in the body only for a specific amount of time and then are removed. Treatments may consist of several visits to the physician to have the seeds placed and removed. This method is used in the treatment of most of the other cancers.

Radiation works by killing cancer cells when they are trying to multiply. The deoxyribonucleic acid (DNA) of cancer cells is more sensitive to radiation than that of normal cells, so the normal cells are able to repair themselves and the cancer cells die.

Cancers treated: Brachytherapy is used for many types of cancer in the body, including prostate, cervical, head and neck, ovarian, breast, lung, gallbladder, uterine, and vaginal cancers, as well as anal/rectal tumors and sarcomas. It can also be used to treat noncancerous conditions such as benign tumors and coronary artery disease. Additionally, brachytherapy can be used in conjunction with other cancer treatments, including chemotherapy and external beam radiation. It can be used as both a curative and a palliative form of treatment.

Why performed: Brachytherapy has been in use since the early twentieth century, and it has been proven to be safe and effective. It allows a higher dose of radioactivity to be used with decreased risk of damage to healthy tissue, quicker healing times, and decreased risk of infection. In breast brachytherapy, for example, the therapy is quicker than external beam radiation, and it only treats a portion of the breast. Brachytherapy often can be performed in five days as opposed to five to seven weeks. The patient has a better cosmetic result and healthy tissue is preserved.

Patient preparation: Before the treatment begins, patients meet with the physician and receive instructions on how to care for themselves after the treatment. The physician will determine what tests should be done prior to brachytherapy, which may include blood tests, electrocardiograms (ECG or EKG), and X rays. The actual prepping of the patient depends on where the seeds are being placed. Typically, a radiation oncologist, a radiation physicist, a dosimetrist, and a radiation therapist are involved in planning the treatment. The radiation oncologist determines the type of treatment needed and is responsible for the overall treatment plan, including the area to be treated and the dose to be delivered. The physicist calculates the dose to be prescribed. The dosimetrist assists in dose calculation and helps in delivering the prescribed dose. The radiation therapist operates the equipment and delivers the dose. Through special computer programs, the dose, duration, and delivery method of the treatment are determined. Without this specific calculation, the cancer cells might receive too little radiation and the normal tissue could receive too much.

Steps of the procedure: The steps of the procedure also vary depending on where the seeds are being placed in the body. The seeds are generally inserted into the site of the tumor through a needle or catheter. Sometimes a device to hold the seeds is placed near the tumor. Often, X rays, ultrasound, computed tomography (CT) scans, or even surgery is used to help position and verify placement of the radioactive material or device.

Some doses are delivered to the patient on an outpatient basis, in which radiation is delivered to the tumor in a short amount of time and then the delivery device is removed and the patient goes home. The patient may return at intervals for more treatment. Alternatively, a patient may spend a couple of nights in the hospital so that the delivery device can remain in place and the radioactivity can be delivered at a continuous rate. These patients are placed in private rooms, usually with limited or no visitors allowed. The hospital staff will continue to take care of the patient, but they limit the amount of time that they spend with the patient in order to keep their radiation exposure low.

A patient may have an intravenous line inserted in order to receive medications. Sedatives or anesthesia may also be used to place the delivery device, again depending on the location of the treatment.

After the procedure: Patients typically can go home after the LDR procedure. The physician will give the patient detailed instructions for self-care at home, which may include limiting contact with pregnant women or children for a limited amount of time so as not to expose them to the radioactivity. The patient may have some pain, swelling, or bleeding at the site of the procedure. Educational materials may be very helpful to the patient and family after the procedure. Side effects and precautions can be outlined. Generally, the patient is to avoid heavy lifting or strenuous physical activity for a few days after the procedure. Sometimes the radiation precautions include instructing the patient to sleep alone for a period of time, to avoid sexual relations for a period of time, and to use tweezers, not bare hands, to pick up any seed that may become dislodged. Instructions on what to do with a dislodged seed are also given.

HDR patients are usually in the hospital for forty-eight to seventy-two hours and then are discharged once the radiation device is removed. They also receive detailed instructions on how to protect family members from exposure and to watch for side effects such as pain and bleeding.

Risks: Like the preparation of the patient and the steps of the procedure, the risks from brachytherapy also vary depending on the area treated. Although relatively safe, brachytherapy is not totally without risks. Patients with permanent brachytherapy seeds continue to give off small amounts of radiation for several weeks. With this type of treatment, there is a risk that the seeds will move out of place. Patients are often told to strain their urine at home in case in seeds do migrate. Patients are given special instructions from their doctor about protecting family members from exposure.

Brachytherapy for prostate cancer can cause sexual dysfunction such as impotence and bowel problems such as diarrhea, although these are not very common. Urinary irritation is a more common side effect because the urine stream becomes obstructed by swelling in the prostate after therapy. A urinary catheter or Foley catheter is placed to allow urine to flow. The prostate usually returns to normal size and the blockage disappears after several weeks, and the catheter can then be removed. Patients may continue to have some urinary burning for a few weeks, but this also resolves.

Results: The physician may order scans or X rays after brachytherapy in order to determine if the treatment was successful. The effectiveness of brachytherapy varies depending on the location of the treatment and the type of cancer that was treated. It has proven to be effective in many types of cancer, especially cervical and prostate cancer. In early prostate cancer, brachytherapy offers ten-year survival rates comparable to surgical removal of the prostate, according to several studies. In general, patients have fewer side effects and a quicker recovery time with this therapy as compared to external beam radiation or surgery. There is also less risk of infection than with surgery. As a result, patients typically have a better quality of life with this procedure, which is easier to tolerate.

Michelle Kasprzak, R.N., B.S.N., O.C.N.

For Further Information

Merrick, G. S., et al. "Long Term Rectal Function After Permanent Prostate Brachytherapy." *Cancer Journal* 13, no. 2 (March/April, 2007): 95-104.

Mitchell, I. "Patient Education at a Distance." *Radiology* 13, no. 1 (February, 2007): 30-34.

Nag, Subir, ed. *Principles and Practices of Brachytherapy*. Malden, Mass.: Blackwell, 1997.

Other Resources

American Brachytherapy Society (ABS)
http://www.americanbrachytherapy.org

American Cancer Society
http://www.cancer.org

National Cancer Institute
http://www.cancer.gov

See also: Afterloading radiation therapy; Anal cancer; Carcinomas; Cervical cancer; Endometrial cancer; Iridium seeds; Mayo Clinic Cancer Center; Neurologic oncology; Radiation oncology; Radiation therapies; Rhabdomyosarcomas; Veterinary oncology

▶ Brain scan

Category: Procedures

Definition: Computed tomography (CT) scan and magnetic resonance imaging (MRI) are two widely used methods of scanning the brain to distinguish normal tissue from abnormal tissue (tumors or masses). The CT scanner uses X rays and a type of ionizing radiation (dye), to acquire images of bone and tissue. MRI uses nonionizing radio frequency signals to acquire its images and is best suited for noncalcified (soft) tissue. Both CT and MRI scanners generate multiple two-dimensional cross-sections, or "slices," of tissue and produce three-dimensional reconstructions. For purposes of tumor detection and identification, MRI is generally superior. However, CT usually is more widely available, faster, and much less expensive, and it may be less likely to require the person to be sedated or anesthetized.

If cancer is suspected, then the CT scan will provide X-ray images of the brain or other internal organs to detect masses or tumors. A dye may be injected into a vein or swallowed to help the organs or tissues show up more clearly. A computer combines the images by "stacking" them on top of each other to offer an exact three-dimensional rendering.

MRI is a procedure using a magnet and radio waves to send a series of detailed images of the brain to a computer. A computer then produces cross-sectional or three-dimensional images for evaluation. A substance called gadolinium may be injected into the patient through a vein. The gadolinium collects around the cancer cells so that they show up brighter in the picture. This procedure is also called nuclear magnetic resonance imaging (NMRI).

Cancers diagnosed: Brain tumor, metastasized cancer

Why performed: Brain scans are ordered by physicians to offer the clearest information available about the brain. The method of scanning depends on the patient's history and examination and the choice by the physician for diagnostic testing.

Patient preparation: If the brain scan involves injecting or ingesting a dye, then the patient may be asked to avoid eating or drinking four hours before the exam. All jewelry must be removed prior to the brain scan.

Steps of the procedure: The patient will be asked to lay down, placing the head in a stabilizer, and remain very still. If contrast (dye) is required, then it will be injected through the intravenous (IV) line that was placed by a radiology nurse or technologist prior to the exam. During the injection, it is normal for patients to experience a warm sensation throughout the body and a metal taste in the mouth. Only the head will be covered by the scanner, and those who experience claustrophobia generally do not have problems with a brain scan.

After the procedure: Patients are not restricted after this procedure and may eat and drive as normal.

Risks: The MRI examination poses almost no risk to the average patient; however, if sedation is necessary, a nurse or technologist will monitor vital signs to avoid excessive sedation. The magnetic field is not harmful to the patient, but metal devices nearby can create malfunction in the MRI. If dye is injected, then there is a rare risk of mild allergic reaction.

The CT scan poses a slight risk of cancer as a result of the exposure to radiation. Studies have shown this risk is equivalent to the amount of radiation to which an average person is exposed in three years from other, unavoidable sources. There is a risk to an unborn fetus; therefore CT scanning is not recommended for pregnant women.

Nursing mothers must wait twenty-four hours after the dye is injected to return to nursing. There is always a slight chance of cancer from radiation exposure, but the benefit of an accurate diagnosis far outweighs the risk.

Results: The brain scan will be read by a neuroradiologist, and the results will be shared with the physician to discuss with the patient.

Robert J. Amato, D.O.

For Further Information

Buthiau, Didier, and David Khayat. *CT and MRI in Oncology*. New York: Springer-Verlag, 1998.
Lee, Howard S., et al. *Cranial and Spinal MRI and CT*. 4th ed. New York: McGraw-Hill Professional, 1999.
Wolbarst, Anthony Brinton. *Looking Within: How X-Ray, CT, MRI, Ultrasound, and Other Medical Images Are Created, and How They Help Physicians Save Lives*. Berkeley: University of California Press, 1999.

See also: Astrocytomas; Brain and central nervous system cancers; Computed Tomography (CT) scan

▶ Breast implants

Category: Procedures
Also known as: Autologous breast implants, saline breast implants, saline-filled breast implants, silicone breast implants, silicone-filled breast implants

Definition: Breast implants are used to reconstruct the natural appearance of one or both breasts following mastectomy for breast cancer. Breast implants may be composed of the patient's own tissue taken from elsewhere on the body (autologous breast implants) or made of artificial substances (saline or silicone breast implants).

Cancers treated: Breast cancer

Why performed: Breast reconstruction is a choice for women following mastectomy. Mastectomy involves surgically removing one or both breasts for the treatment of breast cancer. Breast implants are used to replace breasts that have been removed, to create a symmetrical appearance if only one breast was removed, or to replace the one breast that was removed and enhance the appearance of the remaining breast to improve symmetry. Breast implants are an option to wearing breast prosthetics (removable breast forms).

Patient preparation: Breast implants come in a variety of shapes, sizes, and compositions. The plastic surgeon guides the patient in the selection process. Tissue expanders may or may not be used to stretch the skin in preparation for breast implant placement. In some cases, the tissue expander may be filled with saline and remain in the body, serving as the breast implant.

There are two basic types of artificial implants, saline breast implants and silicone breast implants. Saline breast implants have a silicone outer shell and are filled with saline, a saltwater solution. Saline implants may be prefilled by the manufacturer or filled at the time of surgery and adjusted after surgery.

Silicone breast implants have a silicone outer shell and are filled with silicone, a natural substance. Silicone breast implants may be prefilled with silicone by the manufacturer and nonadjustable, prefilled with silicone and allow for saline insertion at the time of surgery, or prefilled with silicone and allow for saline insertion at the time of surgery and postsurgical adjustments.

Saline implants were approved for use in the United States by the Food and Drug Administration (FDA) in 2000. Silicone implants were approved by the FDA in 2006. Both types of implants are not meant to last a lifetime, may need to be replaced, and have a risk of rupture. Saline implants are advantageous in that ruptures are readily identified because the breast size decreases and the saline solution is absorbed by the body. The size of saline implants can be adjusted easily. Some people believe, however, that saline implants do not look or feel as natural as silicone implants.

Silicone implants have a texture similar to natural breast tissue. While silicone breast implants may look and feel more natural than saline implants, ruptures may not be as easily noticed with silicone breast implants. Following a rupture, the silicone remains near the implant and is not absorbed by the body.

Autologous implants are made of tissue or a tissue flap that is taken from the patient, commonly the abdomen and buttocks. The tissue may contain fat, muscles, blood vessels, and nerves. Autologous implants are a more specialized procedure involving microsurgery and take longer to heal, but they do not have the risk of rupture and do not need to be replaced over time. Some people believe that autologous implants produce the most natural results.

Steps of the procedure: Breast implants may be inserted at the time of the mastectomy or at a later time in another surgery. Patients receiving radiation therapy following mastectomy may need to delay breast reconstruction.

Breast implant procedures do not delay chemotherapy. Breast reconstruction surgery is performed with general anesthesia. Nipple reconstruction may take place following a breast implant procedure.

After the procedure: Patients may spend one to six days in the hospital, depending on the procedure. Patients wear bandages and support garments while healing. Activities may be temporarily restricted, but most activities can be resumed in six to eight weeks.

Artificial implants typically need to be replaced in time. Breast implants should not affect breastfeeding. Special mammography procedures may be needed, however. Breast implants only rarely obscure the detection of new cancer formation.

Risks: The risks of artificial breast implants include rupture, leakage, rippling, infection, and capsular contraction (in which scar tissue surrounding the implants shrinks or hardens). Other risks include the general risks associated with surgery and anesthesia.

Results: The optimal result is symmetrical, natural-appearing breasts.

Mary Car-Blanchard, O.T.D., B.S.O.T.

For Further Information

Poeppl, N., et al. "Does the Surface Structure of Implants Have an Impact on the Formation of a Capsular Contracture?" *Aesthetic Plastic Surgery* 31, no. 2 (March/April, 2007): 133-139.

"Silicone Gel-Filled Breast Implants Approved." *FDA Consumer* 41, no. 1 (January/February, 2007).

Stevens, W. G., et al. "A Comparison of Five Hundred Prefilled Textured Saline Breast Implants Versus Five Hundred Standard Textured Saline Breast Implants: Is There a Difference in Deflation Rates?" *Plastic and Reconstruction Surgery* 117, no. 7 (June, 2006): 2175-2181.

Vázquez, G., and A. Pellón. "Polyurethane-Coated Silicone Gel Breast Implants Used for Eighteen Years." *Aesthetic Plastic Surgery* 31, no. 4 (July/August, 2007): 330-336.

Other Resources

American Cancer Society
http://www.cancer.org

American Society of Plastic Surgeons
http://www.plasticsurgery.org

Breast Implant Safety.org
http://www.breastimplantsafety.org

See also: Breast cancers; Breast reconstruction; Mastectomy; Self-image and body image; Sexuality and cancer

▶ Breast reconstruction

Category: Procedures

Also known as: Breast implants; deep inferior epigastric perforator (DIEP) flap; free flap; gluteal flap; latissimus dorsi flap; pedicle flap; saline breast implants; silicone breast implants; transverse rectus abdominis muscle (TRAM) flap

Definition: Breast reconstruction is a complex procedure performed by a plastic surgeon that restores the appearance of a breast after mastectomy to treat breast cancer.

Cancers treated: Breast cancer

Why performed: Breast reconstruction is performed to reconstruct the size and shape of the breast in a patient who has had a mastectomy. Most women who have had a mastectomy can have breast reconstruction, which may be done either at the time of mastectomy or at a later date. Breast reconstruction may improve the self-esteem and body image of a woman who has had a mastectomy.

Patient preparation: A patient facing a mastectomy who is interested in breast reconstruction probably will be advised to consult with a plastic surgeon experienced in breast reconstruction prior to the mastectomy. Ideally, the breast surgeon and the plastic surgeon work together to develop the best surgical and breast reconstruction strategy for each patient, even if the reconstructive surgery will be done later. Two or more operations probably will be needed to achieve a satisfactory result.

A patient will be given specific instructions prior to surgery. Since smoking can decrease a patient's blood circulation, which is critical to the survival of transplanted tissue, a patient who is a smoker will be given instructions and tips to quit smoking prior to reconstruction procedures that involve the use of transplanted tissue.

Steps of the procedure: There are two basic types of breast reconstruction, implant procedures and tissue flap procedures. A combination of these procedures may also be used. Either type of procedure may be begun either at the same time as the mastectomy (immediate reconstruction) or at a later time (delayed reconstruction).

Saline-filled implants are the most common type of implant used and consist of external silicone shells filled with sterile saline. The use of silicone gel-filled implants has decreased because of concerns of possible health risks if silicone leaks from the implant, although recent research has not found any health dangers associated with their use. Sometimes a one-stage procedure is possible, where the implant is placed behind the pectoral muscle in the chest in the first surgery. For most patients, a two-stage procedure is used in which a tissue expander, like a balloon, is implanted beneath the skin and chest muscle. Over a period of several months, the surgeon injects a saline solution at regular intervals to fill the expander and stretch the chest pocket. At the appropriate time, the expander is removed in a second operation and the permanent implant is put into place.

Tissue flap procedures involve autologous tissue reconstruction and are the more surgically complex option for breast reconstruction. Tissue from the abdomen or back (more commonly), or buttocks or thighs (less commonly), is used. Two types of methods, pedicle flap and free flap, are in use. In a pedicle flap procedure, some of the blood vessels feeding the tissue to be transferred are cut and some are kept intact. The tissue is tunneled beneath the skin to the chest area, where a new breast mound or pocket for an implant is created. In a free flap procedure, the flap of skin, fat, blood vessels, and muscle tissue is disconnected from its blood supply completely and removed from its original location, and intricate microsurgical techniques are used to reattach the tissue flap to new blood vessels near the chest. This procedure typically takes longer to complete than a pedicle flap procedure.

Four main tissue flap procedures are performed: the TRAM (transverse rectus abdominis muscle) flap, the DIEP (deep inferior epigastric perforator) flap, the latissimus dorsi flap, and the gluteal flap.

The TRAM flap procedure uses tissue and muscle from the lower abdominal wall, which may be transferred as a free flap or a pedicle flap. This procedure also results in a tightening of the lower abdomen, or a "tummy tuck." Variations on this procedure use different amounts of abdominal muscle. The use of less muscle for reconstruction may help the patient retain abdominal strength after surgery.

The newer DIEP flap procedure uses skin, fat, and minimal abdominal muscle tissue, and it uses a free flap approach. Patients generally retain more abdominal strength with this type of breast reconstruction.

The latissimus dorsi flap procedure transfers skin, fat, muscle, and blood vessels from the upper back as a pedicle flap, tunneling the tissue under the skin to the front of the chest. The amount of skin and other tissue used in this procedure is generally less than in a TRAM flap surgery, making it useful for reconstructing small and medium-sized breasts or for creating a pocket for a breast implant.

The gluteal flap is a free flap procedure that uses skin, fat, blood vessels, and gluteal muscle tissue from the buttocks to create the breast shape. This procedure is an option for women who cannot use the abdominal site due to thinness or incisions, or for patient preference.

Nipple and areola reconstruction is optional and, if done, is performed as a last step after the patient has healed from the first surgeries. The nipple is reconstructed using tissue from the breast itself or from another part of the patient's body such as the inner thigh. The areola may be created by tattooing the skin to make it match the natural nipple and areola. Saving the nipple from the breast with cancer that is removed (called nipple saving or nipple banking) is sometimes done but is risky because the nipple tissue might contain cancer cells.

After the procedure: A patient will likely feel tired and sore for a week or two after implant reconstruction, and longer, perhaps months, after tissue flap reconstruction. The patient will probably be discharged from the hospital with a surgical drain in place to allow excess fluids to drain from the surgical site. Stitches will be in place after the surgery, but they will most likely be absorbable sutures that will not have to be removed. Scars will fade over time but never go away entirely. It takes about six to eight weeks for the patient to return to normal, depending on the type of procedure performed. A patient will be advised to take it easy during this period and avoid overhead lifting and strenuous physical activity.

Risks: Some risks of breast reconstructive surgery are bleeding, fluid collection, swelling and pain, excessive scar tissue, infection, the death of all or part of the flap, problems at the donor site, fatigue, changes in the affected arm, and the need for additional surgeries to correct problems.

If an infection develops after the implant surgery, then the implant may need to be removed until the infection clears. If an infection develops after flap surgery, then surgical cleaning of the wound may be necessary.

Sometimes local complications occur with breast implants. The most common of these is capsular contracture, which can occur if the scar or capsule around the implant begins to tighten and squeeze down on the soft implant, making the breast feel hard. More surgery may be needed to remove the scar tissue, or the implant may need to be removed or replaced. Rarely, rupture of the implant may occur. Implants may not last a lifetime, so additional surgeries may be needed to replace them.

Breast reconstruction has no known effect on the recurrence of breast cancer, and neither implant nor flap procedures decrease the likelihood of detection of a recurrence of breast cancer.

Results: Breast reconstruction after a mastectomy can improve a woman's appearance and self-confidence. Although the surgeon will try to create a breast shape that matches the other breast closely, a perfect match is not possible, and a reconstructed breast does not have natural sensations. In some cases, surgery on the other breast is performed to improve the match.

Jill Ferguson, Ph.D.

For Further Information

Ahmed, S., et al. "Breast Reconstruction." *British Medical Journal* 330 (2005): 943-948.

Edlick, R. F., et al. "Advances in Breast Reconstruction After Mastectomy." *Journal of Long-Term Effects of Medical Implants* 15 (2005): 197-207.

Farhadi, J., et al. "Reconstruction of the Nipple-Areola Complex: An Update." *Journal of Plastic, Reconstructive & Aesthetic Surgery* 59 (2006): 40-53.

Fentiman, I. S., and H. Hamed. "Breast Reconstruction." *International Journal of Clinical Practice* 60 (2006): 471-474.

Piasecki, J. H., and K. A. Gutowski. "Breast Reconstruction." *Clinical Obstetics and Gynecology* 49 (2006): 401-413.

Serletti, J. M. "Breast Reconstruction with the TRAM Flap: Pedicled and Free." *Journal of Surgical Oncology* 94 (2006): 532-537.

Spear, S. L., and A. N. Mesbahi. "Implant-Based Reconstruction." *Clinics in Plastic Surgery* 34 (2007): 63-73.

Other Resources

American Cancer Society
Breast Reconstruction After Mastectomy
http://www.cancer.org/docroot/CRI/content/CRI_2_6X_Breast_Reconstruction_After_Mastectomy_5.asp

American Society of Plastic Surgeons
Breast Reconstruction
http://www.plasticsurgery.org/patients_consumers/procedures/BreastReconstruction.cfm

Breastcancer.org
Reconstruction
http://www.breastcancer.org/bey_tre_recon_idx.html

Mayo Clinic
Breast Reconstruction After Mastectomy
http://www.mayoclinic.com/health/breast-reconstruction/WO00083

See also: Breast cancers; Breast implants; Mastectomy; Self-image and body image; Sexuality and cancer

▶ Breast Self-Examination (BSE)

Category: Procedures

Definition: The National Breast Cancer Foundation recommends that all women age twenty and older conduct a breast self-examination (BSE) on a monthly basis, in addition to undergoing a clinical breast examination periodically, depending on age and state of health.

Cancers diagnosed: Breast cancer

Why performed: Breast self-examinations are performed by women on their own breasts to detect unusual swellings, lumps, thickenings, or other conditions that may suggest the possibility of a breast disorder, including breast cancer. It is believed that, if performed every month at the same time (in relation to the menstrual cycle), this examination will educate a woman about how her breasts feel normally and will alert her to any sudden changes, thereby facilitating early detection of a precancerous or cancerous mass.

Patient preparation: It is recommended that the examination take place in the shower (where water smooths the skin and makes it easier to detect changes) or lying prone.

Steps of the procedure: Using the left hand to examine the right breast (and vice versa), the woman should, with fingers flat, move gently over every part of the breast in a systematic fashion (vertically up to down or circularly from well beyond the exterial margins inward), starting well above the top margin of the breast and beyond each

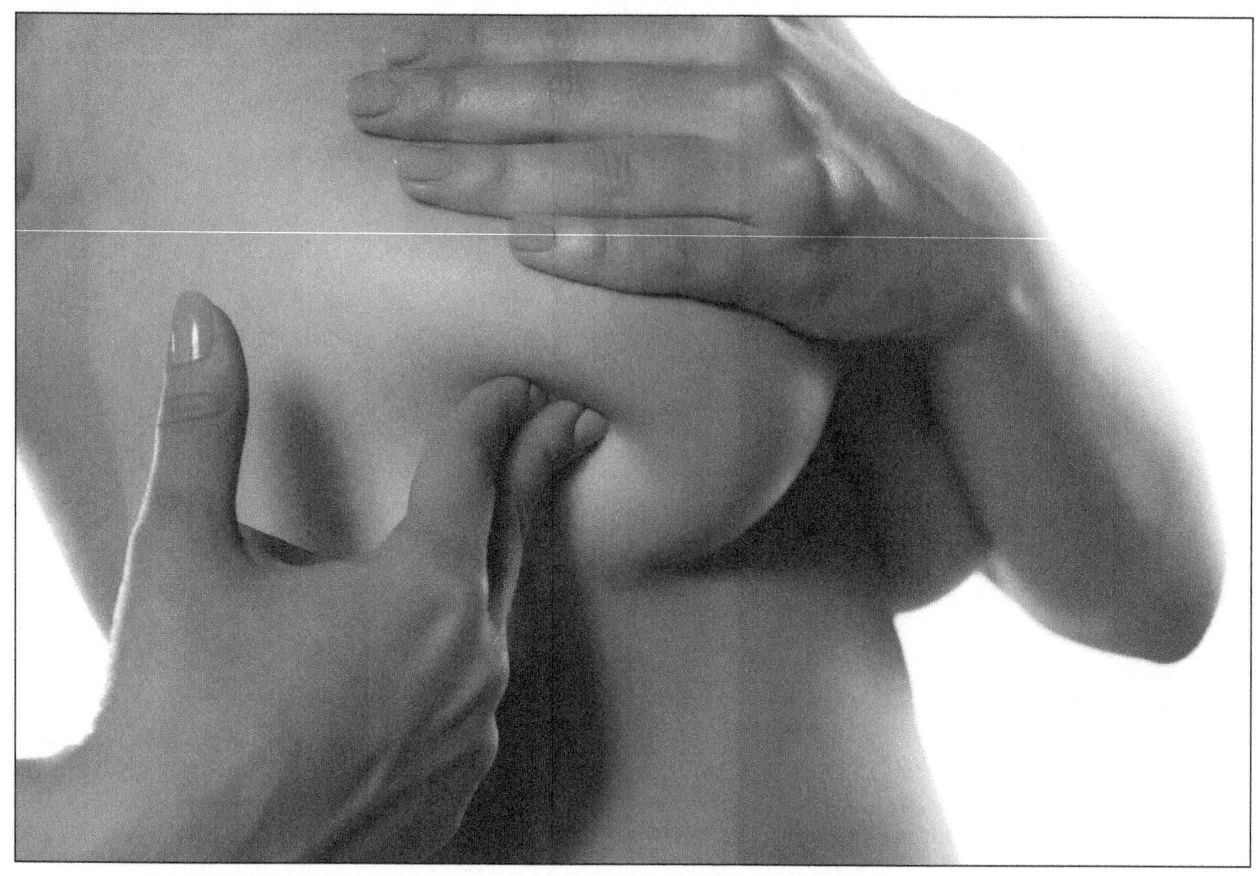

A woman performs a breast self-examination. (iStock)

right and left margin as well. The examination should be conducted three times using light, medium, and heavy pressure. Women must also visually inspect their breasts in a mirror, raising arms overhead and looking at the breasts from all sides. Muscles should be both flexed and relaxed. Women should be particularly alert to any swellings, dimpling of the skin, "orange-peel" (peau d'orange) appearance, discoloration, changes in or discharges from the nipple, lumps no matter how small, or other unfamiliar signs.

After the procedure: If a woman detects a change in how her breasts or nipples feel, then she should promptly schedule an appointment with her physician for follow-up tests.

Risks: There are no risks in performing the examination, and generally such examinations cause no pain.

Results: Women who perform a self-exam become familiar with their own breasts and are able to report abnormalities much earlier than is possible if they wait for an annual clinical examination or mammogram. Early detection of precancerous or cancerous tissue greatly increases not only early treatment but also survival rates.

Christina J. Moose, M.A.

See also: Breast cancer in pregnant women; Breast cancers; Calcifications of the breast; Clinical Breast Exam (CBE); Mammography; Nipple discharge; Palpation; Screening for cancer

▶ Breast ultrasound

Category: Procedures
Also known as: Sonography, ultrasonography

Definition: Breast ultrasound is the use of high-frequency sound waves to produce an image of the breast tissue. The sound waves used are in the range of 20,000 to 10,000,000 cycles per second and are inaudible to the human ear. They are bounced off of the breast tissue and are able to distinguish between solid tumors and fluid-filled cysts. The density and elasticity of tissues affect the velocity of the sound waves traveling through them. Tissues that are denser and less elastic slow the sound waves and appear as shaded areas on the screen image. Tissues that are less dense and more elastic do not interfere with the sound waves and appear as clear areas. The interpretation of the sound wave data is performed by a computer. An advantage of breast ultrasound is that it does not use radiation.

Cancers diagnosed: Breast cancer

Why performed: There are several reasons that breast ultrasounds are performed. After a questionable mammogram, a breast ultrasound may be used to further examine the breast tissue. Some breast conditions may look like a possible cancer on a mammogram but can be identified as benign on ultrasound. For example, breast cysts and some fibroadenomas appear as clear areas on a breast ultrasound, whereas a breast cancer would not. In women under the age of thirty-five, breast ultrasound may be the procedure of choice for screening for breast cancer because younger women have denser breast tissue, which makes it difficult to assess for abnormalities on mammography. Breast ultrasound may also be used to guide a needle biopsy, or needle localization. Ultrasound has proved effective at examining the breasts of women with breast implants. It is often able to illustrate whether the implant has ruptured or not. Mammography does not show fluid leaking from the implant.

Patient preparation: No preparation of the patient is required.

Steps of the procedure: For a breast ultrasound, the patient puts on a hospital gown, which is open in the front, and then lies supine on a table. A pillow is placed under the shoulder of the breast to be scanned. The area to be scanned is uncovered. The patient's arm is placed up over the head, resting on the examination table. The radiology technician or physician uses a transducer (an instrument to transmit and receive sound waves) to scan the breast tissue. A transducer looks like a small cell phone. A gel is used between the transducer and the patient to enhance the transmission of the sound waves for the scan. The transducer is moved slowly and lightly over the breast tissue. Usually, the breast lesion is viewed in several planes, so that its features can be defined. This is accomplished by changing the angle of the transducer in relation to the breast tissue. The images of the breast are printed for further examination.

After the procedure: No additional patient care is required, so the patient can go home.

Risks: There are no known risks of breast ultrasound for the patient. It appears that sound waves are safe for use on human beings. For the physician, however, there is the risk of making an incorrect diagnosis about the presence of breast cancer. Breast ultrasounds do not differentiate microcalcifications (mineral deposits) in the breast tissue. Microcalcifications that are clustered can be a first sign of a developing breast cancer.

The accuracy of breast ultrasounds can vary with the skill of the technician. Once the ultrasound images have been printed, there is no way to determine the angle of the transducer, or to manipulate the images, as can be done with mammograms. Also, breast ultrasound is not as accurate at assessing the whole breast. It is most effective at assessing a small area of breast tissue.

Results: The images of the breast ultrasound demonstrate the different breast tissues, with the ducts appearing darker than the adipose (fatty) tissue between the ducts. The breast ultrasound is most accurate at identifying breast cysts, which are fluid-filled. If on ultrasound an area of the breast appears particularly dense and opaque, then a breast cancer could be present. Breast ultrasound does not differentiate between benign tumors and malignant (cancerous) tumors or growths. As a result, a breast biopsy is required to identify the type of lesion.

Christine M. Carroll, R.N., B.S.N., M.B.A.

For Further Information

Love, Susan M., and Karen Lindsay. *Dr. Susan Love's Breast Book.* Rev. 4th ed. Cambridge, Mass.: Da Capo Press, 2005.

Pagana, Kathleen Deska, and Timothy J. Pagana. *Mosby's Manual of Diagnostic and Laboratory Tests.* 3d ed. St. Louis: Mosby Elsevier, 2006.

Other Resources

American Cancer Society

Mammograms and Other Breast Imaging Procedures
http://www.cancer.org/docroot/CRI/content/CRI_2_6X_Mammography_and_Other_Breast_imaging_Procedures_5.asp

Health A to Z

Breast Ultrasound
http://www.healthatoz/atoz/ency/breast_ultrasound.jsp

Imaginis
Breast Cancer Diagnosis
http://www.imaginis.com/breasthealth/ultrasound_images.asp

Yale Medical Group
Breast Imaging at Yale
http://www.yalemedicalgroup.org/news/dxrad/ymg_breastimaging.html

See also: Breast cancer in children and adolescents; Breast cancer in men; Breast cancer in pregnant women; Breast cancers; Calcifications of the breast; Clinical Breast Exam (CBE); Imaging tests; Mammography; Microcalcifications; Needle biopsies; Premalignancies; Screening for cancer; Ultrasound tests

▶ Breslow's staging

Category: Procedures
Also known as: Breslow thickness, Breslow measurement, Breslow's depth of invasiveness

Definition: Breslow's staging is a test to measure, in millimeters (mm), the vertical thickness (how far a tumor reaches into the skin) of a malignant melanoma tumor. The test was developed by Alexander Breslow (1928-1980), an American pathologist, in the 1970's.

Cancers diagnosed: Melanoma, the most deadly form of skin cancer

Why performed: Once melanoma is confirmed by a skin biopsy, Breslow's staging helps oncologists establish the progress, or stage, of the cancer and whether the cancer has spread. The stage helps oncologists choose the best treatment and determine the best prospects for recovery.

Patient preparation: No special preparation is needed for a skin biopsy.

Steps of the procedure: A skin biopsy is usually done in the doctor's office. A local anesthetic is injected into the area with a small needle. A sample of skin tissue is then removed for examination.

After the procedure: The patient feels no pain and may go home. The skin sample is examined in a laboratory. If melanoma is confirmed, then the sample is subjected to Breslow's staging to help determine prognosis and treatment.

Risks: Small skin biopsies are generally safe and carry only a small risk of bleeding or infection. Sometimes a biopsy may leave a scar.

Results: Early diagnosis is the most effective way of improving the cure rate for patients with melanoma. When laboratory tests confirm melanoma, Breslow's staging classifies the progress of the cancer according to one of five stages. In the first stage, malignant melanoma cells are found only in the outer layer of skin and have not yet invaded the deeper layers or spread. Most patients with melanoma only in the outer layer of skin can be cured with surgery.

The Breslow thickness of a melanoma tumor predicts the approximate five-year survival rate after the tumor is surgically removed.

- Smaller than 1 mm: 95-100 percent
- 1.0-2.0 mm: 80-96 percent
- 2.1-4.0 mm: 60-75 percent
- More than 4.0 mm: 50 percent

In the last stage, the melanoma could be any thickness but has spread to other parts of the body, most likely to the nearest lymph nodes. The majority of patients with melanoma that has spread to nearby lymph nodes cannot be cured with current treatments. The average survival of patients with melanoma that has spread to the lymph nodes is only 7.5 months. Only 5 to 10 percent of patients survive beyond five years.

Wendell Anderson, B.A.

See also: Melanomas

▶ Brief Pain Inventory (BPI)

Category: Procedures

Definition: The Brief Pain Inventory (BPI) is a questionnaire used to measure pain in cancer patients and other patients suffering from chronic pain. The BPI provides information on the intensity of pain (known as the sensory dimension) and the impact of pain on a patient's daily routine (known as the reactive dimension). The BPI was developed in 1989 by Charles Cleeland, M.D., while with the Pain Research group at the University of Wisconsin.

Cancers diagnosed or treated: All cancers that cause chronic or severe sporadic pain

Why performed: The BPI is administered to determine cancer patients' level of pain. Once the level of pain is determined, oncologists work to manage the painful symptoms of cancer and to make patients more comfortable. Pain management is especially important for terminal patients.

Cancer pain appears when a tumor presses against organs, nerves, or bone. Treatments for cancer—such as chemotherapy, radiation therapy, and especially surgery—also can cause pain.

The Veterans Administration and the Joint Commission on Accreditation of Health Care Organizations consider pain the fifth vital sign and require physicians to ask patients about their pain.

Patient preparation: Taking the BPI requires no patient preparation.

Steps of the procedure: The questionnaire for the BPI is usually filled out by the patient. In some cases, a doctor, nurse, or social worker helps by interviewing the patient and recording the answers. Filling out the short version of the BPI takes about five minutes, while the long version takes about ten minutes.

After the procedure: After the patient completes the BPI, it is scored on a scale of 0-10 for both the severity and the impact dimensions of the pain.

Risks: There are no inherent risks involved with the BPI. Its validity has been tested many times, and it has been translated into twenty-five languages. The only possible problem involved with the BPI is a patient's inability or reluctance to report pain accurately.

Results: The results of an individual patient's BPI can be tabulated in a few minutes. The results help oncologists, nurses, and other caregivers develop a pain management plan for the cancer patient.

Wendell Anderson, B.A.

See also: Breakthrough pain; Pain management medications

▶ Bronchography

Category: Procedures
Also known as: Bronchogram, laryngography

Definition: Bronchography is a radiographic evaluation that examines the interior passageways of the larynx, trachea, and bronchi. Bronchography is used somewhat infrequently because of technological advances with computed tomography (CT) scans and bronchoscopy.

Cancers diagnosed: Lung cancers

Why performed: Bronchography is performed to examine structural or functional abnormalities of the lower respiratory tract. Abnormalities that are commonly investigated with bronchography include bronchiectisis, hemoptysis, chronic bronchitis, chronic pneumonia, and tumors.

Patient preparation: The patient is asked to not eat or drink for several hours before the procedure. The patient may also be asked to perform thorough mouth hygiene before the procedure.

Steps of the procedure: The patient is asked to remove all clothing, jewelry, and dentures; to dress in a gown; and to empty the bladder. Vital signs (such as blood pressure and respiratory rate) are taken. The patient is positioned on a table that can tilt in various directions. The patient may also be given a sedative. Next, numbing medication is injected into the back of the patient's throat to prevent gagging. Finally, the physician passes the bronchoscope down the back of the throat into the trachea and bronchi. Contrast dye is released from the bronchoscope as it advances. The dye forms a coating on the lining of the interiors of the bronchi, trachea, and larynx. The physician then takes several X rays from different positions, after which the bronchoscope is removed.

After the procedure: The patient is moved to a recovery room and has vital signs monitored for several hours postprocedure. The patient will not be allowed to eat or drink until the gag reflex has returned. The patient may be asked to gently cough up any remaining contrast dye. Normal diet may be resumed after the procedure. The throat may feel sore after bronchography. A follow-up chest X ray is often performed twenty-four to forty-eight hours after the bronchography to verify the removal of the contrast dye from the airways.

Risks: Risks of the procedure include infection or pneumonia and airway obstruction from the contrast dye in patients with emphysema or chronic obstructive pulmonary disease (COPD).

Results: The contrast dye allows the physician to assess the likely presence or absence of respiratory system abnormalities, such as tumors, in the larynx, trachea, or bronchi. If abnormalities are detected, then the physician will either perform a confirmatory diagnostic procedure or devise a treatment plan based on the specific test results.

Jeremy W. Dugosh, Ph.D.

See also: Adenocarcinomas; Adenoid Cystic Carcinoma (ACC); Bronchial adenomas; Bronchoalveolar lung cancer; Bronchoscopy; 1,4-Butanediol dimethanesulfonate; Carcinoid tumors and carcinoid syndrome; Coughing; Laryngeal cancer; Lung cancers; Pneumonia

▶ Bronchoscopy

Category: Procedures
Also known as: Fiber-optic bronchoscopy

Definition: Bronchoscopy uses a bronchoscope to allow a doctor to see, examine, and biopsy tissues in the respiratory tract and lungs. The procedure is used to check for cancer cells. A bronchoscope is a thin tube equipped with fiber optics or a miniature camera that produces images of the internal airways and lungs.

Cancers diagnosed: Respiratory tract cancer, lung cancer

Why performed: Bronchoscopy is a diagnostic procedure used to view the inside of the airways and lungs. Suspicious tissues are biopsied and examined in a laboratory in order to detect the presence of cancer cells.

Patient preparation: Patients should stop taking aspirin or blood-thinning medication a week before the procedure. Brochoscopy uses local or general anesthesia. Patients receiving general anesthesia should not eat or drink after midnight prior to the day of the procedure. Bronchoscopy is usually an outpatient procedure, and patients should arrange to have someone else drive them home. Patients wear an examination gown, which is removed from the waist up during the procedure, and receive a sedative before the bronchoscopy begins.

Steps of the procedure: Patients receive general or local anesthesia, depending on whether a rigid or a flexible bronchoscope is used. Local anesthesia is injected or sprayed into the throat. Patients receive medication to eliminate secretions and to prevent coughing or gagging. Monitors are placed to measure blood pressure, blood oxygen levels, and heart activity. Oxygen is delivered through a nasal cannula. The bronchoscope is inserted through the nose or mouth. The airways and lungs are inspected. A bronchoalveolar lavage may be performed, which involves inserting sterile fluid to remove mucus or cells for examination. A tissue biopsy is taken by clipping a sample of abnormal tissue. At the end of the procedure, the fluid and bronchoscope are removed.

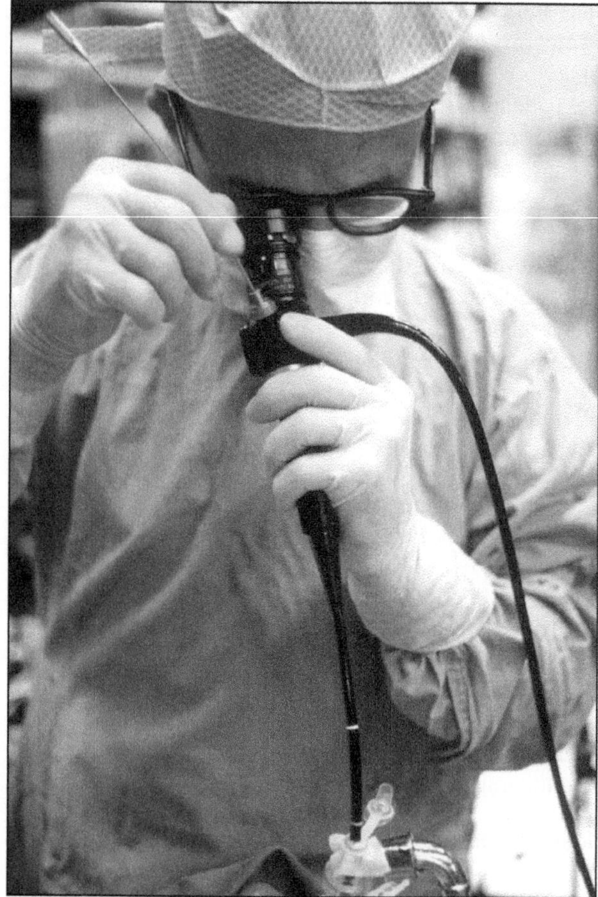

A physician uses a bronchoscope. (National Cancer Institute)

After the procedure: Patients may receive a chest X ray following the procedure to ensure that the lungs were not punctured. Patients should not eat or drink until the anesthesia wears off in order to prevent choking. Patients may be hoarse, experience fever, or cough up small amounts of blood.

Risks: Bronchoscopy is considered a safe procedure. The primary risks are infection and bleeding. There is a slight risk of lung perforation, heart attack, irregular heartbeat, and low blood oxygen.

Results: A healthy respiratory tract and lungs are free of swelling and abnormal growths. Suspicious growths are biopsied to determine whether cancer is present.

Mary Car-Blanchard, O.T.D., B.S.O.T.

See also: Bronchial adenomas; Bronchoalveolar lung cancer; Bronchography; Carcinoid tumors and carcinoid syndrome; Computed Tomography (CT) scan; Coughing; Endoscopy; Gastrointestinal cancers; Hemoptysis; Lambert-Eaton Myasthenic Syndrome (LEMS); Lung cancers; Mesothelioma; Otolaryngology; Pneumonia; Sputum cytology

▶ CA 15-3 test

Category: Procedures
Also known as: Carbohydrate antigen 15-3, cancer antigen 15-3

Definition: CA 15-3 is a transmembrane glycoprotein (carbohydrate-containing protein) found in several tissue types. It is classified as a MUC1 member of the mucin family of proteins. This class of glycoproteins is thought to play a role in reducing cell-to-cell interaction and inhibition of tumor cell cytolysis. The core protein component is identical; the carbohydrate concentration (degree of glycosylation) is the component differentiating between tissue types. Serum/plasma levels are determined by immunoassay.

Cancers diagnosed: CA 15-3 is not an organ-specific marker and has been found at elevated levels in ovarian, prostatic, and lung cancer. Additionally, increased CA 15-3 levels can be found concomitant with benign conditions such as breast or ovarian disease, endometriosis, pelvic inflammatory disease, hepatitis, pregnancy, and lactation.

Why performed: Because CA 15-3 is not sensitive or specific enough to be used as a screening test, its primarily utility is as a tumor marker for monitoring response to therapy and recurrence in breast cancer patients. At least 70 percent of advanced breast cancer cases have tumors that shed CA 15-3. Blood levels typically are proportional to the tumor burden (mass), with higher levels of CA 15-3 indicative of the presence of a larger tumor.

Patient preparation: No special patient preparation is required for accurate CA 15-3 analysis.

Steps of the procedure: A blood sample is collected, typically by venipuncture. The collected serum (or plasma) is tested by immunoassay, which involves capturing the CA 15-3 present in the sample by means of monoclonal anti-CA 15-3 antibodies. A second, detection (labeled) antibody is then introduced, which subsequently binds to the CA 15-3/anti-CA 15-3 complex. The addition of a substrate results in a detectable signal, the level of which is directly proportional to the amount of the CA 15-3 present in the sample.

After the procedure: Pressure should be applied to the venipucture site in order to avoid the development of hematoma (a mass of clotted blood resulting from bleeding under the skin).

Risks: The risks of venipuncture are slight but include excessive bleeding, fainting, hematoma, and infection (always a slight risk any time the skin is broken).

Results: Although each laboratory establishes reference intervals based on the local, normal population, a basic interpretive guideline would place normal at 0-31 units per milliliter (U/mL) and elevated at more than 31 U/mL.

Pam Conboy, B.S.

See also: CA 19-9 test; CA 27-29 test; CA 125 test; Tumor markers

▶ CA 19-9 test

Category: Procedures
Also known as: Carbohydrate antigen 19-9, cancer antigen 19-9

Definition: CA 19-9 is a glycolipid (carbohydrate-containing fat) characterized glycoprotein (carbohydrate-containing protein, or mucin). It is similar to the type A blood group protein, with additional sialic acid residues. CA 19-9 is found in normal fetal cells as well as in the pancreas, salivary ducts, gastric and colonic epithelium, pancreatic and gastric fluid, saliva, and meconium (first stool of a newborn). It is normally removed from circulation by the biliary system. Serum/plasma levels are determined by immunoassay.

Cancers diagnosed or treated: CA 19-9 is elevated in patients with gastrointestinal tract carcinoma, including cancer of the pancreas, stomach, colon, and ovaries. Abnormally high values may also be detected in benign conditions such as acute pancreatitis, cirrhosis, cholecystitis, biliary obstruction, gastric ulcer, pulmonary disease, and chronic hepatitis C and in patients who smoke.

Why performed: Because CA 19-9 is not sensitive or specific enough to be used as a screening test, its primarily utility is as a tumor marker for monitoring response to therapy and recurrence in pancreatic cancer patients. Levels are typically proportional to the tumor burden (mass), with higher levels of CA 19-9 indicative of the presence of a larger tumor. Very elevated levels, defined as more than 1,000 kilounits per liter (kU/L), are highly specific for pancreatic cancer and indicate very advanced disease.

Patient preparation: No special patient preparation is required for accurate CA 19-9 analysis.

Steps of the procedure: A blood sample is collected, typically by venipuncture. The collected serum (or plasma) is tested by immunoassay, which involves capturing CA 19-9 present in the sample by means of monoclonal anti-CA 19-9 antibodies. A second, detection (radiolabeled) antibody is then introduced, which subsequently binds to the CA 19-9/anti-CA 19-9 complex. The addition of a substrate results in a detectable signal, the level of which is directly proportional to the amount of the CA 19-9 present in the sample.

After the procedure: Pressure should be applied to the venipucture site in order to avoid the development of a hematoma.

Risks: The risks of venipuncture are slight but include excessive bleeding, fainting, hematoma, and infection (always a slight risk any time the skin is broken).

Results: Although each laboratory establishes reference intervals based on the local, normal population, a basic interpretive guideline places normal at 0-40 kilounits per milliliter (kU/mL) and elevated at more than 40 kU/mL.

Pam Conboy, B.S.

See also: Bile duct cancer; CA 15-3 test; CA 27-29 test; CA 125 test; Pancreatic cancers; Tumor markers

▶ CA 27-29 test

Category: Procedures
Also known as: Carbohydrate antigen 27-29, cancer antigen 27-29

Definition: Similar to CA 15-3, CA 27-29 is a transmembrane glycoprotein (carbohydrate-containing protein, or mucin) found in several tissue types. This class of glycoproteins is thought to play a role in reducing cell-to-cell interaction and the inhibition of tumor cell cytolysis. The core protein component is identical; the carbohydrate concentration (degree of glycosylation) is the component differentiating between tissue types. Serum/plasma levels are determined by immunoassay.

Cancers diagnosed: CA 27-29 is not an organ-specific marker and has been found at elevated levels in breast, ovarian, colon, stomach, kidney, lung, pancreas, uterus, and liver cancers. Additionally, increased CA 27-29 levels can be found concomitant with benign conditions such as first trimester pregnancy, endometriosis, ovarian cysts, and breast, kidney, and liver disease.

Why performed: Because CA 27-29 is not sensitive or specific enough to be used as a screening test, its primary utility is as a tumor marker for monitoring response to therapy and recurrence in previously treated Stage II and Stage III breast cancer patients. Blood levels are typically proportional to the tumor burden (mass), with higher levels of CA 15-3 indicative of the presence of a larger tumor. Physicians will typically order either CA 27-29 levels or CA 15-3 levels but not both, as they are considered essentially equivalent in diagnostic value.

Patient preparation: No special patient preparation is required for accurate CA 27-29 analysis.

Steps of the procedure: A blood sample is collected, typically by venipuncture. The collected serum (or plasma) is tested by immunoassay, which involves capturing CA 27-29 present in the sample by means of monoclonal anti-CA 27-29 antibodies. A second, detection (labeled) antibody is then introduced, which subsequently binds to the CA 27-29/anti-CA 27-29 complex. The addition of a substrate results in a detectable signal, the level of which is directly proportional to the amount of the CA 27-29 present in the sample.

After the procedure: Pressure should be applied to the venipuncture site in order to avoid the development of a hematoma.

Risks: The risks of venipuncture are slight but include excessive bleeding, fainting, hematoma, and infection (always a slight risk any time the skin is broken).

Results: Although each laboratory establishes reference intervals based on the local, normal population, a basic interpretive guideline for CA 27-29 places normal at 0-32 units per milliliter (U/mL) and elevated at more than 32 U/mL.

Pam Conboy, B.S.

See also: CA 15-3 test; CA 19-9 test; CA 125 test; Tumor markers

▶ CA 125 test

Category: Procedures
Also known as: Cancer antigen 125, CA125, CA-125, CA125-II

Definition: CA 125 is a mucinous glycoprotein that may be elevated in some cancer cells, particularly those associated with ovarian cancer.

Cancers diagnosed: Ovarian cancer, uterine cancer, breast cancer, lung cancer

Why performed: CA 125 serves as a biomarker or tumor marker to determine the presence of cancer. It is generated on the surface of cells and released into the bloodstream. Concentrations of CA 125 often are elevated in ovarian cancer patients.

Patient preparation: No special preparation is necessary.

Steps of the procedure: To determine the level of CA 125 in a patient, blood is drawn from a vein, typically from the inside of an elbow or sometimes from the back of a hand. The site of extraction is first cleaned with an antiseptic. An elastic band is often applied around the upper arm to apply pressure and cause the vein to engorge with blood. After a needle is inserted into the selected vein, blood is collected in a syringe or an airtight vial. Once the blood is collected, the needle is removed and the puncture site is bandaged to stop any subsequent bleeding.

After the procedure: There may be throbbing or bruising around the extraction site.

Risks: The risks involved in collecting blood to ascertain CA 125 levels include the possibility of excessive bleeding, fainting or light-headedness, blood accumulating under the skin (hematoma), and infection around the puncture site. There is always the possibility of multiple punctures being necessary to find a vein that will yield blood.

Results: A CA 125 level greater than 35 units per milliliter (U/mL) of blood is considered to be elevated. In many cases, elevated levels are not an indication of cancer but instead can be attributed to other conditions, such as endometriosis and benign ovarian cysts. The lack of specificity is a key problem when using CA 125 as a cancer marker. In 79 percent of women tested with known ovarian cancers, CA 125 levels were elevated, while the other 21 percent showed no elevated CA 125 concentrations.

The CA 125 test for ovarian cancer is most reliable in women who have gone through menopause. Tracking CA 125 levels periodically over time to determine the rate at which levels fluctuate is much more definitive than a single CA 125 test. Elevated CA 125 levels, particularly in postmenopausal women, indicate the need for further screening that may include ultrasonic imaging, computed tomography (CT) scans, and surgery.

Alvin K. Benson, Ph.D.

See also: CA 15-3 test; CA 19-9 test; CA 27-29 test; Endometrial cancer; Fallopian tube cancer; Fertility drugs and cancer; Ovarian cancers; Ovarian cysts; Ovarian epithelial cancer; Proteomics and cancer research; Tumor markers; Uterine cancer

▶ Carcinoembryonic Antigen Antibody (CEA) test

Category: Procedures
Also known as: Carcinoembryonic antigen antibody test

Definition: Carcinoembryonic antigen antibody (CEA) tests are used primarily to monitor cancer patients to determine whether their disease is recurring and, if so, its stage and extent. CEA is a tumor marker, because anti-CEA antibodies bind to epitopes on carcinoembryonic antigens, allowing CEA quantification in body fluids (primarily serum) and CEA detection on cells or tissue sections by immunostaining.

Cancers diagnosed: Primarily colorectal and gastrointestinal cancers, as well as cancers of the rectum, lung, breast, liver, pancreas, stomach, and ovaries

Why performed: Anti-CEA antibodies are primarily used in the diagnosis of colorectal cancer; they are not recommended for cancer screening, but preoperative determination may assist in staging and surgical treatment planning. After treatment, anti-CEA antibodies may detect recurrence earlier than other techniques. Anti-CEA antibodies are also informative in lung, liver, breast, ovarian, stomach, and pancreatic cancers as they provide prognostic information. Anti-CEA antibodies can also be evaluated in urine (bladder cancer), bronchial lavage fluid (lung cancer), or cerebrospinal fluid (brain tumors) to improve diagnostic accuracy.

Patient preparation: No preparation on the part of the patient is necessary.

Steps of the procedure: The procedure involves a simple blood test and so consists only of the drawing of a blood sample from the patient. When anti-CEA antibodies are used for quantitative determination of CEA in body fluids, a typical solid-phase immunoassay protocol is used. This involves addition of the standards and samples to wells or beads with an adsorbed monoclonal anti-CEA antibody to "catch" and immobilize CEA by high-affinity binding to one of CEA's epitopes. After incubation and washing steps, a second, enzyme-conjugated monoclonal anti-CEA antibody against a different CEA epitope is added. CEA present in the specimen is "sandwiched" between the two different antibodies and serves to bind the enzyme to the well or bead. After washing, colorigenic substrate is added. The rate of color development indicates the activity of the antibody-conjugated enzyme, which is used to infer the CEA concentration in the sample by comparison with known standards.

When anti-CEA antibodies are used to semiquantitatively visualize CEA in immunostaining procedures, the cells or tissues are typically fixed and embedded in paraffin, then sectioned onto glass slides for staining and conventional microscopy. Polyclonal anti-CEA antibodies may be chosen for immunostaining to improve sensitivity.

After the procedure: No special care is needed other than to keep the area of the needlestick clean until it is healed, in order to avoid infection.

Risks: No physical risks or side effects accompany a CEA test, although caution must be used in interpreting results. The CEA test itself poses no risk to the patient. Test results must not be interpreted in isolation to avoid overtreatment or undertreatment.

Results: Standard levels have not been established for CEA tests and vary depending on the patient's age and condition as well as testing methods. Anti-CEA-based assays of CEA in body fluids are difficult to interpret in isolation; serial measurements usually are inspected for recognizable patterns that indicate response to therapy, lack of response to therapy, or recurrence of disease. Because of heterogeneity among anti-CEA antibodies, the same reagents and methods should be used during longitudinal monitoring. In immunostaining procedures, many anti-CEA antibodies recognize antigens shared by members of the CEA family of glycoproteins, resulting in extensive background staining. In particular, cells from the liver and gallbladder often react with anti-CEA antibodies because they contain biliary glycoprotein. Each test report should include a reference range and be interpreted by the consulting physician.

In general, patients with early-stage, small tumors may have low, even normal, CEA levels; later-stage and metastatic disease may yield initially high CEA levels. A subsequent lower CEA level usually indicates reduced tumor activity, whereas a CEA level that rises over time may indicate tumor recurrence.

John B. Welsh, M.D., Ph.D.

See also: Bile duct cancer; Colorectal cancer; Malignant tumors; Pathology; Placental alkaline phosphatase (PALP); Tumor markers

▶ Cardiopulmonary Resuscitation (CPR)

Category: Procedures
Also known as: Basic life support

Definition: Cardiopulmonary resuscitation (CPR) is an emergency procedure performed by health care providers and laypeople that maintains breathing and circulation after a person's heartbeat and breathing cease.

Cancers treated: Can be used to support those with cancer with an advance directive declaring a desire for life support

Why performed: CPR is performed to maintain breathing and circulation and to prevent brain death when a person suffers cardiopulmonary arrest.

Patient preparation: Before beginning CPR, the patient is placed on a flat firm surface in a face-up position. If the patient is found face down, then the patient must be logrolled into a face-up position.

Steps of the procedure: The health care provider makes sure that the patient is unresponsive by tapping the patient on the shoulder and asking, "Are you all right?" The health care provider activates the emergency system, calls for a defibrillator, and begins CPR.

The patient's airway is opened using the head tilt-chin lift maneuver unless a head or neck injury is suspected. To perform this maneuver, the health care provider places one hand on the patient's forehead and applies pressure firm enough to tilt the patient's head back. Next, the health care provider places the fingertips of the other hand

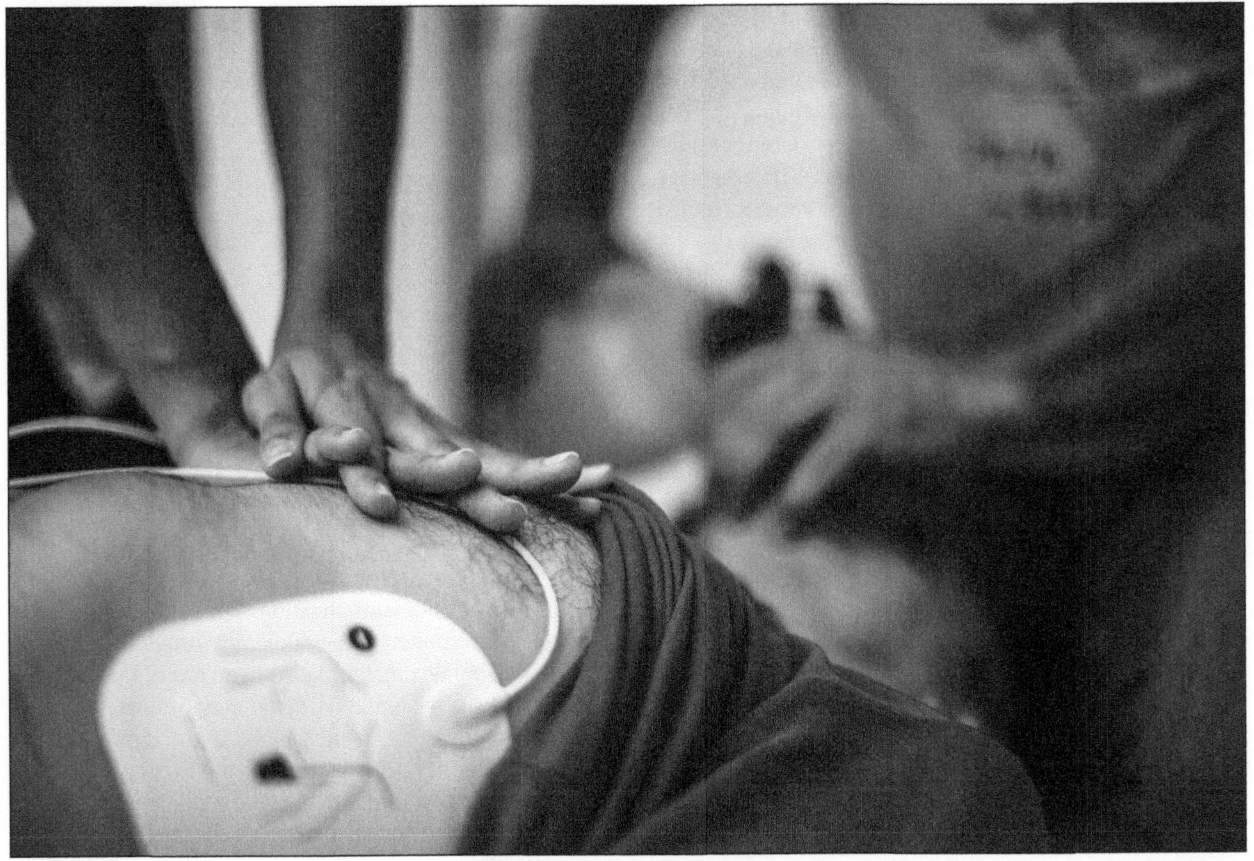

A man receives CPR. (iStock)

under the bony portion of the patient's lower jaw near the chin and then lifts the chin. If a head or neck injury is suspected, then a jaw-thrust maneuver is performed. To perform this maneuver, the health care provider gets into position at the patient's head, rests the thumbs (pointing toward the patient's feet) on the patient's lower jaw near the corners of the mouth, and opens the airway by lifting the lower jaw with the fingertips.

While keeping the airway open, the health care provider looks, listens, and feels for breathing. If no breathing is detected within ten seconds, then the health care provider gives two breaths (each over one second). Each breath should deliver enough volume to make the patient's chest rise.

If the patient has no response, then the health care provider checks to see whether the patient has a pulse. If a pulse is present, then the health care provider continues delivering eight to ten breaths per minute. If no pulse is detected, then the health care provider kneels (or stands, if the patient is in a bed) next to the patient's chest and begins compressions. Chest compressions are begun by placing the heel of one hand on the sternum in the middle of the chest and then placing the heel of the second hand on top of the first. The sternum is depressed 1.5 to 2.0 inches (for an adult), and compressions are delivered at a ratio of thirty compressions to two breaths. Approximately one hundred compressions are delivered each minute. Cycles of thirty compressions and two breaths are delivered continuously until an automated external defibrillator (AED) or standard defibrillator arrives, the patient begins to move, or the advanced cardiac life support team arrives.

When a defibrillator arrives, it is attached to the patient, and the patient's heart rhythm is evaluated. If the heart rhythm is shockable, then the health care providers stand clear of the patient while a shock is delivered. If the patient's rhythm returns to normal and the patient begins to move, then CPR is stopped. Ir the patient's condition remains unchanged, then CPR is continued for five cycles immediately after the shock. The heart rhythm is checked again, and another shock is delivered if the rhythm is shockable. If the rhythm is not shockable, then CPR is resumed while advanced cardiac life support is administered.

After the procedure: During advanced cardiac life support, an endotracheal tube is inserted through the patient's nose or mouth and then advanced into the airway. This tube is used to administer oxygen directly into the patient's lungs. The patient is attached to a portable continuous cardiac monitor, and a large intravenous (IV) catheter is inserted. The IV catheter is used to administer fluids and medications to help establish a normal heart rhythm and maintain blood pressure.

When the patient's heart rhythm begins to stabilize, the patient is transferred to the intensive care unit (ICU). The respiratory therapist attaches the patient to a mechanical ventilator to assist the patient's breathing. The ICU nurses attach the patient to a continuous cardiac monitor and an automatic blood pressure cuff so that they can closely monitor the patient's heart rhythm and vital signs. The nurses also listen to the patient's heart and lungs. A chest X ray is obtained to make sure that the endotracheal tube is in the proper location. A 12-lead electrocardiogram and blood samples are obtained to help determine the cause of cardiac arrest. When the cause is determined, an individualized treatment plan is developed. The length of stay in the ICU depends upon the patient's condition and response to treatment.

Risks: According to the American Heart Association, CPR can double a patient's chance of survival if provided immediately after cardiac arrest. CPR is not without risk, however. It can cause sternal and rib fractures, pneumothorax (collection of air in the chest cavity), hemothorax (collection of blood in the chest cavity), injury to the heart and great vessels, organ laceration, or aspiration of stomach contents into the lungs.

Results: Positive results of CPR are the return of spontaneous breathing and normal heart rhythm without signs of brain damage. When CPR is ineffective, death commonly results.

Collette Bishop Hendler, R.N., M.S.

For Further Information

American Heart Association. "2005 American Heart Association Guidelines for Cardiopulmonary Resuscitation and Emergency Cardiovascular Care." *Journal of the American Heart Association* 112, no. 24 (December 13, 2005).

BLS for Health Care Providers. Dallas: American Heart Association, 2006.

Cardiovascular Care Made Incredibly Visual. Philadelphia: Lippincott Williams & Wilkins, 2007.

Thygerson, A., et al. *First Aid, CPR, and AED*. 5th ed. Sudbury, Mass.: American College of Emergency Physicians/Jones & Bartlett, 2006.

Other Resources

American Heart Association
http://www.americanheart.org

See also: Advance directives; Do-Not-Resuscitate (DNR) order; End-of-life care; Living will

▶ Chemoembolization

Category: Procedures
Also known as: Transcatheter chemoembolization, transarterial chemoembolization (TACE)

Definition: Chemoembolization is a method of treating cancer by introducing chemotherapy drugs directly into a tumor using a catheter placed in an artery that supplies blood flow to the tumor. Chemoembolization works by blocking the flow of healthy blood to the tumor, thereby shrinking the tumor. It is among the category of procedures known as minimally invasive treatments because it targets the tumor and spares healthy tissues.

Cancers treated: Primary liver cancer (hepatoma); other cancers, such as colon cancer, that have spread (metastasized) to the liver. Individuals who have obstruction in vessels of the liver or have liver diseases such as cirrhosis are not usually eligible for chemoembolization. The use of chemoembolization also depends on the number and size of the tumors.

Why performed: Chemoembolization is used primarily for cancer in the liver, whether the cancer is confined to the liver or has spread to the liver from another organ. It is sometimes used in combination with surgery, external radiation therapy, or other cancer treatments. In advanced cancers, chemoembolization is used as a palliative treatment (directed at providing comfort and quality-of-life care) to manage symptoms related to the cancer, such as pain or fluid buildup in organs.

Chemoembolization offers advantages over traditional chemotherapy, since high doses of chemotherapy drugs can be given directly into the tumor rather than systemically. Also, since the blood supply to the tumor (which is needed for tumor growth) is blocked, the chemotherapy drugs can remain in direct contact with the tumor for a longer time than with traditional chemotherapy. The treatment can also be given more often, usually with fewer side effects since the drug is limited to distribution directly to the tumor area and is not circulating throughout the body. Chemoembolization is also more cost-effective than some other cancer treatments such as surgery or conventional radiation therapy.

Patient preparation: A few days prior to the procedure, the patient has blood work to make ensure good liver and kidney functioning. Blood-clotting tests are also done to make sure the patient's blood clots properly.

The patient is usually seen by an interventional radiologist, a medical doctor who is specially trained in treatment and diagnostic procedures using catheters, probes, and image X-ray-guidance. The interventional radiologist will perform the chemoembolization procedure. The physician will also need to know if the patient is taking any blood-thinning medications such as aspirin or coumadin, since they can affect the procedure. The patient is usually admitted to the hospital on the day of the procedure.

Steps of the procedure: An intravenous (IV) line is started in the patient for medication and to provide fluid to the patient throughout the procedure. Although a medication is given through the IV to help the patient to relax, the patient is essentially awake throughout the procedure.

An interventional radiologist performs the procedure under angiography (a special X ray of the arteries and veins) so that the catheter can be placed in the correct vessel that supplies blood to the tumor. A local anesthetic is used to numb the femoral artery area in the groin, where a small incision is made through which the catheter will be inserted. The physician follows the catheter placement via a monitoring screen.

Once the interventional radiologist has threaded the catheter through the artery branches supplying the tumor, the chemotherapy drug used to embolize or block the blood supply is injected through the catheter. The patient may feel a momentary pressure or burning sensation.

After the procedure: After the chemoembolization, a pressure dressing is applied to the groin, and the patient must lie flat for approximately eight hours. Patients may experience pain in the tumor area or groin, and possibly some nausea and fever as a result of the procedure. Since these symptoms may last for up to a week, patients are given pain medications to control symptoms and antibiotics on discharge from the hospital. Usually a one- to two-night stay in the hospital is required so that the patient can be monitored. Most patients can resume normal activities within one to two weeks.

A follow-up computed tomography (CT) scan or magnetic resonance imaging (MRI) is usually ordered by the interventional radiologist one month after chemoembolization in order to assess the continued effectiveness of the treatment on the tumor. Thereafter, a CT scan or MRI is usually done every three months.

Risks: As with any invasive procedure, there are potential risks. Risks of the chemoembolization procedure include infection at the catheter insertion site or blood clots occurring in vessels other than the one supplying the tumor.

Results: Chemoembolization is considered a treatment for liver cancer but should not be considered curative. Although it may be used to treat liver tumors and cause shrinkage and symptom control, studies to date have not suggested chemoembolization as a cure or first-line treatment.

Jo Gambosi, M.A., B.S.N.

For Further Information

Baert, A. L., C. Bartolozzi, and R. Lencioni. *Liver Malignancies: Diagnostic and Interventional Radiology.* New York: Springer, 2003.

Kufe, Donald W., et al., eds. *Holland Frei Cancer Medicine 7.* 7th ed. Hamilton, Ont.: BC Decker, 2006.

VanSonnenberg, Eric, William McMullen, and Luigi Solbiati. *Tumor Ablation: Principles and Practice.* New York: Springer, 2005.

Other Resources

National Cancer Institute
http://www.cancer.org

Society of Interventional Radiology
http://www.sirweb.org

See also: Arterial embolization; Embolization; Hereditary Leiomyomatosis and Renal Cell Cancer (HLRCC); Hereditary non-VHL clear cell renal cell carcinomas; Hereditary papillary renal cell carcinomas; Kidney cancer; Leiomyomas; Liver cancers; Urinary system cancers; Virus-related cancers

▶ Clinical Breast Exam (CBE)

Category: Procedures

Definition: A clinical breast exam (CBE) is a screening test for cancer and other breast conditions intended to detect palpable masses and other indications of possible malignancy at an early stage of progression. A CBE is done by a clinician (physician, nurse practitioner, or physician's assistant). It includes the inspection and palpation of the axillary and supraclavicular lymph nodes and breasts for masses and tenderness, examination for skin changes of the breast, and evaluation for nipple discharge.

Cancers diagnosed: Breast cancer, including cancer in the milk ducts or lobules and cancer that is invasive to surrounding breast tissue; less commonly, breast cancer may originate outside the ducts or lobules, as with inflammatory breast cancer and Paget disease of the breast.

Why performed: Breast cancer is the most commonly diagnosed cancer in U.S. women. It is estimated that in the United States, one out of seven or eight women will develop breast cancer at some time in their lives, and early diagnosis is key to effective treatment. Breast cancer is the second leading cause of cancer death in U.S. women. In 2006, over 212,000 women in the United States were diagnosed with breast cancer.

Positive findings on a clinical breast exam that may be indicative of cancer require further tests. A clinical breast examination can find cancers that are missed by mammography up to 10 percent of the time, and 5 percent of breast cancers are found by the clinical breast examination alone. Mammography is used for screening in women who are forty years and older and diagnostically in younger women who are symptomatic. Clinical breast examination has not been found to be valuable for screening younger women because of limitations posed by their denser breast tissue. Ultrasonography has been used along with clinical breast examination for screening of high-risk young women, as has magnetic resonance imaging (MRI), but this use of MRI is controversial because of its high cost.

Patient preparation: Before conducting a breast examination, the clinician reviews the patient's history and any concerns, including whether she performs breast self-examination (BSE), any history of lumps or nipple discharge, any history of breast surgeries, and family history of breast cancer. Family medical history is most significant if a first-degree relative (or relatives) developed breast cancer while premenopausal. Some women may come for a CBE with a known high risk for breast cancer, including a diagnosis of high-risk status from genetic screening for the *BRCA1* and *BRCA2* genetic defects.

Steps of the procedure: Before the CBE, the clinician informs the patient that many of the steps to be performed are the same ones that she can herself in a self-exam, as the best time to teach BSE is while performing an examination.

Clinical breast examination begins with visual inspection of the breasts. Adequate lighting is important to distinguish subtle changes. Flexation of the pectoral muscles with the patient's hands on her hips, followed by examination of the breasts as the patient lifts her hands high above her head, will help determine the presence of dimpling or retractions, inverted nipples, and other skin changes.

Following visual examination, the lymph nodes should be palpated for any swelling, masses, or tenderness, including those above and below the clavicle and the axillary nodes. It is recommended that this be done while the patient is sitting. Following examination of the lymph nodes, the patient lies supine with her arm high above her head to flatten out the breast tissue and facilitate examination. Palpation should include the full margins of the breast tissue, including the tail of Spence, the area of breast tissue that extends from the upper outer quadrant toward the axilla, which is the site where most malignancies develop. It is important that the entire breast margin be palpated with the flats of the fingers moving in dime-size circles in a systematic fashion so that no area is missed. Common areas that are missed in self and clinical breast exams include the tissue that extends up to the clavicle and the area directly underneath the nipple. Each area should be palpated using light, medium, and then firm pressure.

A well-done clinical breast examination takes at least several minutes. Studies have documented increased success in finding lesions when a minimum of five minutes is spent doing an examination, although studies have also documented that many clinicians spend less than two minutes, an inadequate amount of time, examining the breasts. Patients who are not used to examinations that take longer may be anxious and require reassurance that this is being done in order to be thorough, not as a result of suspicious findings.

When a new breast lump is detected in a patient who is premenopausal, she will often be counseled to wait through one menstrual cycle and then return to the clinic for evaluation. In many cases, the lumps are benign and will spontaneously resolve. If a lump persists, the patient is referred to a breast surgeon who will evaluate the lump using biopsy, mammography, and, for women younger than thirty-five years old, diagnostic breast ultrasound. Mammography can help to evaluate the need for follow-up, but accurate diagnosis of a mass requires biopsy. A biopsy may be done in the office as a needle biopsy (either fine-needle or core needle) or surgically as an excisional biopsy (lumpectomy) that is both diagnostic and may provide treatment. A fine-needle biopsy produces the fastest results, but a negative result for a needle biopsy is nondiagnostic, meaning that because of the high rate of false negatives, further surgical evaluation is needed.

After the procedure: The clinician will reinforce the need for breast self-exam and, for negative examinations, discuss intervals for regular screening mammography and make referrals if necessary. If any positive findings occur, then the need for further testing is discussed. Many patients need help arranging for additional testing, and many clinician offices will assist with scheduling of appointments rather than leaving patients to coordinate care when they may be emotionally distraught by the possibility of a cancer diagnosis.

Risks: Clinical breast examinations are associated with no direct physical risk. False negative results, however, can be misleading and delay diagnosis, while false positive results are very common and can result in invasive testing and significant emotional distress and anxiety as well as expense.

Results: The results of a clinical breast examination may be negative (no findings), in which case no action other than continuation of regular clinical screening and breast self-examination is warranted. Findings that are positive may include a discrete mass, a thickened area, breast tenderness or pain, nipple discharge, and skin changes.

Discrete masses may be fixed or mobile and tender or nontender, and they may be in the breast tissue itself or in the axillary lymph nodes. They are carefully described as to shape, size, and location in the breast, including depth.

A thickened area of breast tissue may be detected bilaterally (in both breasts) or unilaterally (in one breast only). It will be evaluated further but is less likely than a discrete mass to be a cause for concern.

Breast tenderness may be bilateral or unilateral. It may be hormonal and vary over the course of a month, but if associated with skin changes it can be related to infection or possible malignancy. Breast tenderness is common with some hormonal contraception and with pregnancy. Episodic sharp breast pain has been found to be responsive, in many cases, to a decrease in caffeine intake.

Nipple discharge may be bilateral or unilateral and may be clear, reddish or bloody, milky, or greenish. It may occur spontaneously or only with manual expression. It may or may not have an odor. History of recent pregnancy as well as some medications (in particular, many antipsychotics) may cause a bilateral, nonsticky milky discharge called galactorrhea. Bilateral discharge is usually benign. Secretions may be collected on a slide and examined under a microscope to help determine the need for further evaluation, including mammography, other imaging methodologies, and biopsy.

Skin changes may include uneven fullness or flattening, asymmetry that was not previously present, rashes and discoloration, areas of warmth and redness, retraction or dimpling of the skin, inversion of the nipple, crusting and erosion or ulceration of the nipple and areola, and the skin change described as peau d'orange, which looks like the surface of an orange with regularly spaced, shallow pitting. Skin changes are particularly associated with inflammatory breast cancer, which may cause red and swollen skin and a peau d'orange appearance, and Paget disease, which may cause an eroded and/or retracted nipple. Nipple inversion is of clinical concern only if it has not been present previously.

Clair Kaplan, R.N., M.S.N., A.P.R.N. (WHNP), M.H.S., M.T. (ASCP)

For Further Information

Fenton, J. J., et al. "Specificity of Clinical Breast Examination in Community Practice." *Society of General Internal Medicine* 22 (January 9, 2007): 332-337.

Grobstein, Ruth H. *The Breast Cancer Book: What You Need to Know to Make Informed Decisions.* New Haven, Conn.: Yale University Press, 2005.

Knutson, D., and E. Steiner. "Screening for Breast Cancer: Current Recommendations and Future Directions." *American Family Physician* 75, no. 11 (June 1, 2007): 1660-1666.

McDonald, S., D. Saslow, and M. H. Alciati. "Performance and Reporting of Clinical Breast Examination: A Review of the Literature." *CA: A Cancer Journal for Clinicians* 54 (2004): 345-361.

Weiss, N. S. "Breast Cancer Mortality in Relation to Clinical Breast Examination and Breast Self-Evaluation." *Breast Journal* 9, suppl. 2 (May/June, 2003): S86-S89.

Other Resources

American Cancer Society

Detailed Guide: Breast Cancer—Can Breast Cancer Be Found Early?

http://www.cancer.org/docroot/CRI/content/CRI_2_4_3X_Can_breast_cancer_be_found_early_5.asp?sitearea=

Susan G. Komen Foundation

http://cms.komen.org

See also: Breast cancer in children and adolescents; Breast cancer in men; Breast cancer in pregnant women; Breast cancers; Breast Self-Examination (BSE); Calcifications of the breast; Mammography; Needle biopsies; Nipple discharge; Palpation; Screening for cancer

▶ Cobalt 60 radiation

Category: Procedures

Definition: Cobalt 60 is a radioactive isotope that is used to provide radiation therapy during cancer treatment.

Cancers treated: Many cancers, including breast, bladder, oral, and brain cancers

Why performed: Cobalt 60 radiation is used to shrink or destroy tumors or to kill residual cancer cells left after surgical removal of a tumor.

Patient preparation: Patient preparation will vary depending on the type of radiation therapy being administered and the type and location of the cancer. Before therapy is begun, the doctor works with other members of the cancer care team to develop a plan that will provide the maximum dose of radiation to the tumor or cancerous area while creating as little harm as possible to healthy cells in the surrounding area.

Steps of the procedure: Cobalt 60 radiation can be administered in many ways. One way is to use a machine to aim the beam of radiation at the desired area from outside the body. Cobalt 60 can also be administered internally. Small capsules containing cobalt 60 can be inserted into the desired area to release radiation at close range. A device known as a Gamma Knife is a machine that uses 201 separate, stationary beams of cobalt 60 radiation to treat cancers that occur in the brain.

After the procedure: Aftercare varies depending on the type of therapy performed. For most uses of cobalt 60, no specific aftercare is required unless the patient experiences significant side effects.

Risks: The risks of cobalt 60 radiation vary depending on the type of radiation treatment being done, the strength of the radiation dose, the length and frequency of treatment, and the area of the body being targeted. Side effects of cobalt 60 radiation can include fatigue and nausea. If the radiation is delivered from an external source, then the patient may experience skin redness, tenderness, peeling, or discoloration. If the radiation is delivered internally, then there may be soreness around the cite of the delivery device(s).

Results: The way in which success is determined when cobalt 60 is administered depends on the goal of the treatment. If the goal was to eliminate residual cancer cells, such as after surgical tumor removal, then the treatment is usually considered a success if the cancer does not return for five or more years. If the goal of the procedure was to shrink or eliminate a tumor, then success is determined by the presence or absence and size of the tumor.

Robert Bockstiegel, B.S.

See also: External Beam Radiation Therapy (EBRT); Gamma Knife; Radiation oncology; Radiation therapies

▶ Colectomy

Category: Procedures
Also known as: Colon resection, large bowel resection, large intestine surgery

Definition: Colectomy is the surgical removal of part or all of the colon. Either the two remaining ends of the bowel are connected (anastomosis) or the lower end is sealed and the upper end is rerouted to a new opening (ostomy) in the abdomen, forming a stoma. The ostomy may be temporary or permanent.

Cancers treated: Colon cancer

Why performed: For patients at high risk for colon cancer, colectomy is performed to remove precancerous lesions or to prophylatically remove the entire colon, thereby preventing the disease. For patients with colon cancer, colectomy is performed to remove the diseased colon segment with a margin of healthy tissue and all draining lymph nodes, as well as other lesions and involved structures, thereby curing or controlling the disease. For patients with advanced colon cancer, colectomy is performed to manage obstructions, perforations, hemorrhages, or other symptoms.

Patient preparation: Medical tests are completed to plan effective treatment and to evaluate the patient's fitness for major surgery. If an ostomy is needed, then a specialist counsels the patient and helps choose the location for the stoma. For the colectomy, certain patient medications may need to be stopped, the patient's bowel must be cleaned, and the patient's stomach must be emptied.

In an emergency, patient evaluation and preparation may be limited. If the patient's colon is partially obstructed, then the obstruction is relieved before the colectomy. If the patient's colon is completely obstructed, perforated, or bleeding profusely, then the bowel cannot be prepared, and emergency surgery (colectomy or an alternative) is performed once the patient is stabilized.

Steps of the procedure: Colectomy is performed in an hospital. Before the surgery, sensors are placed to monitor the patient's condition. An intravenous (IV) line is started, and an antibiotic is infused. General anesthetic is administered, and a breathing tube is placed. The patient is positioned, a urinary catheter is inserted, and the incision site is prepared.

Colectomy has four steps: opening and evaluation, tissue removal, anastomosis or stoma formation, and inspection and closure. Details vary with the part(s) of the colon involved (ascending, transverse, descending, or sigmoid); why the colectomy is needed (prevention, cure/control, or relief); and the surgical approach chosen (open or laparoscopic). In an emergency, these steps may be reordered or performed as separate procedures.

To begin, the surgeon opens the abdomen with one large incision; four to five small incisions, when using a laparoscope; or a combination of these approaches. Within the abdomen, the surgeon looks for cancer and other abnormalities, then evaluates the colon segment to be removed. If the colon segment cannot be removed safely, then a bypass procedure is performed instead. If the colon segment is removable, then the colectomy continues.

To remove tissue, first the major blood vessels to that colon segment are tied. The colon segment is freed from attachments. The mesentery for that colon segment is clamped and divided; the tied blood vessels are divided and sealed; and then that colon segment is divided and removed, as well as any adjacent tissues that are diseased. All tissues are taken to the laboratory for histopathologic evaluation.

Either the remaining ends of the bowel are connected, forming an anastomosis (colo-colo, colo-rectal, or colo-anal), or the lower end is sealed and the upper end is rerouted. When rerouting, first an ostomy opening is made in the abdomen. The upper end is passed through the ostomy opening; the bowel segment is sized to an appropriate length; and the edge of the cut end is folded back and stitched to the abdomen, forming a stoma.

Finally, the inside of the abdomen is inspected and cleaned, and the incision is closed.

After the procedure: Anesthesia is stopped, and the breathing tube is removed. The urinary catheter and the IV line are kept. If an ostomy was needed, then a clear collection pouch (ostomy appliance) is fitted over the stoma. The patient is transferred to the recovery room and then to a hospital room. Medications are given to control pain and infection. The patient slowly progresses to a normal diet and learns to regulate bowel function. If an ostomy was needed, then it is monitored; once the stoma starts functioning, the patient learns to care for it and to empty and change pouches. At home, the patient follows the physician's instructions about medications, activities, and diet. Additional treatment with radiation therapy, chemotherapy, or both may be recommended.

Risks: Colectomy is moderately safe, with low mortality, but it is riskier in emergencies. The risks relate to anesthesia, infection, and inadvertent damage to structures. Side effects are common, with the most frequent ones being urinary infection, wound infection, and problems related to anastomosis or ostomy. Less frequent side effects are bleeding, perforation, abscess, fecal contamination, incisional hernia, bowel obstructions, and peritoneal seeding.

Results: Long-term outcome varies with patient-specific factors (such as life-threatening condition, disease stage, and overall health) and therapeutic combinations (such as type of radiation therapy, chemotherapy, or both after surgery). Curative removal is possible for many first-time patients, but otherwise recurrence rate is high. Five-year survival is excellent for patients with localized cancer but is poorer for patients with more advanced disease.

Patricia Boone, Ph.D.

For Further Information

Levin, Bernard, et al., eds. *American Cancer Society's Complete Guide to Colorectal Cancer*. Atlanta: American Cancer Society, 2006.

Other Resources

American Cancer Society

Colon and Rectum Cancer Surgery
http://www. cancer.org

Patient Education Institute

Colon Cancer Surgery: Interactive Tutorial
http://www.nlm.nih.gov/medlineplus

Society of American Gastrointestinal and Endoscopic Surgeons

Laparoscopic Colon Resection
http://www.sages.org

See also: *APC* gene testing; Colorectal cancer; Colostomy; Gardner syndrome; Hereditary polyposis syndromes; Pancolitis; Turcot syndrome

▶ Coloanal anastomosis

Category: Procedures
Also known as: Low anterior resection of the rectum; ileal pouch anal anastomosis

Definition: Coloanal anastomosis is the surgical removal of a portion of a diseased rectum or the entire rectum and the attachment of the colon to the remaining rectum or to the anal muscle. This technique preserves anal function so that, in the long term, the process of eliminating stool remains nearly the same.

Cancers treated: Rectal and colon cancer

Why performed: Coloanal anastomosis is performed to treat colorectal cancer or severe dysplasia with inflammatory bowel diseases when other medical therapies have not been effective. It is also performed when a malignant stricture or fistula is suspected.

Patient preparation: Before surgery, the patient's medical status must be optimized by managing malnutrition, treating infection, and correcting anemia and dehydration. In some cases, total parenteral nutrition (tube feeding) may be required before surgery to rest the bowel and reduce symptoms that may be occurring as a result of eating solid foods.

Tests before surgery may include biopsy, endoscopic evaluation, and radiography. Patients should receive thorough education regarding the risks, benefits, and expected outcomes of the proposed surgery. The health care team should discuss the patient's expectations after surgery as well as the care of the temporary ostomy.

One week before the procedure, patients must stop taking anticoagulants, as directed by the physician, to reduce the risk of increased bleeding during surgery. The patient uses a bowel preparation the day before surgery to cleanse the bowel. In many cases, antibiotics are given to reduce the risk of infection. The day before surgery, the patient follows a clear liquid diet and should not eat or drink anything after midnight the evening before surgery.

Steps of the procedure: The procedure is usually performed in two stages. During the first surgery, the diseased portion of the rectum or the entire rectum is removed and the bowel is reconnected to the remaining rectum or the anal muscle. The surgeon also creates a temporary loop ileostomy during the first surgery to divert stool into an external colostomy bag outside the body to allow the bowel to heal. In some cases, the side of the colon is attached to the anus (side-to-end coloanal anastomosis), and a small pouch is created from a section of the colon (about 2 inches long) to store stool until it is eliminated. With the J-pouch coloanal anastomosis procedure, a larger, J-shaped pouch is created. About six to eight weeks after the first surgery, a second surgery is performed to reverse the loop ileostomy and restore anal function. Recent studies have suggested that there is no need for a temporary diverting stoma, so patients should discuss the surgical technique with their surgeon.

After the procedure: Medications are given to manage pain, and an intravenous line delivers fluids and medications as needed. In some cases, nutrients are delivered intravenously until the patient is well enough to take foods orally. A urinary catheter removes urine and is removed about two to three days after surgery. Tubes may be in place to remove fluids and bloody drainage from the wound. Anal leakage is common after surgery and occurs as a result of the stress on the anal muscles during surgery. It may occur for several weeks and can be managed by wearing a cotton pad.

The patient is not able to eat or drink until bowel function is restored, as indicated by the passage of liquid waste. Bowel function usually returns within twenty-four hours up to a few days after surgery. The patient gradually progresses to a clear liquid diet and advances to full liquids and soft, bland foods.

The hospital stay is about five to seven days, depending on the patient's recovery. The patient is encouraged to get out of bed and walk the day after surgery, and activity gradually progresses to several daily walks in the hall.

Before going home, the patient receives instructions from an enterostomal therapy (ostomy) nurse who teaches the patient about caring for the temporary ostomy, obtaining ostomy supplies, and managing potential complications such as stomal blockage. The patient receives specific activity and dietary guidelines. A follow-up schedule is provided, and home care nursing services are scheduled as necessary. The patient can gradually return to regular activities, with a full return to normal activities within five to six weeks after being discharged from the hospital.

Risks: The most frequent complication is pouchitis, an inflammation of the pouch characterized by increased stool frequency, urgency, incontinence, abdominal cramps and pain, and flulike symptoms. Other risks include wound infection, urinary tract infection, poor postoperative anorectal function, stricture of the anastomosis, anal fistula or abscess, and reduced fertility.

Results: Coloanal anastomosis surgery prevents the long-term need for a colostomy bag, maintains anal sensation, and improves continence after the rectum has been removed.

Angela M. Costello, B.S.

For Further Information

Berndtsson, Ina, et al. "Long-Term Outcome After Ileal Pouch-Anal Anastomosis: Function and Health-Related Quality of Life." *Diseases of the Colon & Rectum* 50 (2007): 1545-1552.

Heppell, Jacques. "Surgical Management of Inflammatory Bowel Disease." *UptoDate*, January, 2008.

Huh, Jung Wook, et al. "A Diverting Stoma Is Not Necessary When Performing a Handsewn Coloanal Anastomosis for Lower Rectal Cancer." *Diseases of the Colon & Rectum* 50 (2007): 1040-1046.

Kiran, R., and V. Fazio. "Inflammatory Bowel Disease: Surgical Management." In *Fecal and Urinary Diversions: Management Principles*, edited by J. Colwell, M. Goldberg, and J. Carmel. St. Louis: Mosby, 2004.

Other Resources

American Society of Colon and Rectal Surgeons
http://www.fascrs.org

National Cancer Institute
General Information About Rectal Cancer
http://www.cancer.gov/cancertopics/pdq/treatment/rectal/Patient

National Digestive Diseases Information Clearinghouse (NDDIC)
http://digestive.niddk.nih.gov/index.htm

See also: Colectomy; Colorectal cancer; Enterostomal therapy; Exenteration; Hereditary polyposis syndromes; Ileostomy; Stent therapy

▶ Colonoscopy and virtual colonoscopy

Category: Procedures
Also known as: Endoscopy, CT colonoscopy

Definition: These procedures employ either a colonoscope (a flexible tube inserted into the colon with a light and camera at the tip) or computerized imaging to examine the large intestine for precancerous, cancerous, and other conditions.

Cancers diagnosed: Cancers of the large intestine and rectum, precancerous adenomas, polyps

Why performed: These procedures are intended for the prevention and early detection of colon cancer for people over the age of fifty, or earlier when indicated. They are also a necessary component in the management of inflammatory bowel diseases (Crohn disease and ulcerative colitis) or for individuals who have a family history of polyps or diseases of the large intestine.

Many patients resist the procedure as a result of embarrassment and/or concern over the bowel preparation, which is the same for both traditional and virtual colonoscopy. Neither procedure replaces the need for yearly testing for blood in the feces with a fecal occult blood test (FOBT) or a fecal immunochemical test (FIT). There are several considerations in deciding on the appropriate procedure. Patients should discuss family history of any bowel disease, increasing age, existing medical problems, and other personal issues with a physician when deciding the most appropriate procedure. Both forms of colonoscopy are considered the most thorough and accurate in examining the entire large intestine, but there are differences in how they are performed and what happens if a test is abnormal.

Patient preparation: Patients should not stop taking any medications (such as insulin, aspirin, or blood thinners) to prepare for a colonoscopy unless approved by their physicians. Three days before either procedure, the patient should stop eating a high-fiber diet or taking fiber supplements and iron-containing vitamins or iron tablets. The day before the procedure, all three meals should consist only of clear liquids, such as tea, broth, gelatin, clear juices, tea, or coffee.

The doctor will provide bowel preparation information and laxatives, either tablets or liquid, to take the day before the procedure and possibly again four hours before the procedure. The large intestine must be completely empty and free of all fecal matter in order to clearly see any abnormal growths or changes in the wall of the intestine. The patient may not eat or drink anything after midnight before the procedure unless it is water to take approved medication.

Steps of the procedure: Traditional colonoscopy is usually performed in an outpatient surgery suite. Patients are moderately sedated and given pain medication through an intravenous catheter. It is common for patients to sleep through the procedure, which can take thirty to sixty minutes.

The patient lies on the left side, and a colonoscope is inserted through the anus and rectum. The doctor watches a video screen as the tube is guided through the large intestine. Examination includes visualization during slow withdrawal of the tube, as some growths can be hidden in folds in the intestine. The gastroenterologist is looking at the actual lining of the intestine—not a computerized image.

The following can be done during this procedure: removal of polyps, sampling of abnormal tissue (biopsy), removal of small growths, stopping of small areas of bleeding, laser treatment of abnormal tissue or growths, and the introduction of certain medicines.

Virtual colonoscopy is performed by a radiologist in a radiology suite. No sedation is necessary. The patient is asked to lie on the back on a table. A thin tube is inserted into the rectum introducing air to inflate the large intestine for better visualization. The table passes through the scanner as three-dimensional computerized images of the large intestine are made and immediately viewed on a video screen. The patient is instructed to periodically hold the breath to be sure that the images taken are clear. The procedure is repeated with the patient lying on the stomach and is completed in ten to fifteen minutes.

Identification of anything abnormal might require traditional colonoscopy. Repeat bowel preparation will be necessary if the procedure cannot be performed the same day.

After the procedure: The patient will need to be driven home after traditional colonoscopy, as the sedation used during the procedure makes it unsafe to drive. It can take one to two hours after traditional colonoscopy for the patient to be alert enough to be driven home. There can be some abdominal cramping and feelings of gas. Normal activities can be resumed the following day.

Virtual colonoscopy does not require medication, and patients are free to leave immediately after the procedure. Some cramping might occur following virtual colonoscopy because of the introduction of air during the procedure.

Risks: Perforation and/or infection of the large intestine, while very uncommon, is a possible complication from traditional colonoscopy. The doctor will provide an information sheet that describes what is normal and not normal following colonoscopy. Symptoms that should indicate calling the doctor include bloody diarrhea, blood coming from the rectum, dizziness, fever, severe abdominal pain, and weakness. There is radiation exposure with virtual colonoscopy.

Results: Both procedures are considered the most thorough in examining the entire large intestine. Traditional colonoscopy is better at finding growths smaller than 10 millimeters and has the advantage of permitting biopsies of abnormal growths, removal of polyps, treatment of inflammation or disease, and laser treatment during the examination. Virtual colonoscopy is a much newer procedure and has been widely embraced by those who are fearful of traditional colonoscopy. Traditional colonoscopy is required following virtual colonoscopy if any abnormalities are found. Some studies have found that certain abnormalities on virtual colonoscopy were normal when traditional colonoscopy followed. Studies continue comparing the benefits and drawbacks of each procedure.

Janet R. Green, M.S.P.H.

For Further Information

Cotterchio, M., et al. "Colorectal Screening Is Associated with Reduced Colorectal Cancer Risk: A Case-Control Study Within the Population-Based Ontario Familial Colorectal Cancer Registry." *Cancer Causes & Control* 16, no. 7 (2005): 865-875.

Waye, Jerome D., Douglas K. Rex, and Christopher B. Williams, eds. *Colonoscopy: Principles and Practice*. Malden, Mass.: Blackwell, 2003.

Yee, Judy. *Virtual Colonoscopy*. Philadelphia: Lippincott Williams & Wilkins, 2008.

Other Resources

American Cancer Society
http://www.cancer.org

Mayo Clinic
http://www.mayoclinic.org

National Cancer Institute
http://www.cancer.gov

See also: Adenomatous polyps; Barium enema; Colon polyps; Colorectal cancer; Colorectal cancer screening; Crohn disease; Digital Rectal Exam (DRE); Diverticulosis and diverticulitis; Hereditary mixed polyposis syndrome; Hereditary polyposis syndromes; Inflammatory bowel disease; Juvenile polyposis syndrome; Laxatives; Polypectomy; Polyps; Rectal cancer

▶ Colorectal cancer screening

Category: Procedures
Also known as: Fecal occult blood test (FOBT), immunoassay, or immunochemical, fecal occult blood test

(iFOBT), flexible sigmoidoscopy, double-contrast barium X ray, colonoscopy, or virtual colonoscopy

Definition: Colorectal cancer screening tests are performed to detect abnormalities in the large intestine and rectum. The tests vary in accuracy, ease of performance, and invasiveness.

Cancers diagnosed: Colorectal cancers

Why performed: Early-stage colorectal cancers do not cause symptoms. The treatment of polyps or precancerous lesions can prevent the development of cancer, and the early detection of colorectal cancer can result in a cure. Testing is also performed as surveillance for chronic inflammatory conditions such as Crohn disease, ulcerative colitis, and familial polyposis.

Patient preparation: Preparation varies with the test being performed. FOBT and iFOBT do not require patient preparation. However, FOBT restricts the eating of red meat and the taking of aspirin, ibuprofen, or other nonsteroidal anti-inflammatory drugs (NSAIDs), except acetaminophen, for three days before the samples are taken. Flexible sigmoidoscopy, double-contrast barium X ray, and colonoscopy require that the colon be free of all fecal material so that the lining of the intestine can be visualized. This preparation necessitates taking strong laxatives the day and evening before the examination, eating a clear liquid diet the day before the examination, and not eating any food after midnight of the day of the examination. Some preparation protocols also call for a self-administered enema prior to the procedure.

Steps of the procedure: The fecal occult blood test (FOBT), a test for the presence of blood in the feces, is the simplest test for colorectal cancer and is performed by the patient at home. It is never normal to have blood in the feces, but the presence of blood does not mean cancer. Preparation begins three days prior to the collection of a fecal sample. Patients are instructed to avoid ingesting red meat, beets, other red foods or food containing red dye, aspirin, vitamin C, or iron tablets. The collection kit contains small wooden sticks to obtain stool samples and place on the cards provided. Two samples from different parts of the stool are placed on the card provided and allowed to dry before the card is closed with a flip-over cover (similar to a matchbook). Two samples are required from three separate stool samples on three cards. The cards are then placed in a envelope enclosed with the collection kit and sent to the laboratory. This test is performed yearly beginning at age fifty.

The newer immunoassay (or immunochemical) fecal occult blood test (iFOBT) also detects blood in the feces, but it does not require food or medication restriction prior to sample collection (hence minimizing inaccurate results from lack of proper preparation). Only a single sample is required. There is evidence that the iFOBT might be more accurate at specifically detecting human blood in the stool, but if the result is positive, then further testing is necessary. This test is performed yearly beginning at age fifty.

The double-contrast barium enema is an X ray of the colon and rectum following the introduction of a barium contrast material. After the colon is completely emptied, a barium sulfate solution and air are introduced through the rectum so that the outline of the colon is clear. Following the exam, the patient expels the barium solution and might experience abdominal cramping for up to twenty-four hours. This test should be done every five years unless flexible sigmoidoscopy or colonoscopy is performed.

Flexible sigmoidoscopy allows the visual examination of the rectum and lower third of the intestine with a flexible tube lighted at the end. The physician is able to see a polyp, inflammation of the intestinal walls, or other growths. Biopsies (tiny samples of abnormal tissue) can be taken for diagnosis. This test is quick and has few complications. No sedation is required. The doctor can view only the lower third of the colon, however, so polyps or precancerous lesions beyond this point cannot be seen. If signs of disease are detected, then further testing might be necessary. This test is performed every five years unless double-contrast barium X ray or colonoscopy has been performed.

The most invasive yet most thorough examination for colorectal cancer is colonoscopy. A colonoscope is a flexible tube with a light and a tiny camera at the tip. The patient is usually given "conscious sedation" and sleeps though the procedure. The tube is introduced through the rectum and is passed through the entire colon. Biopsies and removal of polyps are performed as indicated. Virtual colonoscopy uses computerized images to see the entire colon, but biopsies cannot be performed.

After the procedure: Patients have no special instructions to follow after FOBT, iFOBT, virtual colonoscopy, or sigmoidoscopy. Following a colonoscopy, which requires thirty to sixty minutes, the patient will be monitored while waking. Because sedation has been administered, the patient will need to be driven to and from the procedure. Doctors will not allow a patient to drive or go home alone. Patients are told to rest for the remainder of the day and can resume normal activities the next day.

Sometimes gas (air used during the procedure to make it easier to view the colon) is expelled for several minutes or hours following a sigmoidoscopy or colonoscopy.

Risks: The FOBT and iFOBT tests involve no risks, and risks for the double-contrast barium enema and flexible sigmoidoscopy, which require no sedation, are rare. The flexible sigmoidoscopy may, rarely, result in small tears in the colon or rectum. The risks of colonoscopy include bleeding, the possibility of tears in the colon or rectum, and perforation of the colon or rectum. However, these are rare complications. The test should be performed at age fifty and every ten years thereafter if no polyps or other signs of disease are detected.

Results: A negative FOBT result means that no blood was found in the stool samples. A positive test means that blood was found in one or more samples, and further testing will be necessary to determine the source of bleeding. FOBT should be repeated yearly but will not detect polyps or tumors that are not bleeding.

The double-contrast barium enema can miss some small polyps and cancers. Biopsy and polyp removal cannot be performed. Therefore, additional diagnostic procedures might be necessary.

Because sigmoidoscopy examines only the lower third of the colon, polyps or precancerous lesions to that point will be detected and removed; if found, additional procedures (colonoscopy) will be needed. Lesions beyond the lower third of the colon cannot be detected by sigmoidoscopy.

Colonoscopy and virtual colonoscopy are the most sensitive and thorough tests available, although some small polyps and precancerous growths still might be missed.

Janet R. Green, M.S.P.H.

For Further Information

Cotterchio, M., et al. "Colorectal Screening Is Associated with Reduced Colorectal Cancer Risk: A Case-Control Study Within the Population-Based Ontario Familial Colorectal Cancer Registry." *Cancer Causes & Control* 16, no. 7 (2005): 865-875.

Imperiale, T. F., et al. "Fecal DNA Versus Fetal Occult Blood for Colorectal Cancer Screening in an Average-Risk Population." *New England Journal of Medicine* 351, no. 26 (2004): 2704-2714.

Segnan, N., et al. "Randomized Trial of Different Screening Strategies for Colorectal Cancer: Patient Response and Detection Rates." *Journal of the National Cancer Institute* 97, no. 5 (2005): 347-357.

Other Resources

American Cancer Society
http://www.cancer.org

American College of Gastroenterology
Colorectal Cancer Screening
http://www.acg.gi.org/patients/gihealth/colon.asp

National Cancer Institute
Colorectal Cancer Screening: Questions and Answers
http://www.cancer.gov/cancertopics/factsheet/detection/colorectal-screening

See also: Barium enema; Colon polyps; Colonoscopy and virtual colonoscopy; Colorectal cancer; Digital Rectal Exam (DRE); Diverticulosis and diverticulitis; Endoscopy; Fecal Occult Blood Test (FOBT); Hemorrhoids; Immunochemical Fecal Occult Blood test (iFOBT); Polyps; Rectal cancer; Sigmoidoscopy

▶ Colostomy

Category: Procedures
Also known as: Ostomy surgery

Definition: Colostomy is the surgical rerouting of the colon through a new opening (ostomy) in the abdomen, forming a stoma. A colostomy is described by the part of the colon involved (ascending, transverse, descending, or sigmoid); the type of stoma constructed (end-type or loop-type), and the type of ostomy (temporary or permanent).

Cancers diagnosed or treated: Colon cancer, rectal cancer, advanced anal cancer

Why performed: Colostomy is performed to reroute the waste in the colon, either as a temporary diversion or as a permanent new path for waste to leave the body. Temporary diversion may be needed so that newly connected tissues in the lower bowel can heal, to stage an operation for a patient who has a partial obstruction or is too frail to undergo extensive surgery, or in an emergency to relieve an obstructing tumor or to allow an infection to clear before removing diseased tissue. Later, the temporary ostomy may be reversed to restore normal bowel function. Permanent colostomy is needed when the anal sphincter is removed, when the rectum and part or all of the colon are removed and it is not possible or optimal to connect the remaining ends, or when an obstructing tumor cannot be bypassed or an unremovable tumor is likely to obstruct.

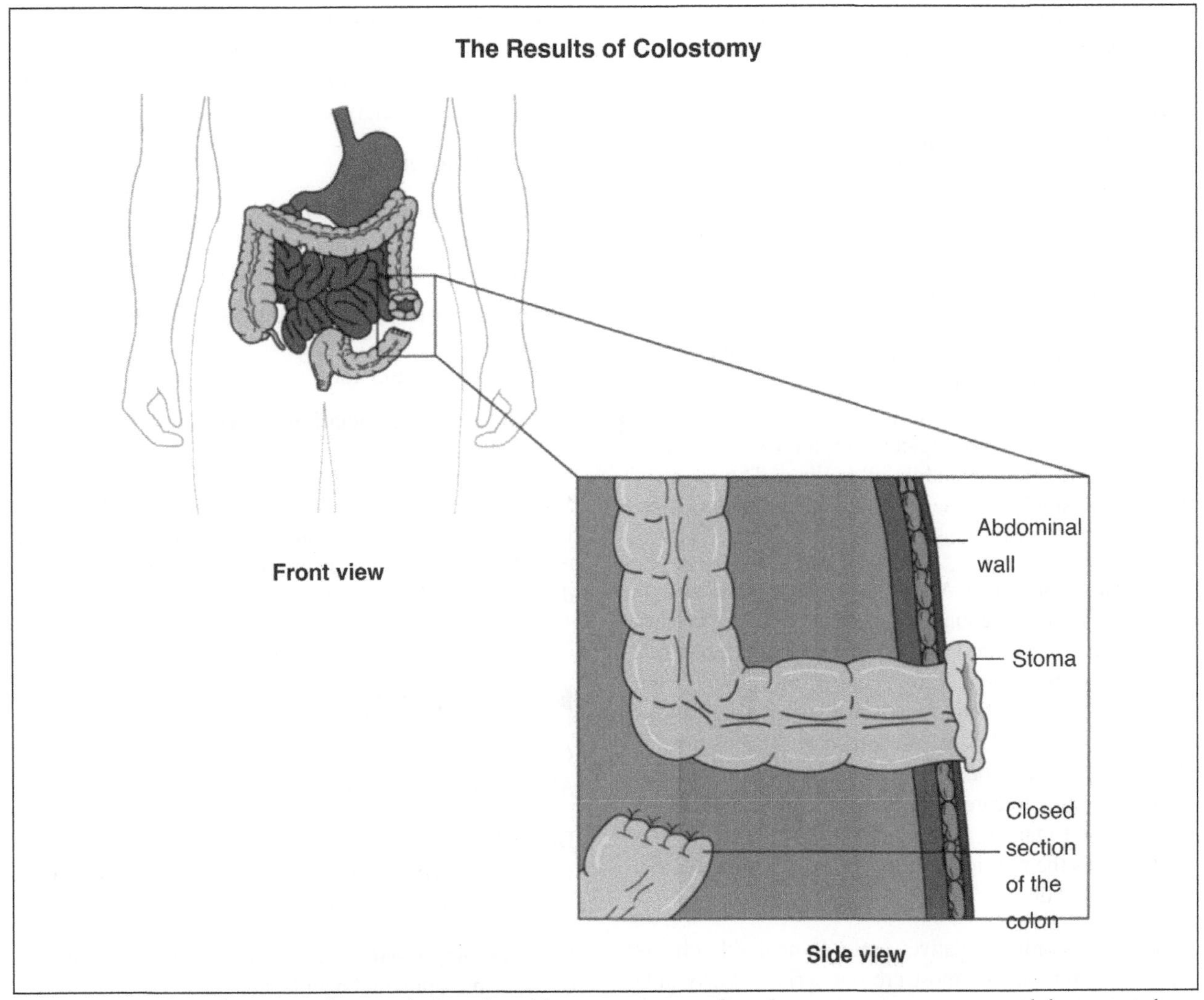

Colostomy is performed to reroute the waste in the colon, either as a temporary diversion or as a permanent new path for waste to leave the body.

Patient preparation: A series of medical tests are completed to plan treatment and to evaluate the patient's fitness for this surgery. A specialist (ostomy nurse or enterostomal therapist) counsels the patient and helps choose the location for the stoma. For the procedure, certain patient medications may need to be stopped, the patient's bowel must be cleaned, and the patient's stomach must be empty. In an emergency, patient evaluation and preparation may be limited.

Steps of the procedure: Colostomy is performed in a hospital as part of or as the first stage of a larger operation. For the procedure, sensors are placed to monitor the patient's condition. An intravenous (IV) line is started, and an antibiotic is infused. General anesthesia is administered, and a breathing tube is placed. The patient is positioned, a urinary catheter is inserted, and the incision sites are prepared.

Most commonly, a colostomy constructs either an end-type or a loop-type stoma. Details for each procedure vary with the larger operation needed, the parts of the bowel involved, and the surgical approach chosen (open or laparoscopic).

With an end-type stoma, this procedure temporarily or permanently connects the upper end of the colon to an opening on the abdomen. First, an ostomy opening is made in the abdomen. The colon is freed from attachments and divided. The upper end is passed through the ostomy opening, the colon segment is sized to an appropriate length, and the edge of the cut end is folded back and stitched to the abdomen, forming an end stoma. The lower end may be totally removed, permanently sealed, temporarily sealed, or temporarily formed into a mucous fistula by connecting it to a second abdominal opening.

With loop-type stoma, this procedure temporarily opens a loop of colon onto the abdomen and constructs either one stoma (end-loop) or two stomas (double-barrel). First, an ostomy opening is made in the abdomen. A loop of colon is freed from attachments and is brought through the ostomy opening. Then, either an end-loop stoma or a double-barrel stoma is constructed. To construct an end-loop stoma, the loop is divided. The lower end is sealed and anchored with one stitch near the ostomy opening, and the cut edge of the upper end is folded back and stitched to the abdomen, forming one stoma. To construct a double-barrel stoma, the loop is slit lengthwise. A small bridge is placed underneath the loop, bisecting the slit and raising the middle of the loop. The edges of the split are stitched to the abdomen on both sides of the bridge, forming two stomas.

After the procedure: After the surgery anesthesia is stopped, and the breathing tube is removed. The urinary catheter and the IV line are kept. A clear collection pouch is fitted over the stoma. The patient is transferred to the recovery room and then to a hospital room. Medications are given to control pain and infection. The ostomy is closely monitored; once it starts functioning, the patient learns how to care for the stoma, empty and change pouches, and manage bowel function. At home, the patient follows the physician's instructions for medications, activities, and diet.

Risks: Colostomy is relatively safe. Stomal side effects are very common, but most are not serious. Early side effects are irritation and leakage. Later side effects are hernia, prolapse, fistula, obstruction, ischemia, necrosis, retraction, separation, and narrowing. When an ostomy is temporary, overall risk includes that of reversing the colostomy.

Results: After colostomy, waste previously collected in the rectum and pushed through the anus now flows through the ostomy into a flat plastic pouch (ostomy appliance) that fits securely over the stoma. Many types and sizes of ostomy appliances are available, depending on the type of colostomy and patient-specific factors. Some patients benefit from minor changes in diet and alterations in clothing. All patients can perform the same activities as before. In recent years, patients' quality of life has greatly improved with advances in ostomy management and stomal care.

Patricia Boone, Ph.D.

For Further Information

Levin, Bernard, et al., eds. *American Cancer Society's Complete Guide to Colorectal Cancer*. Atlanta: American Cancer Society, 2006.

Other Resources

American Cancer Society
Colostomy Guide
http://www.cancer.org

American Society of Colon and Rectal Surgeons
Ostomy
https://www.fascrs.org

United Ostomy Associations of America
http://www.uoaa.org

See also: Colectomy; Coloanal anastomosis; Diverticulosis and diverticulitis; Enterostomal therapy; Exenteration; Gastrointestinal cancers; Hereditary polyposis syndromes; Self-image and body image

▶ Colposcopy

Category: Procedures
Also known as: Colposcopy-directed biopsy

Definition: A colposcopy is a diagnostic procedure in which the cervix is examined using a microscope and any abnormal tissue is biopsied.

Cancers diagnosed: Cervical cancer or its precursor, cervical intraepithelial neoplasia (CIN)

Why performed: Colposcopy is performed as a follow-up to an abnormal Pap smear. It is also performed on a patient exposed to diethylstilbestrol (DES), with repeated inflammation of the cervix or an abnormal-appearing cervix, or with repeated atypical squamous cells of undetermined significance (ASCUS).

Patient preparation: Patients should avoid placing anything in the vagina before the exam—including medicines for yeast infections, douches, and spermicides—and should abstain from sexual intercourse. The physician will provide specific instructions. Some physicians advise patients to take an over-the-counter pain medication, such as ibuprofen.

Steps of the procedure: Colposcopy is performed in the office and takes ten to fifteen minutes. The patient lies on an exam table in the same position as for a Pap smear. A speculum is used to open the vagina and view the cervix.

The physician stains the cervix with acetic acid and iodine using a cotton swab. The physician examines the cervix using a microscope placed about 30 centimeters from the vagina and notes variations in the normally smooth, pink appearance of the cervix, including areas of disordered growth of cells (dysplasia), abnormal patterns of blood vessel growth (punctation), and acetowhite areas (patches of tissue that are white after staining with acetic acid). Biopsies of abnormal areas are taken using biopsy forceps and sent to a laboratory for examination by a pathologist.

After the procedure: The patient may feel mild cramps or pinching and may have dark-colored vaginal discharge after the procedure if biopsies are taken. The physician may recommend that the patient avoid activities such as sexual intercourse, treating for vaginal yeast infections, and douching after the exam.

Risks: There is little risk associated with this procedure; however, heavy vaginal bleeding, foul-smelling discharge, or a high fever should be reported to the physician.

Results: A normal cervix is smooth and pink with no unusual patterns of blood vessels, turns dark with iodine staining, and has only mild acetowhite areas. Abnormal cervical tissue is rough or "humped up," intensely acetowhite, includes patterns of blood vessel growth described as "punctuation" or "mosaic," and is iodine-negative (yellow). The biopsies are graded as CIN I, CIN II, or CIN III, or carcinoma in situ. CIN I findings often resolve themselves and are usually followed with additional colposcopy and Pap smears. CIN II, CIN III, or carcinoma in situ is usually treated.

Michele Arduengo, Ph.D., ELS

See also: Cervical cancer; Conization; Endoscopy; Gynecologic oncology; Hysterectomy; Loop Electrosurgical Excisional Procedure (LEEP); Pregnancy and cancer; Virus-related cancers; Vulvar cancer

▶ Complete Blood Count (CBC)

Category: Procedures
Also known as: Hemogram

Definition: A complete blood count (CBC) is a group of blood tests that provides information about red cells, white cells, and platelets. The tests included are white cell count (WBC); white cell differential (the percentage of each of the white cell types—neutrophils, lymphocytes, monocytes, eosinophils, and basophils); red cell count (RBC); hemoglobin (HGB); hematocrit (HCT); platelet count (PLT); mean corpuscular volume (MCV); mean corpuscular hemoglobin (MCH); mean corpuscular hemoglobin concentration (MCHC); mean platelet volume (MPV); and red cell distribution width (RDW).

The test is performed using whole blood on an automated hematology analyzer. The HCT, MCH, and MCHC are calculated from the measured results of the RBC, HGB, and MCV. MPV is the average size of the platelets. RDW is a calculation based on the red cell indicating the variation in red cell size. A technologist may make a thin smear of the sample on a glass slide, stain it with special dyes, and examine the cells using a microscope.

Cancers diagnosed: All

Why performed: The CBC is a common screening test. It does not determine a specific type of cancer. The results

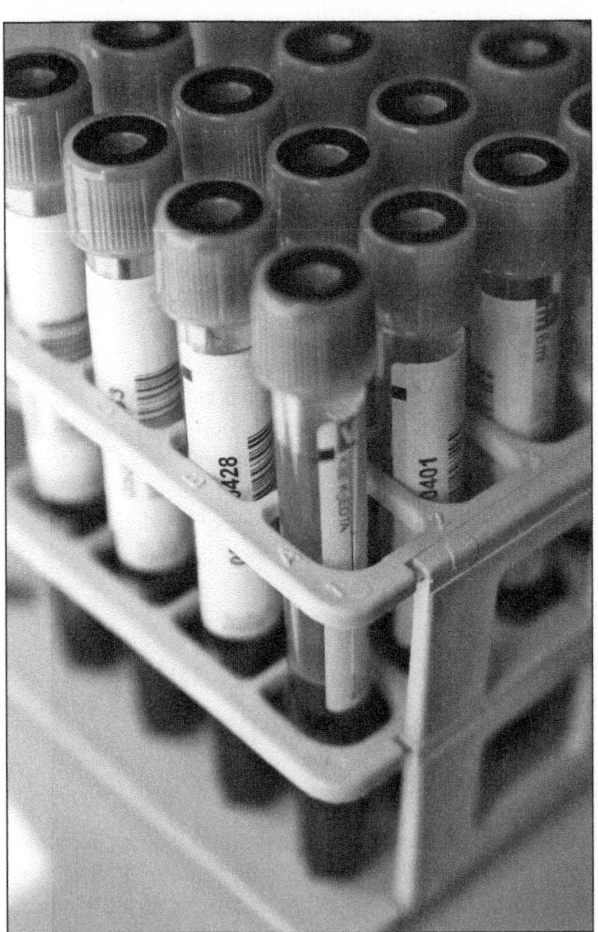

A complete blood count is a common screening test that provides information about red cells, white cells, and platelets. (iStock)

may lead the physician to order other blood tests and imaging studies that determine the presence of cancer. Chemotherapy and radiation treatments may affect any or all of the tests that make up a CBC. Therefore, a CBC or any part of it is used to monitor treatment.

Patient preparation: No special preparation is needed.

Steps of the procedure: A small sample of blood is collected from a vein and placed in a tube. In children, blood may be obtained from a capillary in the heel or finger.

After the procedure: A small gauze or cotton ball is applied at the site of needle insertion. The patient is asked to apply pressure. The person collecting the blood observes the site for bleeding and may apply a bandage. The bandage may usually be removed in thirty to sixty minutes.

Risks: The risks of CBC include bleeding, bruising, hematoma (bleeding under the skin), fainting, light-headedness, or multiple needlesticks to obtain a sample.

Results: Normal CBC levels vary by the patient's sex and age and the analyzer used. Each laboratory establishes a set of normal ranges based on this information. The physician receives a report of the test results with the normal values. CBC results may be higher or lower than normal depending on the type of cancer, treatment, any bleeding, or infectious processes taking place.

Wanda E. Clark, M.T. (ASCP)

See also: Aleukemia; Bone cancers; Cachexia; Childhood cancers; Crohn disease; Embryonal cell cancer; Fanconi anemia; Germ-cell tumors; Hairy cell leukemia; Herpes zoster virus; Hodgkin disease; Lambert-Eaton Myasthenic Syndrome (LEMS); Leukapharesis; Leukemias; Lymphocytosis; Myelodysplastic syndromes; Myeloproliferative disorders; Nephrostomy; Neutropenia; Pneumonia

▶ Computed Tomography (CT)-guided biopsy

Category: Procedures

Definition: A biopsy is needed when a mass has been found on physical examination or from an X ray, magnetic resonance image (MRI), or CT scan. In a CT-guided biopsy, a very thin needle is inserted into the mass while it is being visualized with the CT to withdraw fluid or tissue to be used to determine a diagnosis. CT-guided biopsy can allow a patient to avoid having to go to an operating room to have the biopsy completed. Many oncology patients are unable to tolerate an operation, so this procedure is a valuable diagnostic tool.

Cancers diagnosed: CT-guided biopsy can be used to help diagnose many different masses located in various organs in the body, such as the lung, liver, kidney, and adrenal glands. Solid tumors are frequently biopsied to determine the type of tumor and how fast it is growing. This information will then be used by the oncologist to determine what type of chemotherapy to use and whether radiation would benefit the patient.

Why performed: A biopsy is done to achieve a definitive diagnosis for tumors and masses. In order to ensure that proper treatment is given to the patient, the exact type of cancer must be determined. A mass in the kidney may be kidney cancer or another type of cancer that has spread to that organ. The biopsy can determine what type of cells are present and then what type of therapy would be best to treat that diagnosis. A CT-guided biopsy is done on masses located on internal organs or in deep tissue. Often these masses cannot be felt on examination but are found through imaging.

Patient preparation: This procedure can be done on both an inpatient and an outpatient basis. Preparation will depend on in what organ or area the mass is located. The patient may receive a sedative or pain medication before the procedure and may also be connected to a cardiac monitor to ensure that no cardiac abnormalities occur. The patient may be asked not to eat anything in the eight hours before the procedure. It is important to identify patients who have claustrophobia, as they may experience anxiety with the CT itself and need medication to decrease this anxiety. Patients may have their blood levels monitored to ensure that they have the ability to clot after a biopsy has been completed. Patients should give informed consent prior to having the biopsy done.

Steps of the procedure: The procedure can take as little as twenty minutes to complete. The patient is positioned as comfortably as possible on the back, side, or abdomen to allow for proper access to the area requiring biopsy. The patient should remain in the same position during the whole procedure. A preliminary CT scan is performed to locate the site for needle insertion for the biopsy. Once this site is determined, the skin is properly cleaned and a numbing medication is injected. The biopsy needle is then inserted through the skin into the mass. Another CT

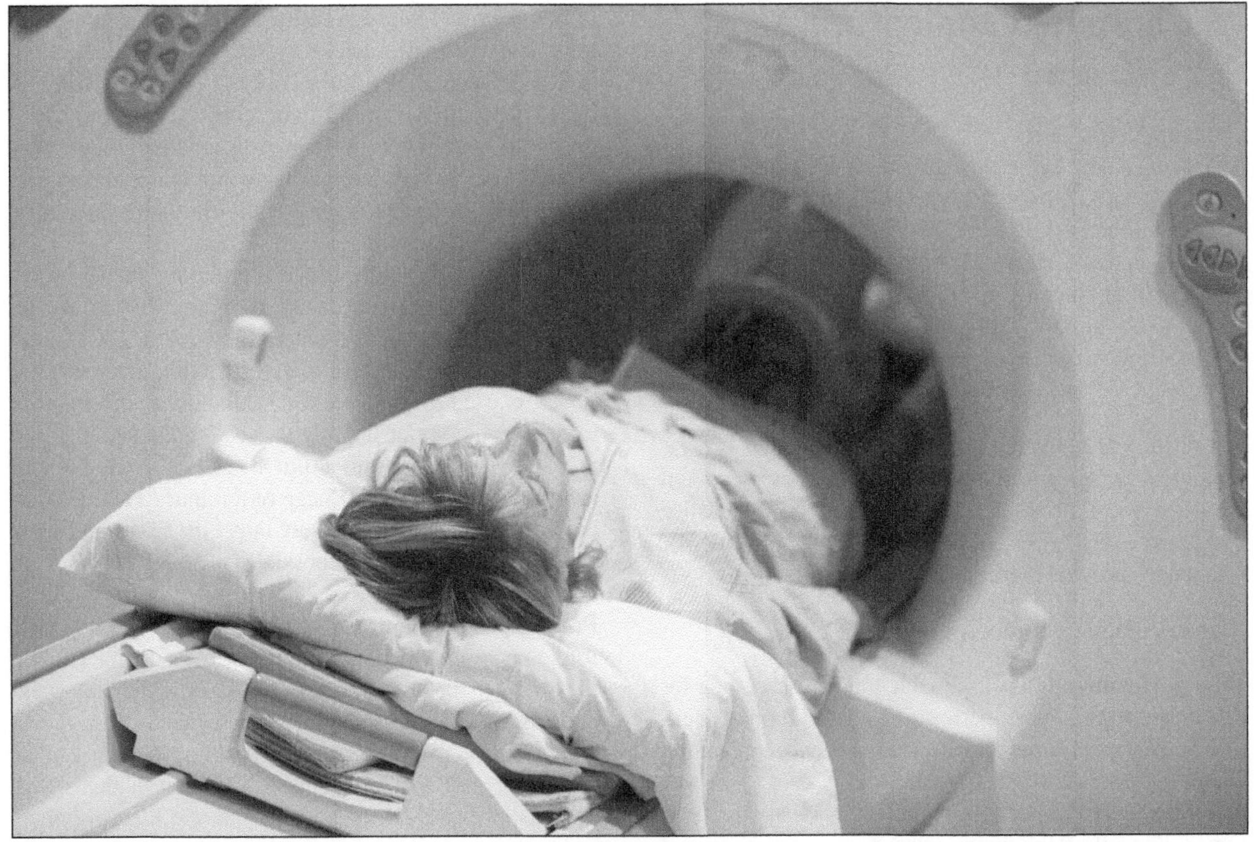

A patient undergoes a CT scan. (iStock)

is done to determine where the tip of the needle is resting. When the tip of the needle is in the correct location, then the biopsy, or sample, is taken and prepared for pathology. After the needle is removed, an additional CT is done to ensure that there are no air bubbles or bleeding.

After the procedure: After completion of the procedure, the patient is monitored either in the hospital or the recovery room for a few hours and then discharged home. The patient may still be drowsy or dizzy from the medication and should not drive.

Risks: CT-guided biopsies are not recommended for patients who have a bleeding disorder or thrombocytopenia. If the patient is or may be pregnant, then special precautions will need to be taken. Risks related to CT-guided biopsies are minimal and include bleeding and infections. It is not recommended that a needle biopsy be done on the spleen because of the tendency of that organ to bleed. There is also a 25 percent risk of a pneumothorax, or collapsed lung, when a biopsy of the lung has been done. Pneumothorax may also occur when biopsies of the liver or adrenal glands have been done.

Results: A preliminary evaluation may be done by the physician prior to sending the sample to pathology. Not all physicians may do so. Many times the sample is sent straight to the pathologist for diagnosis and evaluation. The pathologist will be able to determine what the mass consists of and give a diagnosis so that treatment may begin. If the sample size was not sufficient or the pathologist is unable to determine a diagnosis, then a repeat biopsy may need to be done.

Katrina Green, R.N., B.S.N., O.C.N.

For Further Information

Cooper, Geoffrey M. *The Cancer Book: A Guide to Understanding the Causes, Prevention, and Treatment of Cancer*. Boston: Jones and Bartlett, 1993.

Finn, William G., and LoAnn C. Peterson, eds. *Hematopathology in Oncology*. Boston: Kluwer Academic, 2004.

Klag, Michael J., et al., eds. *Johns Hopkins Family Health Book*. New York: HarperCollins, 1999.

See also: Computed Tomography (CT) scan; Cordotomy; Dukes' classification

▶ Computed Tomography (CT) scan

Category: Procedures

Also known as: Computed axial tomography (CAT) scan, abdominal CT, brain CT, chest CT, contrast CT scan, conventional CT, cranial CT, CT-guided biopsy, electron-beam CT scan, full body CT scan, helical CT scan, lumbosacral CT, multislice CT scan, orbit CT, pelvic CT, spiral CT, thoracic CT, 3D CT, virtual bronchoscopy, virtual colonography, virtual colonoscopy, virtual CT, virtual endoscopy, volumetric CT scan

Definition: A computed tomography (CT) scan is a radiological imaging test used to create cross-sectional slice images of a portion of or the entire body. The slice images are stacked to create three-dimensional images. CT images provide more anatomical detail than X rays.

Cancers diagnosed: Most

Why performed: CT is a valuable tool for screening for cancer, locating tumors, performing guided biopsy, identifying cancer that has spread, staging cancer, planning and monitoring cancer treatment, and checking for cancer recurrence. CT can identify blood vessels that support a tumor, as well as the tumor's shape, size, location, and volume. CT scans are used with procedures to diagnose cancer, such as needle-guided biopsies. They are used in cancer treatments, such as radiofrequency ablation and interstitial therapy.

CT images are archived in computers or printed form. Images are printed on film or with laser imaging. They can be sent and viewed online within a facility and can be compared for changes over time.

Conventional CT was developed in the early 1970's. CT uses controlled amounts of thin, high-energy radiation beams. Images are taken from a variety of angles. A computer calculates information about the images and produces a slice image of a specific area of the body. CT can be taken of the entire body or a specific section. Dye is used to enhance images to show more detail and contrast. The contrast dye can be swallowed, received intravenously, or administered in an enema.

CT has evolved to become faster and to use lower doses of radiation. Spiral or helical CT allows images to be collected quickly. The rapid process helps compensate for movements or breathing that otherwise can blur images. Additionally, spiral CT produces thinner slices of images that show even greater detail. A computer stacks the images to create three-dimensional, rotational pictures of a tumor. Spiral CT is especially useful for imaging liver, lung, and pancreatic cancer.

Recent technology allows doctors to use CT with endoscopy to create virtual endoscopy, virtual bronchoscopy, and virtual colonoscopy or CT colonography. The process uses a computer to create and manipulate three-dimensional images to create a "fly-through" view of an organ, as seen on endoscopy.

CT is used to guide surgeons precisely during procedures. CT is used with needle aspiration biopsy for tumors, such as for breast cancer biopsies. The CT guidance eliminates the need for invasive exploratory surgery.

CT is used to guide certain radiation treatments. For example, interstitial therapy uses CT guidance to insert radioactive material into a tumor. CT is also used to create a three-dimensional image of a tumor to allow external beam radiation to precisely target the tissue and spare as much healthy tissue as possible.

Patient preparation: CT scans may not be appropriate for some people. Patients should let their doctor know if they have diabetes or kidney disease or if they are pregnant. Some facilities conduct a pregnancy test on all women prior to scanning because the radiation can be dangerous to a developing fetus. Children, patients with movement disorders, or patients that are claustrophobic may receive a mild sedative prior to the test. In extreme situations, people may be sedated if they are not able to remain still while the images are taken. Some CT machines may not be used for people that weigh more than three hundred pounds because of size parameters of the machinery. About 5 percent of patients are allergic to contrast dye. Patients should let their doctor know if they are allergic or sensitive to contrast dye, iodine, or shellfish.

CT scans are outpatient procedures performed at a hospital radiology department or freestanding radiology center. Patients will receive instructions prior to their procedure, which vary depending on which procedure is conducted. Patients may be instructed not to eat or drink for several hours before the CT. Some patients need to use an enema or laxatives. Patients may need to drink a liquid contrast agent before arriving at the clinic or upon arriving at the clinic.

Patients wear an examination gown or robe for the procedure. They must remove metal objects that can interfere with the imaging process, such as jewelry, hearing aids, hair clips, glasses, or dentures.

Steps of the procedure: Patients are led into the imaging room. A radiology technologist conducts the CT. Patients lie on a narrow table. The technologist may use positioning devices to help patients maintain specific postures for the test. Head-stabilizing devices may be used for brain scans. Patients may be instructed to change positions throughout the procedure.

During the CT scan, the radiologist technician steps into a room that is separated by a glass partition. The radiologist is in constant contact with the patient via a microphone and intercom system. The radiologist technician operates the CT machine.

To take a CT, the table slides into the doughnut-shaped hole of the scanner. Patients must remain motionless while the images are taken. Patients are instructed to take a deep breath and hold it until they are told to exhale. The CT scanner has an X-ray component that emits beams at specific angles. The beams pass through the body and are detected by equipment on the opposite side. The equipment makes buzzing or clicking noises while the scanner is employed.

Patients receiving a contrast material may have a CT scan first, receive the contrast material, and then receive a final CT scan. An intravenous (IV) line is inserted into the hand or forearm to deliver injected contrast material. Contrast material may be swallowed. An enema is also used to insert contrast material for gastrointestinal-related CT scans. The contrast material may make patients feel temporarily warm or flushed.

The actual CT scan is short, but the preparation and positioning time makes the procedure last from about ten to thirty minutes. Spiral CTs are shorter in length. Patients are asked to wait until it is confirmed that the images are clear. Patients are observed for allergic reactions for a short time following the procedure.

After the procedure: There are usually no aftercare procedures following CT. If the patient has received sedating medication, a friend or relative must drive the patient home.

Risks: Patients may experience an allergic reaction to the contrast dye. The symptoms include hives, shortness of breath, nausea, wheezing, itching, or a bitter taste in the mouth. Severe allergic reaction or anaphylactic shock is a rare risk. Radiation from CT is higher than that of standard X rays. CT is not recommended for pregnant women; the risks to others are minimal.

Results: CT images are read by a radiologist and conveyed to the ordering doctor. The doctor may view the images as well. CT images depict anatomical structures in black, white, and shades of gray. Air, soft tissue, hard tissue, fluids, and the contrast agent show details that otherwise cannot be seen. Abnormal results show different characteristics from what is expected, such as tumors, cysts, cancer metastasis, tumor density, tumor composition, enlarged lymph nodes, or atypical fluid accumulations. In some cases, CT can help differentiate between types of tumors.

Mary Car-Blanchard, O.T.D., B.S.O.T.

For Further Information

Applegate, K. "Pregnancy Screening of Adolescents and Women Before Radiologic Testing: Does Radiology Need a National Guideline?" *Journal of American College of Radiology* 4, no. 8 (August, 2007): 533-536.

Ishikawa, S., et al. "Mass Screening of Multiple Abdominal Solid Organs Using Mobile Helical Computed Tomography Scanner: A Preliminary Report." *Asian Journal of Surgery* 30, no. 2 (April, 2007): 118-121.

Sone, S., et al. "Long-Term Follow-up Study of a Population-Based 1996-1998 Mass Screening Programme for Lung Cancer Using Mobile Low-Dose Spiral Computed Tomography." *Lung Cancer*, August 3, 2007.

See also: Angiography; Bone scan; Brain scan; Bronchography; Computed Tomography (CT)-guided biopsy; Cystography; Ductogram; Endoscopic Retrograde Cholangiopancreatography (ERCP); Gallium scan; Hysterography; Imaging tests; Lymphangiography; Magnetic Resonance Imaging (MRI); Mammography; Nuclear medicine scan; Percutaneous Transhepatic Cholangiography (PTHC); Positron Emission Tomography (PET); Radionuclide scan; Thermal imaging; Thyroid nuclear medicine scan; Urography; X-ray tests

▶ Conization

Category: Procedures

Also known as: Cone biopsy, cold-knife conization, loop electrosurgical excision procedure (LEEP)

Definition: Conization is the surgical excision of an *en bloc* section of the cervix to diagnose suspicious lesions that may be precancerous or overt cancer.

Cancers diagnosed: Precancerous lesions, such as high-grade suspicious intraepithelial lesions (HGSIL) or cervical intraepithelial neoplasia II or III; cervical cancer

Why performed: Conization of the cervix is performed when complete microscopic visualization (colposcopy) of all lesions is inadequate or inconclusive or reveals inconsistent results when compared to a Pap smear. Although a Pap smear and colposcopy detect 58 to 89 percent of all precancerous and cancerous lesions, conization can provide a definite pathological diagnosis. Conization can also be therapeutic if the entire lesion is removed and frank involvement of other organs (vagina, uterus bladder, or rectum) is absent.

Patient preparation: The patient undergoes preoperative evaluation, including blood workups to determine her fitness to undergo surgery and general anesthesia. Patients are instructed to take nothing by mouth the night before the procedure.

Steps of the procedure: After the patient is anesthetized and prepared, the cervix is visualized. Local anesthesia is administered if the patient is not under general anesthesia. The cone base area is determined by applying Lugol's solution. The uterine depth is determined prior to incising. Incision is done in a circular, centrally angled fashion. A suture at the twelve o'clock position of the specimen is placed. Curettage of the remaining ectocervix is done to detect any lesions above the cone tip. Cautery or ligation of any bleeding vessels and vaginal packing is done.

After the procedure: The patient is monitored in the postanesthesia care unit until she is fully awake and ambulatory and her vital signs are stable. Once stable in unit, the patient may be discharged on the same day. Admission for overnight observation is warranted if the patient is unstable or other medical problems need to be managed.

Risks: The most significant risk is miscarriage in women (10 percent) who intend to become pregnant after conization. Only specialists experienced in managing the potential complications should care for these patients. Other risks include excessive intraoperative or postoperative bleeding for as many as ten to fourteen days (30 percent), cervical narrowing as a result of scarring, perforation of adjacent organs, and infertility.

Results: A benign histologic examination of the specimens may reveal increased but orderly normal cell growth within the lesion but no elements of disordered growth of abnormal cells. Histologic examination of the specimens that reveals disordered proliferation and abnormal cellular characteristics is suggestive of cervical cancer.

Aldo C. Dumlao, M.D.

See also: Biopsy; Cervical cancer; Colposcopy; Endoscopy; Gynecologic cancers; Hysterectomy; Loop Electrosurgical Excisional procedure (LEEP); Pap test; Pregnancy and cancer; Vulvar cancer

▶ Continuous Hyperthermic Peritoneal Perfusion (CHPP)

Category: Procedures
Also known as: Intraperitoneal hyperthermic perfusion, intraperitoneal hyperthermic chemotherapy

Definition: Continuous hyperthermic peritoneal perfusion (CHPP) is a procedure that delivers highly heated fluid containing chemotherapeutic agents directly to the abdominal cavity, often during or immediately after abdominal surgery.

Cancers treated: Primary mesothelioma; primary stomach cancers; recurrent or widely spread ovarian cancers; recurrent colon cancer; cancers in the lung, breast, or appendix that have spread

Why performed: The benefits of CHPP are twofold. First, hyperthermia increases cancer cell sensitivity to other treatments (radiotherapy and chemotherapy) and increases the effectiveness of some chemotherapy (such as mitomycin-C) through improved pharmacokinetics. Second, regional administration allows for the direct treatment of errant cancer cells that remain after tumor excision while preserving noncancerous cells.

Patient preparation: Preparation is similar to that of any abdominal surgery. The patient's bowel must be cleansed, and the patient must fast on the day of the procedure. Before surgery and CHPP, intravenous lines are inserted, and general anesthesia is administered. During surgery, the body temperature may be allowed to drop by 3 to 5 degrees Fahrenheit to accommodate impending hyperthermia.

Steps of the procedure: The effectiveness of CHPP is related to the maintenance of a narrow temperature range for a prescribed time, so administration must be monitored closely. First, fluid-delivery tubing and thermometer probes are inserted into the abdominal cavity. Fluid is heated outside the body and is pumped in via catheter to bathe the area, usually at 106 to 108 degrees Fahrenheit, for forty-five minutes to two hours. Then, the fluids are removed with draining tubes.

After the procedure: After CHPP, the patient's incision is closed as with any abdominal surgery. Initial recovery in the intensive care unit (ICU) involves the evaluation of surgical recovery and may require temporary feeding tubes.

Risks: Because surgery and CHPP are often performed together, it is difficult to separate their complications, which include bleeding, infection, and wound-healing problems. Although most normal tissue remains intact to 111 degrees Fahrenheit, the death of normal cells is possible with hyperthermia. Most adverse effects of CHPP are temporary and include local pain, local blood clots, and burns or blisters to the skin, muscles, and nerves. More seriously, damage to blood vessels or to the lungs and heart may occur.

Results: Like systemic chemotherapy, the goal of CHPP is to destroy cancer cells in the peritoneal cavity. Unlike systemic therapy, CHPP aims to eradicate lingering cancer cells directly without affecting normal cells.

Nicole M. Van Hoey, Pharm.D.

See also: Hyperthermic perfusion

▶ Cordectomy

Category: Procedures
Also known as: Vertical hemilaryngectomy, partial laryngectomy

Definition: A cordectomy is a surgical procedure for treating laryngeal cancer. It entails resection of an entire vocal cord, the surrounding soft tissue, and the inner lining of the thyroid cartilage.

Cancers treated: Laryngeal (glottic) carcinoma

Why performed: In defining treatment protocols, the larynx is divided into three anatomical regions: supraglottis, glottis, and subglottis. The distribution of carcinoma among these regions is estimated at 40:59:1. Glottic carcinomas are the most common and readily detected because of the prompt development of symptoms (hoarseness, sore throat, and dysphagia). Early-stage glottic carcinoma can be treated effectively by a single modality, utilizing surgery or radiation. Radiation therapy will provide 85 percent local control for T1 (Stage 1) glottic cancer and local control in 65 percent of T2 (Stage 2) lesions. Vertical hemilaryngectomy (cordectomy) can achieve local control rates of 95 percent for T1 lesions and 80 percent for T2 lesions. Overall, surgery provides better local control, but the potential benefit of radiation therapy has been voice preservation.

Patient preparation: A routine preoperative workup and assessment of anesthetic risks are required. Prior to any surgery for laryngeal cancer, physical examination of the larynx is accomplished with indirect mirror visualization or by direct laryngoscopy. Magnetic resonance imaging (MRI) scans are employed to evaluate tumor size, location, airway patency, and cartilage involvement.

Steps of the procedure: With the patient under general anesthesia, surgical exposure is performed through a traditional transcervical incision. Exposure of the vocal cords is achieved through a laryngofissure approach (a midline incision through the thyroid cartilage).

Carbon dioxide (CO^2) laser cordectomy is now an alternative surgical option. Carried out as an endoscopic procedure, it can be performed on an outpatient basis. The single disadvantage with this procedure is the problem of evaluating free (healthy) tissue margins, especially on frozen section.

After the procedure: With traditional cordectomy, the patient stays in the hospital for a few days so that vital signs, incision site, and respiratory status can be monitored. Patients undergoing laser cordectomy are required to stay only for observation (three to four hours) to detect any signs of airway obstruction. Postoperatively, an adult companion should remain with the patient for the first twenty-four hours.

Risks: The specific risks of cordectomy involve speech problems, airway obstruction, and aspiration. General surgery risks include postoperative infection, scarring, and potential neurologic-vascular compromise to the operative area.

Results: The success of postoperative rehabilitation depends on anatomic and patient factors. The extent of the surgery, the type of reconstruction, and the utilization of radiation are important anatomical factors. Patient factors include motivation, dexterity, and access to speech therapy.

John L. Zeller, M.D., Ph.D.

See also: Electrolarynx; Esophageal speech; Laryngeal cancer; Laryngeal nerve palsy; Laryngectomy; Throat cancer; Tracheostomy

▶ Cordotomy

Category: Procedures
Also known as: Open or closed cordotomy, unilateral or bilateral cordotomy

Definition: Cordotomy is a surgical procedure that disables selected sensory tracts contained within the spinal cord (interruption of the lateral spinothalamic tract). The procedure is commonly performed on patients experiencing severe pain as a result of cancer. Anterolateral cordotomy is effective in relieving unilateral, somatic pain while bilateral cordotomy may be required for visceral or bilateral limb pain. Cordotomy is usually done percutaneously (stereotactic technique) with fluoroscopic guidance while the patient is under local anesthesia. Open cordotomy is not recommended for patients with unstable medical conditions but may be required if percutaneous cordotomy is not feasible or a previous attempt has failed.

Cancers treated: This surgical technique addresses the management of cancer pain that does not respond to oral analgesics.

Why performed: Pain is experienced by up to 75 percent of patients with advanced cancer. Between 25 and 30 percent of these patients report the pain as severe or excruciating. Intraspinal procedures are the last of a long treatment continuum that includes the following:

- systemic regimens utilizing medications and physical therapy
- direct operations for spinal decompression or stabilization
- psychological protocols
- chemotherapy and/or radiation therapy
- regional anesthetics and opioids

The extensive number of available drugs has resulted in adequate control of discomfort from most malignant cancers. For a small number of cancer patients, however, referral for anesthetic or neurosurgical procedures for pain management is still needed.

The optimal candidate for this operation should have unilateral, severe pain in the fifth cervical vertebra (C5) or lower dermatomes that is not treated adequately by less invasive methods. Cordotomy appears to be more effective in the treatment of intermittent shooting pains rather than distressing dysesthesias (burning, prickling pain, or aching). It is indicated for localized, not general, pain and is not usually indicated for pain in the upper torso because of the risk of respiratory complications.

Patient preparation: The procedure is usually done on an outpatient basis. Patients are instructed not to eat or drink anything for five hours prior to the procedure. In cases where open surgery is required, patients should not eat or drink for twenty-four hours prior to the surgery. In both cases, someone should drive the patient to and from the procedure and stay with the patient for at least eighteen to twenty-four hours afterward.

Steps of the procedure: The patient is placed in a supine position with the upper cervical spine in a horizontal position. The patient is given light intravenous sedation. Using local infiltration of anesthesia between the first and second cervical vertebrae, the physician introduces a cordotomy needle in the side of the neck on the side opposite that of the perceived pain. An image intensifier is used to define the point of the dural puncture. Once the needle has been introduced into the subarachnoid space of the spinal cord, a contrast medium is injected to visualize the surrounding anatomy. A special insulated electrode is inserted through the needle. With monitoring, the electrode is directed into the spinal cord.

An electrical cable line is attached to the electrode, and the tip is stimulated with an electrical current. During each stimulation, the patient is closely questioned about sensory changes and motor twitching. In this setting, portions of the spinothalamic tract are destroyed to result in a desired level of analgesia. Disturbances in temperature sensation are usually seen as a result of these cordotomy lesions.

The CT-guided cordotomy technique is similar to this traditional percutaneous method except that the cordotomy electrode needle is inserted with the patient in a computed tomography (CT) machine.

In selected cases, an open cordotomy is needed. The patient is completely anesthetized, placed in a prone position, and undergoes a traditional surgical exposure. A laminotomy is performed at the level of the first and second thoracic vertebrae (T1 and T2), and the spinal cord is directly visualized. Placement of the electrode is accomplished with C-arm fluoroscopy, and disruption of the spinothalamic tract is electrically monitored.

After the procedure: Postoperative care consists of observation for ipsilateral leg weakness, changes in bladder control, significant lower medication requirements, and possible respiratory depression. Hospitalization is usually for one or two days.

Risks: The complication rate from unilateral cordotomy is low, with a mortality rate between 0.6 and 6.0 percent. Bowel incontinence and bladder dysfunction can be seen in 2 to 10 percent of patients. Although information relative to sexual function is difficult to obtain, reports of impotency are rare. Transient hypotension can occur in 2 to 8 percent of cases. Permanent muscle weakness with ataxia (difficulty in walking) can be a major concern in 1 to 6 percent of patients. Respiratory problems are mild and transient, but respiratory failure has been documented in 1 percent of patients. Postcordotomy dysesthetic syndromes (burning distress throughout the entire area that was made analgesic) can occur in 1 to 10 percent of patients. Their pathophysiologic mechanisms are unknown. Open surgical cordotomy seems to be less effective and certainly has a higher risk of complication than do percutaneous techniques.

Results: Cordotomies are performed to treat cancer pain, often from lung or gastrointestinal malignancies. The procedure has been rarely employed in the treatment of lumbar radiculopathy or peripheral neuropathy. The target sites are the lower body as opposed to the upper body in about two-thirds of patients. In the hands of experienced surgeons, the spinothalamic tract can be located in 95 percent of patients. Adequate levels of pain relief are found in as high as 95 percent of patients on discharge from the hospital. At last follow-up, the success rate drops to 84 percent. Review of the literature realistically suggests long-term success rates of 50 to 75 percent. Repeat cordotomies may be necessary in 10 percent of patients.

John L. Zeller, M.D., Ph.D.

For Further Information

Crul, B., L. Blok, and J. van Egmond. "The Present Role of Percutaneous Cervical Cordotomy for Treatment of Cancer Pain." *Journal of Headache Pain* 6, no. 1 (February, 2005): 24-29.

Giller, C. A. "The Neurosurgical Treatment of Pain." *Archives of Neurology* 60 (2003): 1537-1540.

Jones, B., et al. "Is There Still a Role for Open Cordotomy in Cancer Pain Management?" *Journal of Pain and Symptom Management* 25, no. 2 (2003): 179-184.

Loeser, John D., ed. *Bonica's Management of Pain*. 3d ed. Philadelphia: Lippincott Williams & Wilkins, 2001.

Raj, P. Prithvi., ed. *Pain Medicine: A Comprehensive Review*. 2d ed. St. Louis: Mosby, 2003.

See also: Infusion therapies; Pain management medications; Palliative treatment

▶ Core needle biopsy

Category: Procedures

Also known as: Stereotactic (exact) biopsy, Mammotome biopsy, Advanced Breast Biopsy Instrument (ABBI) biopsy

Definition: A core needle biopsy is a procedure in which a sample of a tumor is extracted by using a wide-gauge hollow needle, a Mammotome, or an ABBI. The Mammotome and the ABBI are used for breast biopsies only. A core needle can range in size from 0.25 to 1.0 centimeter in diameter. It has a spring-loaded device that suctions out the tissue sample. The Mammotome suctions in breast tissue and cuts it with a rotating blade. The ABBI extracts a cylinder of breast tissue about the size of the tumor.

Cancers diagnosed: Breast, prostate, kidney, musculoskeletal, and skin cancers

Why performed: Needle biopsies are performed to obtain tissue samples from a tumor that is suspected of being cancerous.

Patient preparation: If a core needle biopsy is performed in a physician's office, then ultrasonic guidance is used to localize the tumor, unless it is palpable. If it is palpable, no radiologic guidance is required.

Needle biopsies that require the use of radiologic imaging to visualize the tumor or that are high risk are performed in an outpatient surgical center or hospital. The preparation for these procedures may include a physical examination, blood work, and possibly an electrocardiogram (EKG). The patient would need to fast for two to four hours before the procedure.

Steps of the procedure: The patient is positioned so that the area to be biopsied is exposed. This area is then scrubbed and disinfected. A local anesthetic is injected into the area.

If the tumor is not superficial, then a small incision (0.125-inch to 0.25-inch long) is made into the tissue above the tumor. The core needle is inserted through the incision, and several tissue samples are taken.

After the procedure: Either a suture (stitch) or Steri-Strip (adhesive paper) is applied to close the edges of the incision. A sterile dressing is applied over the biopsy site. The patient is monitored for one hour after the biopsy.

Risks: The risks of core needle biopsy are bleeding from the biopsy site, local nerve damage, infection, and, for lung biopsies, pneumothorax (collapse of a lung).

Results: The biopsied tissue is sent to a pathologist to be examined under a microscope. The surgeon receives a report that describes the size, shape, and activity of the cells and their nuclei and states whether the tumor is cancerous.

Christine M. Carroll, R.N., B.S.N., M.B.A.

See also: Biopsy; Breast cancer in pregnant women; Calcifications of the breast; Clinical Breast Exam (CBE); Computed Tomography (CT)-guided biopsy; Needle biopsies; Needle localization; Pleural biopsy; Progesterone receptor assay; Stereotactic needle biopsy

▶ Craniotomy

Category: Procedures
Also known as: Brain surgery

Definition: Craniotomy is a surgical procedure in which an incision is made into the skull to gain access to the brain.

Cancers treated: Brain cancers, such as glioma, astrocytoma, medulloblastoma, and ependymoma

Why performed: Craniotomy is performed for cerebral artery aneurysm clipping, arteriovenous malformation repair, increased intracranial pressure control, hematoma drainage, ventricular shunting, and abscess or tumor excision.

Patient preparation: Before surgery, the patient undergoes a computed tomography (CT) scan or magnetic resonance imaging (MRI) of the brain to determine tumor location and size and to evaluate brain tissue swelling. Other routine studies are performed to check for abnormalities and establish a baseline for postoperative comparison. These studies include a chest X ray, an electrocardiogram (EKG), bleeding time, and blood tests to check kidney function, clotting times, white blood cell count, and electrolyte, hemoglobin, and oxygen levels. A blood sample is also drawn to check the patient's blood type in case a transfusion is needed during surgery.

The patient must not eat or drink for at least eight hours before surgery. An intravenous (IV) catheter is inserted for fluids and medications. Depending on the tumor's location, the patient may also receive a bolus dose of an antiseizure medication, such as phenytoin, to prevent seizure activity during and after surgery. An indwelling urinary catheter is also inserted so that urine output can be monitored closely during and after the procedure. Sequential compression devices are applied to the patient's legs and worn during and after surgery to prevent blood clot formation.

Steps of the procedure: Immediately before the procedure, an arterial catheter is inserted into the patient's wrist to monitor blood pressure continuously during surgery. This catheter also permits blood sampling so that oxygen and electrolyte levels can be monitored. A central venous catheter may also be inserted to monitor the patient's fluid status and to administer IV fluids and medications during surgery.

After the patient is anesthetized, the neurosurgeon makes an incision into the skin and the skin is retracted. Next, an incision is made into the muscle and the muscle is retracted. Special tools are used first to make holes in the skull bone and then to cut through the bone to make a bone flap. The bone flap is then separated from the protective layer that surrounds the brain and removed. It is kept moist during the procedure. Next, the neurosurgeon exposes the brain tissue and removes the tumor, if possible. Depending on the tumor location, a ventricular drain may be inserted to prevent hydrocephalus and monitor intracranial pressure. If a ventricular drain is not needed, then an intracranial pressure monitor sensor may be inserted. After the tumor is excised, the neurosurgeon ties off bleeding vessels and then replaces the bone flap and secures it using plates and screws. Next, the neurosurgeon closes the incision and covers it with a sterile dressing. This procedure typically takes several hours.

After the procedure: The patient is transferred to the intensive care unit (ICU) and attached to a monitor that displays heart rhythm, blood pressure, oxygen saturation, central venous pressure, intracranial pressure, and cerebral perfusion pressure. These devices help the ICU nurses monitor the patient's condition closely. The patient may have an endotracheal tube (breathing tube) connected to a mechanical ventilator to assist with breathing or may breathe independently with supplemental oxygen. A patient who is able to breathe without help from a ventilator will be encouraged to breathe deeply and use an incentive spirometer frequently to prevent pneumonia. The head of the patient's bed is maintained at a prescribed elevation based upon the tumor's location. Every two hours, nurses may gently roll the patient to prevent the development of pressure ulcers and pneumonia. If the patient's neurologic status becomes unstable, however, then the patient may be unable to tolerate turning.

Nurses closely monitor the patient's vital signs, respiratory, and neurologic status to detect signs of increased intracranial pressure. If such signs are detected, then nurses administer diuretics, such as furosemide and mannitol, to decrease brain swelling. The patient will also receive a corticosteroid, such as dexamethasone, to combat inflammation. Medications such as codeine will also be administered to control pain. If a ventricular drain was inserted during the procedure, then the nurses will maintain the drain as ordered and closely monitor the type and amount of drainage. Nurses also monitor urine output frequently. A sudden increase in urine output without diuretic use may signal diabetes insipidus, a complication of craniotomy.

During the immediate postoperative period, it is important to keep the patient's environment calm and quiet to minimize anxiety and to avoid increasing intracranial pressure. A drug-induced coma is sometimes necessary to control intracranial pressure that is unresponsive to other therapy; the need is rare, however, following brain tumor resection.

When the patient's condition is stabilized and ventricular drainage is minimal, the ventricular drain is removed and the patient's activity level is increased. The length of hospital stay varies by the tumor location, extent of surgery, and the patient's rate of recovery. Depending on the tumor's extent and location, physical therapy, chemotherapy, or radiation therapy may be needed after surgical recovery.

Risks: There are many risks associated with craniotomy, including increased intracranial pressure, surgical site infection, hydrocephalus, meningitis, intracerebral hemorrhage, air embolism, seizures, stroke, cranial nerve damage, syndrome of inappropriate antidiuretic hormone (SIADH), and diabetes insipidus.

Results: Pathologic examination of the brain tumor specimen reveals the type of cancer.

Collette Bishop Hendler, R.N., M.S.

For Further Information

Greenberg, Mark S. *Handbook of Neurosurgery*. 6th ed. New York: Theime Medical, 2006.

Hickey, Joanne V. *The Clinical Practice of Neurological and Neurosurgical Nursing*. 5th ed. Philadelphia: Lippincott Williams & Wilkins, 2003.

Surgical Care Made Incredibly Visual. Philadelphia: Lippincott Williams & Wilkins, 2007.

Other Resources

American Cancer Society

http://www.cancer.org

See also: Astrocytomas; Brain and central nervous system cancers; Craniopharyngiomas; Neurologic oncology

▶ Cryoablation

Category: Procedures

Also known as: Cryosurgery, targeted cryoablation therapy, ablation therapy

Definition: Cryoablation is a minimally invasive method of treating tumors using extremely cold temperatures to destroy cancer cells or precancerous cells in a localized area. Cryoablation uses liquid nitrogen, alcohol, or an argon gas-based system delivered through probes that are inserted through a small incision in the skin to freeze a particular area of the tumor and kill the cancerous tissue.

Cancers diagnosed or treated: Prostate, kidney, skin, liver, lung, bone, soft-tissue, and pelvic cancers; also being studied for use in certain types of breast tumors and used for some heart rhythm disturbances

Why performed: Cryoablation is often used when a tumor is not operable or removable because of the late stage of the cancer or its difficult location near major blood vessels or other organs not affected by the cancer. It may be used as a primary treatment for some cancers such as prostate cancer or as a palliative treatment for liver or other cancers to relieve pain and control cancer-related symptoms. Progress has been made in treating kidney cancers with cryoablation. Sometimes cryoablation is added to other traditional treatments (radiation therapy or chemotherapy) for cancer. Cryoablation is also used to remove precancerous lesions, such as precancerous moles.

Patient preparation: Minimal preparation is needed for cryoablation. An intravenous (IV) line is started in the patient for sedation, and the patient's blood work is checked. Some physicians may also prescribe an antibiotic as a preventive measure.

Steps of the procedure: The procedure may take one to two hours. If the patient will have cryoablation during an operation as an added treatment for the tumor, then general anesthesia will be used and a hospital stay will be required. Most cryoablation procedures, however, can be done under local anesthesia and require only an overnight stay in the hospital.

An interventional radiologist performs cryoablation using image guidance. A computed tomography (CT) scan, ultrasound, or magnetic resonance imaging (MRI) helps the interventional radiologist guide the probe (usually multiple probes) into the tumor and avoid damage to any healthy tissue surrounding the tumor. A local anesthetic is given in the area overlying the tumor where the probe will enter. The agent used (liquid nitrogen, alcohol, or argon gas) is then delivered through the probes to freeze the tissue.

During freezing, an ice ball or crystals form inside and outside the cell spaces of the tumor tissue. The ice forming inside the cell space leads to cell death by injury to the cell membrane, structures within the cell, or both. Ice that forms outside the cell space, where freezing is slower, causes death by creating a rush of the fluid moving in the space outside the cell. This causes the cell to burst and results in cell death by a deprivation of oxygen to the cell and the cell membrane.

After the procedure: The patient is monitored for a few hours and usually will have to stay overnight in the hospital. A drug such as ibuprofen may be given to relieve a patient's discomfort from having to remain in one position during the procedure.

Although there may be a few restrictions suggested by the physician, most patients can resume their daily activities within one or two days.

Risks: Depending on the type of tumor, side effects from cryoablation vary. The most common minor side effects are pain or bruising at the site, fever, nausea, local infection, fatigue, and temporary low platelet count not requiring transfusion. Most resolve within a week.

Major risks include freezing injury to organs near the tumor, fluid collection within the organ being treated, and puncture of the colon or other organs near the tumor that can result in major bleeding or infection.

For prostate cancer, impotence and loss of bladder control can be a major complication. A more recent cryoablation procedure for prostate cancer, called nerve-sparing cryoablation and focal prostate cryoablation, is being used to reduce the possibility of impotence and urinary incontinence.

Results: The advantages of cryoablation are low complication rates, ability to destroy local tumor tissue with minimal discomfort to the patient, reduction in hospital stay, shortened patient recovery time, less scarring, and lower cost (compared to surgery). It is an especially useful treatment for cancers that are otherwise untreatable and can enhance an individual's quality of life through better symptom control.

For some cancers, such as lung and bone cancer, cryoablation is considered investigational, and health care insurance companies may not cover the procedure.

Jo Gambosi, M.A., B.S.N.

For Further Information

Bahn, Duke, et al. "Focal Prostate Cryoablation: Initial Results Show Cancer Control and Potency Preservation." *Journal of Endourology* 20, no. 9 (2006): 688-692.

Centeno, Arthur S., and Gary Onik. *Prostate Cancer: A Patient's Guide to Treatment*. Omaha, Nebr.: Addicus, 2004.

Chung, Leland. *Prostate Cancer: Biology, Genetics, and New Therapeutics*. Totowa, N.J.: Humana Press, 2001.

VanSonnenberg, Eric, William McMullen, and Luigi Solbiati. *Tumor Ablation: Principles and Practice*. New York: Springer, 2005.

Other Resources

American Cancer Society
http://www.cancer.org

Galil Medical Cryotherapy
http://www.galil-medical.com/galil-medical-cryotherapy.html

See also: Adenoid Cystic Carcinoma (ACC); Basal cell carcinomas; Birt-Hogg-Dubé Syndrome (BHDS); Carcinoid tumors and carcinoid syndrome; Cervical cancer; Dermatology oncology; Eyelid cancer; Hereditary Leiomyomatosis and Renal Cell Cancer (HLRCC); Kidney cancer; Radiofrequency ablation; Skin cancers; Surgical oncology

▶ Culdoscopy

Category: Procedures
Also known as: Flexible culdoscopy

Definition: A culdoscopy is a minimally invasive surgical procedure for visualizing the female pelvic organs through an endoscope (or culdoscope). The endoscope, a rigid viewing tube, is passed through the vagina into the cul-de-sac or retrouterine pouch (the pouch of Douglas), the part of the peritoneal cavity between the rectum and the uterus. The procedure can be used for the diagnosis of diseases such as cancer or the diagnosis of other conditions such as infertility or endometriosis.

Cancers diagnosed: Cancer of the uterus, ovaries, or Fallopian tubes

Why performed: Culdoscopy allows examination of the female pelvic organs and collection of a biopsy (tissue sample) for diagnosing cancer, with minimal discomfort for the patient.

Patient preparation: The procedure is minimally invasive and is usually a hospital procedure with a short stay. Gas distension may be required for visualization but may not be necessary if the procedure is done in the knee-to-chest position. Anesthesia required for the procedure may vary from local or regional to general anesthesia, depending on various factors. If a flexible tube is used, then the patient may stay awake during the procedure. The patient is informed of the risks involved, as well as the benefits of this type of diagnostic procedure.

Steps of the procedure: The patient can be positioned in the knee-to-chest position or lying down (lithotomy) for this procedure. The endoscope, or culdoscope, is inserted into the female pelvic cavity via a small incision or puncture in the top of the posterior (back) vaginal wall. After the surgeon visualizes the pelvic cavity, a tissue sample may be taken and sent to the laboratory to determine the presence of cancer.

After the procedure: The patient may be positioned on her abdomen to help expel any air used in the procedure. The patient is assessed and monitored for bleeding from the vagina. The patient should abstain from sexual intercourse, tampon use, or douches for at least two weeks or until cleared through her health care provider.

Risks: Bowel injury and sepsis are possible risks of culdoscopy. Complications are estimated at 2 percent of patients and include bleeding at the puncture site, infection or peritonitis, or hypersensitivity or allergic reaction to the anesthetic used in the surgery.

Results: Though culdoscopy is still useful as a diagnostic tool, many health care providers have replaced this procedure with a laparoscopy.

Marylane Wade Koch, M.S.N., R.N.

See also: Endoscopy; Fallopian tube cancer; Gynecologic oncology; Pelvic examination; Uterine cancer; Vaginal cancer

▶ Cystography

Category: Procedures

Definition: Cystography is a procedure in which dye is injected into the bladder and X rays are taken to examine the organ.

Cancers diagnosed: Cancers of the bladder and urinary system, prostate cancer

Why performed: Cystography is performed to allow doctors to get a detailed picture of the bladder to check for problems such as cancerous growths.

Patient preparation: Before the procedure, the patient may be asked to refrain from eating solid food for a period of time. The patient may be asked not to drink any fluids or may be asked to drink an increased amount of fluids, depending on the type and purpose of the procedure.

Steps of the procedure: The patient is asked to urinate to empty the bladder as the first step of the procedure. Then a catheter is inserted into the bladder. Through the catheter, a contrast dye is injected into the bladder, until the bladder is full. The patient will experience the feeling of a need to urinate as a result of the fullness of the bladder. Once the dye has been injected, X rays are taken of the bladder. If the patient is male, then a lead shield will be used to protect the testes from the X-radiation. The patient may be asked to move into several different positions to allow for different views of the bladder. Once all the X rays needed have been taken, the catheter is removed and the patient is allowed to expel the dye.

After the procedure: After the procedure, the patient may be advised to drink a large amount of clear fluids for a few days to help flush the dye out of the bladder. Because of the dye, the patient's urine may be an unusual color.

Risks: Some risks are associated with cystography. There is a small risk of infection because of the insertion of the catheter, as well as a small risk of allergic reaction to the injected dye. This procedure is generally not advised for women who are pregnant because exposure to X-radiation can harm the fetus.

Results: The cystography will provide the health care team with detailed pictures of the patient's bladder to use in evaluating the presence of cancerous growths and other bladder problems. Patients generally do not experience any long-term side effects from the procedure.

Robert Bockstiegel, B.S.

See also: Bladder cancer; Cystoscopy; Prostate cancer; Transitional cell carcinomas; Urethral cancer; Urinary system cancers; Urography; Urologic oncology; Urostomy

▶ Cystoscopy

Category: Procedures
Also known as: Cystourethroscopy

Definition: During urination, urine moves from the bladder, through the urethra tube, and to the outside of the body. Cystoscopy uses a cystoscope (a thin tube with a miniature camera and light) to allow a doctor to see, examine, and biopsy abnormal tissues inside the urethra and bladder. This procedure is used to check for possible cancer cells.

Cancers diagnosed: Bladder and urethral cancer; follow-up for renal pelvis and ureter cancer

Why performed: Cystoscopy is primarily a diagnostic procedure used to view the inside of the bladder and urethra. Suspicious tissues are biopsied with a clipper on the end of the cystoscope. The tissue samples are examined in a laboratory for the presence of cancer cells.

Patient preparation: Cystoscopy is performed with general or local anesthesia. Patients receiving general anesthesia should not eat or drink after midnight prior to the day of the procedure. Patients may be asked to provide a urine sample prior to the cystoscopy. The urine sample is tested for the presence of infection. Patients will wear an examination gown for the procedure.

Steps of the procedure: The patient is usually positioned on the back with the knees spread. The lower body is covered with a sheet. The opening of the urethra is cleansed, and a pain-relieving medication is applied. The cystoscope is inserted through the urethral opening and into the bladder. Sterile fluid travels through the cystoscope into the bladder to expand the folds in the bladder and provide the doctor with a good view of the bladder lining. A biopsy is taken of any abnormal-looking tissue. The procedure is short, usually lasting only a few minutes, after which time the fluid and cystoscope are removed. The patient can empty the bladder when the cystoscopy is complete.

After the procedure: Patients may experience a burning sensation while urinating or blood in their urine for about twenty-four hours after the procedure. Antibiotics may be prescribed. Patients should drink plenty of water.

Risks: There is a slight risk of bladder perforation during the procedure or infection following the procedure. Men should contact their doctors immediately if testicular swelling occurs.

Results: A healthy bladder wall appears smooth. Suspicious growths are biopsied to determine whether cancer is present.

Mary Car-Blanchard, O.T.D., B.S.O.T.

See also: Bladder cancer; Cystography; Hematuria; Renal pelvis tumors; Transitional cell carcinomas; Urinary system cancers; Urography; Urologic oncology; Urostomy

▶ Digital Rectal Exam (DRE)

Category: Procedures
Also known as: Rectal exam, prostate exam

Definition: In this procedure, a gloved, lubricated finger is inserted into the rectum to check for abnormalities in the rectal wall. For men, the size and shape of the prostate gland can also be checked for any abnormalities.

Cancers diagnosed: Prostate cancer, rectal cancer, colon cancer

Why performed: A digital rectal exam (DRE) is a simple procedure used to screen for rectal, prostate, and colon cancers. This procedure allows the physician to check for any abnormal thickness or lumps in the rectal wall.

For men, the physician can also check the prostate gland for any unusual characteristics, such as an increase in size or nodules and lumps, since it is located next to the rectum. The benefit of the DRE as a screening tool for prostate cancer is that it can reach a part of the prostate gland where most cancers generally begin. The American Cancer Society recommends that men over age fifty get a DRE annually. High-risk men, defined as those with a family history of prostate cancer or African Americans, should receive DREs yearly beginning at age forty-five. For women, this procedure is usually performed as part of an annual exam.

Patient preparation: No special preparation is needed for this procedure.

Steps of the procedure: A gloved, lubricated finger is inserted into the rectum. There may be slight discomfort during the exam, but this is a quick procedure that generally takes only a few minutes. A stool sample called a fecal occult blood test may also be taken to check for the presence of blood. This test is done to screen for colon cancer.

After the procedure: There are no special instructions, and patients can return to normal activities after the procedure is completed.

Risks: No risks are associated with this exam.

Results: If abnormalities are detected during the procedure, then the physician will recommend additional screening tests, such as a colonoscopy or sigmoidoscopy, which are used to screen for colon cancer. If a problem is suspected with the prostate gland, then a prostate-specific antigen (PSA) blood test, an ultrasound, or possibly a biopsy of the prostate gland may be suggested to screen for prostate cancer.

Vonne Sieve, M.A.

See also: Anal cancer; Anoscopy; Benign Prostatic Hyperplasia (BPH); Carcinomatosis; Colonoscopy; Diverticulosis and diverticulitis; Endorectal ultrasound; Prostate cancer; Prostate-Specific Antigen (PSA) test; Screening for cancer; Sigmoidoscopy; Urologic oncology

▶ Dilation and Curettage (D&C)

Category: Procedures
Also known as: Uterine scraping

Definition: Dilation and curettage (D&C) is used to surgically remove sections of the lining of the uterus and suspicious growths in the uterus in an examination for cancer cells. The lining of the uterus is called the endometrium. "Dilation" refers to manually opening the cervix to access the uterus. "Curettage" refers to using a curette, a surgical instrument, to gently scrape sections of the endometrium away from the uterus.

Cancers diagnosed: Uterine cancer (uterine sarcoma), endometrial cancer (endometrial carcinoma), precancerous cellular changes that can lead to cancer (endometrial hyperplasia), precancerous growths that can change to cancer (endometrial polyps)

Why performed: D&C is performed to diagnose uterine cancer, endometrial cancer, or precancerous cells in the uterus. A D&C obtains tissue specimens for analysis by a pathologist. A D&C may be used if cancer is suspected or if a biopsy is suggestive of cancer but not conclusive. A small tissue sample is obtained in a biopsy, and a larger representation of the uterine tissues is collected with a D&C. Additionally, the tissue specimens may be tested for estrogen and progesterine receptor cells. Increases in these hormones are associated with an increased risk of uterine and endometrial cancer.

Patient preparation: A D&C is a short outpatient procedure performed at a hospital's surgery department or an outpatient surgical center. General anesthesia is usually used, so the patient is not awake. Patients should not eat or drink past midnight prior to the day of the procedure or for seven hours before the D&C. In some cases, spinal or epideral blocks may be used instead of general anesthesia.

On the day of the procedure, the patient provides a urine sample and dons an examination gown.

Steps of the procedure: The patient lies on her back on a surgical table. The patient's knees are spread and her feet are placed in stirrups. The patient's vital signs are monitored, and anesthesia is administered.

The vaginal area and urethra are cleansed. A catheter tube may be inserted into the urethra to collect urine during the procedure. A speculum is inserted into the vagina to separate the vaginal walls. The cervix and vagina are cleansed. Metal devices are used to dilate the cervical opening to allow the doctor to access the uterus.

A curette is an instrument used to remove the lining of the uterus in sections. It has a long narrow handle with a metal loop at the end. The curette is inserted through the vagina and cervix and into the uterus. The doctor uses the curette to gently scrape the lining of the uterus. The tissue specimens are prepared and sent to a pathologist for examination for cancer cells.

When the D&C is complete, the dilating device, speculum, and catheter are removed. The patient is monitored in a postsurgical recovery area until she is alert and is provided with a sanitary napkin to protect her clothing from blood. The patient should not drive and needs to receive a ride home from another person.

After the procedure: Patients may experience menstrual-like cramps or backache and are prescribed pain medication. Bleeding and the passing of small blood clots may occur for a few days following the procedure. Light vaginal bleeding or staining may continue for several weeks. Patients should wear sanitary napkins but should not use tampons. Patients are encouraged to rest for a few days following the surgery and should not participate in sexual intercourse during this time.

Risks: A D&C is considered a low-risk procedure. The risks include those of general anesthesia as well as uterine perforation, cervical laceration, and endometrium scarring. Patients should contact their doctors if they experience heavy bleeding, increased pain, problems breathing, or fever and other signs of infection.

Results: A pathologist examines the tissue specimens for cancerous or precancerous cells. The pathologist's report is conveyed to the doctor.

Mary Car-Blanchard, O.T.D., B.S.O.T.

For Further Information

Engelsen, I. B., et al. "Pathologic Expression of *p53* or *p16* in Preoperative Curettage Specimens Identifies High-Risk Endometrial Carcinomas." *American Journal of Obstetrics and Gynecology* 195, no. 4 (October, 2006): 979-986.

Larson, D. M., et al. "Comparison of D&C and Office Endometrial Biopsy in Predicting Final Histopathologic Grade in Endometrial Cancer." *Obstetrics and Gynecology* 86, no. 1 (July, 1995): 38-42.

Merisio, C., et al. "Endometrial Cancer in Patients with Preoperative Diagnosis of Atypical Endometrial Hyperplasia." *European Journal of Obstetrics & Gynecology and Reproductive Biology* 122, no. 1 (September 1, 2005): 107-111.

Papaefthimiou, M., et al. "The Role of Liquid-Based Cytology Associated with Curettage in the Investigation of Endometrial Lesions from Postmenopausal Women." *Cytopathology* 16, no. 1 (February, 2005): 32-39.

Saygili, H. "Histopathologic Correlation of Dilatation and Curettage and Hysterectomy Specimens in Patients with Postmenopausal Bleeding." *European Journal of Gynaecological Oncology* 27, no. 2 (2006): 182-184.

Wang, X., et al. "Comparison of D&C and Hysterectomy Pathologic Findings in Endometrial Cancer Patients." *Archives of Gynecology and Obstetrics* 272, no. 2 (July, 2005): 136-141.

See also: Colposcopy; Conization; Cryoablation; Endometrial cancer; Gestational Trophoblastic Tumors (GTTs); Giant Cell Tumors (GCTs); Gynecologic cancers; Hysterectomy; Pap test; Uterine cancer

▶ *DPC4* gene testing

Category: Procedures
Also known as: *SMAD4*, *MADH4*

Definition: The *DPC4* gene product maintains normal cell growth rates. Mutations in *DPC4* lead to uncontrolled cell growth and, ultimately, to many cancers, especially those of the gastrointestinal tract and pancreas. Inherited mutations in *DPC4* are one cause of juvenile polyposis syndrome (JPS), an inherited condition that results in a predisposition to colorectal cancer.

Cancers diagnosed: Juvenile polyposis syndrome, familial colon cancer

Why performed: Approximately 20 percent of individuals afflicted with JPS, a condition in which numerous polyps form in the colon, bear mutations in the *DPC4* gene. Other cases may be caused by mutations in *BMPR1A* or other genes. Although polyps resulting from JPS are initially benign, a small proportion may develop into carcinomas. Genetic testing is performed to confirm a diagnosis of patients exhibiting symptoms of JPS and to characterize the *DPC4* mutation causing the disease. Because JPS is an inherited disorder, genetic testing is also often done in previously undiagnosed relatives of JPS patients to determine whether prophylactic treatment is required. Testing is performed at or before age fifteen, the time at which routine screening by colonoscopy is recommended.

Patient preparation: Patients considering genetic testing may meet with a genetic counselor to discuss the benefits and risks of the test and the significance of negative, positive, and inconclusive tests. Material required for genetic testing is obtained from a blood sample or from cheek cells obtained by mouthwash. No special preparation is required.

Steps of the procedure: Samples are sent to a clinical laboratory that offers *DPC4* screening. Deoxyribonucleic acid (DNA) is isolated from the blood sample, and the DNA that encodes *DPC4* is amplified by polymerase chain reaction (PCR) and sequenced using standard methods.

After the procedure: The patient will consult with a physician and/or genetic counselor to discuss the implications of the test results.

Risks: Complications from drawing blood are rare but may include excessive bleeding, hematoma, or infection. Because the information obtained from *DPC4* screening may have significant psychological effects, it is important that patients be offered genetic counseling.

Results: Sequence analysis allows clinicians to identify the specific DNA mutation(s) present in a JPS patient. Once this mutation has been identified, close relatives can be screened to determine if they share the mutation that causes JPS. Routine colonoscopy and polypectomy, beginning at age fifteen, is recommended for those bearing mutations in *DPC4*.

Kyle J. McQuade, Ph.D.

See also: Colorectal cancer; Colorectal cancer screening; Family history and risk assessment; Genetic counseling; Genetic testing; Hereditary cancer syndromes; Hereditary mixed polyposis syndrome; Hereditary polyposis syndromes; Juvenile polyposis syndrome

▶ Ductal lavage

Category: Procedures

Definition: Ductal lavage is a minimally invasive method used to detect gradual changes in breast cells that could indicate a precancerous or cancerous condition. It has been dubbed the "breast Pap smear." The idea dates back to the 1950's, when Dr. George Papanicolaou (1883-1962), the inventor of the Pap smear to detect cervical cancer, first theorized that nipple fluid could be analyzed for precancerous changes.

Cancers diagnosed: Ductal carcinoma in situ (DCIS)

Why performed: According to the American Cancer Society, more than 95 percent of breast cancers originate in the cells lining the milk ducts. Ductal lavage can identify atypical or abnormal changes in breast cells that may fuel cancer development in the future. The test is used to assess women at high risk of breast cancer. It is not intended as a screening tool for breast cancer, nor is it a replacement for mammography.

Patient preparation: No preparation is needed.

Steps of the procedure: A numbing cream is applied to the nipple area. The woman is asked to massage the breast area gently with both hands to help move fluid toward the nipple. A suction device placed over the nipple siphons tiny amounts of fluid from the milk ducts, which helps detect the natural duct openings. Once they are identified, a slender, hollow tube called a catheter is inserted into each duct that produced fluid. Saline flows through the catheter, rinsing out the duct and washing out cells. (*Lavage* is a French word that means "wash" or "rinse.") The fluid containing the cells is then analyzed under a microscope.

After the procedure: The procedure does not usually cause any discomfort. Some women may have a temporary feeling of pressure, tingling, or fullness afterward. No special follow-up care is needed.

Risks: The risks of ductal lavage are rare but may include damage to a milk duct and infection at the site of the catheter insertion. Signs of infection include breast redness, warmth, severe tenderness, and/or persistent fever.

Results: A normal result means that no abnormal cells were detected. In some cases, analysis of the milk duct cells may reveal atypical changes but cannot pinpoint their exact origin in the breast. Not every woman with atypical breast cell changes will develop breast cancer. Experts recommend that the procedure be done along with clinical breast examination and an imaging study, such as mammography.

Kelli Miller Stacy, ELS

See also: Breast cancer in children and adolescents; Breast cancer in men; Breast cancers; Comedo carcinomas; Ductal Carcinoma In Situ (DCIS); Ductogram; Invasive ductal carcinomas; Lobular Carcinoma In Situ (LCIS); Medullary carcinoma of the breast; Microcalcifications; Mucinous carcinomas; Progesterone receptor assay; Tubular carcinomas

▶ Ductogram

Category: Procedures
Also known as: Mammary ductogram, galactogram, galactography, ductogalactography

Definition: A ductogram is an imaging procedure that uses a radio-opaque contrast dye to enhance mammography pictures. A ductogram is used to help identify if cancer is present in the duct of the nipple, which transport breast milk in lactating women.

Cancers diagnosed: Breast cancer, ductal carcinoma in situ (DCIS)

Why performed: A ductogram is used to help determine the source of abnormal nipple discharge and the location of possible cancer. Cancer may cause abnormal nipple discharge. DCIS begins as cancer in the cells that line the ducts. The cancer may remain contained in the nipple or may spread to other parts of the breast. Standard mammography may show small areas of microcalcifications, calcium collections that can be a sign of DCIS. A ductogram creates even better pictures of the suspicious area.

Patient preparation: The patient should not use deodorant or powder on the day of the ductogram. The patient should not express discharge from the nipple before the procedure but should let her doctor know if she does not experience nipple discharge on the day of the procedure. In such cases, the ductogram may need to be rescheduled. The patient should inform her doctor if she is pregnant so that a protective drape will be placed over the abdomen during the procedure.

A ductogram is performed at the radiology department of a hospital or an outpatient radiology center. It is an outpatient procedure that lasts from thirty minutes to an hour. The patient disrobes from the waist up and wears an examination gown for the procedure.

Steps of the procedure: The breast and nipple are cleansed before the procedure. The nipple is sterilized with alcohol. The radiologist identifies which duct is producing abnormal discharge by applying pressure to the nipple to elicit discharge. Local anesthesia may be applied before a blunt-tipped cannula, a small needlelike device, is inserted into the duct. A syringe attached to the cannula delivers the radiopaque contrast dye. The cannula is removed, and mammography images are taken.

After the procedure: A bandage is placed over the nipple. Patients should drink plenty of fluids to help eliminate the dye from the body.

Risks: A ductogram is a low-risk procedure, but pain, infection, or bleeding may occur.

Results: A healthy nipple does not reveal abnormalities. Any abnormalities, such as possible cancer, are highlighted on ductogram images.

Mary Car-Blanchard, O.T.D., B.S.O.T.

See also: Breast cancer in children and adolescents; Breast cancer in men; Breast cancer in pregnant women; Comedo carcinomas; Duct ectasia; Ductal Carcinoma In Situ (DCIS); Ductal lavage; Invasive ductal carcinomas; Invasive lobular carcinomas; Lobular Carcinoma In Situ (LCIS); Nipple discharge

▶ Dukes' classification

Category: Procedures

Definition: Dr. Cuthbert E. Dukes (1890-1977) was a pathologist who developed the classification for operable colon or rectal cancer. He began his studies at St. Mark's Hospital in 1922 and published the Dukes' classification in 1932. Through many years of examining the various clinical stages and prognoses of patients diagnosed with rectal cancer, he was able to develop a pathological classification system that reflected the prognosis based on three categories: A, B, and C. Dukes' classification has been modified to include B1 and B2 as well as C1 and C2. Dr. Vernon Astler and Dr. Fredrick Coller later modified Dukes' classification to include a fourth stage, D.

Cancers diagnosed: Colorectal cancers

Why performed: Patients diagnosed with cancer of the colon or rectum will have treatment and therapy guided by the Dukes' classification system. Patients who have been classified as Stage A may receive more aggressive treatment; those patients classified as Stage D may receive only palliative treatment.

Patient preparation: Dukes' classification is used for a patient who has had a biopsy of the tumor. The biopsy may be obtained surgically or through colonoscopy or a CT-guided biopsy. The patient will have nothing to eat or drink for at least eight hours before any of these procedures. If the cancer is in the lower gastrointestinal (GI) tract, then the patient will have to complete a bowel prep,

Dukes' Stages

Stage	*Description*	*Five-Year Survival Rate (%)*
A	Confined to the lining of the colon	97
B1	Into the thin muscle right below the lining	80
B2	Through the thin muscle right below the lining	80
C1	Limited to bowel wall, with lymph nodes affected	65
C2	Through the bowel wall, with lymph nodes affected	35
D	Distant spread of cancer or inoperable cancer	5

which includes drinking a liquid to cause the stool in the GI tract to be evacuated. If the biopsy will be taken surgically, then the patient may have the skin shaved at the incision site.

Steps of the procedure: The patient will be positioned for comfort. If in the operating room, then the patient will be given general anesthesia. If a sample is to be taken by CT-guided biopsy or colonoscopy, then the patient may be given medications to cause sleepiness and block any pain. Once the patient is positioned and medication is given, the entrance site for the biopsy is cleansed with an appropriate solution. The physician will obtain the biopsy and then place the sample either in a vial with a preservative or on a slide for viewing. The samples will then be sent to the pathologist so that diagnosis and classification can be done.

After the procedure: The patient will be monitored after the procedure for signs of bleeding or pain for a couple of hours. A patient who has completely awakened from the medication-induced sleep and is able to tolerate fluids is able to be driven home by a friend or family member.

Risks: Infections, pain, and bleeding are all risks of obtaining a biopsy for Dukes' classification.

Results: Dukes' classification is based on the pathology of the cancer. A patient will have a biopsy of the disease site and the pathologist will be able to stage the disease based on the defined classification stage. A better prognosis, or five-year survival rate, is directly related to the stage of the disease of the patient. Stage A indicates minimal disease and a high five-year survival rate. Stages B and C indicate that the disease has progressed into the surrounding tissue and the survival rate is decreased. Stage D indicates that the disease has spread, or metastasized, to another site. Stage D is directly related to a poor prognosis or poor chance of five-year survival rate.

Katrina Green, R.N., B.S.N., O.C.N.

See also: ABCD; Breslow's staging; Carcinomas; Gleason grading system; Grading of tumors; Staging of cancer; TNM staging

▶ Electrosurgery

Category: Procedures
Also known as: Electrofulguration, fulguration, medical diathermy, surgical diathermy

Definition: Electrosurgery is the use of electric current to cut, kill tumor cells, or cauterize.

Cancers treated: A variety of cancers, especially those of the skin and mouth

Why performed: Surgeons have many options for removing cancerous growths or tumors. The most traditional method is to use a sharp metal scalpel to cut around the tumor and remove it. This is frequently the method in which surgeons were originally trained and with which they have the most experience. It also is often the most cost effective. There is often significant bleeding during and after this type of procedure, however, and research scientists are always trying to identify new ways to better serve patients. One way that has been developed involves the use of a laser, while another is electrosurgery. Electrosurgery uses an instrument that gives off high-frequency alternating electrical current that heats up cells and allows surgeons to cut with a reduced amount of bleeding. The same equipment can also be used for electrocautery to stop bleeding.

Patient preparation: The required patient preparation depends on the type of electrosurgery being done, as well as on the extent of the procedure. In many cases, the patient will be instructed to prepare in a way similar to preparations for other types of surgeries. This can include avoiding food and liquids for a specified period of time and may involve taking antibiotics to help prevent infection. Patients will generally be specially screened to ensure that they are good candidates for electrosurgery. Individuals with pacemakers or other devices may not be appropriate candidates because of the use of electrical current that flows through the patient's body during the procedure.

Steps of the procedure: Electrosurgery is performed by a surgeon who has had extensive specialized training in using electrosurgical equipment and performing related procedures. The procedure is done using a special generator that takes regular electric current and converts it to electrical current that alternates at a frequency slightly lower than that of AM radio stations. This is done because the electrical current in normal use would result in damage to the patient, including possible nerve or muscle damage and even electrocution. Electrical current of the frequency used by electrosurgical devices is usually considered safe for most individuals, except for those with pacemakers or other implanted devices.

The surgeon uses a special instrument through which the electrical current flows. The surgeon has a number of choices of voltage and frequency, which can be used to achieve various effects, and will usually start with the lowest possible power and increase it until the desired effect is achieved. The tip of the surgical instrument remains cool, but the energy is transferred to the surrounding cells. At low levels, this can cause water to leave the cells and the cells to dehydrate and shrivel. At higher levels, the water inside the cells actually heats enough to boil, but so quickly that it does not have time to escape the cell and the cell actually ruptures. The surgeon can use this instrument to make very thin and precise cuts, to heat tumors to destroy them, or to cauterize cells to stop bleeding, depending on the goal of the procedure.

After the procedure: After electrosurgery, the patient will generally be taken to a recovery room if the procedure was performed under general anesthesia. If there is a wound at an incision site, then it will need to be cleaned and cared for regularly until healing is complete. In many cases, electrosurgery is not the only cancer treatment option being used in a patient's comprehensive cancer care plan. If electrosurgery is used to remove a cancerous growth, then radiation therapy or chemotherapy may still be necessary to kill any cancer cells that remain after the majority are removed surgically.

Risks: Many of the risks associated with electrosurgery are the same or similar to those associated with traditional surgical methods. There is a risk of significant blood loss, pain, swelling, and infection. With electrosurgery, there is also some risk of damage to healthy tissues surrounding the cancerous tissue. Because electrosurgery is usually performed under general anesthesia, there are also the risks associated with anesthesia, such as negative cardiovascular events or allergic reaction. There is some risk of severe burning at a site other than the site of the electrosurgery. Often, smoke is produced during electrosurgery that can be a risk not only to the patient but also to the surgery team if the room is not effectively ventilated.

Results: Results from electrosurgery can vary greatly depending on the type of procedure performed, the area on which the procedure was performed, and other factors. In general, it is believed that electrosurgery can be an effective method for removing tumors or for destroying cancerous growths with less blood loss than traditional surgical methods. For some applications, however, there is concern that electrosurgical techniques may lead to a higher rate of recurrence than other available techniques.

Helen Davidson, B.A.

For Further Information

Dietel, M., ed. *Targeted Therapies in Cancer.* New York: Springer, 2007.

Egan, Tracie. *Skin Cancer: Current and Emerging Trends in Detection and Treatment.* New York: Rosen Publishing Group, 2006.

Lyons, Lyman. *Diagnosis and Treatment of Cancer.* New York: Chelsea House, 2007.

Nathan, David G. *The Cancer Treatment Revolution: How Smart Drugs and Other New Therapies Are Renewing Our Hope and Changing the Face of Medicine.* Hoboken, N.J.: John Wiley & Sons, 2007.

See also: Electroporation therapy; Skin cancers; Urinary system cancers

▶ Embolization

Category: Procedures

Also known as: Vascular embolotherapy; transcatheter embolization; vascular occlusion

Definition: Embolization introduces an agent into the bloodstream to occlude or block a blood vessel that supplies a tumor or organ. This procedure is minimally invasive and can be an alternative to surgery.

Cancers treated: Hepatic (liver) cancer and hepatic metastases; colorectal, pancreatic, and renal (kidney) cancers

Why performed: The purpose of embolization is to shrink a tumor or slow its growth, to redirect blood flow, or to control bleeding. For example, preoperative embolization can reduce blood loss in a subsequent operation, such as liver resection (surgical removal of part of the liver) or nephrectomy (removal of a kidney). Occlusion of blood vessels of the liver to shrink hepatic metastases (cancer that has spread from other parts of the body) is an alternative to surgery when an existing condition, such as cirrhosis, precludes resection. Embolization can be combined with chemotherapy in a procedure called chemoembolization. It involves introducing a chemotherapeutic drug at the tumor site to enhance local concentration of the drug, thereby avoiding systemic side effects. The blood vessel supplying the tumor is then occluded with an embolic agent. In addition, embolization is an alternative to fibroidectomy (removal of uterine fibroids).

Patient preparation: A physician may order diagnostic images based on ultrasound, computed tomography (CT), magnetic resonance imaging (MRI), or X rays to assess the involved organ or site and size of a tumor. In addition, diagnostic tests may be ordered to evaluate the patient's blood and liver and kidney function. Prior to the embolization procedure, the patient is asked about the use of drugs and herbal supplements and about any allergies, such as to contrast media used in imaging. The night before the procedure, the patient may need to abstain from food and liquid for several hours.

Steps of the procedure: A radiologist or other specially trained physician performs the procedure in an interventional suite or, perhaps, in an operating room. A nurse or anesthesiologist sedates the patient and, in some cases, administers general anesthesia. A small incision is made to insert a catheter through the skin into a blood vessel, such as the femoral artery of the leg. The physician threads the catheter through the blood vessel toward the organ or tumor site. A contrast medium or dye is injected into the blood so that angiographic images of the blood vessels can guide the radiologist's progressive threading of the catheter. Sometimes the doctor replaces the initial catheter with a smaller one to move into smaller, branching blood vessels.

When the site is reached, the physician introduces or injects an embolic agent via the catheter and then observes the resulting obstruction of blood flow on a video monitor. Embolic agents can be temporary or permanent. They include metallic coils, gelatin sponge particles or foam, polyvinyl alcohol foam granules, acrylic polymer microspheres, and liquid adhesive (glue). If additional blood vessels need to be embolized, then the physician repeats the process. Embolization can take about thirty minutes to complete, but it may take several hours. At the end of the procedure, the catheter is withdrawn and pressure is applied to the initial incision.

After the procedure: The patient rests horizontally for several hours and usually stays one or more nights in the hospital, mainly for pain control. Some patients experience postembolization syndrome (pain, fever, nausea, vomiting, and fatigue) for a few days or weeks. These symptoms are more likely after embolization of a solid tumor. Many patients resume normal activity within a week. The physician may order follow-up imaging studies to assess the effects of embolization. Sometimes the patient undergoes an operation after the procedure.

Risks: The risks associated with embolization are small when compared to surgery. A few patients, however, may be allergic to the contrast material used for angiography during the procedure. In general, the use of catheters can bruise or damage blood vessels and can introduce infection. If the embolus (plug) occludes the wrong blood vessel, then an unintended interruption of blood flow can damage normal tissue.

Results: Successful embolization alleviates the patient's symptoms and may extend survival time. In some cases, diverting blood deliberately causes hypertrophy (increase in size) of part of the liver, thereby enabling surgery on what was previously an unresectable liver. If embolization is meant to reduce the size of a bulky tumor, then the associated pain becomes more manageable.

Tanja Bekhuis, Ph.D.

For Further Information

Cahill, Bridget A. "Management of Patients Who Have Undergone Hepatic Artery Chemoembolization." *Clinical Journal of Oncology Nursing* 9, no. 1 (2005): 69-75.

"Interventional Radiology for the Cancer Patient." In *Cancer Medicine*, edited by Donald W. Kufe et al. 6th ed. Hamilton, Ont.: BC Decker, 2003. Also available online at http://www.ncbi.nlm.nih.gov/books.

Other Resources

RadiologyInfo
http://www.radiologyinfo.org

Society of Interventional Radiology
Http://www.sirweb.org

Web MD
Embolization: Vascular Lesions
http://www.emedicine.com

See also: Arterial embolization; Carcinoid tumors and carcinoid syndrome; Chemoembolization; Hemoptysis; Hereditary Leiomyomatosis and Renal Cell Cancer (HLRCC); Hereditary non-VHL clear cell renal cell carcinomas; Hereditary papillary renal cell carcinomas; Kidney cancer; Leiomyomas; Liver cancers; Urinary system cancers; Virus-related cancers

▶ Endorectal ultrasound

Category: Procedures
Also known as: Endorectal echoscopy, endorectal ultrasonography, rectal endosonography, transrectal ultrasound

Definition: Endorectal ultrasound (ERUS) is the insertion of an ultrasound transducer through the anus to construct detailed images of the rectal wall and adjacent tissues. ERUS instruments vary in insertion tube design (such as size, flexibility, and view), ultrasound technology (such as frequency, orientation, and scanning), imaging capabilities (such as fiber-optic or electronic and two- or three-dimensional), and configuration (that is, the ultrasound transducer is either mounted on or passed through an endoscope).

Cancers diagnosed: Rectal cancer

Why performed: ERUS may be performed either as a diagnostic procedure to determine tumor boundaries and to assess spread into lymph nodes and pelvic organs or as a surveillance procedure to detect local recurrence.

Patient preparation: A few days before the procedure, the patient may need to stop certain medications, such as aspirin products and blood thinners. The day before the procedure, the patient cleans the rectum, as with an enema.

Steps of the procedure: ERUS is scheduled in a physician's office or other outpatient setting. The patient wears a gown and lies on the side. The patient is awake; if needed, sedation or local anesthetic can be given. First, the physician performs a digital rectal exam. Then, the ultrasound transducer is inserted through the anus into the rectum, and a latex balloon (or alternative for a latex-sensitive patient) covering the ultrasound transducer is inflated. The ultrasound transducer is turned on, sending pulses of sound waves through the balloon into the rectal wall and adjacent tissues. As each pulse of sound waves hits different tissues, some sound waves bounce back and become a gray-scale image on a video monitor. The physician views the images as the ultrasound transducer is moved through the rectum. Tumor dimensions and lymph node sizes are measured. Abnormal tissues are sampled (biopsied) with a fine needle; all tissue samples are taken to the laboratory for cytologic evaluation.

After the procedure: The patient leaves and resumes normal activities, unless sedation or local anesthetic was needed. In the latter case, the patient will need to be driven home by a friend or family member.

Risks: ERUS is relatively safe, with a small risk of these side effects: perforation, bleeding, and infection.

Results: ERUS images are interpreted with criteria developed by Ulrich Hildebrandt and Gernot Feifel in 1985. Boundaries of the tumor in the rectal wall are accurately determined from the thickness and continuity of each layer of the rectal wall. Lymph nodes and pelvic organs are assessed for size, shape, and irregularities. Because cancerous and inflamed tissues look similar in ERUS images, however, cytologic evaluation must verify that abnormalities in lymph nodes or pelvic organs are cancerous.

Patricia Boone, Ph.D.

See also: Anal cancer; Colonoscopy and virtual colonoscopy; Colorectal cancer screening; Prostate cancer; Prostate-Specific Antigen (PSA) test; Rectal cancer; Sigmoidoscopy; Transrectal ultrasound

▶ Endoscopic Retrograde Cholangiopancreatography (ERCP)

Category: Procedures

Definition: Endoscopic retrograde cholangiopancreatography (ERCP) is the X-ray study of the bile and pancreatic ducts using contrast dye injected in the ducts from a tube with a tiny camera at the end (endoscope) inserted down the patient's throat and through the stomach to the duodenum.

Cancers diagnosed: Pancreatic cancer, bile duct cancer, gallbladder cancer

Why performed: ERCP permits a doctor to check for swelling or tumors in the ducts that pass digestive fluids from the gallbladder and pancreas to the stomach, to perform a biopsy, and to remove minor obstructions in the ducts. It may be recommended for patients with a familial history of pancreatic cancer, but it is not used as a routine screening tool for those with an average risk for cancer.

Patient preparation: This procedure is done in an X-ray room. Patients must take nothing by mouth for eight hours prior to the procedure. The doctor may restrict medications such as aspirin, which may increase the risk of bleeding. Patients should report any allergy or sensitivity to anesthetics, dyes, or other medications.

Steps of the procedure: The patient receives a sedative for relaxation and a local anesthetic in the throat to suppress the gag reflex. The doctor helps the patient swallow the endoscope and threads it through the esophagus and stomach into the duodenum, where the common bile duct enters the small intestine. The tube is narrow and flexible and does not interfere with breathing. With the end at the common bile duct, the doctor injects a radiopaque dye and takes an X ray. After removing a biopsy specimen, the doctor removes the tube. The procedure usually takes less than an hour.

After the procedure: To prevent choking, the patient is not given anything to eat or drink until the anesthetic has worn off. After several hours of observation to rule out any complications, the patient may be allowed to return home. Some patients report a sore throat for several days and should eat a soft diet for the next twenty-four hours.

Risks: The risk of complications for ERCP is minor (less than 5 percent) and includes pancreatitis, bleeding, and perforation of the esophagus, stomach, or small intestine. Pain, fever, and chills may indicate an infection. Patients may react to the anesthetic or dye with nausea, hives, blurred vision, dry mouth, retention of urine, or a burning or flushed feeling.

Results: Normal findings show the biliary and pancreatic ducts are of normal size with no obstructions. Abnormal results include narrowing or inflammation of the ducts.

Marcia Pinneau, R.N.

See also: Bile duct cancer; Endoscopy; Gallbladder cancer; Hepatomegaly; Pancreatic cancers

▶ Endoscopy

Category: Procedures

Also known as: Brochoscopy, capsule endoscopy, colonoscopy, colposcopy, cystoscopy, cystourethroscopy, endoscopic retrograde cholangiopancreatography (ERCP), endoscopic ultrasound (EUS), enteroscopy, esophagogastroduodenoscopy (EGD), flexible bronchoscopy, flexible sigmoidoscopy, gastroscopy, hysteroscopy, laparoscopy, laryngoscopy, lower endoscopy, mediastinoscopy, panendoscopy, peritoneal endoscopy, pleuroscopy, proctosigmoidscopy, sigmoidoscopy, thorascopy, upper endoscopy, virtual endoscopy

Definition: Endoscopy is a procedure that involves inserting a thin tube with a viewing instrument inside the body to examine the internal anatomy. There are many types of endoscopes, depending on the purpose of the procedure and the part of the body being examined. Endoscopes may be equipped with lights, fiber optics, ultrasound, lasers, or surgical instruments. Endoscopes may be inserted into the body through small incisions or through natural openings, such as the mouth, vagina, anus, or urethra. Common types of endoscopes include bronchoscopes, colonoscopes, colposcopes, cystoscopes, esophagogastroduodenoscopes, hysteroscopes, laparoscopes, laryngoscopes, mediastinoscopes, sigmoidoscopes, and thoracoscopes.

Cancers diagnosed or treated: Anal cancer, bile duct cancer, bladder cancer, cancer of unknown origin, carcinoid cancer, cervical cancer, colon cancer, colorectal cancer, endometrial cancer, esophageal cancer, gallbladder cancer, laryngeal and hypolaryngeal cancer, liver cancer, lung cancer, cancer of the nasal cavity and parasinuses, metastasized cancer, oral cavity and oropharynngeal cancer, ovarian cancer, pancreatic cancer, prostate cancer, small intestine cancer, stomach cancer, vaginal cancer, uterine cancer

Why performed: Endoscopies are medical procedures used to screen, diagnose, biopsy, stage, treat, and palliatively treat cancer. Endoscopy is used to screen for certain cancers, allowing early detection and treatment. It is used to provide more detailed information about suspicious tissues seen on imaging scans, which then can be biopsied or removed. Endoscopy is used to determine how far cancer has spread to help in staging. In advanced cancer, surgical endoscopy is used for palliative care.

Endoscopes are used in minimally invasive or "keyhole" surgeries. Capsule endoscopy is a newer technology in which a miniature camera and light source are contained in a capsule, which is swallowed. The capsule creates images of the intestine that cannot be reached with standard endoscopy. Virtual endoscopy is another newer technology that uses endoscopy and computed tomography (CT) scans to create three-dimensional images.

Patient preparation: Preparation depends on the type of endoscopy that is being performed. Generally, upper endoscopies use sedation and local or general anesthesia and require fasting. Lower endoscopies use sedation and local or general anesthesia and require fasting, a liquid diet, laxative use, or an enema. Laparoscopic procedures require fasting and general anesthesia. Some endoscopic procedures may use local anesthesia and may not require fasting. Patients receive specific instructions prior to the procedures. Many types of endoscopies are performed as outpatient procedures at hospitals or surgical centers. Some procedures may require a short stay in the hospital.

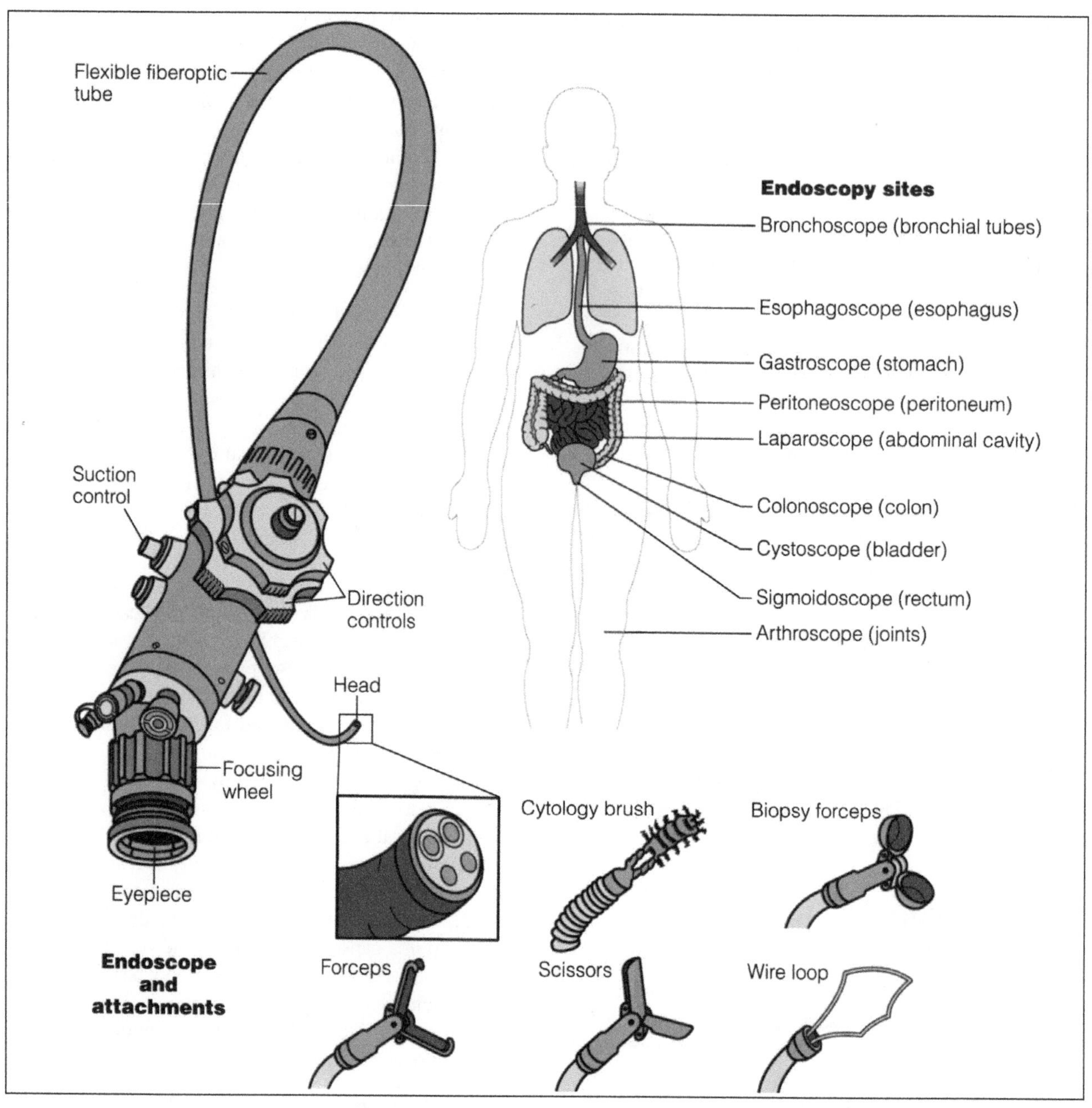

Steps of the procedure: The steps of the procedure depend on the type of endoscopy being performed. An upper endoscopy involves the use of a plastic mouthpiece to keep the mouth open. The well-lubricated endoscope is placed in the mouth and swallowed by the patient. The doctor gently guides the endoscope through the esophagus, stomach, and small intestine by viewing images on a monitor.

A lower endoscopy involves placing a well-lubricated endoscope through the anus and into the rectum and/or colon. The procedure is guided by visual images on a screen.

Laparoscopic endoscopy involves inserting the endoscope through a small incision. Air may be inserted to expand the body cavity to create a better view.

Surgery may be performed with endoscopy. Surgical instruments may be used to take a biopsy. Lasers or surgical instruments may be used to remove small cancerous or precancerous growths.

After the procedure: The patient is observed in the recovery area until alert. Patients receiving outpatient procedures may need another person to drive them home. Some procedures may require a short inpatient stay. Depending on the type of endoscopy, patients may experience discomfort and minimal bleeding. They will receive specific care instructions related to their procedures.

Risks: The risks of endoscopy include pain, bleeding, infection, organ or tissue perforation, and those associated with general anesthesia.

Results: Healthy tissues are free of atypical or abnormal growths. Suspicious tissues may be biopsied during the endoscopy or with a separate procedure. Biopsied tissues or suspicious growths that are removed are tested for the presence of cancerous and precancerous cells.

Mary Car-Blanchard, O.T.D., B.S.O.T.

For Further Information

Ersoy, O., B. Sivri, and Y. Bayraktar. "How Helpful Is Capsule Endoscopy to Surgeons?" *World Journal of Gastroenterology* 13, no. 27 (July 21, 2007): 3671-3676.

Faigel, Douglas O., and David R. Cave, eds. *Capsule Endoscopy*. Philadelphia: Saunders Elsevier, 2008.

Ginsberg, Gregory, et al. *Clinical Gastrointestinal Endoscopy*. Philadelphia: Elsevier Saunders, 2005.

Hara, A. K., et al. "Imaging of Small Bowel Disease: Comparison of Capsule Endoscopy, Standard Endoscopy, Barium Examination, and CT." *Radiographics* 25, no. 3 (May/June, 2005): 697-711.

Hartmann, D., et al. "Capsule Endoscopy: Technical Impact, Benefits, and Limitations." *Langenbecks Archives of Surgery* 389, no. 3 (June, 2004): 225-233.

Pennazio, M. "Capsule Endoscopy: Where Are We After Six Years of Clinical Use?" *Digestive and Liver Disease* 38, no. 12 (December, 2006): 867-878.

Sterman, Daniel, et al. *Thoracic Endoscopy: Advances in Interventional Pulmonology*. Malden, Mass.: Blackwell, 2006.

Wilcox, C. Mel, Miguel Muñoz-Navas, and Joseph J. Y. Sung. *Atlas of Clinical Gastrointestinal Endoscopy*. 2d ed. Philadelphia: Saunders Elsevier, 2007.

Other Resources

American Cancer Society
http://www.cancer.org

American Society for Gastrointestinal Endoscopy
http://www.asge.org

Society of International Gastroenterological Nurses and Endoscopy Associates
http://www.signea.org

See also: Anoscopy; Bronchoscopy; Colonoscopy and virtual colonoscopy; Colposcopy; Culdoscopy; Cystoscopy; Endoscopic Retrograde Cholangiopancreatography (ERCP); Gonioscopy; Hysteroscopy; Laparoscopy and laparoscopic surgery; Laryngoscopy; Mediastinoscopy; Sigmoidoscopy; Thoracoscopy; Upper Gastrointestinal (GI) endoscopy

▶ Enterostomal therapy

Category: Procedures
Also known as: Stomal therapy, stoma care, ostomy care

Definition: Enterostomal therapy is the acute care and rehabilitative treatment of patients who have had an ostomy procedure.

Cancers treated: Colorectal cancer, familial adenomatous polyposis, bladder cancer

Why performed: Enterostomal therapy teaches patients how to care for abdominal stomas (surgically constructed connections between the intestines and the skin). It also includes care for urinary or fecal incontinence and treatment of chronic wounds or pressure ulcers.

A colostomy is a surgically created opening of the colon (large intestine) to divert stool, and an ileostomy is a surgically created opening of the ileum (end of the small intestine) to divert stool. Bypassing or removing part of the intestine or rectum may be necessary in the treatment of colorectal cancer, diverticulitis, or inflammatory bowel disease, especially when there is a blockage. The remaining end of the intestine is brought through the abdominal wall where wastes are excreted through a stoma and collected outside the body in an external pouching system adhered to the skin. The location of the stoma on the abdomen is dependent on where the ostomy was created. In some ileostomy procedures, an internal pouch (called an ileoanal reservoir, ileoanal anastomosis, or "J" pouch), is constructed from the remaining end of the small intestine and connected to the anus to allow normal stool passage via the anal sphincter muscles. Sometimes, a colostomy or ileostomy is temporary, allowing the newly constructed gastrointestinal system to heal when part of these organs have been removed or resected.

A urostomy is a surgical procedure that diverts urine away from the bladder. The ileum or cecum (beginning of the large intestine) is surgically removed and reconstructed into a conduit created for the passage of urine from the kidneys through a stoma in the abdominal wall. The urine is collected outside the body in an external pouching system. A urostomy may be necessary in the treatment of bladder cancer. In some cases when the urinary sphincter muscle does not need to be removed, a "replacement bladder," called an orthotopic neobladder, can be constructed from a section of the intestines and connected to the urethra to allow normal urination.

Patient preparation: Tests performed before ostomy surgery may include X rays, ultrasound, colonoscopy or sigmoidoscopy, blood tests, urine tests, and an electrocardiogram (ECG). Complete bowel cleansing is required beforehand, and the patient will receive specific bowel preparation guidelines. The patient will also receive medication and dietary guidelines, which include following a clear fluid diet. Depending on the type of procedure to be performed, additional tests or patient preparations may be required.

Steps of the procedure: The steps required for enterostomal therapy vary greatly, depending on the type of ostomy that the patient has had. In general, steps include gathering supplies; examining the stoma and condition of the surrounding skin daily and reporting abnormalities to the health care team; cleansing the skin; irrigating the stoma with water either daily or every other day; applying barriers, borders, or pastes to the skin around the stoma and applying the pouch; emptying the pouch when it is one-third full; and changing the pouch as prescribed (every one to three days).

After the procedure: Patients who have had an ostomy wear an external pouching system to collect stool or urine because they cannot control the passage of stool, gas, or urine through the stoma. The pouching system also protects the skin around the stoma. There are a wide variety of pouching systems, and an enterostomal therapy nurse will work with the patient to select a system that meets the patient's preferences and lifestyle.

The stoma is usually swollen and large, but it will reduce in size once it has fully healed, within six to eight weeks after surgery. A nurse will teach the patient how to care for the stoma and skin around the stoma, change the ostomy bag, perform the irrigation procedure, and manage problems or emergencies. The patient will be required to demonstrate these activities independently before being discharged from the hospital. The patient will also receive resources for purchasing ostomy supplies.

The patient does not have feeling in the stoma, but abdominal pain, cramping, bloating, and discomfort are common for a few weeks after the procedure. Pain medication is prescribed as needed.

The patient is usually discharged in three to five days after the procedure, depending on the rate of recovery. Home care enterostomal therapy nursing services will be offered to aid recovery. Regular activities can usually be resumed within six to eight weeks.

After surgery, patients often have concerns about resuming regular activities, returning to work, and engaging in sexual activity. The nurse will discuss these concerns with the patient and can provide referrals to community support resources and other medical specialists as needed.

Risks: As with all surgeries, there are risks associated with ostomy procedures. Complications are rare but may include bleeding, need for further surgery, infection, or scarring. The health care team will discuss the potential risks of the procedure with the patient and his or her family or caregiver.

Results: An ostomy can be a lifesaving surgery, improving symptoms and allowing a patient to enjoy a full range of activities.

Angela M. Costello, B.S.

For Further Information

Aronovitch, Sharon. "Changing a Bowel Diversion Ostomy Appliance: Pouching a Stoma." In *Delmar's Fundamental and Advanced Nursing Skills*. 2d ed. New York: Delmar Learning, 2004.

Other Resources

Canadian Association for Enterostomal Therapy
A Guide to Living with a Colostomy
http://www.caet.ca/booklet_colostomy1.htm.

International Ostomy Association
http://www.ostomyinternational.org

National Association for Continence
http://www.nafc.org

United Ostomy Association, Inc.
http://www.uoa.org

United Ostomy Associations of America
http://www.uoaa.org

Wound, Ostomy and Continence Nurses Society
http://www.wocn.org/patients

See also: Abdominoperineal Resection (APR); Colectomy; Coloanal anastomosis; Colorectal cancer; Colostomy; Diverticulosis and diverticulitis; Gastrointestinal cancers; Gastrointestinal complications of cancer treatment; Ileostomy; Urostomy

▶ Esophagectomy

Category: Procedures
Also known as: Transhiatal esophagectomy, transthoracic esophagectomy, esophagogastrectomy

Definition: Esophagectomy is the surgical removal of part of the esophagus for the treatment of cancer or the relief of cancer symptoms. How much of the esophagus is removed is variable, depending on the location of the malignancy or obstruction. The top part of the stomach may also be removed (a procedure referred to as esophagogastrectomy). After removal of the cancer or obstruction, the stomach is connected to the remaining part of the esophagus, which is restructured into a tube to form a new esophagus.

Cancers diagnosed and treated: Esophageal cancer; high-grade dysplasia with Barrett esophagus; end-stage benign diseases including achalasia, hiatal hernia, and gastroesophageal reflux disease (GERD)

Why performed: An esophagectomy may be recommended as a treatment option for patients with cancer of the esophagus or high-grade dysplasia that occurs with Barrett esophagus. It also may be performed to provide relief of symptoms associated with benign conditions that affect swallowing, such as achalasia, hiatal hernia, and gastroesophageal reflux disease. Esophagectomy is the only surgical treatment currently available for the treatment of esophageal cancer, and it is most successful when performed for patients with early-stage disease.

Because of the complexity of the procedure, an esophagectomy should be performed by an experienced thoracic surgeon at a medical center that specializes in the care of patients with esophageal diseases. Research has shown that patients who undergo an esophagectomy at hospitals with thoracic surgeons who perform large numbers of procedures have improved clinical outcomes and lower mortality rates than do patients who have an esophagectomy at lower-volume hospitals.

Patient preparation: Tests performed before the procedure include a complete cardiac evaluation, esophageal manometry, esophagoscopy with biopsy, endoscopic ultrasound, computed tomography (CT) scan, positron emission tomography (PET) scan, and blood tests. Chemotherapy or radiation therapy may be performed to reduce the size of the tumor before surgery. One week before the procedure, patients must stop taking aspirin and products containing aspirin, ibuprofen, and anticoagulants, as directed by the physician.

Steps of the procedure: General anesthesia is administered. The surgical technique and type of incisions vary, depending on the location and extent of the cancer, the patient's pulmonary function, and the surgeon's recommendations. Surgical techniques include the following:

- transhiatal esophagectomy, in which incisions are made in the abdomen and left side of the neck, but not in the chest
- transthoracic esophagectomy (Ivor-Lewis procedure), in which incisions are made in the chest wall (thoracotomy) and upper abdomen
- triincisional esophagectomy (McKeown esophagectomy), in which incisions are made in the right chest, abdomen, and left side of the neck
- minimally invasive esophagectomy, in which several 1-inch incisions are made between the ribs, a thoracoscope (small video-scope) is used to view the surgical area, and surgical instruments are inserted through the other incisions; this procedure minimizes trauma, decreases postoperative pain, and promotes a shorter hospital stay and a quicker recovery

The esophagus, the tumor or obstruction, and affected lymph nodes are removed. The gastrointestinal system is reconstructed: The stomach is connected to the remaining part of the esophagus. Surgery may last from four to seven hours.

After the procedure: The patient recovers in an intensive care unit (ICU) for twenty-four to forty-eight hours. The patient is intubated to aid breathing and has a chest tube to drain fluid and air. Medications are given to manage pain. A feeding tube is placed in the small intestine (jejunostomy or J-tube) to provide adequate nutrition during the early postoperative period when the patient is unable to eat by mouth. The patient performs deep breathing and coughing exercises to remove lung secretions.

Recovery in the hospital takes about seven days, and full recovery usually occurs within six to eight weeks. The patient is able to advance gradually from clear liquids to soft foods during recovery at home. The J-tube is removed after the esophagus has healed, usually within four weeks after the procedure. The patient's swallowing mechanism is usually restored, as well as the ability to taste food. In some cases, surgical treatment with an esophagectomy may be followed by chemotherapy or radiation therapy.

Risks: The risks of this procedure include leaks from the internal suture line, pneumonia, pulmonary edema, respiratory distress, bleeding, infection, abnormal heart rhythms, pneumothorax (collapsed lung), and persistent pain. The risk of heart attack is rare. Strictures or narrowed areas may occur at the site where the esophagus and stomach were reconstructed, causing difficulty swallowing in 10 to 15 percent of patients. The mortality rate (rate of death) associated with esophagectomy ranges from 3 to 8 percent.

Results: Despite the risks, surgical advancements have improved the long-term success of the procedure. Two-year survival rates for patients who undergo an esophagectomy for the treatment of esophageal cancer range from 35 to 42 percent, and five-year survival rates range from 15 to 24 percent, with higher survival rates in patients with early-stage cancers. Surgery performed for the relief of dysphagia (difficulty swallowing) improves symptoms in 80 percent of patients, according to the American Cancer Society.

Angela M. Costello, B.S.

For Further Information

Ercan, S., et al. "Does Esophagogastric Anastomic Technique Influence the Outcome of Patients with Esophageal Cancer?" *Journal of Thoracic and Cardiovascular Surgery* 129 (2005): 623-631.

Ma, J. Y., et al. "Clinicopathologic Characteristics of Esophagectomy for Esophageal Carcinoma in Elderly Patients." *World Journal of Gastroenterology* 12, no. 8 (2006): 1296-1299.

MacKenzie, D. J., et al. "Care of Patients After Esophagectomy." *Critical Care Nurse* 24, no. 1 (February, 2004): 16-31.

Van Lanshott, J. J., et al. "Hospital Volume and Hospital Mortality for Esophagectomy." *Cancer* 91 (2001): 1574.

Other Resources

American Cancer Society
http://cancer.org

American College of Chest Physicians
http://www.chestnet.org

National Cancer Institute
http://www.cancer.gov

Society of Thoracic Surgeons—Patient Section
http://www.sts.org/sections/patientinformation/

See also: Alcohol, alcoholism, and cancer; Bacteria as causes of cancer; Barium swallow; Barrett esophagus; Candidiasis; Cardiomyopathy in cancer patients; Cigarettes and cigars; Endoscopy; Esophageal cancer; Esophagitis; Fanconi anemia; Gastrointestinal cancers; Gastrointestinal oncology; Hematemesis; Oral and oropharyngeal cancers; Premalignancies; Stent therapy; Stomatitis; Thoracotomy; Upper Gastrointestinal (GI) endoscopy

▶ Exenteration

Category: Procedures

Definition: Exenteration is a major surgical procedure in which the entire contents of a body cavity, such as the pelvis or the orbit (eye socket), are totally removed.

Cancers treated: In female patients, cancer of the reproductive organs such as the uterus, cervix, and Fallopian tubes; in male patients, cancer of the prostate and certain ducts and glands; for both genders, cancer of the rectum and cancers of the eye and surrounding tissues

Why performed: Exenteration of the pelvis in female patients is performed when less radical surgery, chemotherapy, and radiotherapy have failed in the management of advanced and/or invasive cases of vaginal, cervical, uterine, and rectal cancer. Most often, previously treated patients with recurrent cervical cancer undergo the procedure. Cancer that has spread or metastasized is rarely treatable with exenteration; because of characteristic distant metastasis, ovarian cancer does not lend itself to the procedure. In male patients, pelvic exenteration is indicated when prostate and/or rectal cancer is unresponsive to radiation and hormonal therapy and when biopsy demonstrates recurrent cancer and ultrasound shows rectal involvement. Orbital exenteration is indicated for large orbital tumors, or the extension of intraocular tumors, most commonly when squamous and basal cell carcinoma affecting the orbit and its contents are unmanageable by simple removal or irradiation.

Patient preparation: For exenteration of the pelvis, along with laboratory tests, patients are evaluated with pelvic and rectal exams. Imaging procedures include rectal and liver ultrasound, computed tomography (CT) scans, chest X rays, bone scans, and magnetic resonance imaging (MRI) to determine the extent and/or spread of the cancer. Biopsy may confirm a recurrence of cancer. Immediately preceding the operation, the patient is given a bowel prep and antibiotics to prevent postsurgical infection.

In orbital exenteration, a physical exam, history, laboratory tests, and imaging methods such as ultrasound, CT scans, angiography (to examine the orbital blood vessels), and biopsy are employed. Patients may undergo preoperative radiation and/or chemotherapy.

Steps of the procedure: Total pelvic exenteration is an ultraradical surgery comprising total resection (removal) of female reproductive organs (cervix, uterus, tubes, ovaries, and vagina), part of the lower urinary tract (urethra and bladder) and rectum, as well as the muscles that form the pelvic floor.

The process commences with a generous midline (vertical) incision in the abdomen that allows for exploration; during the operation, biopsies may be taken to assess the presence of cancer. If a tumor cannot be found or if pathology shows that the cancer has spread to the pelvic sidewall or has metastasized to the lymph nodes, then the procedure should be discontinued.

If a decision is made to continue, then pelvic blood vessels are clamped and the organs are removed. Before the incision is closed, a urostomy and a colostomy may be performed. A urostomy diverts urine to a small pouch created from the small intestine, which is then connected to the abdominal wall so that urine can pass through a stoma (small opening) for collection. A colostomy attaches the colon to the abdominal wall so that fecal waste may exit the body via a stoma for collection in a small bag.

Variations of pelvic exenteration include anterior exenteration, in which the rectum is left intact, and posterior exenteration, in which the bladder and the urethra are spared. In male patients, removal of the bladder and prostate is called a cystoproctectomy.

In orbital exenteration, the entire contents of the globe are removed, including the eyeball, surrounding tissues, and part of the bony orbit. In certain patients, the eyelids and conjunctiva may be spared. Less radical procedures include evisceration, which spares the extraocular muscles, and enucleation, in which the eye is removed while all other orbital structures are spared.

After the procedure: With pelvic exenteration, a drainage tube is placed into the incision site; there is usually discharge, bleeding, and quite a bit of tenderness and pain for at least a few days. While side effects vary, they often include difficulty with urination, particularly if catheterization is involved. Before the patient is sent home, stitches are removed and a pain medication is prescribed.

After orbital exenteration, the majority of patients experience headache for several days, which may dissipate with the use of pain medications. An ocular ointment containing antibiotics and steroids may also be prescribed.

Risks: With pelvic exenteration, morbidity and mortality depend on the specific procedure and the condition of the patient; the elderly and those with comorbidities are most affected. There is a 30 to 44 percent chance of complications such as kidney failure, fistula formation, and bowel obstruction during the procedure, a mortality rate of 2 to 5 percent, and a five-year survival rate of 23 to 61 percent. The success with rectal anastomosis depends on the degree of resection and concurrent reconstructive procedures; complications such as leaks and fistulas may occur in 30 to 50 percent of cases. Overall, a poor prognosis is associated with recurrence of cancer, a tumor larger than 3 centimeters, involvement of the resection margin or pelvic sidewall, and nodal metastasis.

With orbital exenteration, there may be ear pathology, sinusitis, chronic orbital pain that throbs, orbital cysts, and recurrence of cancer. A five-year survival rate of 64 percent has been observed.

Results: While pelvic exenteration may often be a lifesaving measure, patients should be made aware of postoperative sequelae so as to attenuate the psychological distress related to lifestyle changes such as dealing with permanent catheterization, a colostomy and/or urostomy, and loss of sexual functions. The services of a psychologist and sex therapist may be required. In addition, a variety of postoperative reconstructive procedures are available to support the pelvis and even create a "neovagina" in female patients.

Orbital exenteration will require that the patient adapt to a dramatic change in appearance and loss of eyesight in the affected eye. Wearing an eye patch is a popular option for many patients; after the site has healed, a temporary prosthesis such as a plastic eye may be used. Later, a permanent prosthesis may be attached.

Cynthia Racer, M.A., M.P.H.

For Further Information

Ben Simon, G. J., R. M. Schwarcz, R. Douglas, et al. "Orbital Exenteration: One Size Does Not Fit All." *American Journal* of *Ophthalmology* no. 139, no. 6 (2005): 7-11.

Della Rocca, Robert, Edward H. Bedrossian, Jr., and Bryan Arthurs, eds. *Ophthalmic Plastic Surgery: Decision Making and Techniques.* New York: McGraw-Hill, 2002.

Nemet, A. Y., P. Martin, R. Benger, et al. "Orbital Exenteration: A Fifteen-Year Study of Thirty-eight Cases." *Ophthalmic Plastic & Reconstructive Surgery* 23, no. 6 (November/December, 2007): 468-472.

O'Donovan, Peter J., and Ellis G. R. Downes, eds. *Advances in Gynaecological Surgery.* San Francisco: GMM, 2002.

Rock, John A., and Howard W. Jones III, eds. *Te Linde's Operative Gynecology.* 9th ed. Philadelphia: Lippincott Williams & Wilkins, 2003.

Stolzenburg, J.-U., M. T. Gettman, and E. N. Liatsikis, eds. *Endoscopic Extraperitoneal Radical Prostatectomy: Laparoscopic and Robot-Assisted Surgery*, London: Springer, 2007.

See also: Lacrimal gland tumors; Nasal cavity and paranasal sinus cancers; Urinary system cancers; Vaginal cancer

▶ External Beam Radiation Therapy (EBRT)

Category: Procedures
Also known as: Radiotherapy

Definition: External beam radiation therapy (EBRT) uses a linear accelerator to generate high-energy radiation beams or a machine with a radioactive source, cobalt 60, to kill cancer cells by altering their genetic material.

Cancers treated: Most cancers, with approximately 60 percent of all cancer patients receiving radiation

Why performed: EBRT is performed as a curative treatment alone or in combination with chemotherapy, surgery, and other treatments. EBRT may also be used to treat symptoms or side effects from cancer, such as spinal cord compression and metastases.

Patient preparation: The patient will be referred to a radiation oncologist for a consult visit to determine if external beam radiation therapy is appropriate. Prior to receiving treatment, patients have a simulation using a computed tomography (CT) scanner or other device to visualize the area to be treated. A simulation may take one to two hours. Small marks may be applied to the skin to provide assistance in positioning the radiation beams. The simulation data are used to plan the radiation dose amounts to be given by the linear accelerator. Accurate tumor targeting is the key to protecting normal tissues while killing cancer cells.

Steps of the procedure: The treatment plan will outline the patient position on the treatment table, define the number of treatments to be given, and prescribe the daily total dose to be given. The patient usually has four to six weeks of treatment, five days a week, with two days a week off for normal cells to rest and recover. The patient may need to change into a hospital gown. In the treatment room, the staff will position the patient carefully and then leave the room to program the linear accelerator with the required treatment data. The total time for positioning and radiation administration is about fifteen minutes.

After the procedure: Treatments are generally done on an outpatient basis, and the patient may leave immediately after the daily treatment. Patients are not radioactive following treatments.

Risks: External beam radiation therapy is a local treatment, so risks are generally associated with the site being treated. Skin reactions, similar to sunburn, may occur. Fatigue is often associated with EBRT, but the cause is unknown. There is a risk of a second cancer caused by the radiation. There is also a risk that the radiation will not kill all the cancer cells.

Results: Expected after external beam radiation therapy is expected to kill cancer cells and thus reduce tumor size.

Patricia Stanfill Edens, R.N., Ph.D., FACHE

See also: Afterloading radiation therapy; Brachytherapy; Cervical cancer; Computed Tomography (CT) scan; Medulloblastomas; Radiation oncology; Radiation therapies; Thyroid cancer

▶ Fecal Occult Blood Test (FOBT)

Category: Procedures
Also known as: Stool occult blood, guaiac smear test

Definition: A fecal occult blood test (FOBT) is a simple chemical test on stool (feces) that detects the iron-containing components of hidden or trace amounts of blood. It tests for digestive tract bleeding, a possible indicator of colorectal cancer.

Cancers diagnosed: Colon (large intestine) cancer, rectal cancer, gastric (stomach) cancer

Why performed: Sometimes hidden blood in the stool is the only sign of cancer in its early stages, before symptoms appear. As a result, the FOBT is most frequently used as a colorectal cancer screening test.

Benign (noncancerous) and malignant (cancerous) polyps, tumors, and other tissues that protrude into the intestine can bleed intermittently. The FOBT can detect this abnormal bleeding. It does not diagnose disease. It screens for bleeding that may be caused by gastrointestinal cancer.

Other maladies cause blood loss in the digestive tract and anemia, a low red blood cell count. Therefore, the FOBT is sometimes used to determine the cause of unexplained anemia. It is also used to find the cause of abdominal pain.

Normally, a small amount of blood, a quarter of a teaspoonful or less, leaves digestive tract blood vessels daily and moves into the stool. The FOBT does not react to this small amount of blood. A daily blood loss of at least ten milliliters, or two teaspoonfuls, is required to produce a positive test.

Patient preparation: People who prepare for the FOBT pay attention to their health conditions. They avoid the FOBT when their other situations cause digestive or urinary bleeding, which can produce false positive results. Interfering conditions include anal fissures, gum bleeding after dental procedures, colitis, constipation, diverticulitis, esophagitis, gastroesophageal reflux disease (GERD), gastritis, hemorrhoids, inflammatory bowel disease, menstrual periods, nosebleeds, peptic ulcers, severe throat irritation, and urinary tract infections.

Before FOBT testing, patients restrict certain food, medications, and dietary supplements that can interfere with the test by producing misleading results. They should avoid the following foods for two to three days before the test to prevent false positive results: red meats such as beef, cold cuts, lamb, liver, and processed meats; fish; fruits such as apples, oranges, bananas, grapefruit, grapes, lemons, and melons; poultry; and vegetables such as beets, broccoli, cabbage, carrots, cauliflower, cucumbers, horseradish, mushrooms, radishes, and turnips.

Patients should stop taking the following medications for seven days before the test to prevent false positive results: aspirin and products that contain aspirin; other nonsteriodal anti-inflammatory drugs (NSAIDS), such as ibuprofen and naproxen; colchicine gout drugs; corticosteroids; oxidizing drugs, such as iodine, bromides, and boric acid; and reserpine.

Patients should stop taking dietary iron supplements for seven days before the test to prevent false positive results and should take no more than 250 milligrams of vitamin C per day to prevent false negative results.

Steps of the procedure: Medical facility personnel perform FOBT tests, and patients can do their own testing at home. The manufacturer's instructions must be followed to ensure accurate testing.

A small sample of stool is placed onto a chemically treated test card, pad, or wipe. A chemical solution is added to the sample. The appearance of a blue color indicates a positive result—blood in the stool sample. Absence of blue color indicates a negative result—no blood in the stool sample. In one commonly used test, three stool samples are collected on three-part cards over three days, to better detect intermittent bleeding. The collection cards, pads, or wipes must be protected from heat, light, and chemicals during the collection period.

The American Cancer Society and other medical organizations recommend an annual screening FOBT for all adults beginning at age fifty. They also recommend that others have the test as needed because of personal or family histories of intestinal polyps or colorectal cancer. These organizations emphasize that negative FOBT tests do not replace regular medical checkups, and they recommend regular medical examinations for everyone.

In 2001, immunochemical fecal occult blood test (iFOBTs) became available for detecting blood in the stool. They test for a globelike protein component of blood instead of the iron-containing component detected in the traditional FOBT. They are sensitive and specific for digestive tract bleeding, and they avoid direct stool handling. These new tests have the advantage of eliminating the need to avoid foods, medications, and supplements before testing.

After the procedure: People who receive positive FOBT results have blood in the stool. They undergo specific follow-up testing, such as sigmoidoscopy, colonoscopy, computed tomography (CT) scans, and X rays, to determine the cause. People who receive negative FOBT results follow medical professionals recommendations for regular cancer screening.

Risks: The FOBT is safe and painless and does not cause physical harm, but it is not a foolproof indicator of cancer. Digestive tract bleeding can be intermittent, and negative results can occur in people who have colorectal cancer.

Results: A normal FOBT result is negative, which means that blood is not present in the tested stool sample. An abnormal test result is positive, which means that blood is present in the tested stool sample. Occult blood appears in the stool because of colorectal cancer or other medical conditions. It is important to determine the cause and source of bleeding to diagnose, treat, and resolve the situation.

Susan E. Ullmann, M.T. (ASCP), M.A.

For Further Information

Fishbach, Frances Talaska, with Marshall Barnett Dunning III. *A Manual of Laboratory Diagnostic Testing*. 7th ed. Philadelphia: Williams & Wilkins, 2004.

Pagana, Kathleen Deska, and Timothy J. Pagana. *Mosby's Manual of Diagnostic Laboratory Tests*. 3d ed. St. Louis: Mosby Elsevier, 2006.

Segen, Joseph C., and Joseph Stauffer. *The Patient's Guide to Medical Tests*. New York: Facts On File, 1997.

See also: Anal cancer; Colon polyps; Colorectal cancer; Colorectal cancer screening; Diverticulosis and diverticulitis; Gastrointestinal cancers; Immunochemical Fecal Occult Blood Test (iFOBT); Polyps; Rectal cancer; Screening for cancer; Stomach cancers

▶ Flow cytometry

Category: Procedures

Definition: Cytometry refers to the measurement of the physical and/or chemical characteristics of cells, or, by extension, of other biological particles. Flow cytometry is a process in which such measurements are made while the cells or particles pass, preferably in single file, through the measuring apparatus in a fluid stream.

Cancers diagnosed: Hematological (blood) cancers

Why performed: Flow cytometry is widely used in the clinical setting for a number of cytometry-based procedures, such as immunophenotyping, cell sorting, enumeration of CD34-positive stem cell precursors, enumeration of lymphocyte subsets (B cells, T cells, and natural killer or NK cells), and fetal bleed tests in fetomaternal hemorrhage. The technique is performed on a sample of cells obtained from blood, bone marrow, or other tissue, such as a lymph node. Flow sorting extends flow cytometry by using electrical or mechanical means to divert and collect cells with one or more measured characteristics falling within a range or ranges of values set by the user.

A rapid analysis of a cell sample is possible with an instrument called a cytometer that can count fifty thousand cells per second. Prior to cytometry, cells had to be counted manually under a microscope, a labor-intensive task subject to operator error. Components of a cytometer include a fluidics system, an optical system composed of one or more monochromatic lasers or other light source with filters to serve as an excitation beam, electronics to detect emissions from the cells, and a computer to analyze the data collected.

The flow cytometry technique is widely used for diagnostics and disease monitoring of hematopoietic malignancies. Immunophenotyping of hematological cancers has developed as a clinically valuable but technically complicated diagnostic procedure. It involves a variety of methodological features, in-process strategic judgments, and an extensive knowledge of clinical, morphological, and other laboratory features of the disease processes. A number of various internal quality-control steps are necessary to guarantee reliable results with respect to instrument setup and calibration, selection and validation of monoclonal antibody panels, and process control. The data provide a wide range of hematological information essential for establishing a diagnosis in blood cancers. In leukemias, for example, knowing cell lineage and maturation helps distinguish specific forms of leukemia.

Testing by flow cytometry is performed to distinguish an abnormal population of hematopoietic cells and to determine the cellular lineage of malignant cells, clonality, cellular maturation, and heterogeneity within the cancerous cell populations. Flow cytometric analysis, called immunophenotyping, allows cells to be characterized by their size, complexity, and patterns of expression of surface and cellular markers. Multiparameter flow cytometry is the simultaneous use of multiple fluorochromes, which allows completion of the full diagnostic test with fewer cells, thus reducing the size of the specimen needed.

Immunophenotyping by flow cytometry is used for the initial diagnosis of hematopoietic malignancies, for monitoring the response to treatment administered for the malignancy, and for determining the presence of minimal residual disease that may indicate recurrence of the cancer.

Patient preparation: The specimen, on which the process of cytometry is performed, is generally bone marrow aspirate, although a sample of peripheral blood can also be used. The patient is given instructions by the health care provider based upon the need for a bone marrow procedure versus blood collection.

Steps of the procedure: The procedure of immunophenotyping is based on the ability of hematopoietic cells of different lineages and different levels of differentiation to present specific surface, cytoplasmic, or nuclear markers. These markers, called clusters of differentiation (CD), are molecules on the cell surface, as recognized by specific sets of antibodies, that are used to identify the cell type, stage of differentiation, and activity of a cell.

The procedure of immunophenotyping consists of three main steps: sample preparation, flow cytometric data acquisition, and analysis and interpretation of results. To prepare a sample, cells are labeled with the antibodies tagged by specific fluorochromes, which includes staining with fluorochrome-bound monoclonal antibodies, lysis of red blood cells, and fixation in a formalin-containing reagent. This staining protocol is used for all directly conjugated reagents. A so-called whole blood lysing system is used to prepare immunologically stained leukocytes for flow cytometry analysis. In the process of flow cytometric data acquisition, cells are run through a fluidic stream so that single cells can be analyzed one at a time. Then multiple parameters are collected on each cell and analyzed for forward-angle light scatter, ninety-degree light scatter, and fluorescent signal information from up to six different fluorochromes simultaneously. All data can be stored in the form of list-mode files for later reanalysis.

After the procedure: Patients receive aftercare instructions according to how the sample is obtained. If sedation is used, then limitations and restrictions are communicated to the patient by health care practitioners.

Risks: Potential risks of a bone marrow biopsy and aspirate or blood collection are incorporated into a consent form explained at the facility where the procedure is accomplished and signed by the patient prior to obtaining the sample for analysis.

Results: Data can be analyzed and displayed in a variety of formats, such as single-parameter histograms, dotplots (display of distribution of two antigens on an *x-y* plot), or three-dimensional plots of three antigens. Data are analyzed using a gating strategy, in which specific gates are set around the subpopulations of cells based on common parameters measured on all cells. The quantification of each cell type, its light-scatter properties, its intensity of fluorescence, and certain patterns of surface or cytoplasmic marker expression serve as an indication of hematopoietic abnormalities. The pattern of antigen expression on all the cells is analyzed and compared with the distribution of normal cells. Data interpretation is based on the knowledge of specific cell phenotypes affiliated with certain types of leukemia and lymphomas. Abnormal phenotypes, however, are not always associated with disease progression. Therefore, results of flow cytometric analysis have to be used in conjunction with other diagnostic procedures and clinical evaluations.

Linda August Vrooman, R.N., B.S.N., O.C.N.

For Further Information

Givan, Alice Longobardi. *Flow Cytometry: First Principles*. 2d ed. New York: Wiley-Liss, 2001.

Langdon, Simon P., ed. *Cancer Cell Culture: Methods and Protocols*. Totowa, N.J.: Humana Press, 2004.

McCarthy, Desmond A., and Marion G. Macey, eds. *Cytometric Analysis of Cell Phenotype and Function*. New York: Cambridge University Press, 2001.

Radbruch, Andreas, ed. *Flow Cytometry and Cell Sorting*. 2d ed. New York: Springer, 2000.

See also: Immunocytochemistry and immunohistochemistry; Myelodysplastic syndromes

▶ Gallium scan

Category: Procedures
Also known as: Nuclear medicine scan, radioisotope scan

Definition: A gallium scan is a nuclear medicine imaging study that evaluates specific tissues based upon their uptake of an administered radioactive isotope.

During a gallium scan, the tracer (gallium 67 citrate) is injected into a vein. It travels through the bloodstream into the tissues—primarily the bones, liver, and intestines. It usually takes a few days for the tracer to accumulate in the tissues, so in most cases a scan is done two days after an injection of the tracer and repeated at three days. Areas of increased tracer uptake show up as bright, or "hot," spots on an X ray. Delineated problem areas may be caused by infection, inflammation, or tumor (rapid cell division). The gallium scan was the standard for cancer diagnosis and staging until it was replaced by positron emission tomography (PET) scans. Gallium 67 is often used in conjunction with a bone scan (using technetium 99m phosphate) as "a double tracer" technique to overlay areas of inflammation within organ systems. Gallium is less dependent on blood flow than technetium and may identify foci that would otherwise be missed.

Cancers diagnosed: Major cancers such as lymphoma, malignant bone tumors, and soft-tissue sarcomas; can be used to identify most neoplasms, whether benign or malignant

Why performed: A gallium scan is performed to detect the presence of cancerous tissue. It may be employed to determine whether a cancer has spread (metastasized) to other parts of the body or to monitor the effectiveness of cancer treatment. It can also be used to diagnose inflammatory conditions such as pulmonary fibrosis or sarcoidosis; to monitor the response to antibiotic treatment; to detect an abscess or certain infections, especially in the bones; and to detect an unknown source of infection that is causing a fever.

Patient preparation: Gallium accumulates in the large intestine (colon) before being eliminated in the stool. Patients may need to take a laxative the night before the scan and have an enema one to two hours prior to the scan to prevent gallium in the colon from interfering with pictures being taken of the area. The doctor and radiologist should also be informed of possible pregnancy, breast-feeding activity, and the use of a barium enema within the previous four days or medicine (such as Pepto-Bismol) that contains bismuth, as barium and bismuth can interfere with the test results.

Steps of the procedure: A gallium scan is performed by a nuclear medicine technologist. The scan pictures are interpreted by a radiologist or nuclear medicine specialist.

The arm is cleaned with soap, betadine, and/or alcohol around the injection site. A small amount of the radioactive chemical is then injected through a vein. After administration of the tracer, the patient is brought back to the radiology facility and scans are completed at forty-eight hours and repeated at seventy-two hours.

The protocol for scanning requires the removal of all jewelry. Most clothes are removed, and the patient is provided with a cloth gown or paper covering. The patient lies in a supine position (on the back) upon a table. A large scanning (gamma) camera will be positioned closely above the patient. After the initial injection, the camera will scan for radiation released by the tracer and produce pictures of the tracer in the tissues. These images serve as a baseline to compare subsequent scan data completed in the next two to three days. The camera will move slowly above and around the body. The camera does not produce any radiation, so the patient is not exposed to any additional source of radioactive material. Different positioning may be attempted so that an area of interest can be viewed from different angles. Restricted movement is necessary during each scan to avoid blurring of the acquired images. Often, the patient will be asked to hold his or her breath briefly during some of the scans to minimize chest movement that occurs with respiration. Each scan can take approximately sixty to ninety minutes.

After the procedure: A gallium scan is painless. There are no activity restrictions postscan.

Risks: There is a risk of damage to cells and tissues exposed to any level of radiation, including the low level of radiation released by a radioactive tracer such as gallium. Allergic reactions to radioactive tracers are rare. Most of the tracer will be eliminated from the body (in the urine or stool) within four days. Occasionally, some soreness or swelling can develop at the injection site. These symptoms can be relieved by applying moist, warm compresses to the affected area.

Results: A gallium scan utilizes a special radiographic camera to obtain pictures of certain tissues in the body after a radioisotope makes them visible. The results of the scan are available within forty-eight hours after the scans are completed. The entire process takes approximately five days.

John L. Zeller, M.D., Ph.D.

For Further Information

Hussain, R., D. Christie, V. Gebski, et al. "The Role of the Gallium Scan in Primary Extranodal Lymphoma." *Journal of Nuclear Medicine* 39, no. 1 (1998): 95-98.

Maderazo, E., N. Hickingbotham, C. Woronick, et al. "The Influence of Various Factors on the Accuracy of Gallium-67 Imaging for Occult Infection." *Journal of Nuclear Medicine* 29, no. 5 (1988): 608-615.

Mettler, Fred A., Jr., and Milton J. Guiberteau. *Essentials of Nuclear Medicine Imaging*. 5th ed. Philadelphia: Saunders/Elsevier, 2006.

Ziessman, Harvey A., Janis P. O'Malley, and James H. Thrall. *Nuclear Medicine: The Requisites*. 3d ed. Philadelphia: Mosby Elsevier, 2006.

Other Resources

American College of Radiology
http://www.acr.org

Society of Nuclear Medicine
http://www.snm.org

See also: Burkitt lymphoma; Imaging tests; Nuclear medicine scan; Radionuclide scan

▶ Gamma Knife

Category: Procedures
Also known as: Radiosurgery, stereotactic radiosurgery (SRS)

Definition: The Gamma Knife, not actually a knife, is a large precision system that delivers intensely focused gamma-radiation beams to treat tumors and other problems of the brain and nervous system. It resembles a computed tomography (CT) scanner. Gamma Knife technology was developed by Lars Leskell (1907-1986), a Swedish neurosurgeon.

Cancers treated: The Gamma Knife has been used to treat cancerous tumors in the brain and tumors that originated elsewhere in the body that have spread to the brain. The technology is now being explored to treat cancer of the eye and tumors in the neck, liver, lungs, prostrate, and abdomen.

Why performed: Gamma Knife "surgery" is a noninvasive alternative to traditional open-brain surgery. The precisely focused radiation beams of the Gamma Knife allow surgeons to treat very small, deep-seated tumors without damaging nearby tissue.

Steps of the procedure: Surgeons apply a local anesthetic and use four screws to attach a lightweight frame to the patient's head. The frame prevents the head from moving and allows surgeons to identify the treatment target accurately. With the head frame in place, surgeons take electronic images of the brain to establish the exact size, shape, and location of the target. From the images, surgeons develop a specific treatment plan.

For the treatment, the patient lies on a couch. A helmet is attached to the head frame. The couch slides into the Gamma Knife unit, where radiation destroys the tumor. The patient is awake during the procedure, which lasts from a few minutes to more than an hour, depending on the size and location of the tumor.

After the procedure: When the treatment is completed, the head frame is removed. In most cases, the patient goes home the same day and returns to a normal routine in a day or two.

Risks: Because surgeons make no incisions, the risk of complications from use of the Gamma Knife is low. Some patients feel minor soreness from the head frame. Some patients experience mild headache, dizziness, or nausea, which lasts only a short while.

The dose of radiation outside the target is very low and poses little risk. Occasionally, patients experience swelling in the brain, which is temporary and treatable.

Patient safety: Assisted by computers, a team of neurosurgeons, oncology radiologists, and sometimes a medical physicist carefully pinpoints the exact location of the targeted tumor so that no nearby tissue is affected. The team also calculates the correct dosage of radiation, depending on the patient's size, age, and condition, and on the size and location of the tumor. Of particular importance is the frame that holds the patient's head absolutely still, which medical device engineers have greatly improved.

Results: The effects of radiation treatments take time: weeks, months, or even years.

Wendell Anderson, B.A.

See also: Acoustic neuromas; Astrocytomas; Cobalt 60 radiation; Meningiomas

▶ Gene therapy

Category: Procedures

Definition: Gene therapy is a technique that corrects deleterious, defective, and disease-inducing genes through genetic modifications. Modifications include restoration, substitution, or supplementation of the defective gene. Therapeutic approaches involve introduction of altered genetic material into either normal cells (to develop immunity against cancer) or cancer cells (to combat the disease).

Gene therapy is sometimes aimed at augmenting results from other existing treatment options. It is still in experimental stages, and no gene therapies are available outside clinical trials. However, there are exceptionally large numbers of ongoing clinical trials using gene therapy as their primary clinical approach, and a high percentage of all these clinical trials address cancer-related questions.

How this therapy works: Gene therapy is ideal only for diseases caused by mutations of a single gene. Success with gene therapy depends on multitudes of factors:

- How an altered gene is introduced into the body
- How efficiently the modified (recombined) gene is able to restore or resuscitate normal function
- How specific the targeting of a particular region is
- How sustained the response of the body is
- How low the immunological response of the host is
- The extent to which the other associated risks are eliminated

Special carriers called vectors are used to aid in the transfer of genes. The most commonly used vectors are viruses. Viruses have the remarkable capacity to recognize specific cells and integrate themselves into those cells. Specific classes of viruses called retroviruses have been used extensively in many clinical trials involving gene therapy. However, studies using other types of viruses also abound (such as adenoviruses, adeno-associated viruses, lentiviruses, poxyviruses, and herpesviruses). The reasons for using viruses as vectors are multifold. First, viruses possess a relatively simple genome (genetic composition). Only a handful of genes exist in a viral genome (as opposed to the approximately 30,000 genes, for example, in the human genome), and therefore, it is relatively easy to handle. Second, viruses have evolved ways of surpassing natural barriers that cells put forth. This allows them to gain access across membranes into the cytoplasm as well as to the nuclei of the cells. Third, viruses can be engineered with relative ease to stop replication, gain integration into host deoxyribonucleic acid (DNA), and exit without causing destruction of the host cell. Fourth, viruses have remarkable specificity to infect certain types of cells. This particular characteristic affords greater reliability and hope for better outcomes. However, there are various complications associated with the use of viral vectors, such as host immune response. Therefore, use of nonviral vectors is preferred in certain cases. Numerous types of genes are delivered using viral vectors.

Enhancing host immune responses: Different approaches have been attempted to use gene therapy as a treatment option for patients. Of these, major focus has been on improving the body's immunological responses to cancer. The body's immunological system consists of populations of different kinds of cells (broadly called white blood cells or lymphocytes) whose function is to fight against multitudes of foreign bodies that invade the cells. In cancer patients, however, this immunological response is highly compromised either because of deficiency or improper functioning of lymphocytes. Immune therapy for cancer generally falls under a few specific categories: injection of cytokines (special proteins secreted by the immune system), addition of lymphokine-associated killer cells (LAK cells, which are special immune cells) to existing treatment options, addition of activated peripheral lymphocytes, and infusion of antigen-presenting cells to increase the antigen-recognizing capacity of immune cells. The gene therapy approach employs the idea of enhancing the capacity of normal lymphocytes to become aggressive combatants of cancer by using any of these techniques. Specific retroviruses are manipulated to incorporate certain proteins called T-cell receptors (a kind of lymphocyte), which when introduced into the body produce the required confirmation for lymphocytes to destroy cancer cells. Laboratory (preclinical) experimentation of immunotherapy has been limited by supply of tumor reactive human T cells, but recent research has provided some insight into methodology that could increase this supply and enhance productive research activities. T lymphocytes exert their immunogenicity through secretion of specific proteins called cytokines. Human cells possess different kinds of cytokines, most of which have been used in gene therapy studies. The major advantage of using cytokines in gene transfer studies is that they help not only in tumor destruction but also in eliciting immune memory. Most known cytokines such as interleukins (ILs), interferons (IFNs), granulocyte-macrophage colony-stimulating factors (GM-CSF), and tumor necrosis factor-alpha (TNF) are used in immunotherapy and gene therapy experiments. In fact, cytokines constitute about 25 percent of the genes used in experiments in gene therapy around the world. Preclinical studies using IL-2, IL-12, IL-24, GM-CSF, TNF, and IFN are extremely promising, and all these compounds are used in clinical trials. Cytokines can be delivered using both viral and nonviral modes of entry into the cells. They can be administered directly into tumor cells in vivo (inside cells) or can be engineered with lymphocytes ex vivo (outside cells) and then implanted in stem cells. There are some sporadic reports of vectors themselves contributing to antitumor effects in studies involving cytokine gene transfers. However, gene therapy experiments using cytokines face similar challenges as those of other comparable experiments, where determination of optimal doses of cytokines and elimination of immunosuppressive agents still restrict progress.

Introduction of normal tumor-suppressor cells: Other approaches to gene therapy include replacement of mutated (altered) or deleted genes with healthy copies of genes. For example, a tumor-suppressor gene called TP53 is mutated in a wide array of tumors. The TP53 protein, under normal conditions, suppresses the activation of genes contributing to uncontrolled cell division and proliferation. Replacement of normal, wild type TP53 genes using a retroviral TP53 expression vector is used in gene therapy trials.

Inhibition of oncogenes: An alternative strategy is to alter the oncogene or cancer-inducing gene directly. Genes belonging to the RAS family of oncogenes (such as HRAS, NRAS, and KRAS) and others (such as MYC) are examples of oncogenes. These genes are activated by mutations or modifications that change the composition of their protein products, resulting in the development of cancer. A common approach to inactivate such oncogenes uses a method called antisense technology. A ribonucleic acid (RNA) sequence complementary to that targeted for inactivation is introduced into the cell, then binds and thereby blocks translation of that RNA. Thus, inhibition is ensured at a level before the protein is formed, reducing its opportunities to induce tumor development.

Insertion of suicide genes: Another type of gene therapy involves the transplantation of suicide genes in the body. Suicide genes help convert generally nontoxic substances called prodrugs into physiologically active forms, thereby triggering death of cancer cells. The popular gene and prodrug combination is the herpes simplex virus (HSV) thymidine kinase (HSV-tk)/ganciclovir (GCV). Ganciclovir is a prodrug that is inactive in its dephosphorylated (no phosphate group attached to the protein) form. When it is phosphorylated by HSV-tk introduced through an adenovirus, it attains the capability of inducing so called "death pathways" and triggering cell death. The effect is accentuated by a process called "by-stander effect," whereby surrounding cells receive the toxic metabolites and join the race of combating tumor cells.

Cancer therapy's ultimate goal is complete elimination of cancer cells while leaving noncancerous cells healthy. New possibilities for cancer suicide gene therapy (CSGT) arise from progress in proteomics (study of protein) and genomics.

Aiding antiangiogenesis: Tumors require a copious supply of oxygen for sustenance and access to blood vessels for spread. The process of formation of new blood vessels is called angiogenesis. It is a multistep process that includes proliferation of endothelial cells, cellular migration, membrane degradation, and reorganization of cell cavity or lumen. Some factors that aid in angiogenesis include growth factors such as vascular endothelial growth factor (VEGF), basic fibroblast growth factor, and hepatocyte growth factor (HGF). Gene therapy experiments focus on introducing viruses containing inhibitors of some of these growth factors and attempt to block angiogenesis in tumor cells.

Interaction with other treatment techniques: A commonly employed gene therapy strategy is to insert genes that will facilitate or augment some existing therapeutic intervention. In the case of patients undergoing radiotherapy or chemotherapy, for example, introduction of certain beneficial genes could afford resistance to multiple drugs or protection of bone marrow. Tumor cells have the capacity to efflux drugs, and this capacity is a challenge to overcome in therapeutic procedures. The strategy is to use drug-resistance genes for overcoming drug efflux. A gene that has been approved in protocols for breast and ovarian cancer treatments is multiple-drug-resistance gene (MDR1). This gene is inserted into normal bone marrow to select for cells that are particularly resistant to the specific chemotherapeutic agent in a treatment regimen.

Other approaches: The use of small inhibitor ribonucleic acid (siRNA) technique for silencing oncogenes is gaining momentum in gene therapy studies. Experiments have begun using viral vectors incorporating siRNA in animal models to examine their efficacy in targeting and silencing specific genes. Attempts have also been made to introduce a 47th, artificial chromosome with relevant beneficial genes through a large viral vector.

Using nonviral vectors: The use of viral vectors for delivering specific genes poses some palpable problems such as interaction of the introduced virus with other viruses that it might encounter in the body and nonspecific target stimulation. Therefore, use of nonviral material to transfer genes is preferred in certain cases. Some examples of nonviral vectors are cationic liposomes, polyethylenimines, DNA-liposome complexes, and synthetic polymers. Liposomes are lipid particles possessing the innate ability to traverse cell membranes. The strategy behind gene therapy is to harness this property to deliver desired DNA to cancer cells via lipid-DNA complexes. Naked DNA or plasmids and transposable elements called transposans are other examples of nonviral vectors. Electrotransfer of DNA has been used in experiments as a physical method of transfer of DNA. In this process, the transfer of genetic material is achieved by local application of electric pulses after introducing DNA into the extracellular medium.

Nanomaterials are temperature-sensitive polymers capable of binding and complexing with DNA to form nanorods. The stability of nanorods at physiological temperatures and their capacity to expand when heated make them attractive alternatives to deliver and trap genetic materials. Once inside tumor cells, they disintegrate and make the delivery complete and competent. Both naturally occurring polymers (like chitosans) and synthetic, biocompatible compounds (called propyleneimines) have been used for DNA-binding experiments.

Side effects: Major side effects for gene therapy include host immune responses to foreign genes introduced into the body. Immune responses can include inflammation, allergic reactions, and, rarely, death. It is worth mentioning that gene therapy studies have reported minimal side effects and encouraging responses. The challenge lies in improving efficiency and producing sustainable responses.

Progress and perspectives: Due to its ability to alter genes, which are the basic units of heredity and variation, gene therapy encounters multitudes of social and ethical concerns. The ability to alter genes confers the ability to change the genetic makeup and ultimately the genetic composition of the human population. It might become difficult then to determine what is legitimate and ethical to manipulate. Some of the issues concerning germ-line gene therapy and genetic enhancement are serious concerns and need to be addressed. In the United States, there are stringent procedures and regulations for conducting gene therapy studies and clinical trials. Various government organizations, including the Food and Drug Administration (FDA) and the Recombinant DNA Advisory Committee (RAC), need to provide approval for protocols. However, as with any other approach, the benefits of gene therapy in curing life-threatening diseases have to be weighed appropriately against any possible misuses or abuses of this approach.

Geetha Yadav, Ph.D.
Updated by: Richard P. Capriccioso, M.D.

For Further Information

Anestakis D., Petanidis S., Kalyvas S., Nday C.M., Tsave O., Kioseoglou E., & Salifoglou A. (2015). Mechanisms and applications of interleukins in cancer immunotherapy. *International Journal of Molecular Science*, 16(1):1691-710. http://www.ncbi.nlm.nih.gov/pubmed/25590298

Deming, S. (2015, August). New gene therapy for bladder cancer shows promise. *OncoLog*, 60(8). https://www.mdanderson.org/publications/oncolog/august-2015/new-gene-therapy-for-bladder-cancer-shows-promise.html

Jang, Y.Y., Cai, L., & Ye, Z. (2016). Genome editing systems in novel therapies. *Discovery Medicine*, 21(113):57-64. http://www.ncbi.nlm.nih.gov/pubmed/26896603

Nastiuk, K.L., & Krolewski, J.J. (2016). Opportunities and challenges in combination gene cancer therapy. *Advances in Drug Delivery Reviews*, 98:35-40. http://www.ncbi.nlm.nih.gov/pubmed/26724249

Podajcer, O. L., Lopez, M. V. &Mazzolini, G. (2007). Cytokine gene transfer for cancer therapy. *Cytokine and Growth Factor Reviews*, 18: 183-194. http://www.ncbi.nlm.nih.gov/pubmed/17320465

Other Resources

American Society of Gene Therapy
http://www.asgt.org

Centers for Disease Control and Prevention
National Office of Public Health Genomics
http://www.cdc.gov/genomics

Human Genome Project Information
Gene Therapy
http://web.ornl.gov/sci/techresources/Human_Genome/index.shtml

National Cancer Institute
http://www.cancer.gov

Office of Biotechnology Activities
http://osp.od.nih.gov/office-biotechnology-activities/oba/index.html

See also: Adenoviruses; Family history and risk assessment; Genetic counseling; Genetic testing; Genetics of cancer

▶ Genetic testing

Category: Procedures; Social and Personal Issues
Also known as: Deoxyribonucleic acid (DNA) testing, gene testing, genetic screening, molecular genetic testing

Definition: Genetics Genetic testing is a medical test identifying genetic composition. DNA for genetic testing can be extracted from the cells of many different body fluids or tissues. The majority of genetic tests are completed by using DNA from blood cells. Other sources include cheek lining cells (obtained with swabs or a mouthwash), hair root cells, or the cells in the fluid surrounding a fetus in the womb (amniotic fluid). Gene analysis is accomplished by examining chromosomes, DNA codes, or the proteins produced by genes.

Why performed: Typically, genetic testing is used to find inherited genetic disorders. Genetic testing can determine an individual's genetic composition and can help determine if the tested person has an inherited disorder. Genetic testing can also help establish whether a person can develop genetic diseases or pass them on to subsequent generations.

Sometimes genetic tests are used to assess disease risk. For example, genetic testing can help assess genetic predisposition to colon and breast cancer. The results of this assessment can help determine whether the individual has an increased likelihood of developing these cancers, but does not determine with absolute certainty whether a person will get breast or colon cancer. A person with a negative test (lacking the genetic marker) could still get breast or colon cancer. Conversely, a person with a positive test (possessing the genetic marker) may not get breast or colon cancer. A person with a positive test will, however, have an increased chance of getting breast or colon cancer compared with a person with a negative test.

Many genetic tests are available, and descriptions of most of them are provided by the National Library of Medicine and the National Genome Research Institute. Some of these genetic tests determine chromosomal abnormalities, such as those resulting in Down syndrome, and some identify DNA genetic code changes, such as those occurring with sickle cell anemia. Some of the more common types of tests are described here.

Newborn screening: Infant screening after birth identifies treatable genetic disorders. This type of genetic screening has been practiced for decades in the United States. It is completed on millions of newborns per year, in all 50 states. For example, infants are screened for phenylketonuria, a disorder that causes mental retardation if unrecognized and untreated, and other genetic disorders such as congenital hypothyroidism.

Diagnostic testing: Genetic testing to determine if a particular disease is present is called diagnostic testing. Usually, these types of tests are used to diagnose a disease suspected due to the patient's family health history, personal health history, physical examination, or symptoms.

Carrier testing: Normally, people have two copies of almost all the genes in the body; one copy comes from the father and the other from the mother. Some diseases, known as recessive disorders, will express themselves (cause a disorder) only if both copies of the gene have the disease trait. An example is sickle cell anemia. Carrier testing can determine if a person has one or two copies of the recessive gene. The person who has two copies of the gene with the disease trait will have the disease. The person who has one copy of the gene with the trait and one normal copy of the gene is known as a carrier of the disease. This person does not have the disease itself but carries the disease trait and has a 50 percent chance of passing the trait (gene) to any offspring. This type of testing is useful for individuals with a family history of a genetic disorder. Testing couples who plan to have a child for recessive genetic disorders helps establish their risk of having a child with a genetic disease.

Prenatal testing: Some birth defects and inherited disorders, such as spina bifida and Down syndrome, can be detected with prenatal testing. This type of information can help parents make important decisions regarding the care of a disabled child or the progress of a pregnancy.

Predictive testing: This type of genetic test can determine potential risk for diseases such as colon cancer, breast cancer, ovarian cancer, or hemochromatosis (an iron metabolism disorder resulting in too much iron in the body). For example, the presence of BRCA1 and BRCA2 genes indicate a higher risk of breast and ovarian cancer.

Forensic testing: Forensic testing, such as DNA fingerprinting or paternity testing, is used for criminal investigations or to establish biological parenthood. DNA fingerprinting is accomplished by breaking down DNA into smaller segments. The technique involves using compounds that attack DNA sequences at particular points, splitting the DNA into several fragments. These break points are different in each person because everyone has a unique DNA sequence (unless the person is one of a pair of identical twins). The fragments are lined up and compared with DNA left at crime scenes (and usually with that of people who are not suspects and serve as controls). Matches are very evident visually.

Pharmacogenomics: Genetic testing to determine response to therapy is known as pharmacogenomics. Many tests to predict how effective a medicine will be in a particular person are being developed, and some of these types of genetic tests are available. For example, a medication called trastuzumab treats breast cancer but is effective only when the breast tumors have estrogen receptors. A genetic test determines if a woman's breast tumors have estrogen receptors and, therefore, trastuzumab will help treat them. More tests that predict how a specific person may respond to medications for cancer, asthma, heart disease, and other diseases have entered into development.

Preimplantation genetic diagnosis: In vitro fertilization involves retrieving egg cells (oocytes) from a woman's hyperstimulated ovaries and fertilizing them with sperm in a laboratory. The embryos are cultured in the laboratory until they are three days (morula stage) or five to six days old (late blastocyst-stage). Then the embryos are transferred into the mother's uterus for implantation. Before implantation, a single cell from an 8-cell-stage embryo is removed and screened for specific genetic disorders. Only embryos that lack the specific genetic disorders are implanted.

Direct-to-consumer genetic testing: Some genetic testing laboratories sell genetic tests directly to consumers through print, television, and Internet advertisements. A test for the BRCA1 and BRCA2 genes that have been associated with breast and ovarian cancer was marketed directly to consumers, as were tests for markers for hemochromatosis and cystic fibrosis. Although this type of marketing can raise awareness of the tests, it raises concerns about the accuracy of information presented in advertisements.

One form of direct-to-consumer genetic test arouses particular concern. Some web sites sell genetic tests for aging, behavior, and nutrition. The tests provide genetic profiles that are matched to consumer goods such as creams and dietary supplements. More scientific study is needed to better determine if the commercial pairing of these types of genetic tests with the goods offered provides a significant benefit.

Regardless of the type of direct-to-consumer genetic test, the lack of genetic counseling and the absence of health care professionals in the process raise concerns about how well these genetic tests are interpreted and applied. Often, genetic tests have great implications for not only the person taking the test, but also their relatives. These types of concerns have caused some to advocate more government oversight and regulation of direct-to-consumer genetic testing.

The case of breast cancer genes: A closer look at BRCA1 and BRCA2, the breast cancer genes, provides some background information and shows how testing relates to the science of genetics.

The human body is constantly replacing cells in a process called mitosis. Mitosis is the orderly duplication of cells that ensures each cell has the exact same genetic information. Over the course of many years, some mutations (or changes) in the genetic code can appear, and these changes may result in uncontrolled cell division. When mitosis is not carefully regulated, tumors or cancers can develop. The majority of cancers are due to noninherited changes in the genetic code that occur during life.

However, five to ten percent of all breast and ovarian cancers may have a genetic basis. A person can inherit a mutation in a tumor-suppressor gene, which controls cell division and growth and therefore protects against cancer. From birth, the person who inherits the mutated tumor-suppressor gene does not have carefully controlled cell division. Many factors play a role in determining if the person who inherits the mutated gene will actually develop cancer. People have two copies of every gene (one from the mother and one from the father), and the normal copy of that tumor-suppressor gene may prevent cancer from developing. Additional tumor-suppressor genes may also prevent the development of cancer.

A person inheriting a mutated tumor-suppressor gene has an increased risk of developing cancer but not an absolute (100 percent) risk of getting cancer. The cancer itself is not inherited, but a defective gene that does not adequately protect against cancer is inherited. If a person inherits one of these defective genes and develops cancer, the condition is called hereditary cancer.

Ovarian or breast cancer are regulated by many genes, but two of them have been named and can be found through genetic testing. BRCA1 is short for breast cancer 1 gene, and BRCA2 is short for breast cancer 2 gene. BRCA1 and BRCA2 are tumor-suppressor genes, and they keep cell reproduction from getting out of control. BRCA1 and BRCA2 genes are present in both men and women. If a person inherits a faulty or mutated copy of BRCA1 or BRCA2, that person has an increased risk of developing breast or ovarian cancer, along with a slightly higher risk of developing any type of cancer.

Because half of all genes are inherited from the mother and half are inherited from the father, a mutated BRCA1 or BRCA2 gene can be inherited from either parent. If a person has a faulty BRCA1 or BRCA2 gene, each of the person's children has a 50 percent chance of inheriting the faulty gene. Although inheriting a faulty BRCA1 or BRCA2 gene increases a person's genetic predisposition for breast or ovarian cancer, environmental factors still play a large role in determining whether the person develops breast or ovarian cancer. More mutations in other tumor-suppressor genes need to occur for the person to develop cancer. The causes of the mutations acquired during a lifetime are largely unknown and subject to much speculation and scientific research. One branch of genetic research involves looking not only at the genetic code present in DNA but also into how ribonucleic acid (RNA), another molecule that carries genetic information, may contribute to cancers.

This BRCA1 and BRCA2 example shows how one of the thousands of available genetic tests relates to the science of genetics. It demonstrates the complex relation between genes and disease, and it underscores the necessity of accurate genetic information and competent and caring counseling. As the number of genetic tests continues to grow, it becomes more important to understand the science behind the tests as well as their social implications and applications.

Richard P. Capriccioso, M.D.

For Further Information

Covolo, L., Rubinelli, S., Ceretti, E., & Gelatti, U. (2015). Internet-based direct-to-consumer genetic testing: A systematic review. *Journal of Medical Internet Research, 17(12), e279.*

Institute of Medicine of the National Academies. (2007). *Cancer-related genetic testing and counseling: Workshop proceedings*. Washington, D.C.: National Academies Press.

Schoonmaker, Michele, & William, Erin D. (2013). *Genetic testing: Scientific background and nondiscrimination legislation*. Columbus, OH: Bibliogov.

Sharpe, Neil F., & Carter, R. F. (2006). *Genetic testing: Care, consent, and liability.* Hoboken, N.J.: Wiley-Liss. Kindle edition available.

Update on genetic testing for heart disease. (2012), September 1. *Harvard Heart Letter*. http://www.health.harvard.edu/heart-health/update-on-genetic-testing-for-heart-disease

Other Resources

Center for Disease Control and Prevention
Public Health Genomics Knowledge Base
https://phgkb.cdc.gov/GAPPKB/phgHome.do?action=home

Genetics Home Reference
http://ghr.nlm.nih.gov

Learn.Genetics
Genetic Science Learning Center
http://learn.genetics.utah.edu/content/disorders/screening/

National Institutes of Health
National Human Genome Research Institute
http://www.genome.gov

See also: Cancer education; Epidemiology of cancer; Family history and risk assessment; Gene therapy; Genetic counseling; Hereditary cancer syndromes; Oncology social worker

▶ Gleason grading system

Category: Procedures
Also known as: Gleason score

Definition: The Gleason grading system is the most common system used in the United States to evaluate, or "grade," prostate cancer. The Gleason grade describes the appearance of prostate cancer tissue when observed under a microscope. The grade assigned describes how closely the tumor cells in the prostate tissue resemble normal prostate cells and can predict how quickly the tumor is expected to grow.

Typically, prostate cancer tissue has different patterns within the cells. The first Gleason grade describes the most common pattern. The second Gleason grade is assigned to the next most common pattern of cells in the tissue. Together, these two numbers combined make the Gleason score.

Cancers diagnosed: Prostate cancer

Why performed: Assigning a Gleason grade or score allows the doctor to predict the behavior of the prostate cancer—that is, whether it will be a slow- or fast-growing tumor. This information can have an impact on the treatment choices available to the patient.

Patient preparation: No patient preparation is needed. This evaluation is performed in a laboratory by a pathologist, a doctor who specializes in identifying diseases by examining tissues and cells to determine if cancer cells are present and, if they are, how aggressive the disease may be.

Steps of the procedure: After the patient undergoes a prostate biopsy, the biopsy samples are sent to a pathologist to determine the Gleason grade and score of the prostate cancer tissue.

After the procedure: It may take anywhere from a few days to a couple of weeks to obtain the results. After the results are received, the patient can discuss the best treatment options available based on the type of prostate cancer cells present in the biopsy samples.

Risks: No risks are associated with this procedure.

Results: There are five Gleason grades. Grade 1 appears similar to normal prostate tissue, which means that the tumor is most likely a slow-growing tumor. Grades 2, 3, and 4 reflect increasingly faster-growing tumors. Grade 5 indicates a fast, aggressive prostate cancer.

The Gleason score is determined by adding the two Gleason grades together. The Gleason score is a number between 2 and 10 that reflects how closely the cancer cells resemble normal prostate tissue. In general, a low Gleason score suggests less aggressive tumors and a higher Gleason score suggests more aggressive tumors.

Vonne Sieve, M.A.

See also: Grading of tumors; Prostate cancer; Staging of cancer; Watchful waiting

▶ Glossectomy

Category: Procedures
Also known as: Hemiglossectomy, partial glossectomy

Definition: A glossectomy is a surgical procedure to remove all or part of the tongue.

Cancers treated: Cancers of the tongue

Why performed: A glossectomy is performed to take out the abnormal tissue (tumor) and enough of the surrounding tissue so that the edges, or margins, around the tumor do not contain cancer cells.

Patient preparation: In addition to the usual preoperative preparation (physical examination, blood testing, and consultation with an anesthesiologist), the patient should meet with a speech-language pathologist for a consultation regarding the changes in speech and swallowing that happen when all or part of the tongue is removed. Glossectomies are done in a hospital, and the patient is given general anesthesia. The surgical team will be specialists in head and neck cancer surgeries, including an ear, nose, and throat surgeon, an oral-maxillofacial surgeon, and a plastic surgeon.

Steps of the procedure: Small cancers may require only a biopsy if the surgeon is able to remove enough tissue so that the edges around the tumor have no cancer cells. The tissue is tested tableside during the surgery to determine if the margins are negative (without cancer cells).

If the cancer is small, then the surgeon sews up the tongue or uses a small skin graft to repair the tongue. For larger skin grafts, the skin is frequently taken from the wrist along with the surrounding blood vessels; this type of skin graft is a radial forearm free flap. The graft is sewn into the hole in the tongue, and the blood vessels are connected to supply the graft. A total glossectomy is rarely done. The neck lymph nodes are tested to see if the cancer has spread. If lymph nodes are positive for cancer cells, then additional surgery may be done during the same operation for a limited dissection of the neck.

After the procedure: An inpatient hospital stay of about a week after a glossectomy procedure is expected. A nasogastric tube (from the nose to the stomach) may be used for feeding until food can be taken orally. Subsequent reconstructive surgeries, fitting with prosthetic devices (an artificial tongue), radiation therapy, and rehabilitation therapy may be necessary.

Risks: Possible risks of a glossectomy include bleeding and/or swelling of the tongue, failure of the skin graft, formation of a new opening between the mouth and the skin (a fistula), and difficulty swallowing and talking.

Results: The results depend on the amount of the tongue that was removed; if one-third or more of the tongue remains, then good swallowing and talking function is expected.

Vicki Miskovsky, B.S., R.D.

See also: Arterial embolization; Erythroplakia; Laryngeal cancer; Leukoplakia; Multiple endocrine neoplasia type 2 (MEN 2); Oral and oropharyngeal cancers; Stomatitis

▶ Gonioscopy

Category: Procedures

Definition: Gonioscopy is a procedure used by eye health professionals to examine the interior of the eye to check the drainage angle for growths, problems, and obstructions.

Cancers diagnosed: Cancers of the eye

Why performed: Gonioscopy is performed to allow the doctor to see into the patient's eye to examine the area in which fluid drains in order to check for problems.

Patient preparation: A patient who wears contact lenses will have to remove them.

Steps of the procedure: Gonioscopy is usually performed in a doctor's office, although it can be performed in other settings as well. It is usually performed by an ophthalmologist. The doctor begins by applying eyedrops to the patient's eye to numb it, allowing the doctor and instruments to touch the eye without the patient feeling it. The patient may be asked to lie down or may be asked to rest the head on a headrest if the procedure is performed while the patient is sitting up. The patient is asked to try to refrain from blinking during the procedure.

The doctor uses a special lamp and a special lens to look inside the patient's eye and examine the area between the cornea and the iris. Problems with this area can cause the eye not to drain fluid correctly, which can lead to many eye and vision problems, including eventual loss of vision. In total, gonioscopy usually takes between five and ten minutes for the doctor to perform.

After the procedure: The patient should refrain from rubbing the eye for a period after the procedure. The patient's eye may need to be dilated during the procedure, so he or she may experience loss of vision quality for a few hours afterward.

Risks: In general, no significant risks are associated with gonioscopy. There is a small risk of an allergic reaction to the eyedrops that are used by the ophthalmologist to numb the eye. There is also a very small chance of eye infection.

Results: Gonioscopy allows the doctor to see into the area of the eye where fluid drainage occurs. This can help the doctor see whether normal drainage is occurring or if a growth or other blockage is preventing normal drainage. Normal results for this procedure will show a drainage angle that is wide and open. Abnormal results will show a drainage angle that is blocked or closed.

Robert Bockstiegel, B.S.

See also: Childhood cancers; Computed Tomography (CT) scan; Eye cancers; Eyelid cancer; Genetics of cancer; Ophthalmic oncology

▶ Grading of tumors

Category: Procedures

Definition: The grading of tumors is a system devised to classify malignant tumors. The grade is determined by how aberrant (different from what is expected) the tumor cells are in relation to normal tissue cells when viewed under a microscope. The grading of tumor cells is performed by a medical doctor who specializes in pathology. This system also considers how aggressive the tumor is in regard to growth and metastases (the spread of cancer cells to other organs).

Cancers diagnosed: All

Why performed: Tumors are graded so that physicians have information about the tumor to use in developing a treatment plan for the patient. The higher the grade of the tumor, the more aggressively it is treated. A tumor grade can also give an indication of the likelihood that the cancer can be cured, as well as of the prognosis of the patient.

Patient preparation: Tumor grade is determined by analysis of tissue cells from the tumor. The patient is not directly involved with the grading of the tumor, which is performed by a pathologist.

Steps of the procedure: Specimens (small samples) to be used for grading a tumor are extracted through biopsy (removal of tissue from a tumor) or tissue scraping. An example of a tissue scraping procedure is the Papanicolaou smear (Pap smear), in which cells are scraped from the cervix of the uterus. The tissue samples are then placed in a container with a preservative solution, such as formaldehyde. The pathologist takes thin slices of tumor tissue and prepares slides for viewing under a microscope. Then the slides are examined as to cell structure and growth pattern. Each type of cancer has its own characteristics, although there is a similarity between cells of tumors from similar types of tissue. For example, all sarcomas (cancer of the muscle) are similar no matter the muscle in which they are discovered.

Two important factors identified by the pathologist are histologic grade and nuclear grade. Histologic grade refers to the amount of differentiation between the tumor cells and the cells of the tissue where the tumor resides. Cancer cells that appear quite similar to the tissue cells are low grade, whereas cancer cells that are large and oddly shaped, bearing little resemblance to normal cells, are considered higher grade. Nuclear grade considers the size, shape, and activity of the nucleus of each cancer cell. Nuclei that resemble closely those of normal cells would be low grade. Nuclei that are large and oddly shaped, bearing little resemblance to normal nuclei, would be higher grade. Nuclear grade also considers the relative number of cancer cells that are dividing, as evidenced by the signs of cell mitosis (cell division). In cell mitosis, it is possible to see the genetic material of the cells duplicating and splitting into two cells.

After the procedure: After examining the cancer cells, the pathologist writes a report that describes what the tumor cells look like and the pathologist's impression as to the type and grade of the tumor. Commonly used terms are metaplasia, hyperplasia, and atypical hyperplasia. Metaplasia of cells describes the reversible transformation of normal cells to a slightly different form by injury or stress. It is thought that metaplasia could lead to cancer. Hyperplasia of cells indicates that the cells are reproducing at an abnormally high rate. Atypical hyperplasia signifies that, in addition to the fact that cells are reproducing at a high rate, there are also cells that appear different from normal cells.

Risks: The risk for the grading of tumors is that the pathologist is incorrect in judgments about the tumor cells. The more experience that a pathologist has with a type of tumor cells, the more accurate he or she is likely to be in an assessment of the cells. As a result, pathologists often specialize in certain types of tumors.

Results: The American Joint Commission on Cancer (AJCC) has developed generic (basic) guidelines for the grading of tumors. They are as follows:

- Grade X: tumor cell grade cannot be assessed
- Grade 1: tumor cells appear quite similar to normal cells (low grade)
- Grade 2: moderate differences exist between the tumor cells and normal cells (intermediate grade)
- Grade 3: substantial differences exist between the tumor cells and normal cells (high grade)
- Grade 4: tumor cells bear little or no resemblance to normal cells (high grade)

In practice, variations of this generic tumor grading scale are used. A tumor grading scale has been developed for each type of cancer. For example, prostate cancer is graded by the Gleason scale, which includes grades 2 through 10.

Christine M. Carroll, R.N., B.S.N., M.B.A.

For Further Information

American Cancer Society. "How Are Lung Carcinoid Tumors Staged?" Available online at http://www .cancer.org.

Answers.com. "Tumor Grading." In *Oncology Encyclopedia*. Available online at http://www.answers.com/topic/tumor-grading.

Damjanov, Ivan, and Fang Fan, eds. *Cancer Grading Manual*. New York: Springer, 2007.

National Cancer Institute. "Tumor Grade: Questions and Answers." Available online at http://www.cancer.gov.

See also: Breslow's staging; Gleason grading system; Staging of cancer; TNM staging

▶ Hepatic Arterial Infusion (HAI)

Category: Procedures
Also known as: Regional chemotherapy, intra-arterial chemotherapy

Definition: Hepatic arterial infusion (HAI) is the delivery of chemotherapy treatment directly to the liver by a catheter (thin tube) surgically implanted to the artery leading to the organ; the other end of the catheter is attached to a pump with a chemotherapy drug.

Cancers treated: Tumors of the liver, including colon or rectal cancer that has spread to the liver

Why performed: Liver tumors that cannot be operated on because of their size or location may be treated with HAI. An advantage of this procedure is the high concentrations of the drug sent directly to the liver; since the drug is broken down in the liver, the rest of the body does not suffer the side effects of the chemotherapy.

Patient preparation: The selection of patients who would benefit from HAI is important, and evaluation includes a review of the disease history and a computed tomography (CT) scan looking for metastasized disease in the chest, abdomen, and pelvis. Patients also have a test called hepatic arteriography to look specifically at the arteries leading to the liver.

Steps of the procedure: An incision is made under the right rib cage to place the catheter in the gastroduodenal artery, which joins the arteries to the liver. An incision is also made on the left side of the abdomen where the pump will be implanted. The pump is made of a circle of titanium about 3 inches wide. The pump storage reservoir is filled with sterile water and a blood thinner (heparin), and the pump is turned on. The pump is subsequently filled with the chemotherapy drug, and cycles of two weeks of chemotherapy followed by two weeks of water and heparin are started. The chemotherapy agents delivered by HAI include floxuridine, cisplatin, or doxorubicin.

During the procedure, the surgeon also performs a cholecystectomy (removal of the gallbladder) to prevent chemotherapy from going to the gallbladder.

After the procedure: The pump is refilled as needed with a needle through the skin to the pump reservoir. The pump does not interfere with normal activities.

Risks: There may be technical complications, including infection at the site of pump placement. Most of the systemic side effects of chemotherapy (such as nausea and vomiting) are bypassed with this treatment, but there may be side effects such as abdominal pain and diarrhea.

Results: The use of HAI in inoperable liver tumors shows a higher response rate than does traditional systemic chemotherapy.

Vicki Miskovsky, B.S., R.D.

See also: Cholecystectomy; Liver cancers

▶ Hormone receptor tests

Category: Procedures

Definition: The hormone receptor test is used to determine if a breast tumor is hormone receptor positive. Hormone receptors, present on the surfaces of normal cells, bind to hormones such as estrogen and progesterone to regulate normal cell growth. Many tumors express more of these receptors, however, thus making them more responsive to hormone-dependent cell growth. This is one method the tumor uses to grow at a faster rate than normal. The hormone receptor test analyzes tissue from a breast biopsy for the number of receptors present and will classify the tumor as hormone receptor positive or negative. This information is used to decide the method of treatment for breast cancer.

Cancer diagnosed: Breast cancer

Why performed: If symptoms and screening tests, such as a mammogram, suggest the likelihood of breast cancer, then a biopsy will be performed to determine if the disease is present, the stage of the cancer, and whether the tumor is hormone receptor positive. If the cancer is estrogen receptor (ER) positive or progesterone receptor (PR) positive, it will typically respond well to hormonal therapy. Hormonal therapy will either reduce the levels of estrogen present in the body or prevent the binding of estrogen to the receptors.

Patient preparation: Depending on the type of biopsy planned, the patient may be asked to refrain from eating or drinking the night before any type of surgical procedure. If a needle biopsy is done, then it is advisable to eat lightly prior to the procedure.

Steps of the procedure: A biopsy of the suspicious lump will be further analyzed to determine whether the lump is benign or malignant, the stage of the tumor, and whether it is hormone receptor positive. Tissue samples can be obtained by fine needle biopsy, core (large-needle) biopsy, or open surgical biopsy. The procedure used depends on the size of the tumor, with more invasive methods providing the most conclusive diagnosis and the least invasive method providing more false negatives. A commonly used technique is fine needle aspiration, in which a thin hollow needle is used to take out a small portion of the tumor. Vacuum-assisted or large-gauge needles are used to remove multiple pieces of the tumor. The needle is guided to the tumor using ultrasound imaging, guaranteeing that tissue is removed only from the suspicious region. Needle biopsies are minimally invasive and can be performed in the physician's office with local anesthesia.

Surgical biopsies include incisional biopsies, which remove a small piece of tissue, and excisional biopsies, which remove the entire area of suspected cancer. Surgical biopsies provide the most conclusive diagnosis, with fewer false negatives, but are far more invasive and require a longer recovery time. Once the tissue is removed, it is sent to the laboratory for analysis, where the number of hormone receptors present will be determined.

After the procedure: For a needle biopsy, the opening is very small and little care is needed. It is covered with a small bandage for one to two days, and usual activity can be resumed immediately. If a surgical biopsy was performed, then care of the incision will require coverage with a bandage that can be removed in one or two days. If general anesthesia was used, a friend or relative should drive the patient home. Normal activities can be resumed in one to three days and stitches removed in about one week.

Risks: There is little risk involved in having a biopsy, but the main risk is infection in the area of biopsy, indicated by redness or swelling. A hematoma (collection of blood) may also occur and requires drainage.

Results: The laboratory test will take a few days, after which the physician will discuss whether the suspicious lump is benign or malignant, the stage of the tumor, and the hormone receptor status. About 80 percent of all biopsies in the United States are benign. The results of the hormone receptor test determine whether the tumor will be declared hormone receptor positive. In some practices, a number between 0 and 3 is also given, with 0+ being no receptors present and 3+ having a large number of receptors present. If the tumor has a large number of receptors present, then it is hormone dependent, and hormonal therapies such as antiestrogens will be used. Antiestrogen therapies include tamoxifen and aromatase inhibitors (Arimides, Aromasin, and Femara). Tamoxifen is generally given for premenopausal women, while aromatase inhibitors work better in postmenopausal women. Women whose tumors are hormone receptor positive generally respond very well to antiestrogen therapies and have a better prognosis than those whose tumors are not hormone dependent.

Terry J. Shackleford, Ph.D.

For Further Information

Hunt, Kelly K., et al. *Breast Cancer*. New York: Springer-Verlag, 2001.

Link, John. *Breast Cancer Survival Manual: A Step-by-Step Guide for the Woman with Newly Diagnosed Breast Cancer*. 4th ed. New York: Holt, 2007.

Miller, William R., and James N. Ingle. *Endocrine Therapy in Breast Cancer*. New York: Informa Healthcare, 2002.

Other Resources

American Cancer Society
http://www.cancer.org

BreastCancer.org
http://www.breastcancer.org

M. D. Anderson Cancer Center
http://www.mdanderson.org/diseases/breastcancer

National Cancer Institute
http://www.cancer.gov/cancertopics/types/breast

Susan G. Komen Foundation
http://www.komen.org

See also: Antiestrogens; Estrogen Receptor Downregulator (ERD); Estrogen-receptor-sensitive breast cancer; Hormonal therapies; Progesterone receptor assay; Receptor analysis

▶ *HRAS* gene testing

Category: Procedures
Also known as: v-Ha-ras Harvey rat sarcoma viral oncogene homolog, Harvey murine sarcoma virus oncogene, c-H-ras, HRAS1

Definition: The *HRAS* gene encodes a protein that allows cells to translate extracellular signals into intracellular events that induce cellular growth and division. *HRAS* is overexpressed or mutated to an overactive form in cancer of the bladder and other organs. It is also mutated in individuals afflicted with Costello syndrome, a rare developmental disorder. Symptoms of Costello syndrome include delayed development; distinctive facial features; flexible joints; papilloma around the mouth, nose, and anus; heart abnormalities; and an increased susceptibility to several types of cancer, including rhabdomyosarcoma, neuroblastoma, and transitional cell carcinoma.

Conditions diagnosed: Costello syndrome

Why performed: Costello syndrome is difficult to distinguish from other developmental disorders. Testing for mutations in *HRAS* is a useful method to diagnose Costello syndrome because approximately 80 percent of patients with this disorder have mutations in *HRAS*, while other syndromes are caused by mutations in different genes. Prenatal screening is also available for parents who have children affected with Costello syndrome.

Patient preparation: Patients considering genetic testing may meet with a genetic counselor who will discuss the benefits and risks of the test and the significance of negative, positive, and inconclusive results.

Steps of the procedure: Material required for confirming a diagnosis of Costello syndrome is generally obtained from a blood sample. For prenatal screening, amniotic fluid or chorionic villus sampling is required. Samples are sent to a clinical laboratory that offers *HRAS* screening. Deoxyribonucleic acid (DNA) is purified from the sample, and the DNA that encodes *HRAS* is amplified by polymerase chain reaction (PCR) and sequenced using standard methods.

After the procedure: The patient will consult with a physician and/or genetic counselor to discuss the implications of the test results.

Risks: Complications from drawing blood are rare but may include excessive bleeding, hematoma, or infection. The risk of miscarriage due to chorionic villus sampling is estimated at 1 in 100 to 1 in 200. Because the information obtained from *HRAS* screening may have significant psychological effects, it is important that patients be offered genetic counseling.

Results: Between 10 and 15 percent of individuals with Costello syndrome develop malignant tumors. Once diagnosed, patients should be monitored closely for rhabdomyosarcoma, neuroblastoma, and transitional cell carcinoma.

Kyle J. McQuade, Ph.D.

See also: Gene therapy; Genetic testing; Rhabdomyosarcomas; Neuroblastomas; Transitional cell carcinomas

▶ 5-Hydroxyindoleacetic Acid (5HIAA) test

Category: Procedures
Also known as: HIAA test, serotonin metabolite test

Definition: 5-Hydroxyindoleacetic acid (5HIAA) is the compound that results when the body breaks down (metabolizes) the hormone serotonin.

Cancers diagnosed: Carcinoid tumors

Why performed: Carcinoid tumors release large amounts of serotonin, so doctors look for its metabolite, 5HIAA, in the urine. This test is used to help diagnose and monitor the treatment of these types of tumors.

Patient preparation: Patients are instructed to avoid fruits and nuts in general and, specifically, avocados, bananas, eggplant, kiwis, pineapple and pineapple juice, plums, tomatoes and all tomato products, and walnuts for at least three days before and during this test. These foods can interfere with the test results. In addition, the drugs caffeine, nicotine, acetaminophen (Tylenol), aspirin, cough medicine, diazepam (Valium), ephedrine, heparin, imipramine, isoniazid, levodopa, MAO inhibitors, methyldopa, phenobarbitol, and tricylic antidepressants, as well as herbal and over-the-counter medicines, can interfere with test results.

Steps of the procedure: Generally, a patient provides a twenty-four-hour urine sample, which involves collecting and refrigerating all urine excreted over a twenty-four-hour period. If it is not possible to collect all urine over a twenty-four-hour period, then random urine samples may be collected, but this type of test is not as accurate, because 5HIAA levels can vary throughout the day.

After the procedure: If the test is used as a diagnostic tool and levels of 5HIAA are elevated, leading to a suspicion of a carcinoid tumor, then further tests, such as magnetic resonance imaging (MRI) or a computed tomography (CT) scan, may be performed to determine the existence and location of the tumor. If the test is used as a monitoring tool, then decreasing levels of 5HIAA will indicate that a tumor is responding to treatment, whereas increasing levels indicate that treatment has not been successful.

Risks: 5HIAA levels may be normal even when carcinoid tumors are present; conversely, 5HIAA levels may be elevated though no tumors exist.

Results: Because results vary widely and false negative and false positive results are common, this test does not definitely diagnose carcinoid tumors. The results should be used along with symptoms to determine what further testing is necessary for a diagnosis. As a monitoring tool, the results of this test are used to determine the level of treatment success.

Marianne M. Madsen, M.S.

See also: Carcinoid tumors and carcinoid syndrome; Tumor markers

▶ Hyperthermia therapy

Category: Procedures
Also known as: Thermal ablation, radiofrequency ablation, RFA

Definition: Hyperthermia is a treatment that uses high temperatures to destroy cancer cells directly. Hyperthermia therapy may also be used to raise the temperature of a region of the body to assist other types of cancer treatments, such as chemotherapy or radiation therapy, to be more effective.

Cancers treated: Under study in many cancers, such as breast, cervical, colorectal, kidney, ovarian, and prostate cancers

Why performed: Heat has been shown to ablate (destroy) cancer cells. Hyperthermia therapy also seems to make cancer treatments such as radiation therapy and chemotherapy more effective. While the therapy has been available for years in an experimental mode, recent advances have made the treatment more practical.

Patient preparation: Patient preparation depends on whether hyperthermia therapy is external or internal, such as during surgery; whether heating is local, regional, or whole body; or whether hyperthermia is used as a standalone treatment or to potentiate the actions of chemotherapy or radiation therapy. The level of heat is similar to a fever or a hot bath, but medications may be used to make treatments more comfortable for the patient. When hyperthermia is used during surgery, the patient is generally asleep (under anesthesia), depending on the site being treated.

Steps of the procedure: Hyperthermia therapy may involve local thermal ablation of a tumor using radio waves, ultrasound, or microwaves with a machine from outside the body. Internal hyperthermia therapy uses a probe or needle inserted in the tumor, usually during surgery. Radiofrequency ablation (RFA) uses ultrasound or visualization during surgery to deliver high-energy radio waves to a tumor. Whole-body hyperthermia may use warming blankets or thermal chambers that heat the body. Procedures may be one time, such as during surgery, or daily, as when combined with radiation therapy.

After the procedure: Patients may remain in the hospital if surgery and internal hyperthermia are used. If used in combination with radiation therapy or chemotherapy, hyperthermia treatments are generally outpatient in nature, and the patient may go home after each treatment.

Risks: Side effects depend on the type of hyperthermia therapy but may include pain, infection, bleeding, damage to the skin, and nerve or muscle damage near the treatment site. Whole-body hyperthermia may cause symptoms such as nausea, vomiting and diarrhea, and, rarely, problems with other organs, such as the heart.

Results: Heat may cause cellular changes that kill cancer cells or make cells more susceptible to the effects of chemotherapy and radiation.

Patricia Stanfill Edens, R.N., Ph.D., FACHE

See also: Continuous Hyperthermic Peritoneal Perfusion (CHPP); Fever; Hyperthermic perfusion; Lip cancers; Mayo Clinic Cancer Center; Microwave hyperthermia therapy; Radiation oncology

▶ Hyperthermic perfusion

Category: Procedures
Also known as: Regional perfusion, isolated limb perfusion, hyperthermic isolated limb perfusion, continuous hyperthermic peritoneal perfusion, intraperitoneal hyperthermic chemotherapy

Definition: Hyperthermic perfusion is a delivery system of anticancer drugs in which a warmed solution containing the drugs is directed to a cancerous organ or tissue by passing the solution through the blood vessels of the area or by bathing the tissue or organ in the solution.

Cancers treated: Melanoma, soft-tissue sarcomas, colon cancer, peritoneal carcinomatosis, liver cancer, lung cancer

Why performed: Hyperthermic perfusion is a technique that allows for maximum exposure of the tumor to anticancer drugs while limiting the toxic effects to the entire body. Heating the chemotherapy solution improves the effectiveness of the anticancer drugs.

Patient preparation: To prepare an area for hyperthermic perfusion, it is necessary to temporarily isolate the circulation of the area from systemic circulation. Additionally, in certain types of tumors (such as peritoneal carcinomatosis), cytoreductive surgery is first performed to remove as much visible tumor as possible prior to isolating the area and proceeding with hyperthermic perfusion.

Steps of the procedure: The arms and legs are frequently the regions exposed to hyperthermic perfusion for the treatment of melanoma or for the treatment of sarcoma of soft tissues. Isolating the circulation of an arm or leg is achieved by putting small tubes (cannulas) in the arteries that carry blood to that limb and in the veins that carry blood out from the limb; this process is called cannulating. In addition, a rubber tourniquet is put at the top of the arm or leg to aid in isolating the area. Thermometers are placed at several locations on the limb to monitor the temperature during the procedure.

A perfusion circuit is established by attaching tubing between the artery and vein cannulas and a special type of pump. The pump apparatus includes an oxygenator (to increase the concentration of oxygen in the blood) and a mechanism to heat and cool the perfusion solution.

Heparin (a blood-thinning substance), a special dye, and electrolytes are mixed with the patient's blood and circulated through the isolated area. Heparin is used to prevent blood clots from forming, and the dye is used to monitor the perfusion solution and ensure that it does not escape the intended treatment area. The temperature of the perfusion solution is increased (hyperthermia) as it circulates through the isolated area; the anticancer drugs are added when the solution reaches a prescribed temperature. The temperature of the arm or leg, the rate of flow, and the perfusion pressure are all carefully monitored during the procedure. The circulation of the hyperthermic solution lasts for about one hour, and then the anticancer drug is drained from the treated area and the area is washed out. The whole procedure lasts a maximum of two hours.

Continuous hyperthermic peritoneal perfusion or intraperitoneal hyperthermic chemotherapy uses techniques similar to those used for isolated limb perfusion to deliver a chemotherapy solution to the peritoneal cavity (the space inside the abdomen that has a membrane covering all the organs in the abdomen). Cannulas in the arteries and veins are used with tubing and a pump, and the cavity is sewn shut to create a closed circuit. The entire peritoneal cavity is bathed (perfused) with the warmed chemotherapy solution. Delivering the anticancer drugs directly to the peritoneal cavity allows a much higher dosage of the drugs to be used. As with hyperthermic perfusion of an isolated limb, the procedure for continous hyperthermic peritoneal perfusion lasts about two hours and ends with draining the drug solution and washing out the peritoneal cavity. Other organs, such as the liver and the lungs, can also be isolated with similar methods.

A variety of anticancer drugs are used in hyperthermic perfusion, including mitomycin C, oxaliplatin, melphalan, and tumor necrosis factors (TNFs).

After the procedure: Patients are hospitalized after the procedure and are given low doses of heparin to prevent blood clots. If the procedure has been used for an arm or a leg, then that limb is kept elevated for a few days; the period of hospitalization is approximately three days. The hospitalization period for a more extensive procedure, such as cytoreduction surgery in the peritoneal cavity followed by hyperthermic peritoneal perfusion, is approximately ten days.

Risks: Edema (an accumulation of fluid in tissue) is an expected risk or discomfort from the procedure, but it is most often easily treatable. Severe swelling of an arm or leg to the extent that it interferes with circulation is called compartment syndrome; severe cases of compartment syndrome require amputation of the limb. Other expected risks include temporary toxicity to the bone marrow, inflammation of the veins, and an increased risk of bleeding because of the use of heparin.

Results: Research studies have shown an increased disease-free survival of patients for whom hyperthermic perfusion is used. Results of any therapy, however, are dependent upon many factors, chief among them the stage of the cancer at the time of the therapy.

Vicki Miskovsky, B.S., R.D.

For Further Information

Dollinger, Malin, et al. *Everyone's Guide to Cancer Therapy*. 4th rev. ed. Kansas City, Mo.: Andrews & McMeel, 2002.

Perry, Michael C., ed. *The Chemotherapy Source Book*. 4th ed. Philadelphia: Wolters Kluwer Health/Lippincott Williams & Wilkins, 2008.

Other Resources

National Cancer Institute

Clinical Trials

http://www.cancer.gov/clinical_trials

See also: Continuous Hyperthermic Peritoneal Perfusion (CHPP)

▶ Hysterectomy

Category: Procedures

Also known as: Vaginal hysterectomy, abdominal hysterectomy, total or complete hysterectomy, total hysterectomy with salpingo-oophorectomy, laparoscopic-assisted vaginal hysterectomy, radical hysterectomy

Definition: Hysterectomy is the removal of the female reproductive organs. There are seven different types of hysterectomy. Basic hysterectomy is the surgical removal of the uterus. Total or complete abdominal hysterectomy (TAH) involves the surgical removal of the uterus and cervix. Total hysterectomy with salpingo-oophorectomy is the surgical removal of the uterus, cervix, ovaries, and Fallopian tubes. Vaginal hysterectomy (VH) is the surgical removal of the uterus through the vaginal opening. Abdominal hysterectomy is the surgical removal of the uterus through an abdominal incision. In laparoscopic-assisted vaginal hysterectomy (LAH or LAVH), a laparoscope is inserted through several small incisions in the abdominal-pelvic region, helping guide the surgeon, who then removes the organs through the vaginal opening. Radical hysterectomy is the surgical removal of the uterus, cervix, ovaries, Fallopian tubes, surrounding lymph nodes, surrounding muscles and ligaments, and the superior portion of the vagina.

Cancers treated: Ovarian, uterine, abdominal, Fallopian tube, and cervical cancers; for certain types of breast cancer, a complete hysterectomy or oophorectomy may be required if the type of tumor is estrogen sensitive.

Why performed: In addition to the treatment of cancer, hysterectomy may be performed for abnormal bleeding or hemorrhaging, endometriosis, pelvic pain, dysmenorrhea, ovarian cysts, ovarian tumors, fibroid tumors, prolapsed bladder, prolapsed uterus, bleeding cervical polyps, pelvic floor reconstruction, hyperplasia, abdominal mass, and pelvic inflammatory disease (PID). Hysterectomy may also be advised for patients with colon, bladder, or rectal cancers to help increase their long-term survival.

Patient preparation: Many patients find that doing their own research and getting a second opinion give them valuable information. They may ask their health care professionals for informational pamphlets from Krames Communication or the American College of Obstetricians and Gynecologists. Prior to having a hysterectomy, most patients undergo some of the following procedures: a Pap test and other laboratory tests, pelvic examination, hormone therapy, biopsy, ultrasound, hysteroscopy, electrocardiography (EKG), computed tomography (CT), magnetic resonance imaging (MRI), colposcopy, laparoscopy, colonoscopy, dilation and curettage (D&C), and myomectomy. Some patients have tried Kegel exercises to help strengthen the pelvic muscles or have worn a pessary.

Patients should stop smoking one week prior to surgery. They should bring a list of questions and a complete list of all medications, including vitamins, herbal remedies, and any over-the-counter medications, to the preoperative (pre-op) examination in order to find out which medications they can take or which ones they will need to stop taking prior to surgery.

A pre-op evaluation by a doctor or surgeon includes a chest X ray and laboratory work. The results of the pre-op tests have the potential to postpone or cancel any surgery. The risks versus the benefits of the surgery are evaluated. Patients should follow their physician's pre-op instructions to help ensure the best possible outcome for the surgery. The night before the surgery, they should have nothing to eat or drink after 6:00 p.m. and should take a shower and wash the hair with antibacterial soap.

Steps of the procedure: The morning of the surgery, the patient is given a hospital gown to wear. No personal clothing will be allowed. All jewelry must be removed as to not interfere with heart monitors and other medical electrical devices. All makeup and nail polish must be removed for the observation process, helping to verify oxygen levels. The patient should not use any lotions, deodorants, or perfumes, as they make it difficult for surgical personnel to adhere EKG chest leads, attach monitors, and secure bandages onto the body. A bladder catheter may be inserted for urinary drainage purposes. General anesthesia is required for this surgery. The anesthesiologist will talk to the patient before surgery.

Four incision styles may be used. Vertical incision involves a visible external incision for an abdominal hysterectomy, approximately 6 inches long, extending upward from the symphysis pubic bone to the navel. For horizontal incision (also known as transverse incision or bikini cut), a 6-inch-wide, visible, horizontal incision is placed approximately 1 inch above the pubic bone. Vaginal incision requires an incision through the superior portion of the vagina. LAVH requires approximately four small incisions in the abdominal/pelvic area and an incision in the superior portion of the vagina.

Four main abdominal muscle layers are cut in order to remove the uterus: rectum abdominis, external oblique, internal oblique, and transverse abdominis. If the ovaries are removed, then the ovarian ligament, suspensory ligament, and broad ligament are also severed.

The number of internal dissolvable stitches and the number of external staples to close the incision depend on the complexity of the surgery. The physician may also change the staples to Steri-Strips around five to ten days after the surgery (post-op).

After the procedure: The initial recovery time is six to eight weeks; however, the complete healing process takes six to twelve months. The patient should take showers, not baths, until the doctor approves of the latter. The patient should also take pain medication as directed, walk for exercise, and drink plenty of liquids. The body endures many physical, emotional, and hormonal changes after a hysterectomy. Weight-lifting restrictions, sexual relationship concerns, anemia, post-op bleeding, adhesions, and blood clots are issues that the doctor should discuss with the patient.

The patient should understand the post-op instructions and call the medical facility if fever, nausea or vomiting, severe pain anywhere in the body, difficulty breathing, or hemorrhaging occurs. It is normal to have a slightly bloody vaginal discharge up to fourteen days post-op as a result of the healing process and sutures dissolving and falling out.

Menopause is a life-altering stage. The patient will need to educate herself about hot flashes, night sweats, hormone replacement therapy (HRT), vitamin and mineral supplements, and herbal remedies.

Risks: The risks of hysterectomy may include bleeding, blood transfusions, adhesions, pain, surgical and post-surgical complications, nausea or vomiting, blood clots (thrombosis), abscess, cellulitis, infections, nerve injury, bowel injury, intestinal injury, bladder injury, prolapsed bladder, prolapsed rectum, twisted bowel, gas pain, adverse reaction to anesthesia, and death.

Results: Hysterectomy may result in the removal of cancers, the stopping of menstrual and irregular bleeding, a decrease or elimination of pain, and repair of the bladder or bowel. Menopause is the direct result of a hysterectomy, as menstrual flow will permanently cease. Hot flashes, night sweats, vaginal dryness, osteoporosis, cardiovascular (heart) disease, memory loss, dry skin, xerostomia (dry mouth), dry eyes, and decreased sexual libido can occur.

Suzette Buhr, R.T.R., C.D.A.

For Further Information

Dennerstein, Lorraine, Carl Wood, and Ann Westmore. *Hysterectomy: New Options and Advances*. New York: Oxford University Press, 1995.

Jones, Marcia L., Theresa Eichenwald, and Nancy W. Hall. *Menopause for Dummies*. 2d ed. New York: Wiley, 2006.

Litin, Scott C., Jr., ed. *Mayo Clinic Family Health Book*. 3d ed. New York: HarperCollins, 2003.

Porter, Robert S., ed. *The Merck Manual of Women's and Men's Health*. 2d ed. New York: Simon & Schuster, 2006.

Other Resources

BestHealth, Wake Forest University Baptist Medical Center
http://www.besthealth.com

University of Michigan Comprehensive Cancer Center
http://www.cancer.med.umich.edu

See also: Cervical cancer; Choriocarcinomas; Dilation and Curettage (D&C); Endometrial cancer; Endometrial hyperplasia; Fallopian tube cancer; Fertility drugs and cancer; Gestational Trophoblastic Tumors (GTTs); Granulosa cell tumors; Gynecologic cancers; Gynecologic oncology; Hereditary leiomyomatosis and Renal Cell Cancer (HLRCC); Hormone Replacement Therapy (HRT); Hot flashes; Hystero-oophorectomy; Laparoscopy and laparoscopic surgery; Leiomyomas; Leiomyosarcomas; Pap test; Salpingectomy and salpingo-oophorectomy; Sexuality and cancer; Uterine cancer; Vaginal cancer

▶ Hysterography

Category: Procedures
Also known as: Hysterogram

Definition: Hysterography is a diagnostic procedure that uses contrast dye to enhance X-ray images of the interior of the uterus.

Cancers diagnosed: Uterine cancer, endometrial cancer

Why performed: Hysterography is a diagnostic procedure that is used to help identify uterine and endometrial cancer. Hysterography allows a doctor to analyze the interior lining of the uterus to check for possible cancerous growths, such as uterine sarcoma or endometrial cancer.

Patient preparation: The preferred time to receive a hysterography is after the last day of menstruation and prior to ovulation, to prevent interrupting a pregnancy. Routine laboratory tests for sexually transmitted diseases (STDs) and pregnancy are conducted before the procedure.

Hysterography is an outpatient procedure performed at a radiology department. Patients may receive pain medication, a mild sedative, or antibiotics prior to the procedure. Patients don an examination gown and wear nothing below the waist. The procedure can usually be completed in about fifteen to forty-five minutes.

Steps of the procedure: Patients lie on their backs on an examination table during the procedure. The patient's knees are spread and the feet are placed in stirrups. A speculum is inserted into the vagina to separate the vaginal walls. The cervix is cleansed. A thin catheter is inserted through the cervical opening. Contrast dye is delivered to the uterus through the thin tube.

The doctor views the contrast dye as it fills the uterus by watching images on a fluoroscopy screen. X rays are taken during the process. Patients may be repositioned to allow X rays to be taken from various angles.

When the hysterography is complete, the catheter and speculum are gently removed. Patients are monitored for a short time for allergic reaction or bleeding.

After the procedure: Patients may experience menstrual-like cramps or light bleeding for a few days following the procedure. Patients should not use tampons and douches or participate in sexual intercourse for two days. Patients may receive pain medication or antibiotics. Patients should contact their doctor if they experience heavy bleeding, infection, allergic reaction, breathing problems, or increased pain.

Risks: The risks of hysterography include allergic reaction to the contrast dye, infection, or prolonged bleeding.

Results: A healthy uterus has no abnormal growths or tissues. Suspicious or cancerous-appearing growths are biopsied in a separate procedure to confirm a diagnosis of cancer.

Mary Car-Blanchard, O.T.D., B.S.O.T.

See also: Endometrial cancer; Endoscopy; Gynecologic cancers; Gynecologic oncology; Hysterectomy; Hystero-oophorectomy; Hysteroscopy; Oophorectomy; Pelvic examination; Salpingectomy and salpingo-oophorectomy; Uterine cancer

▶ Hystero-oophorectomy

Category: Procedures
Also known as: Total abdominal hysterectomy and bilateral salpingo-oophorectomy

Definition: Hystero-oophorectomy is the surgical removal of the uterus and both the right and left Fallopian tubes and ovaries.

Cancers treated: Invasive cervical carcinoma Stage I to IIA, endometrial carcinoma, uterine leiomyomas

Why performed: Hystero-oophorectomy is the primary treatment and staging modality for malignant cancers amenable to resection arising from any of the three tissue layers of the uterus. Benign tumors of the uterus such as fibroids (leiomyomas) that do not regress with time, that degenerate, or that bleed excessively are also an indication. The ovaries are often removed simultaneously in postmenopausal women in order to prevent possible degeneration of cells into ovarian cancer. In premenopausal women undergoing hystero-oophorectomy, the ovaries are removed when they are at high risk for developing estrogen-stimulated cancers such as breast and endometrial cancers.

Patient preparation: The patient undergoes preoperative evaluation for any coexisting diseases to determine her fitness to undergo surgery and general anesthesia. Patients are instructed to take nothing per mouth the night before the procedure.

Steps of the procedure: After the patient is anesthetized, in the lithotomy position, surgically prepped and draped, a transverse or vertical incision is made above the pubic bone. The incision is taken down to the pelvic cavity. The uterine and ovarian vessels are identified, dissected, and separated from the ureters, and the bladder is separated from the uterus. The supporting ligaments and dissected vessels of the Fallopian tubes, ovaries, uterus, and cervix are then isolated, cut, and ligated, and the vaginal and cardinal ligament stumps are sutured together. A laparoscopic approach may be similarly done, except that the uterus, Fallopian tubes, and ovaries are removed vaginally.

After the procedure: The patient is monitored in the postanesthesia care unit until she is fully awake and vital signs are stable. Once the patient is stable in the unit, she may be discharged to the gynecologic ward for postoperative monitoring. Once the patient is stable, ambulatory, voiding, and eating, she may be discharged after a few days.

Risks: The most significant risks of the procedure are deep vein thrombosis, pulmonary embolism, perforation of the bladder or bowel, and accidental ligation of the ureters.

Results: A gross and microscopic examination of large masses may reveal central necrosis and hemorrhage and increased growth of uterine cells but no elements of disordered growth of abnormal cells. Microscopic examinations that reveal disordered proliferation and abnormal uterine or cervical cells are suggestive of uterine cancer or invasive cervical cancer.

Aldo C. Dumlao, M.D.

See also: *BRCA1* and *BRCA2* genes; Breast cancers; Fallopian tube cancer; Gynecologic oncology; Hormonal therapies; Hot flashes; Hysterectomy; Oophorectomy; Salpingectomy and salpingo-oophorectomy

▶ Hysteroscopy

Category: Procedures
Also known as: Uterine endoscopy

Definition: Hysteroscopy uses a type of endoscope to allow a doctor to see, examine, and biopsy abnormal tissues or growths inside the uterus, the part of the female reproductive system where a fertilized egg develops. The procedure is used to check for cancer cells and remove suspicious tissue, precancerous tissue, or cancerous growths.

A hysteroscope is a thin tube with a viewing instrument and a light. There are different types of hysteroscopes, depending on whether the procedure is for diagnosis or treatment purposes. The tube may be flexible or rigid. It expands like a telescope. A hysteroscope can contain fiber optics that produce images on a video screen. It can also contain tubes for inserting gas or fluids and surgical instruments.

Cancers diagnosed or treated: Uterine cancer, uterine sarcoma, endometrial cancer, precancerous growths

Why performed: Hysteroscopy is used as a diagnostic or a treatment procedure. It is used to view the inside of the uterus to detect possible cancerous growths, such as uterine sarcoma and endometrial cancer. Suspicious tissues are biopsied. A biopsy entails removing tissue, mucus, or fluid samples with thin surgical instruments that are inserted through the hysteroscope. The tissues are examined for cancer cells in a laboratory. For small cancers, removing the cells helps to treat the cancer.

Patient preparation: The preferred time to receive a hysteroscopy is after the last day of menstruation and before ovulation, to prevent interrupting a pregnancy. Routine laboratory tests, including blood and urine tests, are conducted before the hysteroscopy. A pregnancy test, Pap smear, and sexually transmitted disease (STD) testing may be performed as well.

A hysteroscopy is an outpatient procedure performed in a doctor's office, outpatient surgical center, or hospital. Hysteroscopy uses local anesthesia, general anesthesia, paracervical nerve block, or mild sedation. It can be performed with no anesthesia in select individuals. Patients receiving general anesthesia should not eat or drink after midnight prior to the day of surgery.

On the day of the hysteroscopy, patients are requested to empty their bladder before the procedure begins. Patients wear an examination gown with nothing on below the waist.

Steps of the procedure: Patients lie on their backs with their knees spread and feet placed and secured in stirrups. Patients receive anesthesia, and their vital signs are monitored during the procedure. A catheter may be inserted through the urethra and into the bladder to collect urine.

A speculum is inserted into the vagina to separate the vaginal walls, allowing the doctor to see the cervix (opening to the uterus). The doctor may dilate the cervical opening with a device; some hysteroscopes are narrow enough to fit through the cervical opening without requiring dilation.

The hysteroscope is inserted in the vagina, moved through the cervix, and advanced to the uterus. Gas or sterile fluid may be used to expand the uterus and provide the doctor with a good view. The gas or fluid is delivered through a tube in the hysteroscope. Fluid is preferred in some cases because it washes mucus from the uterine walls, allowing the mucus to be collected for biopsy and creating a clearer image.

The doctor views the walls of the uterus, looking for any signs of abnormality, such as an irregular growth, fibroid, or polyp. A biopsy is taken of any abnormal or suspicious tissue or growths. At completion of the hysteroscopy, the gas, fluid, catheter, and hysteroscope are removed.

After the procedure: Patients are monitored in the recovery area. Patients are discharged when they are awake and alert. Patients should have another person drive them home.

Mild cramping or pain may occur for about eight hours after the procedure. Light bleeding may occur for a couple of days.

Risks: Rare complications of hysteroscopy include infection; prolonged bleeding; uterine, bowel, or bladder perforation; and fluid absorption into the bloodstream. Patients should contact their doctor if they develop a fever, severe pain, unusual discharge, or heavy bleeding.

Results: A healthy uterus has no abnormal growths or tissues. Suspicious growths are biopsied to determine whether cancer is present.

Mary Car-Blanchard, O.T.D., B.S.O.T.

For Further Information

Bettocchi, S., et al. "What Does 'Diagnostic Hysteroscopy' Mean Today? The Role of the New Techniques." *Current Opinions in Obstetrics and Gynecology* 15, no. 4 (August, 2003): 303-308.

Donnez, Jacques, ed. *Atlas of Operative Laparoscopy and Hysteroscopy*. 3d ed. New York: Informa Healthcare, 2007.

Fuller, Arlan F., Jr., Robert H. Young, and Michael V. Seiden. *Uterine Cancer*. Hamilton, Ont.: BC Decker, 2004.

Luesly, David M., Frank Lawton, and Andrew Berchuck, eds. *Uterine Cancer*. New York: Informa Healthcare, 2005.

Mayo Clinic. *Mayo Clinic: Guide to Women's Cancers*. New York: Kensington, 2005.

Pasic, Resad P., and Ronald Leon Levine. *A Practical Manual of Hysteroscopy and Endometrial Ablation Techniques: A Clinical Cookbook*. New York: Informa Healthcare, 2004.

Valle, R. F. "Development of Hysteroscopy: From a Dream to a Reality, and Its Linkage to the Present and Future." *Journal of Minimally Invasive Gynecology* 14, no. 4 (July/August, 2007): 407-418.

Other Resources

American Cancer Society
http://www.cancer.org

National Cancer Institute
http://www.cancer.gov

National Women's Health Information Center
U.S. Department of Health and Human Services
http://womenshealth.gov

See also: Endometrial cancer; Endoscopy; Gynecologic cancers; Gynecologic oncology; Hysterectomy; Hysterography; Hystero-oophorectomy; Oophorectomy; Pelvic examination; Salpingectomy and salpingo-oophorectomy; Uterine cancer

▶ Ileostomy

Category: Procedures
Also known as: End ileostomy, loop ileostomy, separated loop ileostomy, continent ileostomy

Definition: An ileostomy is a procedure that creates an opening on the abdomen (stoma) from a segment of the latter portion of the small bowel (ileum). An ileostomy can be permanent (end ileostomy) or temporary (loop ileostomy).

Cancers treated: Colorectal and small bowel cancer; metastatic pelvic cancer, including vaginal, cervical, ovarian, and prostate cancers

Why performed: The ileum may sometimes become diseased and may cause symptoms of bowel obstruction, bleeding, or nutrient malabsorption. Potentially life-threatening or premalignant conditions such as severe inflammatory bowel disease involving the ileum and colon (Crohn disease, ulcerative colitis) are also managed with the use of ileostomy. Because the ileum absorbs many essential nutrients relative to the rest of the small bowel, preservation of disease-free regions is paramount. An ileostomy is performed primarily in order to divert digested material for excretion in cases where the colon or rectum is diseased or otherwise unusable. It is also done in order to permit healing of the remaining, but usable, colon to be used later in reestablishing continuity between the small and large bowel. This is also done after two bowel ends are newly rejoined (anastomosis) to allow the bowel to rest and expedite healing. The ileostomy is located before the anastomosis to prevent digested material from stimulating the joined ends from unnecessary contractions.

Patient preparation: Surgical risk assessment is conducted through a general physical examination, medication review and revision, electrocardiography (EKG) and chest X ray, and pulmonary function tests as needed.

Other considerations include ensuring that the patient is adequately nourished and hydrated beforehand. Bowel preparation by a gradual decrease in food and liquid intake and enemas is carried out at least twenty-four hours prior to the procedure.

The decision to undergo the procedure should be accompanied by active patient participation. The patient must be thoroughly briefed regarding the care of and implications of a permanent ileostomy in the event that reattachment to the distal bowel is not possible. If the procedure is agreeable to the patient, then the position of the stoma is discussed and marked on the patient's abdomen prior to the procedure.

Steps of the procedure: After the patient is positioned and the surgical site is sterilized, a mid-abdominal incision is made and carried down to the abdominal cavity. The length of the small and large bowel is examined for viable and nonviable regions. Any diseased sections are excised, with the undiseased ends reattached. Any additional abdominal cavity procedure such as lymph node dissection and resection is carried out.

The construction of the ileostomy will depend on the severity of disease (the presence of disease-free colon for reattachment in a separate procedure). A permanent end ileostomy is constructed by dividing the remaining ileum from the colon, preserving as much bowel as possible. Both ends are closed with staples or sutures. The thin membrane containing the bowel's blood vessels (mesentery) at the proximal ileal end is cut to allow manipulation; the vessels directly supplying it are preserved. Another abdominal incision is made over the previously marked area, through which 6 centimeters of ileum is pulled. The stapled end is cut, and a spigot is fashioned by suturing the ileum onto the skin at three points. This prevents the fluid and electrolyte imbalance of ileostomy dysfunction caused by partial stoma obstruction.

A temporary loop ileostomy is constructed in a similar manner as an end ileostomy except that both ends of the ileum are used, with the distal end nonfunctional in excretion. In addition, interruption of the mesentery is minimal because of the need for both ends to be supplied adequately with blood.

After the procedure: The patient is allowed to recover consciousness in a postanesthesia care unit before going to the surgical ward. Recovery time can reach ten to twelve days, with resumption of normal activity by four to eight weeks. Maintenance of the ileostomy involves becoming familiar with frequent changing of the different parts of the ileostomy appliance, such as the skin barrier and the ileostomy bag. With the absence of the colon as a water-reabsorbing and storage apparatus for digested food, the patient must empty the collection bag frequently and be more aware of the amount and type of food and drink consumed, especially during exercise and hot weather.

Risks: The risks of bleeding, impaired healing, and infections are always present. Meticulous adherence to surgical technique prevents most of these complications. Long-term risks for the duration of the ileostomy include obstruction from food particles or bowel adhesions, fistulas, infection, and dehydration from increased ileostomy fluid output.

Results: An ileostomy is not directly curative for cancer, but it is a helpful procedure in restoring the patient's continence and a semblance of normal bowel function at a later time through anastomosis of ileum to colon or rectum. While the position of an ileostomy allows for easy cleaning and draining of the ileostomy appliance and does not interfere greatly with daily routines and activities, one of the most important patient considerations to be made is that of self-image after ileostomy.

Aldo C. Dumlao, M.D.

For Further Information

Bernstein, Charles N. *Inflammatory Bowel Disease Yearbook 2004*. London: Remedica, 2004.

Gislason, Stephen J. *Food and Digestive Disorders: Irritable Bowel Syndrome, Crohn's Disease, Celiac Disease, Ulcerative Colitis, Ulcers, Reflux and Motility Disorders*. Sechelt, B.C.: Environmed Research, 2003.

Williams, Simon J. *Medicine and the Body*. London: Sage Publications, 2003.

See also: Coloanal anastomosis; Colorectal cancer; Enterostomal therapy; Gastrointestinal complications of cancer treatment; Hereditary polyposis syndromes

▶ Imaging contrast dyes

Category: Procedures

Cancers diagnosed: Imaging contrast dyes are used in radiographic studies to help physicians diagnose cancers that affect the brain, lungs, gastrointestinal tract (esophagus, pancreas, liver, stomach, small intestine, colon, and rectum), genitourinary system (kidneys, ureters, and bladder), and reproductive organs (endometrium/uterus, ovaries, and prostate), and to observe cancer spread (metastasis) to other parts of the body.

Why performed: Imaging contrast dyes (contrast materials, agents, or media) enhance the visualization of internal organs and structures in radiographic studies for diagnosis and treatment. Contrast-enhanced studies highlight differences between normal and abnormal conditions in solid organs, the vascular system, and the gastrointestinal and genitourinary tracts. These chemical substances do not permanently discolor organs and can enhance X-ray images of the body. Imaging contrast dyes alter the way X-rays pass through the body, thereby producing more detailed images than non-contrast-enhanced studies.

Various imaging contrast dyes are used and the particular dye employed depends on the desired medical imaging modality. Iodine-based and barium sulfate compounds are the most common types of contrast medium for enhancing X-ray-based imaging techniques, such as radiography, fluoroscopy, ultrasonography, computed tomography (CT), nuclear magnetic resonance imaging (MRI), and intravenous pyelogram (IVP). Iodinated contrast can be injected into veins or arteries, within intervertebral discs or spinal fluid, and other body cavities. These compounds enhance images of the gastrointestinal tract, vasculature, soft tissue, brain, and breasts. Barium-sulfate, which is usually used to examine the gastrointestinal tract, is the most common oral or rectal contrast material and is available as a powder, liquid, paste, or tablet.

An IVP is an iodine-based contrast study, which characterizes the anatomy, size, and shape of the urinary system. The kidneys excrete these compounds from the bloodstream and concentrate them in the ureters and bladder. However, an IVP is not used when kidney cancer is suspected as other techniques, such as ultrasound and CT imaging studies, yield more detailed information. Contrast agents are also used in MRI (refer to Gadolinium Dyes and Technetium Isotopes).

Patient preparation: Imaging contrast dyes are generally safe medications, but they may carry a risk of rather uncommon allergic or adverse reactions. Prior to their procedure, patients should inform their physicians about: previous reaction to imaging contrast dyes, severe allergies, and reactions to food, drugs, preservatives, or animals; medications and herbal supplements; and recent illnesses, surgeries, or medical conditions (asthma, hay fever, cardiovascular disease, diabetes, kidney diseases, pheochromocytoma, myeloma, thyroid disorder, or sickle cell anemia).

Kidney function tests should be obtained a month before contrast-enhanced studies in those patients with reduced kidney function. Premedication with antihistamines and corticosteroids is recommended for patients with a history of mild to moderate reactions to intravenous imaging contrast dyes. Patients with diabetes who are scheduled for contrast-enhanced studies should not take metformin on the day of the examination and 2 days afterwards to minimize contrast-induced kidney damage.

Prior to studies, female patients should always inform their healthcare providers about current or possible pregnancy or breast feeding. Imaging contrast dyes are avoided during pregnancy to minimize risk to the fetus. If contrast enhanced studies become necessary, pregnant patients should discuss their healthcare providers about potential risks and benefits of the contrast-enhanced examination.

Patients will be advised not to eat in the preceding hours of oral barium studies. Patients may find the taste of barium suspensions somewhat unpleasant, but tolerable. If rectal contrast is indicated, patients will be prescribed a bowel preparation.

Iodinated studies may cause patients to experience a warm, flushed sensation and a transient metallic taste.

Steps of the procedure: Imaging contrast dyes can be administered orally, rectally, and intravenously. Injection methods depend on the accessibility of veins and medical conditions.

After the procedure: Imaging contrast dyes are absorbed by the body or excreted in urine or feces. Increased fluid intake facilitates removal of the contrast material from the body. Changes in normal bowel movement patterns and white discoloration of feces typically occur with barium studies for the first 12 to 24 hours.

Risks: Contrast-enhanced studies may be associated with minor physiological disturbances or rare, severe life-threatening situations. Radiological departments are equipped to address serious allergies or other reactions to contrast dyes. Patients should notify their physicians about severe and persistent side effects.

Mild side effects of iodine-based contrast materials include nausea, vomiting, headaches, itching, skin flushing, rash, or hives. Moderate side effects include severe rash or hives, wheezing, palpitations, changes in blood pressure, and shortness of breath. Severe side effects include difficulty breathing, throat swelling, convulsions, low blood pressure, and cardiac arrest.

Mild side effects of barium-sulfate contrast materials may include nausea, vomiting, diarrhea, stomach cramps, and constipation. Patients who are at greater risk include those with a history of asthma, cystic fibrosis, dehydration, or intestinal blockage or perforation.

Patients with kidney diseases are at risk for developing contrast-induced kidney damage, in which preexisting kidney function may worsen.

Results: Imaging contrast dyes used in examining arteries in the body (MRI or CT angiogram) show normal vasculature and the abnormal tumor-induced blood vessel formation common to some cancers. An IVP can show abnormalities of the renal pelvis and ureters, including cancers.

Barium enemas can screen for colorectal cancer in instances when a colonoscopy is contraindicated. The large colon will have normal shape without blockage if there is no cancer. Abnormal findings may include polyps (growths from the lining of the colon), intestinal inflammation, and structural abnormalities such as areas of narrowing (strictures) or small pouches in the lining of the colon (diverticulosis).

An upper gastrointestinal series is an oral barium study that assesses the esophagus, stomach, and duodenum (upper part of the small intestine). A normal result shows no changes in the structures and movement, but concerning results include abnormal movement, enlarged veins in the esophagus, masses, scars, strictures, swelling, and ulcers (break in the gastrointestinal lining).

Jason F. Lee, MD, MPH
Miriam E. Schwartz, MD, MA, PhD

For Further Information

American College of Radiology. (2015). *Manual on Contrast Media* (Vol. 10.1). Retrieved from http://www.acr.org/quality-safety/resources/contrast-manual

Lisle, D. (2012). *Imaging for students* (4th ed.). Boca Raton, FL: CRC Press. Excellent how-to book that shepherds medical students through the theory and techniques of medical imaging.

Rose, T., & Choi, J. (2015). Intravenous imaging contrast media complications: The basics that every clinician needs to know. *The American Journal of Medicine*, 128(9): 943-949.

Thomsen, H., & Webb, J. (Eds.). (2014). *Contrast media: Safety issues and ESUR guidelines* (3rd ed.). Germany: Springer-Verlag Berlin Heidelberg.

Other Resources

American Cancer Society: X-rays and other radiographic tests
http://www.cancer.org/treatment/understandingyourdiagnosis/examsandtestdescriptions/imagingradiologytests/imaging-radiology-tests-xrays

American College of Radiology. ACR Appropriateness Criteria®
http://www.acr.org/Quality-Safety/Appropriateness-Criteria

Food and Drug Administration: Radiography
http://www.fda.gov/Radiation-EmittingProducts/RadiationEmittingProductsandProcedures/MedicalImaging/MedicalX-Rays/ucm175028.htm

RadiologyInfo.org, produced by the American College of Radiology and the Radiological Society of North America
http://www.radiologyinfo.org

▶ Imaging tests

Category: Procedures
Also known as: Radiology tests

Definition: Imaging tests are procedures that use a source of energy to evaluate specific internal structures of the body and obtain a visual representation of such structures using special equipment. The energy sources used for these procedures may be magnetic fields, radio waves, radioactive particles, sound waves, or X rays. Imaging tests include computed tomography (CT) scans, magnetic resonance imaging (MRI), radiography (X rays) with and without contrast studies, mammography, radionuclide imaging, and ultrasonography.

Imaging tests are distinguished based on the manner by which the bodily structure is viewed. CT scans use a concentrated beam of X rays to obtain multiple views of such structures; the images are then processed in a computer to provide a three-dimensional composite for easier analysis and interpretation.

MRI uses magnetic force to align hydrogen atoms of the body in one direction. A burst of radiofrequency waves is then applied, causing a change in alignment. Signals are emitted by the hydrogen atoms as they return to their original orientation. A computerized scanner detects and converts these signals into two- or three-dimensional images for analysis and interpretation.

Radiography utilizes X rays, high-energy electromagnetic waves in small doses, to obtain images of body structures. Modified types of X-ray studies employ dyes as contrast agents to view structures that regular X-ray techniques do not visualize; the contrast agents can outline or fill in structures and can provide better radiographic imaging. These modified studies include upper gastrointestinal (GI) series (barium swallow), examining the lining of the esophagus, stomach, and upper part of the small intestines; lower GI series (barium enema), analyzing the colon and rectum linings; intravenous pyelography (IVP), viewing the urinary tract (kidney, ureters, and bladder); angiography inspecting arteries such as those in the heart and brain; and lymphangiography, investigating the lymph vessels and lymph nodes.

Mammography employs X rays for examining the breasts to screen for breast disease in the absence of symptoms and for diagnosis when breast abnormalities are detected by screening. The images are available either on X-ray photographic films or in digital form electronically stored in a computer.

Radionuclide imaging (nuclear scan) uses radioactive tracers to obtain images from within the body; radioactive emissions are picked up by a computerized external detector, and the processing of these signals provides images of the internal body structures. Examples of radiopharmaceuticals include gallium 67, used to detect bone marrow, lung, and lymph node tumors; technetium 99, employed in whole-body scans to evaluate metastasis of various primary cancers; thallium 201, utilized in detecting breast cancers, thyroid tumors, and lymphomas; and iodine 123 and iodine 131, used to detect thyroid cancers and neuroendocrine tumors such as carcinoid tumors. Depending on the disease, the tissues affected absorb more or less of the radioactive tracers; the nuclear scans can locate tumors and identify cancer spread.

Ultrasonography employs high-frequency sound waves to produce images of internal body structures. During the procedure, the sonographer uses a small handheld transducer that generates sound waves. Internal body organs reflect these sound waves back to the transducer, and a computer processes these signals into images. Ultrasound scans show the size and shape of organs as well as blood flow in some cases; abnormalities in the organ structures and blood flow can be observed if present.

Cancers diagnosed or treated: Almost all types of solid cancers, including those of the breasts, brain and spinal cord, thyroid, bones, gastrointestinal organs (esophagus, stomach, pancreas, liver, colon, and rectum), reproductive organs (ovaries, prostate, and testes), soft tissues (muscles, tendon, and fat), and urinary tract organs (bladder, ureters, and kidneys); hematological cancers such as Hodgkin disease and non-Hodgkin lymphoma

Why performed: Imaging tests are performed in cancer management for many reasons, including screening for the presence or absence of cancer in people who have no symptoms, diagnosing cancer, obtaining image-guided biopsy, staging cancer or evaluating tumor spread, planning a cancer treatment (such as assessing the specific site of a tumor prior to radiation treatment), and evaluating cancer treatment to determine if it is working or whether a tumor has recurred.

Patient preparation: The type of imaging test and use of contrast material will dictate the patient preparation. For example, patients may be instructed not to eat or drink several hours before a CT scan, radionuclide imaging, special X-ray procedures, or ultrasound is performed. If a contrast dye will be used, and depending on what part of the body will be evaluated, then the patient may need to drink the liquid contrast, may need an intravenous (IV) catheter for injection, or may use an enema. The radioactive material for nuclear scans is given by mouth or by injection through an IV line. Standard X rays and mammograms do not require special preparation. The best time for a mammogram is about one week following a menstrual period, when the breasts are least likely to be sensitive. For pediatric patients, the parents need to be counseled on proper preparations for the imaging tests so that the patients' anxiety may be reduced. In emergency cases, preparation for imaging procedures may not be possible.

Steps of the procedure: Imaging tests are often done on an outpatient basis in a hospital or clinic radiology department. The type of radiology test and use of contrast material will dictate the procedure. Generally, the patient will be asked to use a medical examination gown or to undress to expose the body part that needs to be studied. Metallic objects that can interfere with imaging tests will be removed, if possible. The patient may be asked to sit, stand, or lie down depending on the body structure that needs to be evaluated. A certified radiology technologist will guide patients through the steps of the procedure. A radiologist may be present if there is a need to perform a biopsy or provide an intervention; the radiologist will provide the final radiological report with the evaluation and analysis of the images.

Patients undergoing CT scans lie on a flat table attached to a CT scanner that looks like a large doughnut-shaped machine. The table can slide in and out of the hole in the scanner. The X-ray tube and detector are rotated around the patient while images are obtained. The detector takes numerous snapshots of the X-ray beam, and these image slices are processed by a computer to provide the three-dimensional CT scan image.

Patients undergoing MRI scans lie flat on a table that can slide back and forth in the opening of the cylindrical or tunnel-type MRI scanner. The cylinder encloses the patient, causing a feeling of claustrophobia in some patients. During the procedure, the machine makes loud thumping or banging noises that represent the magnetic fields turning on and off. Earplugs or headphones can be used during the procedure. Patients who have metallic implants such as pacemakers, surgical clips or staples, and implanted pumps, IV catheters, or ports for medications should thoroughly discuss the risks and benefits of MRI scans with their physicians. Tattoos and cosmetics can affect MRI images; thus, it is important to inform the radiology technologist about them before the procedure.

Standard radiographic studies are straightforward. The patient will be examined for the specific body structure that is being evaluated, such as the chest or abdomen. Modified X-ray studies using contrast agents such as barium swallow, barium enema, IVP, angiography, and lymphangiography will require provision of the contrast material via oral, injection, or rectal routes prior to the procedure. Angiography and lymphangiography will require diet restriction to only liquid oral intakes before the test; the contrast agent will be injected through an IV line just before the X-ray procedure. Restriction of food intake (no food or drink) for eight to twelve hours prior to barium swallow, barium enema, or IVP will be required; a series of X rays of the upper GI, lower GI, and urinary tract will be obtained during the procedure.

Mammography screening requires exposure of the breasts (undressing from the waist up to the breasts) and removal of jewelry from the neck. Deodorants, ointments, creams, perfumes, and powders should not be used on the day of the mammogram, as these substances can interfere with the breast imaging. The breasts are placed one at a time on a flat surface and compressed during the X-ray imaging; the patient has to hold her breath during this procedure. Additional views of the breasts will be obtained if there is suspicion of breast disease.

Radionuclide imaging requires a patient to lie on a table while the nuclear scanner moves back and forth examining the nuclear activity in the patient's body. Prior to the procedure, a radioactive tracer will be provided to the patient through oral intake or IV injection (for example, two hours before a bone scan or a few days before a gallium scan). The radiopharmaceuticals emit gamma rays during the procedure; these signals are detected by a special gamma camera and transformed by a computer process into a two- or three- dimensional image showing where the tracers are absorbed by the body to a greater or lesser degree.

Ultrasonography is a straightforward examination in which the patient lies flat on a table. The ultrasonographer passes a transducer over the body structure (such as the liver, kidneys, gallbladder, or uterus) that is being evaluated. A gel is applied to the surface of the body above the structure; the gel has a dual purpose—to lubricate the skin to prevent friction and discomfort as well as to improve the transmission of sound waves. In some cases, the transducer is shaped as a probe (as in vaginal ultrasound or prostate evaluation through the rectum). The transducer will be covered with gel before its insertion into the vaginal tract or anorectal passage. These procedures are not painful, but they can cause discomfort and a feeling of pressure.

After the procedure: Generally, no aftercare is required for the imaging tests discussed, and patients can return to normal activities immediately after the procedures. Patients who used contrast dyes may be monitored after the imaging tests to ensure that they have no adverse reactions to the agents used. Patients who ingested radioactive tracers should drink plenty of fluids to aid in their excretion; flushing of the toilet immediately after voiding can also decrease the risk of exposure to radioactivity. Removal of the gel used in ultrasonography is done by the ultrasound technician.

Risks: Strict guidelines are practiced by radiology departments to decrease the risk of radiation exposure in imaging tests. The risk of exposure to X rays is generally exceeded by the benefits. The amount of radiation is low enough that adverse reactions are rare. Mammography also uses such low levels of X rays that any risk from radiation exposure is minimal. CT scan exposure to radiation is higher than that of a standard X ray, but the level of exposure is still low and should not cause adverse effects. The risks of nuclear medicine scans are also minimal. The amount of radiopharmaceuticals used exposes patients to an amount of radiation that is similar to or lower than that of a conventional X ray. The radiotracers are passed out of the body quickly (within a few hours or days); increased fluid intake can facilitate rapid excretion. Close proximity to children and sexual activity should be discussed with the patient's health care team; depending on what radiotracer was used, these activities may be restricted for a short time. Ultrasound is considered free of risks. MRI also poses no risks and does not produce adverse physical effects; however, the effects of MRI on an unborn child are unknown.

Although radiation exposure in imaging tests is minimal and should not produce adverse effects, pregnant patients and mothers who are breast-feeding should discuss the risks and benefits of the imaging tests with their physicians, especially patients who will require ingestion of contrast dyes and radioactive materials. The abdominal region of pregnant patients is protected with a radiation shield when imaging tests are performed during mammography and radiography. Patients who have renal failure or who are allergic to contrast agents and radiopharmaceuticals should also discuss the use of these substances and other imaging test options with their physicians. Patients who have surgically implanted devices such as cardiac pacemakers, surgical aneurysm clips, and other metallic implants in the eyes or ears should inform their physicians about these devices. Because of the strong magnetic field involved, MRI is absolutely contraindicated when these metallic devices are present. If a biopsy or other invasive techniques are performed, then the risks will include infection and bleeding at the site of intervention.

Results: Normal results will show no structural abnormalities in the imaging tests. Abnormal findings will include masses, tumors, abnormal presence of blood or fluids, enlarged organs, and structural anomalies (such as unusual shape, size, borders, or function). The radiologist determines whether the structures are normal or abnormal and will send a formal report to the physician about these findings.

Alex B. Cantrell, B.A., and
Miriam E. Schwartz, M.D., M.A., Ph.D.

For Further Information

American Cancer Society. *Imaging.* Atlanta: Author, 2007.

Beers, Mark H., et al., eds. *The Merck Manual of Medical Information, Second Home Edition.* Whitehouse Station, N.J.: Merck Research Laboratories, 2003.

Brinton Wolbarst, Anthony. *Looking Within: How X-Ray, CT, MRI, Ultrasound, and Other Medical Images Are Created and How They Help Physicians Save Lives.* Berkeley: University of California Press, 1999.

D'Amico, Anthony V., Jay S. Loeffler, and Jay R. Harris, eds. *Image-Guided Diagnosis and Treatment of Cancer.* Totowa, N.J.: Humana Press, 2003.

Hayat, M. A., ed. *Cancer Imaging, Volume 1: Lung and Breast Carcinomas.* Oxford, England: Elsevier Academic Press, 2007.

_______. *Cancer Imaging, Volume 2: Instrumentation and Applications.* Oxford, England: Elsevier Academic Press, 2007.

Kevles, Bettyann. *Naked to the Bone: Medical Imaging in the Twentieth Century.* New Brunswick, N.J.: Rutgers University Press, 1997.

Other Resources

American Cancer Society
http://www.cancer.org

National Cancer Institute
http://www.cancer.gov

See also: Angiography; Bone scan; Brain scan; Bronchography; Computed Tomography (CT)-guided biopsy; Computed Tomography (CT) scan; Cystography; Ductogram; Endoscopic Retrograde Cholangiopancreatography (ECRP); Gallium scan; Hysterography; Lymphangiography; Magnetic Resonance Imaging (MRI); Mammography; Nuclear medicine scan; Percutaneous Transhepatic Cholangiography (PTHC); Positron Emission Tomography (PET); Radionuclide scan; Thermal imaging; Thyroid nuclear medicine scan; Urography; X-ray tests

▶ Immunochemical Fecal Occult Blood Test (iFOBT)

Category: Procedures
Also known as: Fecal immunochemical test (FIT)

Definition: An immunochemical fecal occult blood test (iFOBT) is a method for the qualitative detection of a minute amount in the feces of otherwise invisible blood from the lower gastrointestinal tract.

Cancers diagnosed: Colorectal cancers

Why performed: The iFOBT is a screening test for bleeding associated with cancer of the colon and rectum.

The bleeding may be attributable to conditions other than cancer such as polyps and adenomas, which when discovered and removed early can significantly reduce the risk of cancer.

Although the incidence of colorectal cancer has decreased in the United States since the 1980's, the colon is still the third most common site of all cancers. The decrease in cancer cases is attributed to screening for fecal occult blood. The immunochemical fecal occult blood test uses an antibody specific for human globins and is more specific than the traditional guaiac test, which detects the heme subunit of mammalian hemoglobin and requires the patient to adhere to dietary and medication restrictions three days prior to testing.

Patient preparation: The patient collects the specimen at home. No dietary or medication restrictions are required prior to sample collection. Blood from hemorrhoids, menstrual blood, or open wounds may invalidate the screening for fecal occult blood. Because bleeding from polyps or other potential lesions is typically intermittent, the patient may be asked to perform collection on three consecutive days.

Steps of the procedure: Two collection procedures are available, depending on which manufacturer provides the diagnostic kit. Both require the patient to follow the instructions provided with the kit.

One company provides a collection paper that is taped to the toilet seat and onto which the feces is deposited. The patient unscrews the sampling device from the collection tube and randomly pierces the specimen with the grooved end of the device in at least five different sites of the feces. The sampler is then screwed in the collection tube and tightened. The patient shakes the tube to mix the specimen with the buffer solution in the collection tube.

The second manufacturer provides two sampling pads that are inoculated with a sampling of toilet water collected after a bowel movement and brushed on the test card provided.

After collection, the sample from either kit is sent to the clinical lab and the results are reported to the ordering physician.

After the procedure: Positive results are often followed by an endoscopic evaluation such as a colonoscopy.

Risks: One of the risks in iFOBT is a false result because of improper sample collection, as patients may have an understandable aversion to handling a fecal sample. However, an adequate and carefully collected sample is the first critical step in detecting colorectal bleeding, which may be the first sign that the individual is facing disease. Early detection and treatment is the key to the prevention of colorectal cancer.

Results: The iFOBT is a screening test. Positive results must be evaluated and followed by a physician to determine the source of the bleeding. Gastrointestinal bleeding may be the result of diverticulitis, colitis, polyps, or colorectal cancer.

Jane Adrian, M.P.H., Ed.M., M.T. (ASCP)

See also: Asian Americans and cancer; Colonoscopy and virtual colonoscopy; Colorectal cancer; Colorectal cancer screening; Digital Rectal Exam (DRE); Fecal Occult Blood Test (FOBT); Gastrointestinal cancers; Hereditary polyposis syndromes; Medicare and cancer; Polyps; Premalignancies; Primary care physician; Screening for cancer; Small intestine cancer

▶ Immunoelectrophoresis (IEP)

Category: Procedures

Also known as: Gamma globulin electrophoresis,- immunoglobulin electrophoresis

Definition: Immunoelectrophoresis (IEP) is a semiquantitative method used in clinical and research laboratories to determine the levels of three major immunoglobulins in the blood: immunoglobulin M (IgM), immunoglobulin G (IgG), and immunoglobulin (IgA). This test is often replaced by the quantitative immunofixation (IFE) test in clinical laboratories for diagnostic purposes.

Cancers diagnosed: Multiple myeloma, chronic lymphocytic leukemia, Waldenström macroglobulinemia

Why performed: An IEP test is often performed when the immunoglobulins are increased in a serum protein electrophoresis test.

Patient preparation: The IEP test may be performed on urine, cerebrospinal fluid (CSF), or the serum obtained from a blood specimen collected by routine venipuncture.

Steps of the procedure: The specimen is placed in a well on a slide prepared with a semi-solid gel. An electric current is passed through the gel. The current causes the different serum proteins to separate according to their varying electric charges. An antiserum is placed in a trough alongside the separated immunoglobulins. The antibodies in the antisera attach to the specific immunoglobulins. This reaction is measured, and relative quantities of IgM, IgG, and IgA per deciliter of patient serum are reported to the ordering physician.

After the procedure: The physician may order an immunofixation test to further quantify the IgM, IgG, and IgA.

Risks: There are no risks to this procedure other than those associated with specimen collection. Because the IEP test results may be applied to a large number of conditions, follow-up tests are necessary for a differential diagnosis.

Results: While some cancer diagnoses are associated with elevated immunoglobulins, increased immunoglobulins can also suggest recent vaccinations or treatment with hydralazine, isoniazid, phenytoin (Dilantin), procainamide, oral contraceptives, methadone, steroids, therapeutic gamma globulin, or tetanus toxoid and antitoxin. Consequently, immunoelectrophoresis test results must be interpreted in the context of the patient's history and clinician judgment.

IEP test results demonstrating elevated or decreased IgM, IgG, or IgA levels may indicate a wide variety of conditions.

Increased IgM may point to Waldenström macroglobulinemia, an increased secretion of IgM caused by malignant lymphocytes, chronic infections such as hepatitis, mononucleosis, and autoimmune diseases such as rheumatoid arthritis. Decreased IgM may suggest acquired immunodeficiency (HIV/AIDS), immunosuppression caused by steroids, or leukemia.

Increased IgG may indicate chronic liver disease, autoimmune diseases, hyperimmunization reactions, or chronic infections, such as tuberculosis or sarcoidosis. Decreased IgG can indicate Wiskott-Aldrich syndrome, HIV/AIDS, or leukemia.

Increased IgA can point to chronic liver disease, chronic infections, or inflammatory bowel disease. Decreased IgA is seen in ataxia-telangiectasia, low blood protein (hypoproteinemia), and drug-induced immunosuppression.

Jane Adrian, M.P.H., Ed.M., M.T. (ASCP)

See also: Chronic Lymphocytic Leukemia (CLL); Lactate Dehydrogenase (LDH) test; Multiple myeloma; Protein electrophoresis; Waldenström Macroglobulinemia (WM)

▶ Infusion therapies

Category: Procedures
Also known as: Central line infusions, intravenous therapy, parenteral therapy

Definition: Infusion therapy is a medical procedure for the insertion of fluid, medication (such as chemotherapy, pain medications, or antibiotics), and nutrients or vitamins into the body. Fluid can be inserted either through a vein (intravenously), into a muscle (intramuscularly), into the tissue of the spinal cord (intraspinally), or under the skin (subcutaneously). Infusion therapies for cancers are typically used for pain medications, chemotherapy, and antibiotics.

Cancers treated: Cancers that require chemotherapy or pain management, as directed by a physician

Why performed: Infusion therapy is performed to provide the rapid delivery of medication, fluid, or nutrients to a patient.

Patient preparation: Patients are requested to remain hydrated before and after infusion therapy, particularly when administered chemotherapy. Sugar consumption should be limited during this time frame. Many patients are recommended to participate in a low-impact stress relief program while undergoing infusion therapy.

Steps of the procedure: Infusions can be performed in a clinical setting or at home. A catheter (a thin plastic tube that covers a needle) is typically inserted into either the hand or the arm of the patient. Once the catheter has been inserted, the needle is removed and the tube remains. The fluid to be inserted is administered at a predefined rate (either "pushed" at intervals or steadily) from an infusion bag that contains the solution. The type of catheter used depends upon the length of infusion time.

An intravenous port can also be inserted into the patient's chest to provide easy access for infusion therapy, if the therapy is required frequently.

After the procedure: Infusion therapy is typically an outpatient procedure. Patients should pay close attention to the injection site to watch for possible infusion-related reactions. Any unexpected or serious reactions should be reported to a doctor immediately. Chemotherapy can cause a variety of side effects following administration, particularly nausea and fatigue.

Risks: Infusion therapy can lead to skin reactions including rash, bruising, burns, and tenderness, as well as fluid leakage at the site of injection. Furthermore, infusion therapy has a risk of sepsis, infection, occlusion of the catheter (partial or complete obstruction), and overdose. Chemotherapy can cause hair loss, fatigue, nausea, diarrhea, and fever.

Results: Infusion therapies provide an effective, direct administration of fluids into the vascular system of the body.

Anna Perez, M.Sc.

See also: Antidiarrheal agents; Antifungal therapies; Antiviral therapies; Autologous blood transfusion; Biological therapy; Bone Marrow Transplantation (BMT); Chemotherapy; Colony-Stimulating Factors (CSFs); Gene therapy; Hemolytic anemia; Hepatic Arterial Infusion (HAI); Herbs as antioxidants; HIV/AIDS-related cancers; Home health services; Interleukins; Leukapharesis; Lymphangiography; Magnetic Resonance Imaging (MRI); Monoclonal antibodies; Neurologic oncology; Pneumonectomy; Prevention; Stem cell transplantation; Topoisomerase inhibitors; Transfusion therapy; Transitional care; Tyrosine kinase inhibitors

▶ Intensity-Modulated Radiation Therapy (IMRT)

Category: Procedures

Definition: Intensity-modulated radiation therapy (IMRT) is a cancer treatment that allows the precise delivery of higher doses of radiation to the cancer while protecting the normal tissue surrounding the tumor.

Cancers treated: Cancers of the breast, head and neck, lung, prostate, liver, female reproductive system, and brain; lymphomas

Why performed: IMRT enables radiation oncologists to deliver radiation to areas of the body that may be difficult to treat, or to reach tumors that may be located near vital organs and that cannot be treated surgically. Since IMRT allows higher doses of radiation to be given directly to the tumor and avoids normal tissue, there are fewer side effects than with traditional external radiation therapy.

IMRT provides a more precise, conformed radiation dose to be delivered to the tumor area by controlling the intensity of the radiation beam within a given area. Radiation beams can be turned on or off or can be blocked during treatment, varying the beam intensity across the targeted field. The radiation beam or beams may be moved hundreds of times, with each beam having a different intensity. Using IMRT allows for lower doses of radiation to be delivered to one area of the tumor while higher doses may be delivered to another area.

Patient preparation: There are no special preparations prior to IMRT treatment.

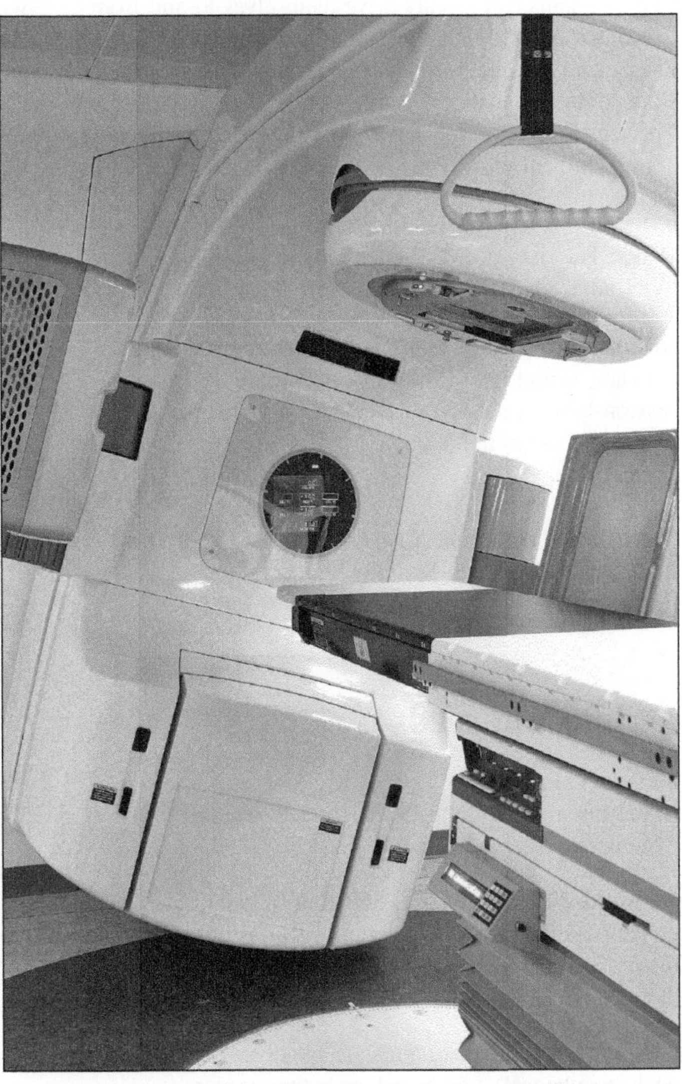

An intensity-modulated radiation therapy scanner. (iStock)

Steps of the procedure: Approximately one to two weeks prior to treatment, a radiation oncologist evaluates the patient. A staging computed tomography (CT) scan is done to identify the three-dimensional shape of the tumor. This information is used to plan the dose and shape of the radiation beam(s) for treatment. Other tests may also be needed.

The radiation oncologist works with a dosimetrist, who calculates the dosage, and a medical physicist to ensure that the radiation is delivered to the exact tumor area location. The area where the beam will be directed is usually temporarily tattooed on the patient's skin with ink, which will help the radiologist each time the IMRT is given to the patient. IMRT usually takes fifteen to thirty minutes.

After the procedure: IMRT is given on an outpatient basis. Patients can usually drive themselves to and from treatment. After IMRT, the patient may experience some fatigue and, depending on the area of treatment, may have some redness on the skin over the area being treated. These effects are temporary and will subside a few weeks after treatment ends. Patients may also want to discuss taking vitamin supplements with their physician.

Risks: The risks of IMRT affecting normal tissue and arteries adjacent to the tumor are minimal.

Results: The goal of IMRT is to reduce tumor size and alleviate symptoms. IMRT involves multiple treatment sessions over a number of weeks or months, depending on the success of the results.

Jo Gambosi, M.A., B.S.N.

See also: Mayo Clinic Cancer Center; Medulloblastomas; Memorial Sloan-Kettering Cancer Center; Radiation therapies

▶ Iridium seeds

Category: Procedures
Also known as: Iridium 192, high-dose-rate (HDR) or temporary brachytherapy

Definition: Iridium seeds are high-dose radiation sources temporarily placed into a tumor site in order to stop the growth of cancer cells or to relieve symptoms without damaging normal tissue.

Cancers treated: Breast, prostate, gynecologic, head and neck, esophageal, lung, rectal, and other cancers

Why performed: Internal radiation used to kill cancer cells at the site of a tumor provides effective local cell death and discourages regrowth. Using iridium seeds delivers a higher dose of radiation directly to the tumor, protects normal tissue, and allows outpatient care with shorter, more comfortable treatments and fewer side effects.

Patient preparation: Before the procedure, patients will have imaging studies such as X rays, a computed tomography (CT) scan, ultrasound, or magnetic resonance imaging (MRI) to decide where the iridium seeds should be placed to work best. Patients may have other tests such as blood work or electrocardiography (EKG). If seeds are to be placed in the prostate, then an enema and bowel cleansing routine is used. Some sites require only local anesthesia, while others may require general anesthesia and surgery. Patients should receive clear directions from a doctor or nurse based on the site of treatment before the procedure.

Steps of the procedure: A treatment plan is developed by the doctor and the radiation therapy staff. A needle, catheter, or balloon catheter is placed in the site when patients are either asleep or the area has been numbed to ensure that there is no pain. An iridium seed is sent through the catheter by a computerized machine called a high dose remote afterloader; it is left in the tumor for a few minutes and then removed. Treatments can be once or twice a day and the number varies by site.

After the procedure: Once all treatments are complete, the catheters will be removed gently, usually without difficulty or discomfort. It is safe for patients to be around others, including children and pregnant women, because no radiation remains in the body.

Risks: The side effects depend on the site treated but may include urinary symptoms, rectal symptoms, fatigue, eating problems, shortness of breath, pain, redness, and swelling.

Results: Iridium seeds for high-dose brachytherapy appear to be as effective as other methods of prostate cancer treatments. Their use in the treatment of breast cancer is newer, but early data show control of cancer cells at the local site equal to that of other treatments. Other diseases report equally effective results with good local control as compared to other treatments.

Patricia Stanfill Edens, R.N., Ph.D., FACHE

See also: Afterloading radiation therapy; Brachytherapy; Neurologic oncology; Radiation oncology

▶ Ki67 test

Category: Procedures
Also known as: Ki67 proliferation index

Definition: The Ki67 protein is present in actively dividing cells. It is expressed during all phases of the cell cycle, except for G0 (known as the resting phase). The Ki67 test detects Ki67 in tumors using an immune-based assay, which identifies the dividing cells.

Cancers diagnosed or treated: Primarily breast and prostate cancers

Why performed: High Ki67 levels correlate with more aggressive tumors. Characterizing the proliferation rates of tumors via Ki67 expression can help determine what kind of treatment a patient should receive. The Ki67 test can also be used to examine whether a patient has responded to therapy by evaluating changes in cellular proliferation.

Patient preparation: A biopsy is performed to obtain tumor tissue for the Ki67 test. Biopsies can be done either with a needle or through surgery, depending on the size and location of the tumor. If general anesthesia is required for surgery, then the patient must fast prior to the biopsy.

Steps of the procedure: Tumor tissue collected from the biopsy will be sliced very thin and then fixed to a microscope slide. Ki67 will be detected by a method called immunohistochemistry, in which antibodies are used to bind to tumor cells expressing Ki67, and then the cells are stained with a colored reagent to identify Ki67+ cells. The tumor sample is examined under a microscope, where cells are counted using an eyepiece grid. Approximately five hundred to two thousand cells are counted and marked as either Ki67+ or Ki67−.

After the procedure: After a needle biopsy, pressure will be applied at the injection site to stop bleeding. For an open biopsy requiring general anesthesia, the patient will have blood pressure and pulse monitored prior to discharge from the hospital. Transport home must be provided. Open biopsies may also require bed rest for up to twenty-four hours after the procedure, and heavy lifting should be avoided for at least two weeks to allow the incision to heal.

Risks: Because the Ki67 test is an *ex vivo* assay (meaning "outside of the body"), the only risks are those associated with the biopsy, which include bleeding and infection. Open biopsies may also have risks associated with the surgery (such as scarring) and the anesthesia (such as allergic reactions and changes in blood pressure or heart rate).

Results: Results are reported as a percentage using this equation: ([number of Ki67 + cells / total number of tumor cells] × 100). There is no established cutoff to define a high Ki67 proliferation index, but approximately 20 to 30 percent is a common result to be deemed positive.

Elizabeth A. Manning, PhD.

See also: Biopsy; Immunocytochemistry and immunohistochemistry; Tumor markers

▶ Lactate Dehydrogenase (LDH) test

Category: Procedures
Also known as: Lactic acid dehydrogenase, L-lactate: NAD + oxidoreductase

Definition: Lactate dehydrogenase (LDH) is a ubiquitous intracellular enzyme that catalyzes the interconversion of pyruvate and lactate. In oncology it is used as a serum marker of cell damage or turnover. The enzyme is a tetramer of H (heart) and/or M (muscle) subunits, allowing five possible isoenzyme forms: LDH-1 (H4), LDH-2 (H3M1), LDH-3 (H2M2), LDH-4 (H1M3), and LDH-5 (M4).

Cancers diagnosed: Malignancies causing effusions, germ-cell tumors, and other tumors with high cell turnover

Why performed: Serum LDH is elevated in many non-neoplastic diseases. In oncology, its concentration may be determined to estimate the stage of disease and prognosis in several cancers, such as non-Hodgkin lymphoma, myeloma, disseminated melanoma, and metastatic prostate carcinoma. The ratio of serum LDH to LDH concentration in pleural, peritoneal, or pericardial effusions can help distinguish benign from malignant processes; high LDH concentrations in effusion fluid suggest the presence of cancer. Because the five isoenzymes have characteristic relative abundances in different tissues, determination can assist in the diagnosis of several tumors.

Patient preparation: No fasting or other special preparation on the part of the patient is necessary for this simple blood test.

Steps of the procedure: After the blood sample is collected, serum is isolated by centrifugation and the activity of the enzyme is measured in either the forward direction (oxidation of lactate and NAD+ to pyruvate, NADH, and H+) or the reverse direction. In the forward reaction, the rate of appearance of NADH can be followed spectrophotometrically because it strongly absorbs ultraviolet (UV) light at 340 nM; NAD+ does not. The enzyme activity is calculated by comparing the rate of NADH appearance in the patient sample to rates obtained from standard preparations. If the cause of elevated LDH cannot be determined by other means, then the isoenzymes can be separated by electrophoresis, with LDH-1 (all H subunits) migrating fastest, followed in order by LDH-2 through LDH-5. LDH can also be visualized in tissue sections by immunohistochemistry.

After the procedure: No special aftercare is required other than monitoring the blood collection site for signs of infection until healed.

Risks: There are no risks to the patient. High false positive rates are seen in patients with other systemic illnesses.

Results: Abnormally high LDH values and abnormal isoenzyme patterns are seen in many different diseases and must be interpreted in the light of the clinical history and other laboratory results. Results for enzyme activity obtained with different methods are not interchangeable. In oncology, abrupt increases in LDH indicate an unfavorable prognosis in terminally ill patients. The LDH-1 isoenzyme is reliably elevated in germ-cell tumors (teratoma, seminoma, or ovarian dysgerminoma) and can serve as a tumor marker. In leukemia, lymphoma, and multiple myeloma, LDH-3 and LDH-4 are often elevated. Elevated LDH-5 in colorectal cancer is strongly associated with poor survival.

John B. Welsh, M.D., Ph.D.

See also: Germ-cell tumors; Multiple myeloma; Non-Hodgkin lymphoma; Paracentesis; Testicular cancer; Tumor markers

▶ Laparoscopy and laparoscopic surgery

Category: Procedures
Also known as: Keyhole surgery, minimally invasive surgery (MIS), pinhole surgery

Definition: Laparoscopy is a procedure that allows doctors to look inside the abdominal or pelvic cavities using a small tube attached to a camera and video monitor. This procedure has been used since 1973 to diagnose and to treat various conditions, including certain types of cancer.

Cancers diagnosed or treated: Cervical, colorectal, gallbladder, kidney, liver, ovarian, pancreatic, prostate, stomach, and uterine cancers

Why performed: There is some evidence that laparoscopy may involve less risk than open abdominal surgery because it uses only a small incision in the abdomen. Although the procedure can take longer than conventional surgery, some studies report that patients recover more quickly from laparoscopy and have a lower risk of infections.

Patient preparation: No food or liquids are allowed for twelve hours before the procedure, and medical staff will ensure that the patient's bladder and colon are empty. The hospital may provide specific instructions to help patients prepare for the procedure.

Steps of the procedure: Patients usually are given general anesthesia, but sometimes other types of anesthesia may be used. Following anesthesia, when the patient is unconscious, the abdominal area is cleaned and shaved. A small tube (catheter) may be inserted through the urethra into the bladder to collect urine that may be discharged during the procedure. A cannula may be inserted through the vagina into the uterus of a female patient to help doctors move the uterus and ovaries and obtain a better view of other organs. Then a short incision (0.5 to 1.0 inch) is made, usually in the navel area. A hollow needle is inserted into this incision, and gas (either carbon dioxide or nitrous oxide) is slowly pumped through the needle. The gas inflates the abdominal cavity, lifting it away from the organs, to allow doctors to see the organs clearly. Next, a thin tube (a laparoscope) is inserted through the incision into the abdominal cavity. A camera located on the eyepiece of this tube transmits images to a video monitor, enabling the surgeon to see into the abdominal and pelvic areas. Other small incisions may be made in the abdomen to insert instruments used to remove organs or collect tissue samples. In some cases, the surgeon also may be assisted by a robotic arm. When the procedure is finished, the scope is removed and the gas is released from the abdominal cavity. The incision is closed, usually with stitches that dissolve within several days.

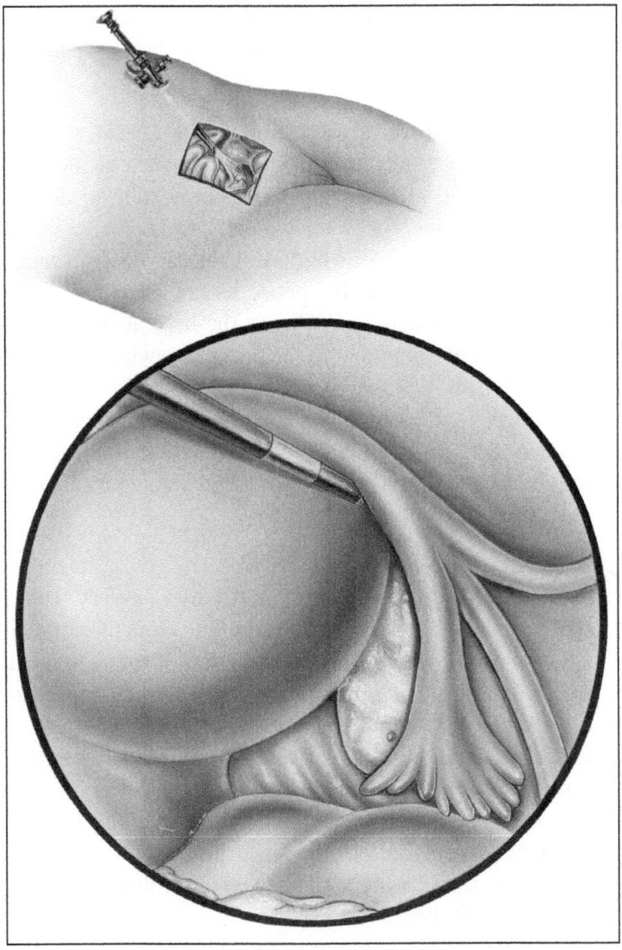

Laparoscopy. (iStock)

New hand-access devices can now enable surgeons to place a hand into the abdomen during laparoscopy and use it for different functions, which used to be possible only with open abdominal surgery.

After the procedure: Depending on the procedures performed and their outcomes, patients either return home or remain in the hospital. Patients may feel some abdominal bloating or shoulder pain, caused by the effects of the gas on the diaphragm. Patients should contact their doctor if they experience bleeding, redness, swelling, or discharge at the incision site or if they develop a fever, hoarseness that lasts more than a few days, or severe abdominal pain.

Risks: The risks and benefits of this procedure are still being studied. The laparoscopic procedure is technically complex for the surgeon because it involves restricted vision, a limited working area, and hand-eye coordination when working with the instruments. The risks for the patient may include infection in the abdominal cavity, damage to internal organs, failure to remove the cancerous tissue or organs completely, or damage to blood vessels that causes internal bleeding. Patients with existing lung problems may not be able to tolerate the increased carbon dioxide in the abdominal cavity.

Deciding whether to use laparoscopy rather than open abdominal surgery to diagnose and treat certain cancers (for example, ovarian cancer) should be made according to the patient's overall risk factors as determined by additional tests, such as ultrasound. Open abdominal surgery allows the doctor to look inside organs for tumors and to remove cancerous organs or tissue during the same procedure. There are concerns that laparoscopy may limit doctors' ability to completely detect and or remove such tissue, and it is important that patients discuss these concerns with their doctors. Research shows that the length of hospital stay and risk for infection are reduced with laparoscopy, but also that the success of the procedure is dependent upon the training and skill of the surgeon.

Results: The results of laparoscopy vary according to the procedures performed and the type and stage of cancer. The scar from the incision is very small and should heal quickly, depending on the patient's general health.

Amy J. Neil, M.S., M.A.P.

For Further Information

Hamad, G. G., M. T. Brown, and J. A. Clavijo-Alvarez. "Postoperative Video Debriefing Reduces Technical Errors in Laparoscopic Surgery." *American Journal of Surgery* 194 (2007): 110-114.

Huscher, C. G., et al. "Laparoscopic Versus Open Subtotal Gastrectomy for Distal Gastric Cancer: Five-Year Results of a Randomized Prospective Trial." *Annals of Surgery* 241, no. 2 (2005): 232-237.

Meadows, Michelle. "Robots Lend a Helping Hand to Surgeons." *FDA Consumer* 36 (2002).

Shehzad, K., et al. "Current Status of Minimal Access Surgery for Gastric Cancer." *Surgical Oncology* 16, no. 2 (June 6, 2007): 85-98.

Other Resources

WebMD

Laparoscopic Abdominoperineal Resection
Laparoscopic Proctosigmoidectomy
Prostate Cancer: Laparoscopic Prostate Surgery
Risks of Hysterectomy
Surgery to Treat Colorectal Cancer
http://www.webmd.com

See also: Abdominoperineal Resection (APR); Biopsy; Cholecystectomy; Colectomy; Colorectal cancer; Colostomy; Culdoscopy; Endoscopy; Exenteration; Fallopian tube cancer; Gastrointestinal oncology; Hematologic oncology; Hereditary Leiomyomatosis and Renal Cell Cancer (HLRCC); Hysterectomy; Hystero-oophorectomy; Hysteroscopy; Infertility and cancer; Kidney cancer; Liver biopsy; Liver cancers; Mediastinal tumors; Medical oncology; Mesothelioma; Oophorectomy; Ovarian cancers; Ovarian cysts; Pancreatic cancers; Pediatric oncology and hematology; Pheochromocytomas; Pleural biopsy; Prostatectomy; Salpingectomy and salpingo-oophorectomy; Splenectomy; Surgical biopsies; Urinary system cancers

▶ Laryngectomy

Category: Procedures
Also known as: Hemilaryngectomy, vertical partial laryngectomy, total laryngectomy

Definition: Laryngectomy is the surgical removal of some or all of the larynx (voice box). Total laryngectomy removes the entire structure, whereas partial laryngectomy involves removal of only sections of the larynx.

Cancers treated: Primary or recurrent cancer of the larynx, tumors metastasized to the larynx from other parts of the body

Why performed: Laryngectomy is performed when tumors and cancers prevent normal larynx function and threaten to invade other tissues of the head and neck. Partial laryngectomy is performed for early-stage cancers (T1 and T2 stages). Total laryngectomy is performed for advanced cancers (stages T3 and T4) and when cancer recurs after radiation therapy or more conservative surgical treatments.

Patient preparation: Apart from the usual presurgery blood and heart tests, patients may undergo a battery of other tests. To determine the extent of spread and permit staging of the cancer, patients will undergo computed tomography (CT) or magnetic resonance imaging (MRI) scans. They may have chest X rays to rule out the spread of cancer in the lungs and barium swallows to determine if the cancer has invaded the esophagus. Patients will also have tests to determine if they have sufficient lung function to cough; coughing is necessary to remove secretions from the airway and prevent aspiration of food and liquids into the lungs. Patients undergoing total laryngectomy will meet with a speech therapist before the surgery to discuss options for artificial voice restoration. Some patients may undergo radiation therapy prior to surgery.

Steps of the procedure: Following anesthesia, the surgeon will make an incision into the trachea at the base of the throat and insert a tracheostomy tube to deliver air into the lungs. An extensive incision is created in the neck, and the cancerous region of the larynx is excised. In total laryngectomy, the entire larynx is removed and the end of the trachea is sewn to the hole at the base of the throat. The opening into the throat is sewn shut, which means that the esophagus no longer has any connection to the airway. Depending on the extent of the cancer, patients undergoing partial or total laryngectomy may also require removal of portions of the esophagus, thyroid gland, or lymph nodes.

After the procedure: Patients will stay in the intensive care unit (ICU) for one to two days after surgery. Tubes will be inserted in the neck to drain fluid from the surgical site, which will prevent blood clots from forming that can impair healing. Patients will still have the tracheostomy tube in place to help them breathe. In partial laryngectomy, once swelling in the airway has subsided, the tube is removed and the hole at the base of the throat is sealed. In total laryngectomy, this hole, called a stoma, remains permanently open after tube removal. Patients who have undergone total laryngectomy breathe through the stoma for the rest of their lives.

For several days after surgery, patients will also have a tube threaded through a nostril and down the esophagus to permit the delivery of liquids and nourishment into the stomach. This tube will stay in place until the swelling in the throat subsides and the patient is able to swallow without aspirating.

Patients usually spend seven to ten days in the hospital, although convalescence continues at home and may take many weeks. During the hospital stay, partial laryngectomy patients will learn new swallowing techniques to prevent aspiration. Total laryngectomy patients will begin working with a speech therapist on an alternative method of voicing.

Risks: Laryngectomy patients are at risk for pulmonary embolism, heart attack, and stroke. Risks related to the surgery include infection, impaired wound healing, tissue necrosis, and respiratory problems as a result of aspiration or narrowing of the airway. Aspiration pneumonia is a common postsurgical complication of partial laryngectomy until the patient relearns how to swallow. Total laryngectomy patients are not at risk for aspiration because the throat is no longer connected to the airway; however, they may still experience problems swallowing because of impaired motility or narrowing of the esophagus. A common complication of total laryngectomy is development of a pharyngocutaneous fistula, which is an opening that causes saliva to drain from the throat into the neck. Fistulas increase the risk of infection and hemorrhage from carotid artery rupture.

Results: The primary goal of laryngectomy is to eliminate the cancer, with secondary goals of retaining voice function and swallowing capability. Cure rates after laryngectomy depend on the cancer location and stage and whether metastasis to the neck has occurred. Generally, cancers detected at the T1 and T2 stages have cure rates of 80 to 95 percent. For advanced cancers, cure rates are 25 to 50 percent. Cure rates at any stage are lower if laryngectomy must be performed because cancer has recurred.

Partial laryngectomy patients who experience ongoing difficulties with aspiration may require either total laryngectomy or placement of a gastrotomy feeding tube. When one or both vocal cords are preserved, the voice will be functional but altered. Total laryngectomy patients must undergo postsurgery therapy to learn new ways of voicing. These patients must also learn to how care for their stomas to prevent infection and entry of foreign materials into the lungs.

Pamela S. Cooper, Ph.D.

For Further Information

Casper, Janina K., and Raymond H. Colton. *Clinical Manual for Laryngectomy and Head/Neck Cancer Rehabilitation*. 2d ed. San Diego, Calif.: Singular, 1998.

Lawson, Glenda. "Upper Airway Problems." In *Medical-Surgical Nursing*, edited by Wilma J. Phipps et al. 7th ed. St. Louis: Mosby, 2003.

National Cancer Institute. *Laryngeal Cancer (PDQ) Treatment*. Washington, D.C.: Author. Available online at http://www.cancer.gov.

Other Resources

American Cancer Society
http://www.cancer.org

International Association of Laryngectomees
http://www.larynxlink.com

See also: Cordectomy; Electrolarynx; Esophageal speech; Laryngeal cancer; Oral and maxillofacial surgery; Throat cancer

▶ Laryngoscopy

Category: Procedures
Also known as: Autoscopy, laryngeal endoscopy

Definition: Laryngoscopy is the visual examination of the voice box (larynx) using a long-handled mirror or rigid or flexible tube (indirect) or a laryngoscope (direct).

Cancers diagnosed or treated: Cancer of the larynx

Why performed: Indirect and direct laryngoscopy are both diagnostic. Direct laryngoscopy is used for close-up, comprehensive examination, biopsy, and surgery.

Patient preparation: Indirect laryngoscopy is performed in the doctor's office and requires no advance preparation. Patients must remove dentures just prior to the examination. Direct laryngoscopy is performed under anesthesia, so the patient must not eat or drink several hours beforehand. Blood tests may be required several days before the procedure to confirm that anesthesia poses no risk.

Steps of the procedure: For indirect laryngoscopy, the patient sits facing the physician. The physician sprays a topical anesthetic on the patient's tongue and throat prior to inserting the mirror or rigid telescope into the mouth. If a flexible fiber-optic tube is used for viewing, then the nose is sprayed with topical anesthetic/decongestant before the physician threads the tube through a nostril and into the throat.

In direct laryngoscopy, the patient is anesthetized lying face up to allow insertion of laryngoscope into the throat. Anesthesia is delivered via a line inserted into a vein. The throat and larynx are sprayed with topical anesthetic prior to insertion of a small breathing tube followed by the laryngoscope.

After the procedure: Laryngoscopy is usually performed on an outpatient basis. If extensive surgery is also performed, however, then an overnight hospital stay may be necessary. Patients who have biopsy or surgery with laryngoscopy may experience hoarseness, and slight bleeding is normal. After surgery, patients may be advised not to smoke, to rest the voice, and to avoid coughing or throat clearing.

Risks: Laryngoscopy is a generally safe procedure. Rare complications of direct laryngoscopy are excessive swelling or spasm of the larynx, which are medical emergencies if breathing is hindered. The most common side effects caused by laryngoscope insertion are sore throat, gums, lips, or tongue. Tongue numbness may occur, but feeling usually returns in a few weeks. Rarely, introduction of the laryngoscope may chip a tooth.

Results: Normal vocal cords are symmetrical and move freely. If cancer is present, then cord movement may be reduced or absent on one side or cords may appear asymmetrical. Normal tissues appear pink and smooth. Raised, irregular white or red lesions or ulcerated, bleeding masses are suspicious. Biopsy and pathology are necessary to determine whether lesions are cancerous.

Pamela S. Cooper, Ph.D.

See also: Cordectomy; Endoscopy; Gastrointestinal cancers; Laryngeal cancer; Laryngeal nerve palsy; Otolaryngology; Throat cancer

▶ Laser therapies

Category: Procedures

Definition: Laser therapies use light amplification by the stimulated emission of radiation (LASER) instead of or in addition to other treatment options. Some laser therapies are widely accepted, while many are still considered experimental.

Cancers treated: Many types of cancers, including skin, eye, colon, lung, esophageal, vaginal, and liver cancers

Why performed: There are many reasons that laser therapy may be performed on a cancer patient. Some laser therapies are done in place of surgery, with the goal of destroying some or all of a tumor. In other cases, laser therapy may be used to shrink a tumor to provide relief from symptoms and improve quality of life. Laser therapy may also be done to activate photosensitizing chemicals in cancer cells to start a chemical reaction that kills the cells.

Patient preparation: The patient preparation required for laser therapy varies depending on the procedure being performed. The patient may be required to avoid eating or drinking fluids for a certain amount of time or may be given antibiotics to help prevent infection. A patient undergoing photodynamic laser therapy will be given a photosensitizing chemical a specified number of hours or days before the procedure is scheduled to be performed. The photosensitizing chemical is usually injected but can be applied topically in some cases.

Steps of the procedure: The actual steps differ depending on the type of procedure; the type of laser used; the size, type, and extent of the cancer; and the preferences of the surgeon performing the procedure. The first step of photodynamic therapy is usually to expose, or mostly expose, the tumor or area of cancerous cells, or to introduce the laser to the area using an endoscope. This is necessary because many of the lasers used to activate photosensitizing chemicals cannot travel safely through thick amounts of skin, tissue, or membrane. Therefore the laser must be very near the cells that it is going to activate. The laser is then directed toward the tumor or cancerous area and turned on for a short period of time. The endoscope or other instrument is then removed. This procedure can be repeated as necessary.

When the laser is being used to shrink a tumor, the laser light must also be able to reach the tumor without having to travel through normal, healthy cells that would be damaged. This is often achieved using an endoscope. The endoscope is introduced to the area of the tumor, and the laser is directed. The beam from the laser heats up the tumor cells to a point hot enough to kill them. After the desired amount of cancer cells have been killed, or it is no longer feasible to treat additional cells without harming surrounding healthy tissue, the endoscope is removed.

Laser surgery is generally done in much the same way as traditional surgery; however, instead of a scalpel, the surgeon uses a laser to make cuts. Lasers are preferable to scalpels in some cases because of their ability to make very thin, fine cuts, allowing the surgeon to work with increased precision. The laser beam also tends to seal and sterilize blood vessels as it cuts, reducing the chances of infection and minimizing bleeding. Laser surgery requires extremely specialized, often very costly equipment, and it requires that the surgeon have significant training to perform it.

After the procedure: After a patient has received photosensitive chemicals to treat the cancer, it is necessary for the patient to stay out of the sun. Although the photosensitizing chemicals are generally left mainly in the cancer cells after a few days, enough residual chemicals may be present in the rest of the body to make the skin extremely sensitive to sunlight. In some cases, the patient may be required to avoid sunlight for as long thirty days or more. Aftercare for other forms of laser therapy varies depending on the way in which the therapy was performed and the area that was treated. Aftercare for many procedures will be similar to aftercare for similar surgical procedures performed to the same area.

Risks: The risks associated with laser therapy vary. Procedures in which a laser is used to shrink or destroy a tumor, as well as those in which a laser is used to cut out all of or a portion of the tumor, have the risks normally associated with surgical procedures, which can include swelling, bleeding, infection, pain, and some risk of damage to surrounding tissue. Specific risks are also associated with the use of a laser to activate photosensitive chemicals; however, they are usually considered mild and vary depending on the type of laser and chemical used.

Results: The result expected from laser therapies varies depending on the type of laser treatment performed, the type and extent of the cancer being treated, and the goals of the treatment. When laser therapy is done instead of surgical procedures, patients often experience less swelling and bleeding and are less likely to develop an infection. Laser procedures, however, may not last as long as other types of treatments and may need to be repeated.

Helen Davidson, B.A.

For Further Information

Lyons, Lyman. *Diagnosis and Treatment of Cancer*. New York: Chelsea House, 2007.

Vij, D. F., and K. Mahesh, eds. *Medical Applications of Lasers*. Boston: Kluwer Academic, 2002.

Watson, Tim, ed. *Electrotherapy: Evidence-Based Practice*. 12th ed. New York: Churchill Livingstone, 2008.

Waynant, Ronald W. *Lasers in Medicine*. Boca Raton, Fla.: CRC Press, 2002.

See also: Colorectal cancer; Coughing; Electroporation therapy; Electrosurgery; Endotheliomas; Esophageal cancer; Eye cancers; Liver cancers; Lung cancers; Ophthalmic oncology; Penile cancer; Rothmund-Thomson syndrome; Skin cancers; Vaginal cancer

▶ Leukapharesis

Category: Procedures
Also known as: Apheresis, hemapheresis

Definition: Leukapharesis is a process of filtering whole blood to remove stem cells or white blood cells.

Cancers treated: Most forms of leukemia, lymphoma, and myeloma

Why performed: Because high-dose chemotherapy destroys normal blood-producing stem cells in the bone marrow, these cells must be replaced in order to restore blood cell production. Stem cell transplantation is often performed to support high-dose chemotherapy as a treatment option for many forms of leukemia, lymphoma, and myeloma. Autologous transplant means that a patient donates his or her own blood cells for reinfusion after chemotherapy; allogeneic transplant means that a donor supplies blood cells for infusion into another person.

Patient preparation: Donors and patients undergo a complete blood count to determine the number of platelets, red and white blood cells, and hemoglobin levels. The collection of stem cells and white blood cells is usually performed on an outpatient basis. For the treatment of some blood and lymphatic cancers, a donor may be injected for five days with a drug to stimulate the production and release of large numbers of stem cells and white blood cells from the marrow into the bloodstream.

Steps of the procedure: An intravenous catheter is inserted into the donor. Blood passes out of the patient and circulates through a cell separator machine. The fraction of the blood containing stem cells or white cells is separated via centrifugation from the blood that is not required for the transplant; the latter blood fraction is then remixed and returned to the donor through the catheter. When a patient's own stem cells are used, they may be frozen and stored until needed; stem cells from a donor can be collected when they are needed.

After the procedure: Donors are generally free to leave the clinic after the procedure. Patients receiving treatment may leave after their marrow begins producing sufficient new blood cells and treatment complications have been addressed.

Risks: Patients may experience temporary light-headedness and numbness or tingling of the nose, lips, or fingers. Possible complications include bleeding at the needle site, clotting in blood vessels, and similar complications. Because the procedure involves skin penetration and open access to blood vessels, infection is a risk.

Results: Stem cells infused into the bloodstream of a patient receiving chemotherapy will travel to the marrow of certain bones and stimulate the production of cells that eventually mature into healthy blood cells, replacing the normal cells that are lost during high-dose chemotherapy.

Terry A. Anderson, B.S.

See also: Autologous blood transfusion; Bone Marrow Transplantation (BMT); Leukemias; Lymphomas; Myeloma; Myeloproliferative disorders; Pheresis; Transfusion therapy

▶ Limb salvage

Category: Procedures
Also known as: Limb sparing

Definition: Limb salvage surgery includes all surgical procedures designed to accomplish removal of a malignant tumor and resection of the limb with an acceptable oncologic, functional, and cosmetic result.

Cancers treated: Soft-tissue neoplasias (malignant fibrous histiocytoma, fibrosarcoma, liposarcoma, rhabdomyosarcoma, synovial sarcoma); bone malignancies (osteosarcoma, chondrosarcoma, adamantinoma, Ewing sarcoma)

Why performed: In the recent past, most sarcomas were treated by amputation. Tumor recurrence, metastasis, and a generally dismal prognosis had been powerful deterrents to any progress in the surgical treatment of such tumors. Since the late 1980's, however, limb salvage has all but replaced amputation as the treatment of choice for sarcomas of the extremities. This dramatic change came about as a result of two important developments: effective chemotherapy and precision imaging technology. Today, up to 85 percent of extremity sarcomas are treated with limb salvage surgery.

Limb salvage surgery (LSS) can result in survival rates and disease-free intervals that equal those previously achieved with amputation. The presumed functional and psychological advantages of LSS over amputation, however, have yet to be established. LSS appears to offer the possibility of better psychological functioning with a more intact body image, but it is more complex and demanding than amputation and is associated with increased morbidity. The duration of surgery is longer. Infection, pain, and other complications are more common with LSS. Barriers to limb salvage include major vascular involvement, incasement of a major motor nerve, and a pathologic fracture of the involved bone.

Patient preparation: Both imaging studies and biopsy results are used to stage bone and soft-tissue sarcomas. Staging of the tumor influences preoperative chemotherapy or radiation treatments and allows the surgeon to begin planning the limb salvage procedure. The preoperative treatment period provides an opportunity for the surgeon to meet with the patient and family to discuss the choice of the surgical treatment. Treatment by amputation remains a viable and sometimes preferable option and should be openly discussed with the patient in an unbiased manner. Currently, every patient with a malignant tumor of the extremity should be considered for LSS if the tumor can be excised with an adequate tissue margin resulting in a limb worth saving. A limb worth saving needs an acceptable degree of function and cosmetic appearance with a minimal amount of pain, and it needs to be durable enough to withstand the demands of normal daily activities.

Steps of the procedure: Surgical treatment of musculoskeletal neoplasms of the extremities is complex and varied. Tumors occur in all anatomic locations of the extremity and, therefore, surgical procedures must be tailored to the anatomic location. Three principles are involved in any operation for extremity sarcomas: excision of the tumor, skeletal reconstruction, and soft-tissue reconstruction. Obtaining an adequate surgical margin takes precedence over all other considerations. If an adequate surgical margin can be achieved only with an amputation, then the patient must be so informed and must understand that to do less will compromise the chances for long-term survival.

After the procedure: The rehabilitation process is performed by a multidisciplinary team. Steps in the process include a preoperative physical examination of limb function and disability. Pretraining of the patient is necessary to reduce the rehabilitation time and to lessen the emotional stress following surgery.

Age, surgical site, use of allograft bone, the implementation of soft-tissue flap coverage, residual function of associated joints, the possibility of joint reconstruction, use of appropriate orthoses and/or splints, and palliative care will influence, modify, and direct physical and occupational therapies.

Risks: LSS is an extensive series of procedures involving masses of soft tissues, bones, and joints. In contrast to ordinary orthopedic procedures, in which the goal is to solve a local problem with minimal exposure and damage, limb salvage deliberately damages many anatomic areas and may cause the following problems:

- bone and joint damage
- muscle damage
- skin damage
- nerve damage (due to mobilization of major nerves and direct damage resulting from radiotherapy and neurotoxic agents)
- vascular damage (vessel damage and spasm during surgical exploration and excision of major vessels as a result of tumor involvement)

• damage to the lymphatic system (resulting in chronic swelling and limb edema)
• scars (pain, dysesthesias, restricted range of movement)
• infections (in 18.7 percent of cases)
• effects of cancer treatments (radiotherapy, chemotherapy)

Radiotherapy damages the skin, subcutaneous tissues, and muscles, causing fibrosis, decreased tissue elasticity, and contractures. Radiation can result in increased bone fragility and the additional risk of fractures. Chemotherapy may cause chronic weakness and fatigue. It requires repeated hospitalizations, which make it difficult to maintain the intensity and continuity of a rehabilitation program.

Results: Limb-sparing surgery is now widely accepted as a treatment option for extremity sarcomas. Numerous reports confirm low recurrence rates after tumor resection with adequately wide margins. Studies about functional loss following such procedures are limited.

John L. Zeller, M.D., Ph.D.

For Further Information

DeVita, Vincent, Jr., Samuel Hellman, Steven A. Rosenberg, et al., eds. *Cancer: Principles and Practice of Oncology*. 7th ed. Philadelphia: Lippincott Williams & Wilkins, 2005.

Malawer, Martin, and Paul H. Sugarbaker, eds. *Musculoskeletal Cancer Surgery: Treatment of Sarcomas and Allied Diseases*. Washington, D.C.: Kluwer Academic, 2001.

Schwartz, Herbert S., ed. *Orthopaedic Knowledge Update: Musculoskeletal Tumors 2*. 2d ed. Rosemont, Ill.: American Academy of Orthopaedic Surgeons, 2007.

Schwarzbach, M., Y. Hormann, U. Hinz, et al. "Results of Limb-Sparing Surgery with Vascular Replacement for Soft Tissue Sarcoma in the Lower Extremity." *Journal of Vascular Surgery* 42, no. 1 (July, 2005): 88-97.

Skinner, Harry B., ed. *Current Diagnosis and Treatment in Orthopedics*. 4th ed. New York: Lange Medical Books/McGraw-Hill, 2006.

Other Resources

American Academy of Orthopedic Surgeons
http://www.aaos.org

See also: Amputation; Bone cancers; Fibrosarcomas, soft-tissue; Hyperthermic perfusion; Orthopedic surgery; Rhabdomyosarcomas; Sarcomas, soft-tissue; Self-image and body image; Surgical oncology; Synovial sarcomas

▶ Linear accelerator

Category: Procedures
Also known as: Linac, radiation therapy machine

Definition: A linear accelerator (linac) is a machine that can produce high-energy X rays and electrons that are used to kill cancer cells and shrink tumors. A linear accelerator's beam is shaped and sized to treat the tumor and protect surrounding normal tissue.

Cancers treated: Most solid-tumor cancers, such as breast, colorectal, prostate, and brain cancers; leukemia and lymphoma; cancer symptom management

Why performed: External radiation used to kill cancer cells at the site of the tumor provides effective local cell death and discourages regrowth.

Patient preparation: A computed tomography (CT) scan or other radiology test is done to determine the tumor site to be treated. The doctor, a radiation oncologist, reviews the patient's chart and marks the tumor site. This information is loaded into a treatment-planning computer that calculates how much radiation the patient is to receive. The calculations are then programmed into the linear accelerator. The treatment planning may take several hours. Patients may also be fitted with positioning devices that help to hold the body still during treatment.

Steps of the procedure: Treatments on the linear accelerator are usually given once a day for four to six weeks. Treatments are not usually given on Saturday and Sunday in order to allow normal cells to recover. Depending on the site being treated, patients change into gowns or wear street clothes. The patient is carefully positioned on the treatment table or chair by the staff. The staff leaves the room, but an intercom allows the patient to call for help if needed. The treatment is painless and takes just a few minutes, during which the patient must lie still. The equipment is noisy, the machine rotates around the patient, and the treatment table may move. Treatments are usually on an outpatient basis, and patients return home each day.

After the procedure: Once all treatments are complete, the patient will see a doctor to determine the status of the tumor and plan any necessary follow-up treatment. It is safe for the patient to be around others, including children and pregnant women, because no radiation is in the body.

Risks: Side effects depend on the site treated and may include redness and skin irritation, urinary symptoms, diarrhea, fatigue, eating problems, shortness of breath, and hair loss at the treatment site.

Results: External radiation from a linear accelerator provides effective local control of cancer cells. As part of a comprehensive plan of care, radiation therapy can lead to a cure.

Patricia Stanfill Edens, R.N., Ph.D., FACHE

See also: Accelerated Partial Breast Irradiation (APBI); Acoustic neuromas; Colorectal cancer; External Beam Radiation Therapy (EBRT); Intensity-Modulated Radiation Therapy (IMRT); Radiation oncology; Radiation therapies; Stereotactic Radiosurgery (SRS); Veterinary oncology

▶ Liver biopsy

Category: Procedures
Also known as: Liver needle biopsy, fine needle aspiration biopsy, laparoscopic liver biopsy, transvenous or transjugular liver biopsy

Definition: A liver biopsy is the removal of a small sample of liver tissue through a needle or surgically. The tissue sample is examined in the laboratory for the presence of cancer cells.

Cancers diagnosed: Liver cancer

Why performed: A liver biopsy is performed to diagnose liver disease and assess the degree of liver damage (disease staging). It may be performed when a liver abnormality is found during an ultrasound, computed tomography (CT) scan, magnetic resonance imaging (MRI) test or nuclear scan. It may also be performed to determine the cause of unexplained jaundice (yellowing of the skin) or abnormal results of liver function blood tests.

Patient preparation: One week before the procedure, patients must stop taking aspirin and products containing aspirin, ibuprofen, and anticoagulants, as directed by the physician. A blood test will be performed before the procedure to evaluate the patient's blood and platelet count and clotting ability of the blood. Patients must not eat or drink for eight hours beforehand.

Steps of the procedure: In fine needle aspiration biopsy, an intravenous (IV) line is inserted into a vein in the patient's arm to deliver medications. In many hospitals, a sedative is given to the patient before the procedure (conscious sedation), so that the patient is awake but relaxed and able to respond to the physician's instructions during the procedure. The patient lies on the back, with the right hand above the head, remaining as still as possible during the procedure. The biopsy site is cleansed, and a local anesthetic is injected into the area where the needle will be inserted. A small incision is made on the right side of the chest, near the rib cage. Ultrasound is often used to guide the biopsy needle that is placed through the incision into the liver. The physician may ask the patient to hold his or her breath for up to ten seconds while the needle is placed in the liver. A small sample of liver tissue is removed through the needle for analysis in a laboratory.

During a laparoscopic biopsy, a laparoscope (a small camera on a thin tube) is inserted into a small abdominal incision. The laparoscope transmits magnified images of the liver onto a video monitor to guide the physician as laparoscopic instruments are inserted through additional small abdominal incisions to remove tissue samples from one or more parts of the liver. General anesthesia is usually used with this type of biopsy. A laparoscopic biopsy may be used when a tissue sample is needed from more than one area of the liver or when a larger tissue sample is needed.

During a transvenous biopsy (also called transjugular biopsy), a catheter (thin tube) is inserted into a vein in the neck and guided to the liver. A biopsy needle is inserted through the catheter to collect the sample of liver tissue. This technique is not common, but it may be used for certain high-risk patients, including those who have a blood-clotting disorder, fluid in the abdomen, or liver failure or who are morbidly obese.

After the procedure: The patient stays in a recovery room and lies on the right side for four to six hours after the procedure. Pain medication may be prescribed, if needed, to relieve minor discomfort or pain in the shoulders or back. The patient should not drive or operate machinery for eight hours after the procedure. Depending on the physician's instructions, the patient may be required to stay on bed rest at home for eight to ten hours after the procedure. The patient should avoid vigorous physical activity and heavy lifting, as directed by the physician. The patient may feel discomfort at the incision site and in the right shoulder for a few hours to a few days after the procedure. For one week after the biopsy, the patient should avoid aspirin and products containing aspirin, ibuprofen, and anticoagulants, as these medications decrease blood clotting, which is necessary for healing. The patient may take acetaminophen (Tylenol) to relieve pain as needed after the procedure.

Risks: With ultrasound guidance, liver biopsy is a relatively safe procedure, with a 0.6 percent risk of complications. Although rare, the complications of a liver biopsy include puncture of the lung or gallbladder that may result in bile leakage, internal bleeding, and infection. The risk of death (mortality rate) of the liver biopsy procedure is approximately 1 in 10,000 to 12,000.

Results: The tissue sample that was removed during the procedure may be benign (noncancerous) or malignant (cancerous). The type of cancerous cells and extent of disease will help guide the patient's treatment.

Angela M. Costello, B.S.

For Further Information

Grant, A., and J. Neuberger, for the British Society of Gastroenterology. "Guidelines for the Use of Liver Biopsy in Clinical Practice." *Gut* 45, suppl. 4 (1999): IV1-IV11.

Scheuer, Peter J., and Jay H. Lefkowitch. *Liver Biopsy Interpretation*. 7th ed. Philadelphia: Elsevier Saunders, 2006.

Siegel, C. A., et al. "Liver Biopsy 2005: When and How?" *Cleveland Clinic Journal of Medicine* 72, no. 3 (2005): 199-224.

Other Resources

American Liver Foundation
http://www.liverfoundation.org

American Society for Gastrointestinal Endoscopy (ASGE)
http://www.askasge.org

International Foundation for Functional Gastrointestinal Disorders
http://www.iffgd.org

National Digestive Diseases Information Clearinghouse (NDDIC)
http://digestive.niddk.nih.gov/index.htm

See also: Alcohol, alcoholism, and cancer; Biopsy; Chemoembolization; Computed Tomography (CT) scan; Gastrointestinal oncology; Hemochromatosis; Hepatitis B Virus (HBV); Hepatitis C Virus (HCV); Hepatomegaly; Laparoscopy and laparoscopic surgery; Liver cancers; Needle biopsies; Oncogenic viruses; Risks for cancer; Surgical biopsies; Virus-related cancers

▶ Lobectomy

Category: Procedures
Also known as: Pulmonary lobectomy, lung lobe removal

Definition: Lobectomy is the surgical removal of a lobe of a lung.

Cancers treated: Lung cancer

Why performed: Lobectomy is a surgical procedure used to treat lung cancer when the tumor is limited to one area of the lung. It may also be used to treat bronchiectasis, tuberculosis, lung abscess, localized fungal infections, or blebs associated with emphysema.

Patient preparation: Before surgery, studies are performed to check for abnormalities and establish a baseline for postoperative comparison. These studies include a chest X ray, electrocardiogram (ECG), bleeding time, and blood tests to check kidney function, electrolytes, hemoglobin, oxygen levels, and white blood cell count. Pulmonary function tests are performed to evaluate lung function. A blood sample is also drawn to check the patient's blood type in case a transfusion is needed during surgery. The patient must not eat or drink for at least eight hours before surgery, and an intravenous (IV) catheter is inserted for fluids and medications. An indwelling urinary catheter may also be inserted so that urine output can be monitored closely during and after the procedure.

Steps of the procedure: When the patient arrives in the operating suite, an arterial catheter may be inserted to monitor the patient's blood pressure and oxygenation. After the patient is anesthetized, the surgeon makes an incision into the chest cavity. When the chest cavity is entered, the lung collapses. The surgeon locates and ties off sources of bleeding, spreads the ribs, and exposes the area of the lung for removal. The surgeon removes the affected lung lobe and repairs the vessels and lung passages from where it was removed. The surgeon inserts one or two chest tubes to drain fluid and reexpand the lung. Then, the surgeon closes the chest cavity and applies a sterile dressing.

After the procedure: The patient is typically transferred to the intensive care unit (ICU) and attached to a monitor that displays heart rhythm, blood pressure, and oxygen saturation. These devices help the ICU nurses closely monitor the patient's condition. The patient receives supplemental oxygen and IV fluids. The nurses check the chest tube drainage frequently to monitor for excess bleeding. The patient is encouraged to turn, cough, breathe deeply, and use an incentive spirometer to prevent pneumonia. Sequential compression devices are attached to the patient's legs to help prevent blood clots.

Risks: The risks of lobectomy include surgical site infection, pneumonia, hemorrhage, and respiratory failure.

Results: Pathologic examination of the lung specimen reveals the type of cancer.

Collette Bishop Hendler, R.N., M.S.

See also: Bilobectomy; Bronchoalveolar lung cancer; Esophagectomy; Lung cancers; Mesothelioma; Pleural effusion; Pleurodesis; Pneumonectomy; Surgical biopsies; Thoracoscopy; Thoracotomy

▶ Loop Electrosurgical Excisional Procedure (LEEP)

Category: Procedures
Also known as: Large loop excision of the transformation zone (LLETZ), large loop excision of the cervix (LLEC), loop cone biopsy of the cervix

Definition: Loop electrosurgical excisional procedure (LEEP) is a procedure that may be used to excise or cut away abnormal, possibly precancerous cells (cervical intraepithelial neoplasia) on the surface of the cervix as indicated by the results of a Pap test.

Cancers diagnosed or treated: Cervical intraepithelial neoplasia or dysplasia (CIN), abnormal cell changes on the surface of the cervix

Why performed: A LEEP removes abnormal, possibly precancerous cells indicated by results of a Pap test and seen on colposcopy (a noninvasive device used to see inside the cervix) on the surface of the cervix. A LEEP may also be used as a diagnostic procedure when abnormal cells are suspected high in the cervical canal and are not visible using a colposcope.

Patient preparation: While there is no standard preparation needed for a LEEP, the patient should consult with her doctor or provider. A LEEP is not performed while a patient is menstruating.

Steps of the procedure: The patient, unclothed from the waist down, draped with a cloth or paper, lies on an exam table as for a typical pelvic exam with feet raised in stirrups. A speculum is inserted in the vagina to allow the physician to see inside the vagina and cervix to guide the colposcope to the area where the abnormal cells are located. A tube is attached to the speculum to remove any smoke caused by the procedure. Then an electrosurgical dispersive pad is placed on the thigh, which allows the electric current to return safely. The physician will attach a single-use disposable loop electrode to the generator hand piece. A vinegar (acetic acid) or iodine solution will be used to prepare the cervix, allowing the physician to assess the extent of the abnormal cells. If a cervical block or anesthetic will be used to numb the cervix, then a pain medication will be administered beforehand. Once the local anesthetic or block is injected into the cervix, the electroloop is generated and the wire loop will pass through the surface of the cervix. Finally, an electrosurgical generator sends a painless electrical current that cuts away the affected cervical tissue as the loop wire moves through the cervix, causing the abnormal cells to burst. The procedure takes about ten to twenty minutes to complete.

After the procedure: The patient may go home following the procedure. While rare, complications may include mild cramping, mild discomfort or pain, bleeding, heavy vaginal discharge, or strong vaginal odor. The patient should report any significant side effect to her doctor. The patient is typically advised not to engage in sexual intercourse for four weeks following the procedure. Ibuprofen (Motrin, Advil) may be taken for cramping. The patient is advised not to lift heavy objects, douche, or use tampons for four weeks following the procedure and is advised to take showers instead of baths to reduce the risk of infection. The patient's doctor will make a follow-up appointment to perform a colposcopy to check that all abnormal cells have been removed and perform a Pap test to confirm this.

Risks: The LEEP is very safe. The benefits of treating potentially precancerous cells with the procedure outweigh its minimal risks. Those risks may include heavy bleeding, bleeding with clots, severe abdominal cramping, fever, foul-smelling discharge, incomplete removal of abnormal tissue, cervical stenosis (narrowing of the cervix), infection, and possibly cutting or accidental burning of normal tissue if the patient moves during the procedure.

Results: Typically, the patient returns to normal activity within one to three days after the LEEP. The doctor will disclose the results of the histologic specimen obtained from the LEEP regarding whether invasive cancer may have developed deep in cervical tissue. A follow-up appointment is made to perform a colposcopy to confirm that all abnormal cells have been removed, a Pap test is repeated to confirm their removal, and the patient is advised to return on a regular basis for Pap tests to track the possible recurrence of abnormal cervical cells.

Susan H. Peterman, M.P.H.

See also: Afterloading radiation therapy; Antiviral therapies; Benign tumors; Biological therapy; Birth control pills and cancer; Carcinomas; Carcinomatosis; Cervical cancer; Colposcopy; Conization; Diethylstilbestrol (DES); Endometrial cancer; Exenteration; Fertility drugs and cancer; Gynecologic cancers; Human papillomavirus (HPV); Hysterectomy; Hystero-oophorectomy; Infectious cancers; Pap test; Pelvic examination; Pregnancy and cancer; Vaccines, preventive; Vaginal cancer; Virus-related cancers

▶ Lumbar puncture

Category: Procedures
Also known as: Spinal tap

Definition: Lumbar puncture is the insertion of a needle between two vertebrae in the lower back (lumbar region) into the spinal canal in order to obtain a sample of cerebrospinal fluid (CSF) for analysis.

Cancers diagnosed or treated: Cancers of the central nervous system (brain and spinal cord), such as meningeal carcinomatosis

Why performed: Although usually used for diagnosing disease, sometimes the procedure is used to provide a mechanism for the introduction of medications to treat disease, to introduce agents for further study of possible disease, or as actual treatment for some disease. Lumbar puncture results are used to help diagnose diseases such as meningitis, subarachnoid hemorrhage, Guillain-Barré syndrome, and multiple sclerosis. In addition, dyes for myelograms or anesthetics for pain relief may be introduced using lumbar puncture.

Patient preparation: A computed tomography (CT) scan or magnetic resonance imaging (MRI) scan is sometimes completed prior to lumbar puncture, but these scans are not always indicated. Certain blood tests are taken to compare the results from the blood to the results from the cerebrospinal fluid collected during the lumbar puncture, including serum chemistry panels (glucose) and complete blood counts (white blood cell count). Ideally, medications such as aspirin, ibuprofen, or other antiplatelet agents should be discontinued forty-eight to seventy-two hours before an elective lumbar puncture.

Steps of the procedure: The patient is placed on his or her side with knees drawn up toward the chest and back flexed toward the legs. Sterile procedure is completed, including sterile gloves, alcohol swabbing, iodine preparation, and isolation of the puncture area with sterile towels or paper drapes. The health care professional performing the procedure palpates (feels) the spine to locate the best position to insert the needle in the patient's lower back. In adults, the spinal cord extends down to the first lumbar vertebra (five lumbar vertebrae are present, with the highest on the back labeled as number 1), so the health care professional locates an area below vertebral1, usually between the third and fourth lumbar vertebrae or the fourth and fifth lumbar vertebrae. Infants require a 14-15 insertion area since the spinal cord terminates at a lower level in infants than in adults. A local anesthetic with a tiny needle is used to numb the insertion site for the larger lumbar puncture needle.

After the procedure: The patient should lie flat on the back for about two hours following the procedure. Rising too fast after a lumbar puncture can increase the risk of the most frequent complication of an lumbar puncture, a positional headache.

Risks: A headache that changes with position is the most frequent complication, occurring in about 25 percent of cases. These headaches usually resolve with rest and hydration. Uncommon complications include damage to nerves in the head and facial region that typically resolve within four months. Rare complications include tumors and cysts that form in the area of the needle insertion site.

People with leukemia may have an increased risk of hematoma (clot) formation at or near the insertion site of the lumbar puncture needle. Lenworth N. Johnson and Michael A. Meyer have reported in *Neuro-ophthalmology*

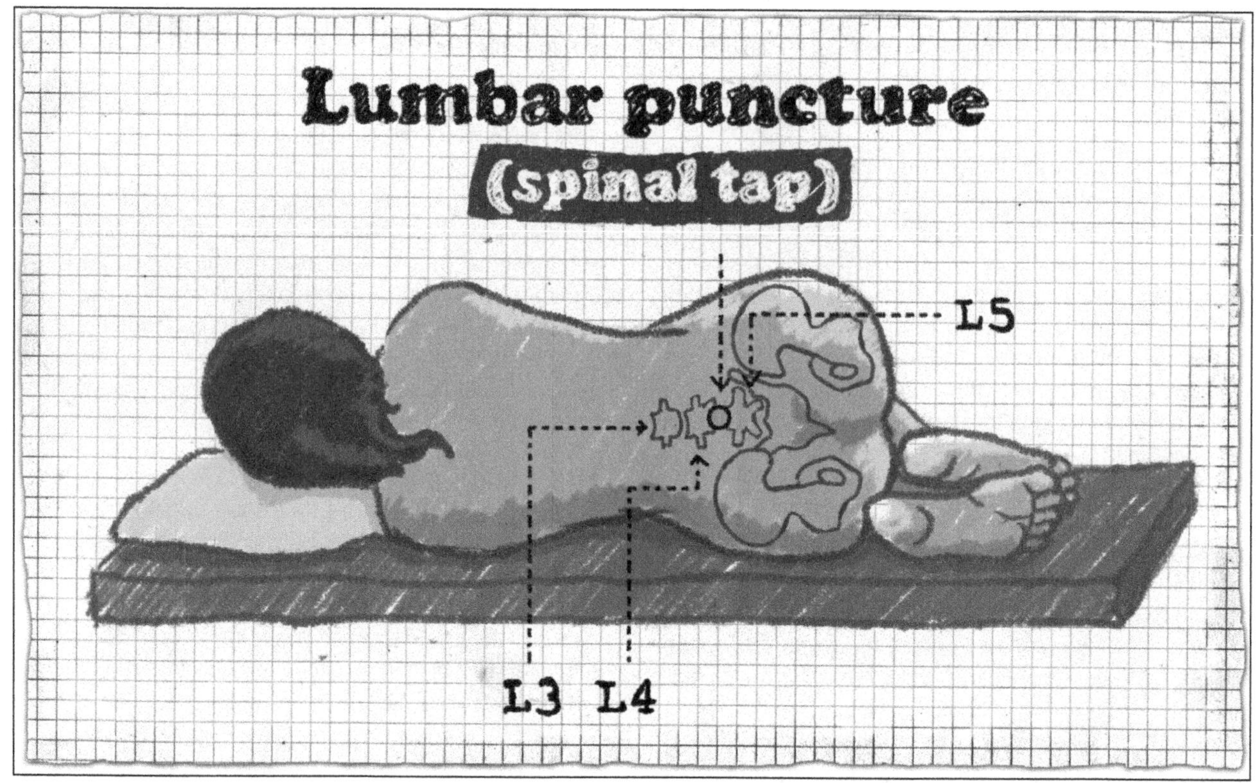

A lumbar puncture. (iStock)

(2005) that leukemia patients who have a traumatic lumbar puncture can suffer contamination of the CSF with cancer cells, and the median survival time of these patients can be reduced in this situation.

The gravest complication of a lumbar puncture is herniation of the brain stem, where the lower portion of the brain is suddenly pulled down by the pressure release of opening the spinal canal to remove fluid. This can happen if a brain tumor or growth has increased pressure in the spinal canal, since the fluid in the spinal canal is physically in contact with fluid surrounding the brain (hence the term "cerebrospinal fluid," with "cerebro" referring to the brain). This rare occurrence is minimized by screening with neurological and ophthalmologic examinations and CT/MRI scanning as indicated.

Results: Normal cerebrospinal fluid is clear and colorless. Sometimes, blood discolors the CSF, giving it a reddish color. If blood is present, then it can indicate a very serious condition known as subarachnoid hemorrhage. Usually, if blood is present in the CSF, then the blood comes from what is known as a "traumatic tap," resulting from the inadvertent puncture of small blood vessels with the lumbar puncture needle. A traumatic tap is not usually a serious problem, but the blood source requires identification. Four or five small tubes of CSF are collected from a typical lumbar puncture. Blood from a traumatic tap diminishes from the first tube collected to the last tube collected. Other tests can be completed to help determine the source of blood found in a lumbar puncture.

Laboratory tests routinely completed on CSF include protein, glucose, and white and red blood cell counts. Cultures and studies for bacteria, fungi, and viruses may be completed. Cells found in the CSF may be microscopically examined to determine if cancers of the brain or spinal cord are present. The pressure of the fluid as it initially drains out of the spinal canal, called the opening pressure, is measured, as is the closing pressure at the end of the procedure. Elevated pressures can indicate tumors or masses in the cranial cavity.

Richard P. Capriccioso, M.D.

For Further Information

Fischbach, Frances Talaska, and Marshall Barnett Dunning III. *A Manual of Laboratory and Diagnostic Tests*. 7th ed. Philadelphia: Lippincott Williams & Wilkins, 2004.

Johnson, Lenworth N., and Michael A. Meyer. "Lumbar Puncture." In *Neuro-ophthalmology: The Practical Guide*, edited by Leonard A. Levin and Anthony C. Arnold. New York: Thieme Medical, 2005.

Pagana, Kathleen Deska, and Timothy J. Pagana. *Mosby's Manual of Diagnostic and Laboratory Tests*. 3d ed. St. Louis: Mosby Elsevier, 2006.

Other Resources

WebMD

Lumbar Puncture
http://www.webmd.com/brain/Lumbar-Puncture?page=1

See also: Acute Lymphocytic Leukemia (ALL); Blood cancers; Carcinomatous meningitis; Leptomeningeal carcinomas; Medulloblastomas; Meningeal carcinomatosis; Nuclear medicine scan; Pineoblastomas; Retinoblastomas

▶ Lumpectomy

Category: Procedures
Also known as: Breast-conserving surgery, partial mastectomy

Definition: A lumpectomy is breast-conserving surgery and is the most common form of breast surgery performed for cancer. It is usually done as an inpatient procedure, or as "day surgery," under general or local anesthesia, when a lump or mass is found in only one section of the breast by physical examination, mammogram, ultrasound, or magnetic resonance imaging (MRI) of the breast. During a lumpectomy, the lump and some of the surrounding normal-appearing breast tissue are removed and the margins between the lumpectomy and the rest of the breast are examined for any residual tumor.

Cancers diagnosed or treated: Breast cancer

Why performed: A lumpectomy is performed to remove cancer as a breast-conserving method; it is also sometimes called partial mastectomy, as opposed to complete removal of the breast, known as mastectomy. Patients may not be candidates for lumpectomy and radiation if they have more than one cancer in the same breast, have a connective tissue disease such as lupus or vasculitis, are pregnant, or have already had radiation to the same breast.

Sentinel node biopsy may also be performed on the same day of the operation in order to examine the lymph nodes in the armpit or axilla of the breast affected for the presence of cancer that may have spread from the primary lump or site in the breast to the lymph nodes.

Patient preparation: Lumpectomy is usually preceded by a breast biopsy performed by a radiologist or breast surgeon that confirms the presence of breast cancer and in most cases tells the surgeon the type of breast cancer present. This latter information allows the surgeon to decide on the need for the surgery and the type of operation necessary.

Patient instructions are NPO (from the Latin *nulla per os*, or "nothing by mouth") after midnight on the day before the surgery. If sentinel node biopsy is performed in conjunction with lumpectomy, then the patient will need to be injected with radionuclide the day before the breast surgery. The injection is usually done around the nipple or areola by a nuclear medicine physician or radiologist. In the operating room the next day, the surgeon then uses a probe that is sensitive to small doses of gamma radiation emitted by the radiotracer to identify and remove the main draining node or nodes in the axilla, thereby eliminating the need to sample all the nodes in the axilla and thus reducing the risk of lymphedema, a swelling of the affected arm that can occur after full axillary node dissection.

Steps of the procedure: If the lump cannot be felt, then a procedure to mark the location of the mass will be performed, usually in the radiology suite the morning of the surgery. A thin wire or needle is inserted using mammography or ultrasound to guide the radiologist, depending on if the lesion was visible on prior mammogram or ultrasound. This is called a breast needle (or wire) localization. The surgery itself lasts about an hour. After general anesthesia is given, the surgeon will make a curved incision in the breast, usually in the form of a smile or frown which follows the contour of the breast in order to minimize scarring. After the lump and the surrounding breast tissue are removed with a scalpel, a drain may be left in place to collect excess fluid or blood, and the surgeon will then close the wound with stitches and apply a sterile dressing over the wound.

After the procedure: The patient will awake in the recovery room and may be required to stay overnight, depending on many factors, including the procedure itself, the general health of the patient, and how easily the patient recovers from anesthesia.

Risks: The risks of general anesthesia are the same regardless of the procedure; patients who have any questions about anesthesia or any part of the operation should discuss these issues with their referring physician or health care provider. There may be some loss of sensation in the affected breast, and the breasts may not match in size and shape after the surgery, which may or may not be acceptable to the patient.

Results: Once the pathology results are back, the doctor will review the pathology report and discuss the next steps, including the need for additional therapy.

Lumpectomy is usually, but not always, followed by radiation therapy to eliminate any possibility of microcancers (cancer that are too small to identify by physical examination or radiologic means). If the margins are not clean of cancer, then a second operation, called a reexcision, may be necessary.

Debra B. Kessler, M.D., Ph.D.

For Further Information

Benedet, Rosalind. *Understanding Lumpectomy: A Treatment Guide for Breast Cancer*. Omaha, Nebr.: Addicus Books, 2003.

Dewar, J. A., R. Arriagada, S. Benhamous, et al. "Local Relapse and Contralateral Tumor Rates in Patients with Breast Cancer Treated with Conservative Surgery and Radiotherapy." *Cancer* 76 (1995): 2260-2265.

Giulano, A., D. M. Kirgan, J. M. Guenther, et al. "Lymphatic Mapping and Sentinel Lymphadenectomy for Breast Cancer." *Annals of Surgery* 220 (1994): 439-442.

Reiber, A., K. Schramm, G. Helms, et al. "Breast-Conserving Surgery and Autogeneous Tissue Reconstruction in Patients with Breast Cancer: Efficacy of MRI of the Breast in the Detection of Recurrent Disease." *European Journal of Radiology* 13 (2003): 780-787.

See also: Accelerated Partial Breast Irradiation (APBI); Biopsy; Breast cancers; Breast Self-Examination (BSE); Breast ultrasound; Clinical Breast Exam (CBE); Lumps; Mammography; Mastectomy; Needle biopsies; Needle localization; Sentinel Lymph Node (SLN) biopsy and mapping; Stereotactic needle biopsy; Surgical biopsies; Surgical oncology; Wire localization

▶ Lymphadenectomy

Category: Procedures
Also known as: Lymph node dissection

Definition: Lymphadenectomy is the surgical removal of lymph nodes. It is used to diagnose and treat almost all types of cancers because lymph nodes are found throughout the body and are one of the first places to which cancer spreads. Lymphadenectomy is an especially common procedure in diagnosing and treating breast cancer because of the number of lymph nodes located near the breast.

Cancers diagnosed and treated: Most, especially breast cancer

Why performed: The lymphatic system is part of the immune system, which helps keep the body free of disease. Lymph is a clear, yellowish fluid that oozes out of blood vessels and is carried in channels throughout the body. Eventually it is funneled back into a vein and reenters the blood circulatory system. Interspersed along the lymph channels are about six hundred enlarged areas called lymph nodes.

Lymph nodes filter bacteria, viruses, and cancer cells out of the lymph. These undesirable cells are then destroyed by white blood cells (lymphocytes) stored in the lymph nodes. There are many lymph nodes in the head and neck, another large cluster near the breast and under the armpit, and another group in the groin. When bacteria, viruses, or cancer cells overwhelm lymph nodes, the nodes swell and can be felt on the surface of the body. For example, when the lymph nodes behind the ears and along the throat are enlarged, people often say they have "swollen glands," although lymph nodes are not true glands.

Lymph nodes can be surgically removed either as a diagnostic tool or as a therapeutic procedure to treat cancer. In a lymph node biopsy, several samples of lymph node tissue are removed and examined under the microscope to see if they contain cancer cells. Based on the results of the biopsy, full removal of some nodes (a lymphadenectomy) may be performed.

One newer approach to lymphadenectomy aimed at preventing unnecessary surgery involves identifying sentinel nodes and removing them first. Sentinel nodes are the first nodes to which lymph travels after it leaves the area where cancer is present. They provide an early warning that the cancer has begun to spread. The location of sentinel nodes is determined before surgery by lymphangiography and other imaging tests. Lymphangiography involves slowly injecting a fluorescent dye into the lymphatic system and tracing its progress using X rays.

If no cancer is found in the sentinel nodes, then the cancer probably has not spread to the lymphatic system and no additional nodes need to be removed. If cancer has spread to the sentinel nodes and beyond, then lymphadenectomy becomes a treatment for cancer and lymph nodes suspected of containing malignant cells are surgically removed.

Patient preparation: Before a lymphadenectomy, various tests such as a lymphangiogram (dye injected into the lymphatic system) and other imaging scans are done to locate the cancer, determine where it is likely to have spread, and indicate to the surgeon which lymph nodes should be removed.

The patient is prepared for major surgery. In addition to tests to locate the cancer, the patient is given standard preoperative blood and liver function tests, meets with an anesthesiologist, and is required to fast for about eight hours before surgery.

Steps of the procedure: Lymphadenectomy is usually performed under general anesthesia in a hospital. An incision is made in the appropriate area, and lymph nodes and surrounding tissue are removed. Often the sentinel lymph nodes or a sampling of other lymph nodes are removed and examined under a microscope while the patient is still on the operating table. The condition of these nodes then dictates how much other tissue the surgeon will remove. Temporary drains are inserted under the skin to remove excess lymph that accumulates, and the incision is closed.

After the procedure: This procedure normally requires a hospital stay. The length of stay and the recovery period depend on the number of nodes removed and the general health of the patient. The patient may feel temporary numbness or a tingling or burning sensation in the region where the lymph nodes were removed. Radiation therapy or chemotherapy may be given after lymphadenectomy to help kill any cancer cells that remain in the body.

Risks: All surgery carries the risk of bleeding, infection, and allergic reaction to anesthesia. Nevertheless, the greatest risk related to lymphadenectomy is the development of lymphedema after the operation. Lymphedema occurs when the lymphatic system is overwhelmed by large amounts of lymph. The lymph seeps into the surrounding tissue and causes swelling. About 15 percent of individuals have mild lymphedema, with 1 to 2 percent reporting severe swelling. Postoperative radiation therapy increases the risk of developing lymphedema.

Results: For diagnostic lymphadenectomy, if no malignant cells are found in the removed lymph nodes, then it is unlikely that cancer has spread beyond the primary tumor. If lymph nodes are enlarged and malignant cells are found, then there is a high chance that the cancer may metastasize. Therapeutic lymphadenectomy may slow cancer but does not, by itself, cure it. The success of this treatment depends on the stage of the cancer and how many lymph nodes are involved.

Martiscia Davidson, A.M.

For Further Information

Khatri, Vijay P., ed. *Lymphadenectomy in Surgical Oncology*. Philadelphia: Saunders, 2007.

Leong, Stanley P. L. *Selective Sentinel Lymphadenectomy for Human Solid Cancer*. New York: Springer, 2007.

Sato, K., R. Shigenaga, S. Udea, et al. "Sentinel Lymph Node Biopsy for Breast Cancer." *Journal of Surgical Oncology* 96, no. 4 (September 15, 2007): 322-329.

Other Resources

BreastCancer.org
Lymph Node Removal
http://www.breastcancer.org/treatment/surgery/lymph_node_removal/index.jsp

WebMD Cancer Health Center
Lymph Node Biopsy
http://www.webmd.com/cancer/lymph-node-biopsy

See also: Axillary dissection; Biopsy; Breast cancers; Lumpectomy; Lymphangiography; Lymphangiosarcomas; Lymphedema; Lymphocytosis; Lymphomas; Metastasis; Sentinel Lymph Node (SLN) biopsy and mapping; Surgical oncology

▶ Lymphangiography

Category: Procedures

Definition: Lymphangiography is the injection of a dye or radioactive material into the lymphatic system so that the location and condition of lymph nodes and lymph vessels can be determined using X rays.

Cancers diagnosed: Most often used to determine the location of sentinel lymph nodes in breast cancer or to determine the condition of lymph nodes prior to biopsy or removal; sometimes used to diagnose lymphomas

Why performed: The lymphatic system is part of the immune system. It consists of a network of channels that carries lymph, a clear, yellowish fluid, and about six hundred nodes, or enlarged spaces. The lymph nodes trap bacteria, viruses, and cancer cells so that they can be destroyed by

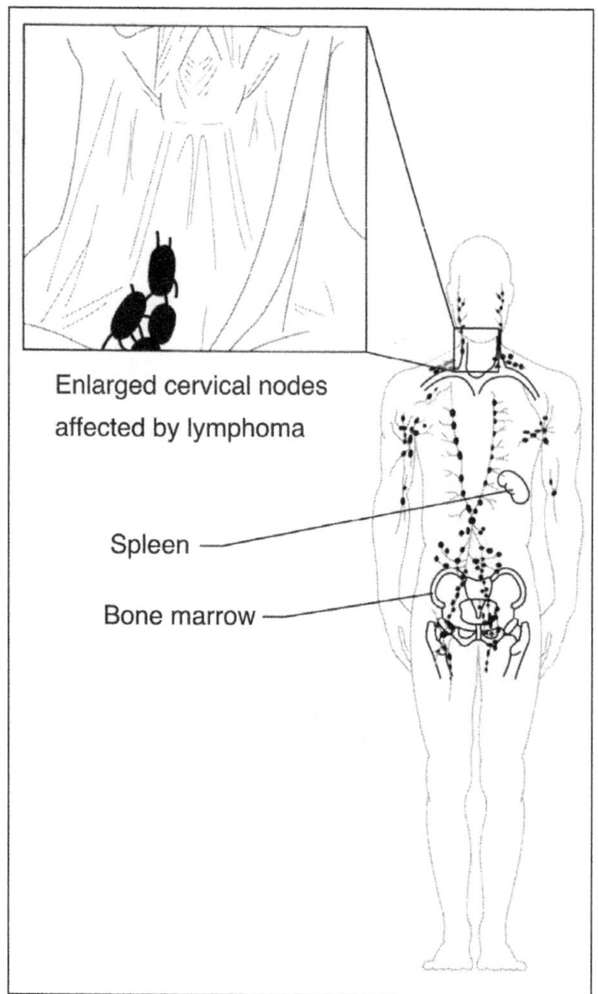

Major nodes of the lymphatic system; enlarged nodes can be caused by lymphomas and other cancers.

white blood cells stored in the nodes. Lymph nodes are one of the first places to which cancer spreads, so knowing if there are cancer cells in the nodes is important in staging and treating all cancers.

Lymphangiography helps the surgeon determine where to biopsy or which lymph nodes to remove. The sentinel nodes are the first nodes through which lymph flows after it passes the primary tumor. In some women with breast cancer, the sentinel node is located using lymphangiography and then removed. If no cancer is found, then no additional nodes need to be removed, thus reducing the amount of surgery that the patient needs.

Patient preparation: Minimal preparations are needed for lymphangiography. The patient may be asked not to drink for several hours before the test, since the lymphangiography takes up to seven hours and requires that the patient remain still.

Steps of the procedure: A dye is infused into the hand or foot. The dye enters the lymph system and highlights the lymph channels and nodes. The dye may cause a mild burning feeling. It enters the body very slowly, and the patient must remain still during this time.

After the procedure: The site where the dye was infused is cleaned and closed. The patient's urine may be bluish for several days. Dye can remain in the body for up to two years.

Risks: Allergic reaction to the dye and infection at the infusion site are the main risks.

Results: From this test, the physician can tell if the lymph nodes are swollen or clogged, a condition that may indicate cancer. The surgeon can also determine which nodes are sentinel nodes.

Martiscia Davidson, A.M.

See also: Biopsy; Breast cancers; Cystography; Embolization; Imaging tests; Lymphadenectomy; Lymphangiosarcomas; Lymphedema; Lymphocytosis; Lymphomas; Metastasis; Sentinel Lymph Node (SLN) biopsy and mapping; Testicular cancer; X-ray tests

▶ Magnetic Resonance Imaging (MRI)

Category: Procedures

Definition: Magnetic resonance imaging (MRI) is a noninvasive and pain-free diagnostic imaging test performed using powerful magnets and radio waves rather than ionizing radiation. The magnets cause the protons in the hydrogen ions found in the body's water to arrange themselves in a certain way in relation to the magnetic field. Once the protons are aligned, the radio waves are bounced off the tissues. This is the "resonance" part of the test. The signals that return to the scanner are analyzed by computer. An MRI takes slicelike images of the body, but it is able to acquire these images in several planes, so that it provides three-dimensional images. MRI can provide high image resolution and significant detail. Consequently, it provides more information than computed tomography (CT).

Most MRI machines consist of a large cylinder, called a bore, with a thick casing around it. The magnets

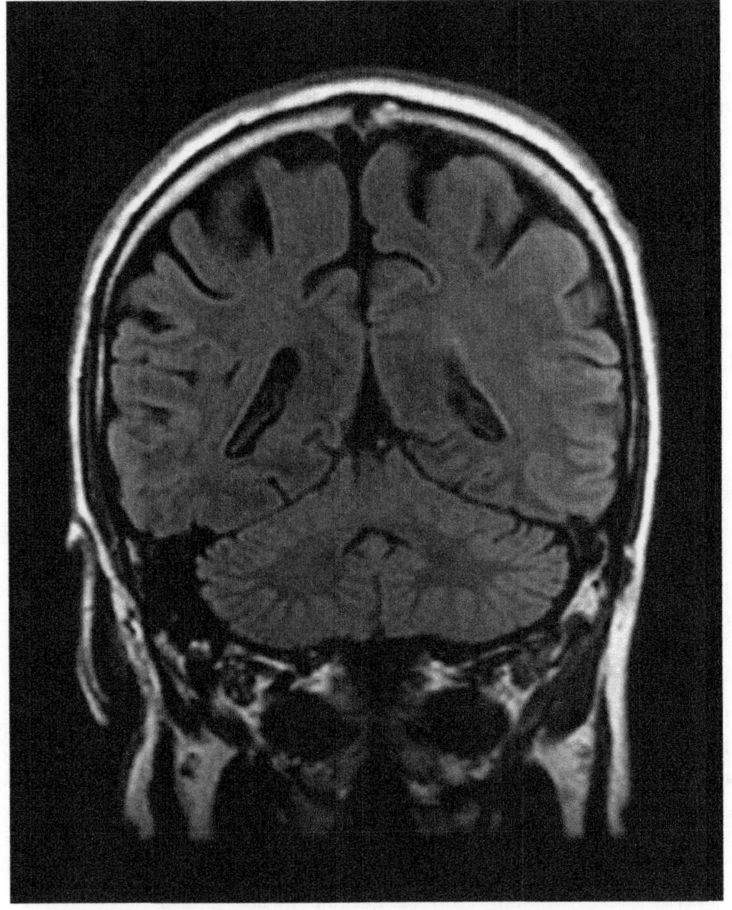

An MRI allows doctors to see soft tissues in the brain. (iStock)

surround the patient when he or she is being scanned. Open MRI units have been developed, but they are not available everywhere. In open MRI machines, the magnets do not surround the patient, as there are gaps in the magnets. This change does affect the quality of the images created to some degree, but it also permits the scanning of very obese patients and those with claustrophobia (fear of closed spaces).

In order to receive a clear image, several types of magnets are used in an MRI machine: resistive magnets, permanent magnets, superconducting magnets, and gradient magnets. Resistive and superconducting magnets consist of coils of wire around a cylinder. They become magnetic only when electrical current is passed through them. Superconducting magnets are bathed in liquid helium, which is extremely cold at a temperature of –452.4 degrees Fahrenheit. This greatly decreases the resistance of the wire coil. As a result, superconducting magnets require a great deal less electrical current to magnetize. A permanent magnet is always a magnet and requires no electrical current to flow through it. The gradient magnets are very low-strength magnets and are used to localize the magnetic field to the portion of the body being examined.

There are several drawbacks to MRI. A large percentage of patients are excluded from MRI testing because the test cannot be performed if the patient has any metal in or on the body or if he or she is on any machinery for monitoring or life support. Patients with pacemakers, cochlear implants, clips in the brain, artificial heart valves, older vascular stents, intrauterine devices, metal plates or screws, surgical staples, implanted drug infusion ports, and recently replaced artificial joints should not have MRIs. Patients who are on a ventilator, a cardiac monitor, or an infusion pump or in traction should not have an MRI.

Another drawback is that the patient must lie perfectly still during the exam in order for the imaging to be clear. An MRI can be difficult for a patient with claustrophobia because the scan is performed with the part to be examined in the center of the tube. Another drawback is that extremely obese patients cannot be scanned by the closed scanner if they are too large for the bore. In addition, MRIs usually are not performed on pregnant patients because there has not been enough research done to ensure the safety of the fetus.

Cancers diagnosed: An MRI can diagnose most kinds of cancer. It can be used to assess the blood vessels, lungs, liver, heart, stomach, large and small intestines, biliary tract, kidneys, brain and nerves, spleen, pancreas, male testes and prostate, female uterus and ovaries, and the pelvic, knee, and hip bones. To identify structures in the abdomen, it is helpful to use oral contrast, such as liquid barium, and/or intravenous dyes, such as gadolinium. MRI is particularly effective at evaluating tumors in the central nervous system, spine, joints, extremities, breasts, and liver.

Why performed: An MRI is performed to evaluate abnormalities in body tissue. These abnormalities include tumors, congenital abnormalities, vascular abnormalities, tissue inflammation, infection, bleeding, and edema.

Patient preparation: Before an MRI, a patient must remove all metal from the body, such as jewelry, watches, belt buckles, hearing aids, removable dental work, and hairpins. The clothing must have no metal on it, such as zippers or metal decorations. The patient is also asked to empty the pockets prior to the MRI. Since the MRI uses a strong magnet, any metal objects could become projectiles once the MRI is turned on, potentially causing injury to the patient. The patient may be asked to wear hospital pajamas if there is metal on the clothing. The patient is asked to remove any makeup before the MRI because the iron in some makeup can be affected by the MRI. Also, medication patches should be removed prior to an MRI because the procedure can cause a burn on the site of the patch.

The patient is often given earplugs because the MRI scanner makes loud noises. It is essential that the patient lie still while in the scanner, so he or she may be given a sedative prior to the test. This is more likely if the patient has claustrophobia or is confused. Positioning devices are used to keep the body part to be scanned in a stationery position. If the patient is to receive contrast dye, then an intravenous line will be inserted into the arm. The patient may be given a liquid contrast to drink before the test. For some parts of the body, small coils are positioned by the area to be scanned. These devices enhance the radio waves and thus improve the MRI images.

Steps of the procedure: For an MRI, the patient lies on a table in the center of the MRI machine. Foam blocks and straps may be used to position the patient. If intravenous contrast is to be used, then it will be injected at this time.

Once the patient is positioned, the table slides into the bore of the MRI. The MRI scanner is turned on and the scan is performed. The scan usually includes several runs and can take from fifteen to forty-five minutes depending on what part of the body is being scanned and the reason for the scan. There is a microphone in the room with the MRI machine so that the patient can communicate with the technician. The patient may be given prism glasses to wear so that he or she can see the MRI technician.

After the procedure: After the procedure, there is no special follow-up care required unless the patient has received a sedative prior to the MRI. In this case, the patient will need to be driven home.

Risks: There are few risks associated with an MRI, unless the person has metal on or in the body or there are metal objects in the room where the test is performed. There is a small risk that a patient might be allergic to the radioactive dye, if it is used.

Results: The MRI yields multidimensional computer images of the tissue being examined. A radiologist who reviews these images is able to differentiate between cancer, edema, infection, bleeding, and inflammation. The patency of blood vessels can also be exhibited. MRI is particularly effective for examining the central nervous system.

Christine M. Carroll, R.N., B.S.N., M.B.A.

For Further Information

Westbrook, Catherine. *MRI in Practice*. 3d ed. Malden, Mass.: Blackwell, 2005.

Huettel, Scott, et al. *Functional Magnetic Resonance Imaging*. Sunderland, Mass.: Sinauer Associates, 2004.

Pagana, Kathleen Deska, and Timothy J. Pagana. *Mosby's Manual of Diagnostic and Laboratory Tests*. 3d ed. St. Louis: Mosby Elsevier, 2006.

Other Resources

How Stuff Works

How MRI Works

http://health.howstuffworks.com/mri.htm

Neurosciences on the Internet

Use of Functional Magnetic Resonance Imaging to Investigate Brain Function

http://www.neuroguide.com/gregg.html

Radiology Info

MRI of the Body

Http://www.radiologyinfo.org/en/info.cfm?pg=bodymr&bhcp=1

WebMD

Magnetic Resonance Imaging (MRI)

http://www.webmd.com/a-to-z-guides/magnetic-resonance-imaging-mri

See also: Angiography; Bone scan; Brain scan; Bronchography; Computed Tomography (CT)-guided biopsy; Computed Tomography (CT) scan; Cystography; Ductogram; Endoscopic Retrograde Cholangiopancreatography (ERCP); Gallium scan; Hysterography; Imaging tests; Lymphangiography; Mammography; Nuclear medicine scan; Percutaneous Transhepatic Cholangiography (PTHC); Positron Emission Tomography (PET); Radionuclide scan; Thermal imaging; Thyroid nuclear medicine scan; Urography; X-ray tests

▶ Mammography

Category: Procedures
Also known as: Breast X-ray

Definition: Mammography is a radiographic procedure used to examine internal breast tissue for possible abnormalities. Three types of mammograms are performed: screening mammogram, diagnostic mammogram, and digital mammogram.

In a screening mammogram, X-ray images of the breast are recorded on X-ray film (conventional method) or electronically (digital method). The recommendation for screening mammograms is once every two years for those women who are forty to forty-nine years old and once every year for women fifty years old and above. Patients with a family history of breast cancer, however, should have the first mammogram before forty years of age and should continue to have them yearly. Also, regardless of age, patients who have been diagnosed as having breast cancer should have a mammogram yearly.

In a diagnostic mammogram, a series of X-ray images of the breast from various angles are recorded on X-ray film (conventional method) or electronically (digital method). Diagnostic mammograms are used to diagnose lumps that a woman feels during self-examination or a health care provider detects during a clinical breast examination if other unexpected symptoms—such as change in breast shape or size, or occurrence of nipple discharge, breast pain, or thickening of breast skin—are present. During a diagnostic mammogram, more X rays are taken than during a screening mammogram in order to get views from many angles. A diagnostic mammogram may be required if the patient has breast implants in order to be able to view breast tissue that can be hidden by the implant.

In a digital mammogram, X-ray images of the breast are recorded electronically and are stored on a computer. The images can then be manipulated via computer software for further evaluation. The average dose of radiation used is lower than that for film mammography. In terms of cancer detection, no differences between digital imaging and traditional film imaging have been found for the general population. Digital mammography is considered preferable, however, for those women who are under the age of fifty, have dense breasts, or are premenopausal or perimenopausal.

In addition, the National Cancer Institute (NCI) is supporting research to develop new procedures for detecting breast tumors. Technologies currently being investigated are magnetic resonance imaging (MRI) and positron emission tomography (PET). Other methods being investigated are those to detect genetic markers for breast cancer, which involve analysis of blood, urine, or fluid aspirated from the nipple.

Cancers diagnosed: Breast cancer

Why performed: In the United States, the most frequently occurring cancer for women is breast cancer. By age eighty, approximately one of every nine women will develop this cancer. Mammography allows for the screening and early detection of breast-tissue abnormalities. Statistics indicate that use of mammography can result in detection of breast cancer one to two years before it can be detected by breast self-examination. Early detection of breast cancer improves the chances for successful treatment of this form of cancer.

Patient preparation: The patient should shower or bathe prior to the mammogram and should not use deodorant, body lotions, sunscreens, creams, powders, or perfume on the chest or underarms, as they may cause "artifacts" (false images) to appear on the X-ray image.

Steps of the procedure: Patients who have breast implants should mention that fact when making the mammogram appointment. Both the technologist who performs the mammogram and the radiologist who interprets the mammogram must have experience in working with implants.

Prior to undergoing mammography, the patient will be asked if she has undergone any type of breast surgery, as this may affect the way in which the X-ray films are interpreted. She will then be asked to remove all clothing and jewelry from the waist up. The patient will be given a short gown and asked to put it on so that it opens in the front.

The procedure begins with the radiologic technologist placing one of the breasts on a platform and lowering a plastic plate onto the breast until it is flattened as much as possible. This allows for the successful X-ray visualization of as much breast tissue as possible. The technologist then positions the X-ray machine, stands behind a protective barrier, and takes the image. A front-view X ray (from the upper surface down) and a side-view X ray of the breast will be taken. Next, the technologist repeats this procedure with the other breast. While the patient may feel uncomfortable when the breast is being flattened, this discomfort is short in duration.

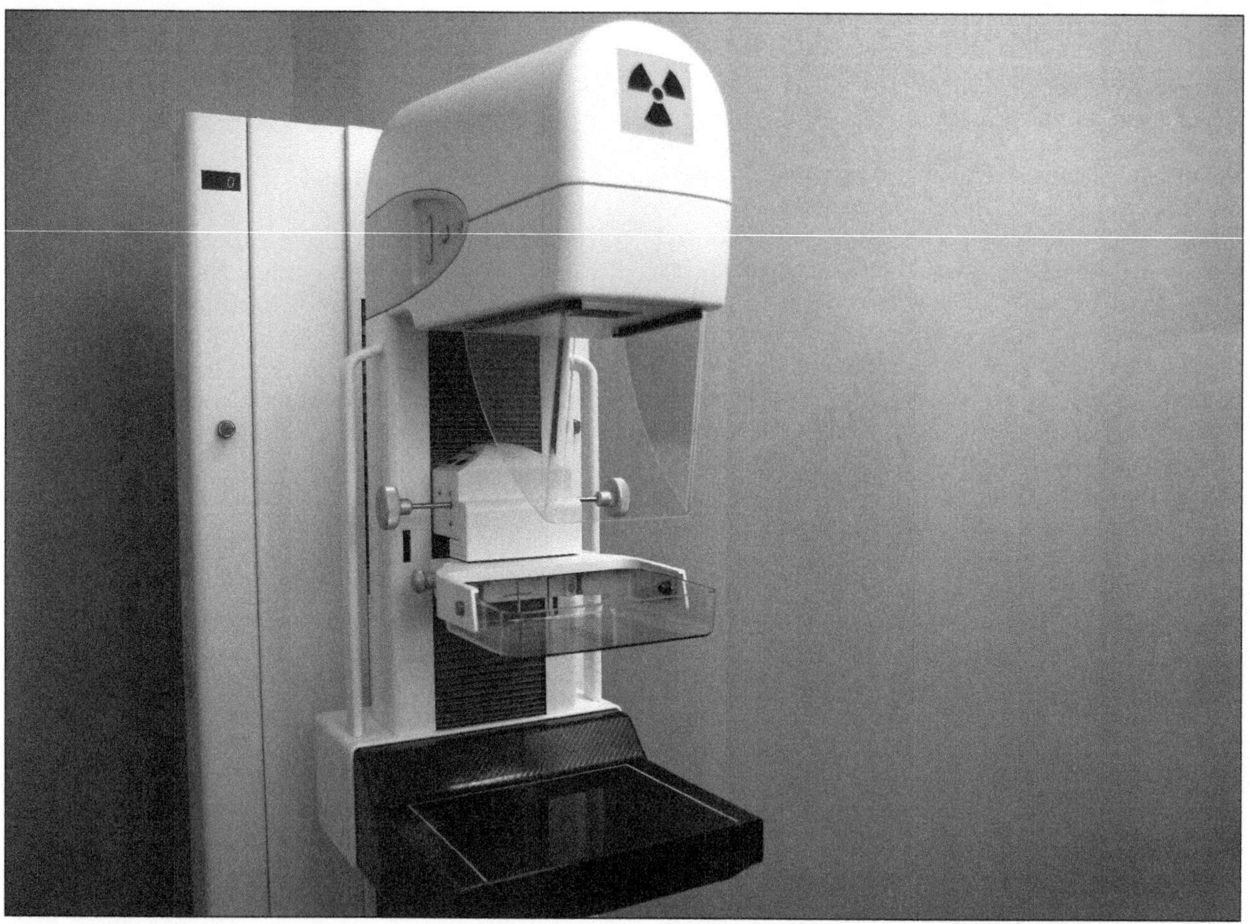

Women are advised to have mammograms once every two years between ages forty and forty-nine and once every year after reaching the age of fifty. (iStock)

After the procedure: The patient will be asked to wait while the X-ray films are developed and then viewed by a radiologist to make sure that none of the images need to be retaken. Once this has been confirmed, the patient will be allowed to redress and use deodorant.

The patient should ask how long it will take to get the results of the mammography and whether those results will be sent to the patient as well as to the doctor. She may also want to ask where the "films" will be stored, so that they can be retrieved if the patient moves out of the area and needs to have future mammograms performed at another location. This is important because the new radiologist may use those earlier images as a reference to determine if there have been any changes in breast tissue over time.

Risks: Mammography uses low-dose radiation and is considered to be very safe. Patients who are pregnant or think they may be pregnant, however, should not have a mammogram. A pregnant woman should not be exposed to X rays because of the possible risk to the fetus.

The safety and reliability of mammograms are mandated by a federal law called the Mammography Quality Standards Act (MQSA). This law requires that all mammography facilities in the United States meet stringent quality standards, including those for the medical physicist, who tests the mammography equipment; the technologist, who takes the mammogram; and the radiologist, who interprets the mammogram. The facilities must also maintain certification by the Food and Drug Administration (FDA) and undergo an annual inspection.

Results: A normal result means that the X-ray films revealed no obvious signs of breast cancer. In certain instances, however, breast cancer may still be present. This false negative result is more common for those women with breast tissue that is more dense, as is typical for younger

Categories of the Breast Imaging Reporting and Database System (BI-RADS)

Category	*Assessment*	*Follow-up*
0	Need additional imaging evaluation	Additional imaging needed before a category can be assigned
1	Negative	Continue annual screening mammography (for women over age 40)
2	Benign (noncancerous)	Continue annual screening mammography (for women over age 40)
3	Probably benign	Receive a 6-month follow-up mammogram
4	Suspicious abnormality	May require biopsy
5	Highly suggestive of malignancy (cancer)	Requires biopsy
6	Known biopsy—proven malignancy (cancer)	Biopsy confirms presence of cancer before treatment begins

women. The more dense the breast tissue, the more difficult it is to visualize abnormal spots on the X-ray image.

An abnormal result means that something has been identified that needs to be looked at more closely. The abnormality may be an unusual-looking area of breast tissue or a type of cyst or lump. Even the presence of a lump, however, does not necessarily indicate cancer. A lump can be either benign (noncancerous) or malignant (cancerous). Therefore, additional testing—such as a diagnostic mammogram, ultrasound, or biopsy—may be required to determine if the abnormality is the result of breast cancer. The most common type of biopsy is known as a needle biopsy. This procedure consists of inserting a small-gauge needle into the area in question and removing a small tissue sample. That sample is then sent to a laboratory for determination if any cancerous cells are present. An abnormality that is interpreted as breast cancer when none is present is called a false positive result. Like the false negative result, it is more common for younger women. It is also more common for those women who have a family history of breast cancer, have had a previous breast biopsy, or are taking estrogen.

The American College of Radiology (ACR) has established a system for uniform reporting of mammogram results called the Breast Imaging Reporting and Database System (BI-RADS) that consists of seven categories. Radiologists and physicians use it to help determine appropriate patient care.

Cynthia L. De Vine, B.A.

For Further Information

Lanyi, M. *Mammography: Diagnosis and Pathological Analysis*. New York: Springer, 2003.

Pisano, E. D., C. Gatsonis, E. Hendrick, et al. "Diagnostic Performance of Digital Versus Film Mammography for Breast-Cancer Screening." *New England Journal of Medicine* 353 (October 27, 2005): 1773-1783.

Qasee, A., et al. "Screening Mammography for Women Forty to Forty-nine Years of Age: A Clinical Practice Guideline from the American College of Physicians." *Annals of Internal Medicine* 146, no. 7 (April 3, 2007): 511-515.

Other Resources

American Cancer Society
http://www.cancer.org

American College of Radiology
http://www.acr.org/index.asp

National Breast and Cervical Cancer Early Detection Program
http://www.cdc.gov/cancer/nbccedp/index.htm

National Cancer Institute
Cancer Information Service
http://cis.nci.nih.gov

National Women's Health Information Center
http://www.womenshealth.gov

Susan G. Komen Breast Cancer Foundation
http://www.komen.org

See also: Accelerated Partial Breast Irradiation (APBI); Breast cancer in children and adolescents; Breast cancer in men; Breast cancer in pregnant women; Breast cancers; Breast implants; Breast ultrasound; Calcifications of the breast; Childbirth and cancer; Clinical Breast Exam (CBE); Comedo carcinomas; Duct ectasia; Ductal carcinoma In Situ (DCIS); Ductal lavage; Ductogram; Estrogen-receptor-sensitive breast cancer; Fibroadenomas; Fibrocystic breast changes; Hormone Replacement Therapy (HRT); Invasive ductal carcinomas; Invasive lobular carcinomas; Lobular Carcinoma In Situ (LCIS); Lumpectomy; Medullary carcinoma of the breast; Microcalcifications; Needle biopsies; Needle localization; Nipple discharge; Peutz-Jeghers Syndrome (PJS); Phyllodes tumors; Tubular carcinomas; Wire localization

▶ Mastectomy

Category: Procedures
Definition: A mastectomy is the surgical removal of a breast.

Cancers diagnosed or treated: Breast cancer

Why performed: A mastectomy is performed to remove a breast that has been affected by cancer. It is very important to remove all the cancerous tissue so that the cancer cannot spread to other parts of the body. Many women diagnosed with breast cancer have the option to choose between mastectomy and breast-conserving surgery (lumpectomy) plus radiotherapy. These women should consider many factors before making a decision. Mastectomy is usually recommended for certain types of patients, including women who have previously had radiotherapy to the affected breast, women with two or more areas of cancer in the same breast, women with connective tissue diseases (such as scleroderma) that make them inappropriate candidates for radiotherapy, and male breast cancer patients. Male breast cancer is relatively rare (men account for less than 1 percent of breast cancer cases) but its treatment, including mastectomy, is the same as it is in women.

Women believed to be at moderate or high risk of developing breast cancer may choose to have one or both breasts removed prophylactically to prevent, rather than to treat, breast cancer. It is believed that preventive mastectomy reduces the chance of developing breast cancer by 90 percent or more in women with a BRCA1 or BRCA2 gene mutation (mutations that make them more susceptible to breast cancer), or in those with a strong family history of the disease.

Patient preparation: The patient will probably meet with the surgeon a few days before the surgery. The surgeon will want to know about any medications the patient is taking that could interfere with surgery. A routine blood workup, urinalysis, and an electrocardiogram (ECG) may be performed a few days before the surgery. Patients will normally be instructed not to eat or drink for at least eight hours before surgery.

If the patient is to have a sentinel lymph node biopsy during the procedure, a small amount of a radioactive substance and a blue dye will be injected into the area several hours before surgery. Sentinel lymph nodes are the first lymph node to which cancers usually spread from primary tumors.

Steps of the procedure: There are five types of mastectomy: 1) A partial mastectomy (also called breast-conserving surgery) only removes the cancerous part of the breast. 2) A total (or simple) mastectomy involves removal of all of the breast tissue. The surgeon may also remove some of the lymph nodes from under the arm to see if the cancer has spread. 3) A skin sparing or nipple sparing mastectomy removes the entire breast, but leaves most of the skin over the breast, or the nipple and circle around it (areola) intact. 4) A modified radical mastectomy involves removal of all breast tissue plus all lymph nodes from under the arm. 5) A radical mastectomy involves removal of all breast tissue and all lymph nodes from under the arm, plus the muscles from the chest wall. This procedure was the most commonly performed type of mastectomy in the past, but it is rarely performed today.

Mastectomy is performed under general anesthesia. A diagonal or horizontal cut is made across the breast, and the breast tissue is removed. Small nerves are cut between the breast tissue and the skin area.

To determine whether cancer has spread to the axillary lymph nodes under the arm, most patients will have a procedure known as sentinel lymph node biopsy. A small amount of radioactive liquid and/or a blue dye are injected into the breast. This allows the surgeon to identify the draining lymph nodes for the area—the ones most likely to contain cancer cells if the cancer has started to spread. There are usually one to five sentinel lymph nodes. They will absorb the radioactive tracer (which can be detected with a gamma probe) and may have also be stained with the blue dye. These lymph nodes are removed and tested with a procedure known as axillary lymph node dissection to see whether they contain cancer cells. If a sentinel lymph node contains cancerous cells, then more lymph nodes will need to be removed. If the sentinel nodes are cancer-free, then it is very unlikely that the cancer has spread to other lymph nodes. In this case, the patient can avoid the potential side effects of full lymph node surgery.

Breast reconstruction may be done after the tissue is removed. A plastic or rubber drainage tube will most likely be inserted to drain fluid from the wound area before the incision is closed up with stitches. A pressure dressing is placed over the wound area to minimize oozing after the surgery.

After the procedure: The patient will experience short-term pain and swelling and will have a scar. Possible complications include wound infection. The patient will most likely have one or more drainage tubes coming from the wound area to drain blood and tissue fluid to prevent them from collecting and causing swelling or infection. These tubes will be removed several days after the surgery. Occasionally, fluid collects around the wound after the tubes have been removed and needs to be drained.

The extent of the surgery will determine the length of hospital stay, but it will probably be three days or less. Reconstruction may extend the hospital stay. After going home, the patient will need considerable rest. Lifting or carrying of heavy objects should be avoided, and the patient should not drive for a few weeks. Gentle exercises may be recommended to relieve pain and stiffness and to encourage circulation to the area.

Many patients experience a pulling sensation near or under the arm after a mastectomy. Patients may experience phantom breast sensations such as unpleasant itching, "pins and needles," pressure, or throbbing after a mastectomy. One study showed that more than one-third of the patients experienced such sensations and that the incidence was similar whether or not the patient had had breast reconstruction. These sensations are believed to be caused by the cutting of small nerves during the procedure and are similar to phantom pains that can occur after limb amputations.

Undergoing a mastectomy can be an emotional time for a patient. Patients may find it helpful to talk to others who have been through the operation, both before and after the surgery. If a breast reconstruction procedure is not done at the time of the mastectomy, then the patient can use a prosthesis inside her bra to provide the shape of a breast.

Risks: A mastectomy is normally a safe and effective operation. There are extremely rare risks associated with the use of general anesthesia. In rare cases, hematoma (an accumulation of blood in the wound area) or seroma (an accumulation of clear fluid in the wound area) may occur. Both of these conditions will get better on their own, or a doctor can drain them.

Removing lymph nodes can sometimes lead to fluid buildup and swelling in the affected arm, which can cause pain and tenderness in the arm and hand. This condition, called lymphedema, can start immediately after the surgery, or months or years later. It is more likely to occur if all of the lymph nodes and vessels are removed. Lymphedema cannot be cured, but the symptoms can be reduced by early recognition of the condition and careful management. Other possible side effects of lymph node removal are limitation of arm and shoulder movement and numbness of the upper arm.

Results: Mastectomy has results similar to those of lumpectomy plus radiation. With single mastectomy, double mastectomy, or lumpectomy plus radiation, around 80 percent of women were still alive 10 years after their diagnosis. The earlier the cancer is caught, the greater the odds of long-term survival.

Jill Ferguson, PhD
Updated by: Stephanie Watson

For Further Information

American Cancer Society. (2016). Surgery for Breast Cancer. Retrieved from http://www.cancer.org/cancer/breastcancer/detailedguide/breast-cancer-treating-surgery.

Kurian, A. W., Lichtensztajn, D. Y., Keegan, T. H., Nelson, D. O., Clarke, C. C., & Gomez, S. L. (2014). Use of and mortality after bilateral mastectomy compared with other surgical treatments for breast cancer in California, 1998-2011. *JAMA*, 312: 902-914.

National Cancer Institute. (2015). Male Breast Cancer Treatment-for health professionals (PDQ). Retrieved from http://www.cancer.gov/types/breast/hp/male-breast-treatment-pdq.

National Cancer Institute. (2013). Surgery to Reduce the Risk of Breast Cancer. Retrieved from http://www.cancer.gov/types/breast/risk-reducing-surgery-fact-sheet.

UpToDate. (2013). Patient information: Surgical procedures for breast cancer—Mastectomy and breast conserving therapy (Beyond the Basics). Retrieved from http://www.uptodate.com/contents/surgical-procedures-for-breast-cancer-mastectomy-and-breast-conserving-therapy-beyond-the-basics.

Other Resources

American Cancer Society
Surgery for Breast Cancer
http://www.cancer.org/cancer/breastcancer/detailedguide/breast-cancer-treating-surgery

Imaginis: The Breast Cancer Resource
Mastectomy
http://www.imaginis.com/breasthealth/mastectomy.asp

National Cancer Institute
Surgery to Reduce the Risk of Breast Cancer
http://www.cancer.gov/cancertopics/factsheet/Therapy/preventive-mastectomy

See also: Breast cancers; Breast implants; Breast reconstruction; Lumpectomy; Lymphedema; Mammography

▶ Mediastinoscopy

Category: Procedures
Also known as: Thoracoscopic mediastinal biopsy

Definition: Mediastinoscopy is an endoscopic procedure used to examine the mediastinum (space between and in front of the lungs). Compared to open-chest surgery, which requires one 6-inch to 8-inch incision, mediastinoscopy uses several small, 1-inch incisions to access the mediastinum, thereby minimizing trauma, decreasing postoperative pain, and promoting a shorter hospital stay and a quicker recovery.

Cancers diagnosed or treated: Sarcoidosis, lung cancer, lymphoma, Hodgkin disease, myasthenia gravis, mesothelioma, mediastinal or neurogenic tumors, thymomas

Why performed: Mediastinoscopy is performed with a biopsy to evaluate abnormal mediastinal tissue, lymph nodes, inflammation, or infection. It can be used as a staging procedure to evaluate non-small-cell lung cancer.

Mediastinoscopy is also used to remove malignant lymph nodes and mediastinal tumors. Benign and malignant mediastinal tumors that are not removed can interfere with the normal function of the organs in the mediastinum, including the aorta, vena cava, heart, and pericardium.

Patient preparation: Tests may include a chest X ray, computed tomography (CT) scan, and magnetic resonance imaging (MRI). One week before the procedure, patients must stop taking anticoagulants, as directed by the physician. In general, patients must not eat or drink for eight to ten hours before the procedure.

Steps of the procedure: A sedative may be given before the patient receives general anesthesia. A mediastinoscope (small videoscope) is inserted under the sternum through a small incision at the base of the neck. The mediastinoscope is manipulated, and images of the abnormal area are displayed on a computer screen to guide the surgeon during the procedure. CT may also be used during the procedure. Other surgical instruments are inserted through two or three small chest incisions, and a tissue sample is removed.

After the procedure: The hospital recovery is about one to two days, and some patients may be able to go home the day of the procedure. Before going home, the patient receives a follow-up schedule and aftercare instructions. The patient can generally return to normal activities within three to four weeks after discharge.

Risks: The risks of mediastinoscopy include bleeding, infection, allergic reaction to the anesthetic, blood vessel damage, a tear in the esophagus, laryngeal nerve injury that can cause permanent vocal hoarseness, or collapse of a lung (pneumothorax). The overall complication rate is reportedly low, at under 2.5 percent, with major complications under 0.5 percent and mortality under 0.5 percent.

Results: The biopsy tissue is examined for malignancy, inflammation, or infection. The type and extent of disease will help determine the patient's treatment.

Angela M. Costello, B.S.

See also: Bronchoalveolar lung cancer; Endoscopy; Lung cancers; Mediastinal tumors; Mesothelioma; Pneumonectomy; Surgical biopsies; Thoracoscopy

▶ Microwave hyperthermia therapy

Category: Procedures
Also known as: Heat therapy

Definition: Microwave hyperthermia therapy is a procedure in which microwaves are used to heat an area in which cancer is present. It is considered an experimental therapy and is not widely available, and it is usually used in combination with radiation therapy or chemotherapy.

Cancers treated: A wide variety of cancers, including prostate, breast, bladder, lung, and liver cancers

Why performed: Microwave hyperthermia therapy aims either to kill tumor cells or to make them more susceptible to other cancer treatments.

Patient preparation: Patient preparation for microwave hyperthermia therapy depends on the area in which the therapy will be done and whether the therapy will be localized or regional. Patients should discuss carefully with their cancer care team the possible outcomes of the therapy and what the realistic outcome expectations are.

Steps of the procedure: In localized hyperthermia, a rod containing coils that produce microwaves is introduced to the tumor. The rod is then turned on and the microwaves heat up the tumor cells. The tumor cells may be heated to such an extent that they die, or they may be heated only to an extent that makes them more susceptible to chemotherapy drugs. It is very difficult to heat only the tumor cells, and normal cells surrounding the tumor may also be affected.

In regional microwave hyperthermia therapy, a device that produces microwaves is aimed at a region, such as an arm or leg. The machine is then started and produces microwaves that heat the entire region. In this case the cells are heated enough to make chemotherapy drugs more effective but not enough to kill the cells.

After the procedure: If the microwave hyperthermia is administered in conjunction with chemotherapy or radiation, then the patient will experience the effects that he or she usually experiences after such therapy. The patient may experience temporary feelings of pain or discomfort from the procedure.

Risks: Microwave hyperthermia therapy is considered an experimental procedure. The risks will depend on the specific procedure being performed but may include pain, infection, swelling, blood clots, and nerve or muscle damage.

Results: The goal of microwave hyperthermia therapy is usually to improve the effectiveness of chemotherapy drugs or radiation therapy. In these cases, the results of the treatment may be hard to define because many other things can also affect the effectiveness of such treatments. The results will also vary depending on the area in which the tumor is located, the extent of the cancer, and whether the procedure was done on a localized or regional area.

Helen Davidson, B.A.

See also: Bladder cancer; Breast cancers; Chemotherapy; Hyperthermia therapy; Liver cancers; Lung cancers; Prostate cancer; Radiation therapies; Radiofrequency ablation

▶ Mohs surgery

Category: Procedures
Also known as: Mohs micrographic surgery

Definition: Mohs surgery is a surgical technique for precisely excising malignant cutaneous tumors. It was developed in the 1930's by Dr. Fredric Mohs. In 1969, Dr. Mohs reported the use of the technique for excising basal cell carcinomas and squamous cell carcinomas and claimed a five-year cure rate of 100 percent. Subsequent data and studies led to the validation of the technique within the surgical community. Mohs surgery is now commonly used for the resection of malignant and nonmalignant tumors in cosmetically sensitive areas such as the face and neck, hands, and genitalia.

Cancers treated: Basal cell carcinomas, squamous cell carcinomas

Why performed: With Mohs surgery, the tumor can be surgically excised with precision, maintaining the best surgical and cosmetic outcome. Accurate tumor margin assessment and high cure rates are achievable with this technique. In addition, Mohs surgery allows the patient to be spared the unnecessary removal of normal tissues, ultimately providing a more functional and cosmetically optimal outcome.

Patient preparation: The patient is screened for allergies to numbing medicines such as lidocaine. The surgical site is prepped in a sterile fashion. Local anesthesia is typically used, and the patient's wound is covered between surgical stages.

Steps of the procedure: Mohs surgery is typically performed under local anesthesia by a dermatologist trained in the procedure in an outpatient setting. The procedure typically takes between two and four hours and is generally very well tolerated, with a low incidence of postsurgical complications.

During the procedure, the tumor, along with a small area of clinically normal-appearing skin around the tumor, is excised. The tissue is then immediately processed by a histology technician, and the margins are evaluated by the surgeon. Mohs micrographic diagrams are used to map out the tissue for the histology technician and the surgeon. If the microscopic margins are positive, then their precise locations are noted on the Mohs map and tissue is resected only from that area. This process is repeated in stages until the entire tumor is removed and clear margins are seen.

Following the complete resection of the tumor, the defect is either closed immediately using various surgical repair techniques or allowed to close by secondary intention. The type of closure depends on the type of defect and the preference of the surgeon.

After the procedure: The patient should be provided with thorough wound care instructions before discharge.

Risks: The risks of Mohs surgery include allergy to the numbing medication, scarring, pain, and infection.

Results: The procedure ideally results in the complete clearing of the tumor in question. The patient should be counseled that recurrence is always a possibility.

Sarah Kasprowicz, M.D.

See also: Basal cell carcinomas; Bowen disease; Dermatofibrosarcoma protuberans (DFSP); Dermatology oncology; Penile cancer; Squamous cell carcinomas

▶ Needle localization

Category: Procedures
Also known as: Wire localization, stereotactic (exact) localization

Definition: Needle localization is a procedure that is used to mark a nonpalpable mass (one that cannot be felt) prior to biopsy (removal of a piece of tissue). It is most commonly associated with breast biopsies. Needle localization is performed by a radiologist or surgeon using ultrasound, mammography, or magnetic resonance imaging (MRI) to view the tumor.

Cancers diagnosed: Breast cancer

Why performed: Since the breast mass is not palpable, the surgeon needs a way to find the tumor in order to biopsy it. The wire serves as a marker for the tumor.

Patient preparation: Needle localization is associated with surgical and core needle breast biopsy. Usually, this procedure is performed in a radiology office or a breast biopsy room. For a surgical biopsy, within a month before the procedure, the patient has a preoperative physical examination, routine blood work, and possibly an electrocardiogram (EKG). Also, she will have to fast after midnight the day of the procedure. For core needle biopsy, the patient needs to fast only for two to three hours before the procedure.

Steps of the procedure: First, the mass is localized. When ultrasound is used, the transducer (used to transmit and receive sound waves) is held to the side of the mass while the needle is inserted. With mammography, it is necessary to use special mammography plates with a screen or a small door in them, so that the needle can be inserted while the breast is compressed. MRI imaging requires the use of a special attachment through which the needle can be inserted.

A local anesthetic is injected over the tumor. Either a thin wire or a needle is then inserted into the tumor. The position of the wire or needle is verified with the radiologic imaging being used.

After the procedure: The biopsy is performed either in an operating room (for a surgical biopsy) or in the biopsy room (for a core needle biopsy). The wire or needle is removed with the breast tumor.

Risks: There is a slight risk of bleeding or infection after this procedure.

Results: The surgeon is able to localize the nonpalpable breast tumor by the presence of the wire and then to remove it. Pathology will be performed on the tissue sample to determine whether it is cancerous.

Christine M. Carroll, R.N., B.S.N., M.B.A.

For Further Information

Rosen, Paul Peter, and Syed A. Hoda. *Breast Pathology: Diagnosis by Needle Core Biopsy*. 2d ed. Philadelphia: Lippincott Williams & Wilkins, 2006.

Rubin, Eva, and Jean F. Simpson. *Breast Specimen Radiography: Needle Localization and Radiographic Pathologic Correlation*. Philadelphia: Lippincott-Raven, 1998.

Other Resources

eMedicine
Breast Needle Localization
http://www.emedicine.com/Radio/topic911.htm

WebMD
Breast Biopsy
http://www.webmd.com/breast-cancer/guide/breast-biopsy

See also: Biopsy; Breast ultrasound; Magnetic Resonance Imaging (MRI); Mammography; Needle biopsies; Stereotactic needle biopsy; Ultrasound tests; Wire localization

▶ Nephrostomy

Category: Procedures
Also known as: Percutaneous nephrostomy (PCN), nephropyelostomy

Definition: Nephrostomy is a procedure in which an opening is made and a nephrostomy tube (catheter) is placed into the kidney to drain urine to outside the body.

Urine is collected into a bag attached to the nephrostomy tube. The procedure is done either through a surgical incision or percutaneously (through the skin).

Cancers treated: Ovarian, cervical, colon, and other cancers of the pelvic area

Why performed: Tumors may cause a blockage of one or both of the ureters, the tubes that normally carry urine from the kidneys to the bladder. The blockage causes a backup of urine into the kidneys, creating a great risk of infection and kidney damage that cannot be repaired. The insertion of nephrostomy tubes prevents the backup of urine. Nephrostomy tubes may also be placed during a diagnostic procedure called an antegrade pyelogram, which is done to determine the location of the blockage. In some cases, the nephrostomy tubes are inserted to allow the placement of anticancer drugs directly into the kidney. Nephrostomy tubes are also used for other conditions that affect the urinary tract.

Patient preparation: Nephrostomy is usually performed on hospitalized patients. Some patients may have the procedure done without admission to a hospital. Preparation for the procedure may vary depending on the patient's condition, the physician's practice, and the facility. Generally, the patient must not have anything to eat or drink for four to eight hours before the procedure. The physician may ask the patient to temporarily stop or adjust the dose of some medications, including aspirin, blood thinners, and diabetes medications. Laboratory tests such as a complete blood count (CBC), coagulation tests, urinalysis, and urine culture for bacteria may be done before the procedure. The physician discusses the procedure, including the type of local anesthetic used, sedation, risks, and aftercare. The patient gives the physician permission to perform the procedure by reading and signing a consent form. Before signing the form, the patient may ask the physician questions to clarify anything that the doctor has said or any part of the consent form that the patient does not understand.

Steps of the procedure: An intravenous (IV) line is inserted, usually in the patient's arm or hand, to provide fluids, antibiotics, pain medication, and sedation. Nephrostomy is generally performed in the interventional radiology department by an interventional radiologist or urologist. The patient lies on the stomach and remains awake, although medication is given that may cause drowsiness. Monitoring of blood pressure, heart rate, and oxygen level is done throughout the procedure. Imaging procedures such as ultrasound, computed tomography (CT), or fluoroscopy are used to visualize the area. These procedures are done before and during insertion of the nephrostomy tube to guide the physician in placing the tube.

The site where the tube will be inserted is sterilized. A medication such as lidocaine (Xylocaine) is given to numb the skin and tissues. A small incision is made, and a needle is inserted into the kidney. Contrast dye is injected for visualization, and the nephrostomy tube is inserted. The needle is removed. A dressing is placed over the site, and the nephrostomy tube is connected to a drainage bag. The tube site is on the right or left side of the back near the waistline, depending on which kidney is blocked. If both kidneys are blocked, then the physician will insert tubes for each kidney.

After the procedure: The patient is taken to the recovery room or back to the hospital room. A nurse will monitor the patient for any changes in blood pressure, heart rate, or breathing. The nurse monitors the urine output by measuring the urine collected in the bag. The bag may be attached to the patient's leg by use of straps that are provided. Before discharge, the physician and/or a nurse will give the patient instructions on caring for the nephrostomy site, emptying the bag, monitoring the urine output, and noting signs of complications. Patients may need others to assist them in caring for the site and emptying the bag once they are home. In addition to the urine drained through the nephrostomy tube, the patient will still need to urinate. If only one tube is placed but the other kidney works normally, then the urine from that kidney still passes into the bladder. If nephrostomy tubes are placed in both kidneys, then there may still be drainage of some urine into the bladder.

Risks: The risks of nephrostomy include bleeding, infection, blood clots in the nephrostomy tube or bladder, and dislodgement of the nephrostomy tube.

Results: The placement of nephrostomy tubes will alleviate the backup of urine in the kidneys or allow treatment to be given. Although their use is normally for a short time, in some cases the blockage cannot be removed and the nephrostomy tubes remain in use permanently. In these cases, the tubes are replaced periodically.

Wanda E. Clark, M.T. (ASCP)

For Further Information

Berman, Joel. *Understanding Surgery: A Comprehensive Guide for Every Family*. Wellesley, Mass.: Branden Books. 2001.

Nurse's Five-Minute Consult: Treatments. Philadelphia: Lippincott Williams & Wilkins, 2007.

Other Resources

National Institutes of Health
Caring for Your Nephrostomy Tube
http://clinicalcenter.nih.gov/ccc/patient_education/pepubs/percneph.pdf

See also: Cervical cancer; Kidney cancer; Ovarian cancers; Renal pelvis tumors; Urinary system cancers; Urologic oncology; Urostomy

▶ Nuclear medicine scan

Category: Procedures
Also known as: Radionuclide scan, positron emission tomography (PET) scan, single photon emission computed tomography (SPECT) imaging

Definition: A nuclear medicine scan detects electromagnetic radiation, usually gamma rays, emitted from an injected radioactive tracer than has been taken up by an organ in the body to be studied, with the goal of producing an image.

The most common radioisotope used is technetium 99m, known as the workhorse of nuclear medicine, whose gamma rays are absorbed by a sodium iodide crystal detector. Interaction of the gamma rays with the crystals results in production of a pulse of fluorescent light proportional in intensity to the energy of the gamma ray. The light is amplified and converted into an electrical signal by the photomultiplier tubes. The electrical signal is then fed to a computer, which analyzes the pulse height and generates an image of the distribution of the radiotracer in the body or organ under study. An array of these crystal detectors attached to a collimator, along with the photomultipliers and computer, is called a gamma camera. The gamma camera is used to scan the patient. The pattern of uptake of radiotracer in the organ or whole body under study varies depending on the disease process.

Multiple gamma cameras are sometimes used to generate a three-dimensional view of an organ; this particular type of nuclear medicine scan is called single photon emission computed tomography (SPECT) imaging.

The exceptions to the use of technetium in nuclear medicine scanning include gallium scanning, which uses gallium as the radionuclide; some thyroid imaging that uses radioactive iodine; indium-labeled white cell studies and cerebral perfusion scans; some cardiac imaging that uses thallium; the Schilling test, which uses cobalt-labeled vitamin B_{12}; and PET scanning, which uses antimatter or positron emission instead of a gamma emitter.

PET imaging utilizes fluorodeoxyglucose (FDG) labeled with F-18, a positron emitter. The F-18-labeled FDG is preferentially taken up by cancer cells because of their increased metabolic rate and therefore increased need for sugar compared to normal cells. The scanner used in PET imaging is not the gamma camera but a separate scanner based on coincidence detection of the annihilation photons resulting from positron decay. PET scanning is often combined with computed tomography (CT) performed at the same time.

Cancers diagnosed: All types of cancers, both primary and secondary (metastatic), can be diagnosed using nuclear medicine scans; for PET scans, the cancers more commonly diagnosed are lymphoma (Hodgkin and non-Hodgkin), esophageal cancer, lung cancer, head and neck cancers, colorectal cancer, pancreatic cancer, renal cancer, breast cancer, thyroid cancer, and melanoma.

Most cancers are identified as a result of their increased uptake of the radiotracer. Others are identified as a result of their lack of uptake, called photopenia, as can be seen in some liver tumors evaluated with HIDA or sulfur colloid. For HIDA scans, differentiation among primary hepatic tumors is performed because of increased uptake seen in focal nodular hyperplasia but not hepatic adenoma, which appears photopenic. In sulfur colloid liver-spleen scans, hepatic adenoma is again seen as a cold defect because of the lack of Kupffer cells (the phagocytic or "sweeper" cells in the liver that form part of the reticuloendothelial system) compared with focal nodular hyperplasia, which has either normal or increased colloid uptake as a result of the presence of Kupffer cells. Macrophages in the spleen function similarly. A type of benign hepatic tumor known as a cavernous hemangioma is often diagnosed by increased uptake of radiotracer on red blood cell scans in a pattern that is virtually pathognomonic. For bone scans, metastatic disease from prostate and breast as well as osteosarcoma and osteiod osteoma are most commonly diagnosed as a result of increased radiotracer activity from osteoblastic activity of the cancer cells (that is, increased bone turnover caused by the cancer cells). Multiple myeloma, on the other hand, is photopenic on bone scans. For iodine scans, thyroid cancer of both primary and secondary types is identified because of the increased uptake of radioiodine. In some cases, such as thyroid cancer, the scan and the treatment can be combined using radioactive iodine. Carcinoid tumor and medullary carcinoma of the thyroid are diagnosed with somastatin receptor imaging called indium DTPA-labeled octreotide, and pheochromocytomas are diagnosed with iodine-labeled metaiodobenzylguanidine (MIBG).

Why performed: Nuclear medicine scans (bone scan, iodine scan, HIDA scan, red blood cell scan, sulfur colloid scan, octreotide scan, PET scan) are used to diagnose primary and secondary cancer. They are also used to diagnose various ailments depending on the type of scan, including but not limited to the following: acute and chronic cholecystitis and evaluation for postoperative leaks following cholecystectomy (HIDA or DISIDA scan); gastrointestinal bleeding (red blood cell pertechnetate scan); goiter, hypothyroidism versus hyperthyroidism, and evaluation for ectopic thyroid tissue (thyroid scan); hyperparathyroidism caused by parathyroid adenoma (parathyroid scan); Meckel's diverticulum (Meckel's pertechnetate scan); pernicious anemia and malabsorption as a result of sprue (Schilling test); testicular torsion, testicular trauma, orchitis, and epididymitis (testicular pertechnetate scan); bone fractures, Paget disease, prosthesis evaluation, reflex sympathetic dystrophy, bone infarction, and bone infection (bone scan); kidney obstruction, renal transplant rejection, and renal artery stenosis (renal scan); infectious and inflammatory disorders of the lungs, abdomen, pelvis, genitourinary tract, and bone, including acquired immunodeficiency syndrome (AIDS), sarcoidosis, and fever of unknown origin, among others (gallium scan); infection (indium-labeled white blood cells); cardiomyopathy-myocarditis and ejection fraction of the heart, often performed after doxorubicin chemotherapy for breast cancer (MUGA scan); coronary artery disease, coronary artery bypass graft surgery evaluation, valvular heart disease, and risk stratification following myocardial infarction (myocardial perfusion imaging, radionuclide ventriculography, cardiac SPECT, cardiac PET); pulmonary embolus (lung or V/Q scan); gastrointestinal bleeding, portal hypertension, and gastric emptying (sulfur colloid scan); normal pressure hydrocephalus, cerebral spinal fluid leaks, and surgical shunt patency (indium-labeled DTPA cisternography); evaluation for brain death (DTPA cerebral blood flow study); stroke (HMPAO cerebral perfusion imaging with SPECT); identification of seizure focus, evaluation for Alzheimer's disease versus other forms of dementia and depression, Parkinson's disease, and drug addiction (brain SPECT and brain PET).

Patient preparation: Patients are asked to fast at least four hours prior to most scans, especially DISIDA scans and PET scans. For thyroid imaging, patients should stop thyroid medication (synthroid) and avoid CT contrast intravenous dye for one month prior to the scan, as both synthroid and CT contrast dye will interfere with the scan results. Cisternography requires the injection of indium-labeled DTPA radiopharmaceutical into the lumbar subarachnoid space by lumbar puncture, also called spinal tap, prior to scanning. The Schilling test requires the patient to collect urine for twenty-four hours after injection of the radiotracer labeled vitamin B^{12}, and the urine is then evaluated. The patient also receives an intramuscular injection of nonlabeled vitamin B^{12} as part of the test, prior to the urine collection.

Steps of the procedure: The radioisotope is prepared by the technologist and injected into a peripheral vein by the radiologist or nuclear medicine physician. For white blood cell scans and some red blood cell scans, a small amount of blood is withdrawn from the patient and labeled with the radioisotope and is then reinjected prior to scanning. The patient is then placed on the back on a table under a gamma camera connected to a computer. Scan time is variable depending on the procedure but usually takes about one hour.

After the procedure: The scan is generated by the computer attached to the detector and read by the radiologist the same day. The patient will need to contact his or her doctor for the radiology report and for follow-up treatment.

Risks: Minor pain or bruising at the injection site may occur. If the patient is pregnant, then the scan should be avoided if possible, since the radiation dose, although small in most cases, is not negligible. Radioactive iodine should not be administered to a pregnant patient because of the risk to the fetus as the radioiodine crosses the placenta with significant exposure to the fetal thyroid, causing cretinism. Radioiodine is also excreted in human breast milk, and nursing should be stopped following diagnostic or therapeutic studies performed using radioiodine.

Results: The results of a nuclear medicine scan are dependent on the type of scan performed and the reason for the study. Their use in detecting tumors helps the cancer care team stage the cancer and develop a treatment plan.

Debra B. Kessler, M.D., Ph.D.

For Further Information

Mettler, Fred A., Jr., and Milton J. Guiberteau. *Essentials of Nuclear Medicine Imaging*. 5th ed. Philadelphia: Saunders/Elsevier, 2006.

Sandler, Martin P., R. Edward Coleman, and James A. Patton, eds. *Diagnostic Nuclear Medicine*. 4th ed. Philadelphia: Lippincott Williams & Wilkins, 2003.

Wahl, Richard L., ed. *Principles and Practice of Positron Emission Tomography*. Philadelphia: Lippincott Williams & Wilkins, 2002.

See also: Brain scan; Cold nodule; Gallium scan; Imaging tests; Positron Emission Tomography (PET); Radionuclide scan; Thyroid nuclear medicine scan; X-ray tests

▶ Ommaya reservoir

Category: Procedures
Also known as: Implanted intrathecal device, intraventricular device

Definition: An Ommaya reservoir is a device surgically placed under the scalp that allows administration of drugs, such as chemotherapy, directly into the cerebrospinal fluid (CSF), bypassing the blood-brain barrier. It may also be used to sample CSF.

Cancers treated: Brain and related nervous system lesions, any brain metastasis

Why performed: Blood vessels that provide blood to the brain filter out drugs and other substances, preventing them from reaching the brain and cerebrospinal fluid. This blood-brain barrier also blocks chemotherapy from reaching cancer cells in the brain and CSF. With the surgical placement of an Ommaya reservoir under the scalp, drugs may be delivered directly to tumors or metastases. In some cases, the Ommaya reservoir has been used to drain cystic lesions in the brain.

Patient preparation: The Ommaya reservoir, a small dome-shaped device with an attached tube, is placed by a neurosurgeon during surgery. The patient is under general anesthesia, so there is no pain. An area of the head is shaved and an incision is made in the skin. The tube, or catheter, is inserted through a small hole made in the skull and threaded into a hollow space, or ventricle, which holds CSF.

Steps of the procedure: After the surgical site heals, a physician or specially trained nurse may access the device to remove CSF or to administer chemotherapy or other drugs. This procedure may be done in the hospital or specialty outpatient clinic. Accessing the device is a sterile procedure. The skin over the device is cleansed, and then a sterile needle is used to pierce the dome and instill the chemotherapy or drug. The needle is withdrawn and pressure is applied to the needle site to control any bleeding.

After the procedure: The patient should report any symptoms such as headache, unusual sleepiness, stiff neck, nausea, and vomiting immediately. Any usual side effects of chemotherapy administration may occur. It is important to observe the area over the Ommaya reservoir for signs of infection, such as redness and warmth at the needle site. Patients may go home between treatments with the device in place and may continue normal activities.

Risks: The risks associated with an Ommaya reservoir are generally related to blockage of the tube or infection.

Results: The patient may expect that chemotherapy and other drugs reach the necessary site of action with minimum pain.

Patricia Stanfill Edens, R.N., Ph.D., FACHE

See also: Chemotherapy; Infusion therapies; Medulloblastomas

▶ Oophorectomy

Category: Procedures
Also known as: Ovariotomy, ovariectomy, bilateral oophorectomy, preventive or prophylactic bilateral oophorectomy (PBO), prophylactic oophorectomy, laparoscopic oophorectomy

Definition: Oophorectomy is the surgical removal of both ovaries as a treatment for ovarian cancer or metastasized cancer. The two ovaries are the part of the female reproductive system that produces egg cells (ova) and releases hormones, including estrogen. Both ovaries may be removed as a preventive measure for women with a high risk of ovarian cancer or breast cancer. Oophorectomy may be used for patients with estrogen-sensitive breast cancer to prevent its recurrence.

Cancers treated: Ovarian cancer, metastasized cancer, preventive treatment for patients at high risk for ovarian or breast cancer, treatment for estrogen-sensitive breast cancer

Why performed: Both ovaries are removed with an oophorectomy to help treat ovarian cancer. Most ovarian cancers develop in the epithelial cells that cover the outside of the ovary. Ovarian cancer can also develop in the germ cells (the cells that produce eggs) or in the stromal cells (the cells inside of the ovary that produce estrogen and progesterone).

Ovarian cancer can spread to other parts of the body. Other parts of the female reproductive system such as the Fallopian tubes, which transport eggs to the uterus for fertilization, may be removed in a surgery termed a bilateral salpingo-oophorectomy. Oophorectomy is used to treat metastasized cancer that originated elsewhere in the body and has spread to the ovaries.

Women with the *BRCA1* or *BRCA2* gene mutations have a high risk for breast cancer and gynecologic cancer. A preventive bilateral oophorectomy (PBO) is used to remove both ovaries of women with a family history and high risk of ovarian cancer. A PBO is usually performed after a woman has experienced childbirth or at about the age of thirty-five. Research has shown that PBO does reduce the risk of ovarian cancer for high-risk women.

Research shows that PBO before the age of forty can significantly reduce the risk of breast cancer for women with the *BRCA1* or *BRCA2* gene mutations. Oophorectomy may also be used as a preventive treatment for premenopausal women with estrogen-sensitive breast cancer. Removing both ovaries removes the main source of estrogen in the body and can help to prevent estrogen-sensitive cancer cells from growing.

Patient preparation: Patients receive laboratory and blood tests prior to surgery. X rays or ultrasound images may be taken to help plan the procedure. Patients should eat a light dinner and not eat or drink after midnight on the day prior to the surgery. In some cases, preparations may be used to empty the colon.

Steps of the procedure: Oophorectomy for the treatment of cancer uses general anesthesia and an open surgical method. A vertical incision is made on the abdomen. The abdominal muscles are spread apart to allow the surgeon access to the ovaries. The vertical incision allows the surgeon to view the abdominal cavity for disease or cancer. After both ovaries are removed, the incision is closed and bandaged.

A horizontal incision may be used to remove both ovaries if cancer is not present. A horizontal incision is associated with less scarring and bleeding. A laparoscopic oophorectomy may also be used if cancer is not present, in cases of preventive surgery.

Laparoscopic oophorectomy is guided by images produced by a laparoscope, a narrow tube with a light, viewing instrument, and miniature camera. The laparoscope is inserted through small incisions in the abdomen. Surgical instruments are inserted through the laparoscope to remove the ovaries. Because laparoscopic surgery is minimally invasive and uses only small incisions, it is associated with less pain, less bleeding, fewer complications or infections, a shorter hospital stay, and a quicker recovery time.

After the procedure: The patient remains in the hospital for three to five days and returns to regular activity levels in about six weeks. Patients receiving open surgery may experience discomfort from having the abdominal muscles moved during the procedure. Patients receiving laparoscopic surgery may remain in the hospital for a night or two and resume regular activities sooner.

Patients who have both ovaries removed are no longer able to become pregnant and therefore experience "surgical menopause." Those without cancer may receive hormones to help ease the risk of medical complications and menopausal symptoms. Symptoms of menopause may be greater in women experiencing surgical menopause than in women with naturally occurring menopause.

Patients with ovarian cancer usually receive chemotherapy following oophorectomy. Chemotherapy uses medication, or a combination of medications, delivered over a period of time to help kill any remaining cancer cells. Radiation therapy is rarely used.

Risks: The surgical risks of oophorectomy include infection, bleeding, blood clots, and damage to other organs. Some women experience decreased sex drive and decreased orgasm. Bilateral oophorectomy increases the risk of cardiovascular disease, osteoporosis, and thyroid cancer. Hormone therapy can help reduce the risk.

Results: Normal results are removal of both ovaries without complications and no findings of cancer. Abnormal results include removal of both ovaries with findings of cancer, metastasized spread, or complications.

Mary Car-Blanchard, O.T.D., B.S.O.T.

For Further Information

Fader, A. N., and R. G. Rose. "Role of Surgery in Ovarian Carcinoma." *Journal of Clinical Oncology* 25, no. 20 (July 10, 2007): 2873-2883.

Kauff, N. D., and R. R. Barakat. "Risk-Reducing Salpingo-oophorectomy in Patients with Germline Mutations in *BRCA1* or *BRCA2*." *Journal of Clinical Oncology* 25, no. 20 (July 10, 2007): 2921-2927.

Parker, W. H., et al. "Elective Oophorectomy in the Gynecological Patient: When Is It Desirable?" *Current Opinion in Obstetrics and Gynecology* 19, no. 4 (August, 2007): 350-354.

See also: *BRCA1* and *BRCA2* genes; Breast cancers; Fallopian tube cancer; Gynecologic oncology; Hormonal therapies; Hot flashes; Hysterectomy; Hystero-oophorectomy; Salpingectomy and salpingo-oophorectomy

▶ Oral and maxillofacial surgery

Category: Procedures

Also known as: Mouth surgery, maxillectomy, laryngectomy, neck dissection

Definition: Oral surgery and maxillofacial surgery are general terms for surgery of the mouth (oral) and of the upper jaw and face (maxillofacial). Specially trained dentists, known as oral and maxillofacial surgeons, perform this type of surgery. Otorhinolaryngologists (ear, nose, and throat specialists) also perform certain oral and maxillofacial surgeries, as do cosmetic, or plastic, surgeons. Surgeons use oral and maxillofacial surgery to treat a wide range of injuries, defects, and diseases.

Cancers treated: Oral or mouth cancer, including cancer of the lips, mouth, gums, salivary glands, tongue, face, neck, jaws, and hard and soft palates (roof of the mouth)

Why performed: In treating cancer, doctors use oral and maxillofacial surgery most often to destroy or remove cancerous tumors. In some cases, doctors use oral and maxillofacial surgery to repair or reconstruct parts of the jaw and other boney structures of the face and throat to help patients speak or swallow better, or to restore a patient's appearance following surgery or an injury.

Patient preparation: What happens before oral and maxillofacial surgery to remove or destroy a tumor depends on its location. Patients who are undernourished because chewing or swallowing is difficult, owing to the site of the tumor, receive fluids intravenously to build up their strength before the operation. Generally, patients are instructed not to eat or drink anything eight hours before the procedure. Because various general and local anesthetics are used during the surgery, patients should inform their doctors of substances to which they are allergic. Surgeons sometimes perform oral and maxillofacial surgery in an operatory, so patients need to arrange for a ride home after the procedure. Nurses help hospital patients prepare for their surgery.

Steps of the procedure: Because tumors can develop in so many sites in the mouth and face, and because surgeons may either destroy or remove the tumor, surgical procedures vary widely. For example, surgeons remove early-stage tumors of the tongue with a laser instrument operated directly through the mouth. In cases where the cancer has spread to the neck lymph nodes, a common occurrence, surgeons remove the affected lymph nodes, a procedure know as a neck dissection. Following this primary surgery, surgeons may have to perform additional operations to restore normal function to the patient's neck, shoulder, or other nearby parts of the body. In some cases, surgeons perform secondary surgery to restore nerve function. In many cases, oral and maxillofacial surgery disfigures the patient's face or neck. When that happens, surgeons perform restorative, or reconstructive, surgery to restore the patient's appearance. Such secondary surgery includes the use of tissue flaps to restore soft tissue, skin grafts, bone grafts, and prostheses (metal or plastic parts to replace original body parts).

Whatever the type of surgery, patients receive, as needed, a combination of anesthetics, medicines that put the patient to sleep, relax the patient, and block pain.

After the procedure: Following surgery, care varies for each patient depending on the type of surgery and the location and extent of the cancer. Some patients may return home several hours after surgery. Others may have to stay in the hospital for several days. Postoperative care and rehabilitation may include additional surgery, speech therapy, dietary guidance, and psychological counseling.

Risks: The risks from oral and maxillofacial surgery include harmful reactions to anesthetics and medications, wound infection, excessive bleeding, and slow healing, which are common to most surgeries. More specifically, oral and maxillofacial surgery can adversely affect a variety of body functions, including speaking, chewing, swallowing, and controlling the flow of saliva. These risks depend on the size and location of the tumor. Sometimes when destroying or removing a tumor, surgeons destroy or remove surrounding tissue or structures in the mouth. In addition, some patients disfigured by oral and maxillofacial surgery experience psychological problems because of the change in their appearance. Coupled with a severe illness or aggressive treatment, a changed look creates mental and social problems for some patients.

Results: Typically, the earlier oral cancer is detected and treated, the better the chances of survival. When a tumor is destroyed or removed in the early stages of the cancer and the cancer has not spread, the five-year relative survival rate for patients is about 81 percent; the five-year relative survival rate for all stages of oral cancer is about 59 percent, according to the American Cancer Society. This does not mean, however, that five-year survivors are cancer-free or that the cancer will not reappear.

Wendell Anderson, B.A.

For Further Information

Hupp, James R., Edward Ellis, and Myron R. Tucker. *Contemporary Oral and Maxillofacial Surgery*. 5th ed. Philadelphia: Elsevier Health Sciences, 2008.

Parker, James N., and Philip M. Parker, eds. *The Official Patient's Sourcebook on Lip and Oral Cavity Cancer*. San Diego, Calif.: Icon Health, 2005.

Wray, David, et al. eds. *Textbook of General and Oral Surgery*. New York: Churchill Livingstone, 2003.

Other Resources

American Association of Oral and Maxillofacial Surgeons
http://www.aaoms.org

Oral Cancer Foundation
http://www.oralcancerfoundation.org

See also: Cordectomy; Electrolarynx; Erythroplakia; Esophageal speech; Glossectomy; Laryngeal cancer; Laryngectomy; Oral and oropharyngeal cancers; Throat cancer

▶ Orchiectomy

Category: Procedures

Also known as: Radical orchiectomy, inguinal orchiectomy, bilateral orchiectomy, unilateral orchiectomy, orchidectomy

Definition: Orchiectomy is a surgical procedure to remove one or both of the testicles in men with testicular or prostate cancer.

Cancers treated: Testicular cancer, prostate cancer

Why performed: Orchiectomy is used to remove one or both testicles as a treatment for testicular cancer. The testicles are the male sex organs that produce sperm and the hormone testosterone. The testicles are located in the scrotum. Nearby lymph nodes may also be removed at the time of orchiectomy. Artificial testicles may be placed at the time of surgery or in a later reconstructive procedure. Radiation therapy and chemotherapy for treatment of testicular cancer may follow orchiectomy. Orchiectomy may be the only treatment needed to cure early-stage testicular cancer.

A radical or inguinal orchiectomy includes removing one or both testicles and the spermatic cord. The spermatic cord is removed to prevent the cancer from spreading to the lymph nodes and the kidneys. An inguinal orchiectomy involves removing the testicles through an incision in the groin area, rather than directly through the scrotum.

Orchiectomy may be used to remove both testicles in men with prostate cancer. The growth of prostate cancer cells requires testosterone, and removing the testicles eliminates the source of this hormone. Without testosterone, the prostate tumor decreases in size, and symptoms are relieved. Orchiectomy does not cure prostate cancer, but it can help prolong the lives of men with advanced prostate cancer.

Patient preparation: Patients having both testicles removed will not be able to father children after orchiectomy. Patients with one testicle should be able to do so. Patients can choose to bank their sperm in case they wish to father children in the future. It is recommended that men with one testicle consider sperm banking as a precaution in case the second testicle needs to be removed in the future.

Orchiectomy can be an outpatient or inpatient procedure. It can be performed at an outpatient surgical center, urology clinic, or hospital surgery department. General anesthesia is most frequently used, in which the patient is not awake. Epidural anesthesia may be used, in which the patient is awake but does not feel anything from the waist down.

Prior to surgery, the patient receives standard blood and urine tests. The patient is advised not to take blood-thinning medications in the two days before the surgery and should not eat or drink for eight hours before the procedure. The patient uses a special antibacterial soap to wash his genitals and groin before surgery. Orchiectomy takes about forty-five minutes to an hour.

Steps of the procedure: The patient lies on his back on the surgical table. The patient is anesthetized, and vital signs are monitored throughout the surgery. The surgeon makes a 3- to 4-inch incision in the lower abdomen. The surgeon moves the testicles up through the inguinal canal and out through the incision. After removal of the testicles and spermatic cord is complete, the area is closed with sutures and bandaged.

After the procedure: The patient is observed in a recovery area until he is alert. He may stay overnight in the hospital or have another person drive him home. The patient receives medication for mild to moderate pain. Bed rest is recommended for a day.

The patient should wear a jock support or support briefs for two to three days and should not participate in strenuous activities for two to four weeks. Pain may be experienced in the abdomen or scrotum for several weeks. The patient should contact his doctor if he experiences increased pain, bleeding, or signs of infection.

Risks: Orchiectomy is considered a low-risk procedure. The risks include infection, bleeding, abscess formation, nerve injury, bladder damage, and the general risks associated with anesthesia. Removing both testicles causes changes in testosterone levels that increase the risk of hot flashes, erectile dysfunction, loss of sexual interest, loss of muscle mass, gynecomastia (enlarged breasts), and osteoporosis.

Results: Removing a cancerous testicle cures the cancer in the testicle. In the case of prostate cancer, removing the testicles prevents the cancer cells from using testosterone and slows the growth of the cancer while reducing symptoms.

Mary Car-Blanchard, O.T.D., B.S.O.T.

For Further Information

Bohle, A. "Long-Term Followup of a Randomized Study of Locally Advanced Prostate Cancer Treated with Combined Orchiectomy and External Radiotherapy Versus Radiotherapy Alone." *International Brazillian Journal of Urology* 32, no. 6 (November/December, 2006): 739.

Cheung, W. Y., et al. "Appropriateness of Testicular Cancer Management: A Population-Based Cohort Study." *Canadian Journal of Urology* 14, no. 3 (June, 2007): 3542-3550.

Mikkola, A., et al. "Ten-Year Survival and Cardiovascular Mortality in Patients with Advanced Prostate Cancer Primarily Treated by Intramuscular Polyestradiol Phosphate or Orchiectomy." *Prostate* 67, no. 4 (March 1, 2007): 447-455.

Ondrus, D., et al. "Nonseminomatous Germ Cell Testicular Tumors Clinical Stage I: Differentiated Therapeutic Approach in Comparison with Therapeutic Approach Using Surveillance Strategy Only." *Neoplasma* 54, no. 5 (2007): 437-442.

Pectasides, D., D. Farmakis, and M. Pectasides. "The Management of Stage I Nonseminomatous Testicular Germ Cell Tumors." *Oncology* 71, nos. 3/4 (July 17, 2007): 151-158.

Sheinfeld, Joel. *Testicular Cancer: An Issue of Urologic Clinics*. Philadelphia: Saunders, 2007.

Sokoloff, M. H., G. F. Joyce, and M. Wise. "Urologic Diseases in America Project: Testis Cancer." *Journal of Urology* 177, no. (June, 2007): 2030-2041.

Other Resources

American Cancer Society
http://www.cancer.org

See also: Cryptorchidism; Prostate cancer; Sertoli cell tumors; Testicular cancer

▶ Palpation

Category: Procedures
Also known as: Manual examination, feeling, probing, touching, manipulation

Definition: Palpation is the careful manual examination of the size, shape, firmness, consistency, texture, tenderness, or location of some body part or organ. Health care professionals use palpation during a physical examination for screening and diagnostic purposes.

Cancers diagnosed: Cancers of the breast, prostate, uterus, ovaries, liver, abdomen, pancreas, skin, bladder, lower colon and rectum, or lymph nodes

Why performed: Despite the technological advances in health care diagnostics, health care providers still acquire valuable information through direct interaction with the patient. By providing a physical examination, providers can screen patients for possible abnormalities. Sometimes cancer can be discovered through palpation of various body parts or organs. For example, a provider can use palpation to screen for cancers of the breast, prostate, uterus, ovaries, liver, abdomen, pancreas, skin, bladder, lower colon and rectum, or lymph nodes. A woman can use palpation in her monthly breast examination to detect lumps or thickening tissue that could indicate cancer.

Palpation is a noninvasive procedure that is less costly than procedures involving technology and can be a highly reliable initial step. When an abnormality is discovered, further diagnostics are performed to diagnose the cancer and determine treatment alternatives.

Patient preparation: Patient preparation depends on the type of palpation procedure. The patient should receive a thorough explanation of what is involved in the examination. Any anticipated discomfort should be disclosed to the patient, and any patient questions should be answered prior to the examination. Successful physical palpation depends of the skill of the provider and a thorough preparation of the patient.

Steps of procedure: The steps of the procedure depend on the area palpated during the physical examination.

After the procedure: The patient should be informed of any possible discomfort, tenderness, or soreness that may occur after the examination, which is generally minimal with palpation. Though palpation does not provide a definitive diagnosis, the practitioner can provide immediate feedback to the patient about cancer possibilities and make plans for further tests.

Risks: One advantage of palpation as a means of screening for cancer and other health care problems is that there is little risk of an adverse event to the patient. Palpation usually results in minimal and/or short-term discomfort for the patient.

Results: A skillful practitioner can use palpation as an effective way to screen a patient for cancer. Immediate follow-up plans can be made for further diagnostics without waiting for the return of other test results.

Marylane Wade Koch, M.S.N., R.N.

See also: Breast Self-Examination (BSE); Clinical Breast Exam (CBE); Digital Rectal Exam (DRE); Fibroadenomas; Gynecologic cancers; Pelvic examination; Screening for cancer; Testicular Self-Examination (TSE)

▶ Pancreatectomy

Category: Procedures
Also known as: Pancreatoduodenectomy, Whipple procedure, distal pancreatectomy, total pancreatectomy

Definition: Pancreatectomy is a surgical procedure done to remove all or part of the pancreas.

Cancers treated: Pancreatic cancer

Why performed: Pancreatectomy is done to remove all or part of the pancreas. This procedure may be performed when trying to cure the cancer by removing all of it, or it can be done as palliative care to reduce or prevent symptoms from cancer that has already spread to other areas.

Patient preparation: The first step of patient preparation is a thorough evaluation by the cancer care team to ensure that the patient is a good candidate for a pancreatectomy. It is a very difficult procedure that usually has a long recovery time, and it is not appropriate for many individuals. The procedure is appropriate only for individuals who have cancer that is expected to be fully removable by the procedure. As few as 10 percent of individuals diagnosed with pancreatic cancer are good candidates for this surgery. In some cases, pancreatectomy may also be appropriate as a palliative treatment.

Some patients receive radiation or chemotherapy before pancreatectomy. This may be done in an attempt to shrink the tumor to make complete removal more likely. It may also be done before the procedure, because the high risk of complications and long recovery time often mean that necessary additional treatments cannot begin until many weeks after the surgery. In the days before the procedure, patient preparation is generally similar to that for other major surgical operations. Patients may be instructed to avoid food or liquids for a certain amount of time before the procedure or be given antibiotics or other medications to help minimize the risk of complications.

Steps of the procedure: Three main types of pancreatectomy are performed. Which one is performed depends on where the cancer is located and the extent of the cancer's spread. If the goal is palliative, then the procedure performed will depend on the symptoms being treated or prevented. The three types of procedures differ in the amount and section of the pancreas that is removed.

The most common type of procedure is known as a pancreatoduodenectomy, also called the Whipple procedure. During this procedure, the surgeon removes the head of the pancreas (the part closest to the small intestine). The surgeon also usually removes the duodenum, the gallbladder, and part of the bile duct. In some cases, the surgeon removes part of the stomach as well. The part of the pancreas that remains is then surgically connected to the patient's small intestine.

Another procedure in which only part of the pancreas is removed is known as a distal pancreatectomy. When performing this procedure, the surgeon removes only the tail end (the thinner end) of the pancreas. In some cases, the spleen is also surgically removed at the same time. This procedure is appropriate only when the tumor is relatively small and localized in the distal end of the pancreas.

When the entire pancreas is removed, the procedure is known as a total pancreatectomy. When this is done, the surgeon takes out all of the pancreas and usually the spleen. This procedure is used when the cancer is located within the body of the pancreas.

After the procedure: Pancreatectomy is a major surgical procedure and usually requires a prolonged hospital stay. Most patients remain in the hospital for two or more weeks after the procedure. During this time, the patient is carefully monitored to check for complications such as infection and bleeding. If the surgery was done using an open technique, then the wound requires care and monitoring. Patients who did not receive chemotherapy or radiation therapy before the pancreatectomy generally receive it as soon as it is feasible after the surgery. If the entire pancreas, or a very large portion of the pancreas, was removed, then the patient may be given a regimen of medications to take to correct insulin and other imbalances if the pancreas no longer produces sufficient quantities for good health.

Risks: There are many significant risks associated with pancreatectomy. According to the American Cancer Society, when a pancreatoduodenectomy is performed by an extremely skilled and experienced surgeon at a hospital or center where the health care team is very experienced in the procedure, 2 to 5 percent of patients die as a direct result of complications of the surgery. When the procedure is performed by a less experienced surgeon at a small hospital that may not be prepared for possible complications, up to 15 percent of patients may die. Nonfatal complications from the procedure are very common. They can include infection, bleeding, and leakage at one of the points a surgical connection was made.

Results: The results from pancreatectomy vary depending on the type of procedure performed and the extent to which the cancer has spread to other areas of the body. For patients who had cancer that is considered completely removable through the pancreatectomy, the five-year rate of survival is about 20 percent.

Robert Bockstiegel, B.S.

For Further Information

DeVita, Vincent T., Jr., Samuel Hellman, and Steven A. Rosenberg, eds. *Cancer: Principles and Practice of Oncology—Pancreatic Cancer*. Philadelphia: Lippincott Williams & Wilkins, 2006.

Lowy, Andrew M., Steven D. Leach, and Philip Philip, eds. *Pancreatic Cancer*. New York: Springer, 2008.

Riess, H., A. Goerke, and H. Oettle, eds. *Pancreatic Cancer*. New York: Springer, 2008.

Suda, Koichi, ed. *Pancreas: Pathological Practice and Research*. New York: Karger, 2007.

Other Resources

American Cancer Society
http://www.cancer.org

Pancreatica
http://www.pancreatica.org

See also: Alcohol, alcoholism, and cancer; Bile duct cancer; Cholecystectomy; Endocrine cancers; Endocrinology oncology; Endoscopic Retrograde Cholangiopancreatography (ERCP); Gallbladder cancer; Islet cell tumors; Multiple endocrine neoplasia type 1 (MEN 1); Pancreatic cancers; Pancreatitis; Percutaneous Transhepatic Cholangiography (PTHC)

▶ Pap test

Category: Procedures
Also known as: Pap smear, Papanicolaou test, gynecological exam

Definition: A Pap test is the removal of microscopic cells from the cervix, the opening between the vagina and uterus in females, for laboratory evaluation.

Cancers diagnosed: Cervical cancer

Why performed: The Pap test is a diagnostic procedure performed for early detection of cervical cancer. The test can also detect abnormal, noncancerous cells and certain vaginal infections. Cervical cancer has been linked to certain strains of the human papillomavirus (HPV), which is sexually transmitted. These viruses can be detected with current Pap test technology. According to guidelines from the American College of Obstetricians and Gynecologists, a female patient should have the first Pap test within three years of having sexual intercourse

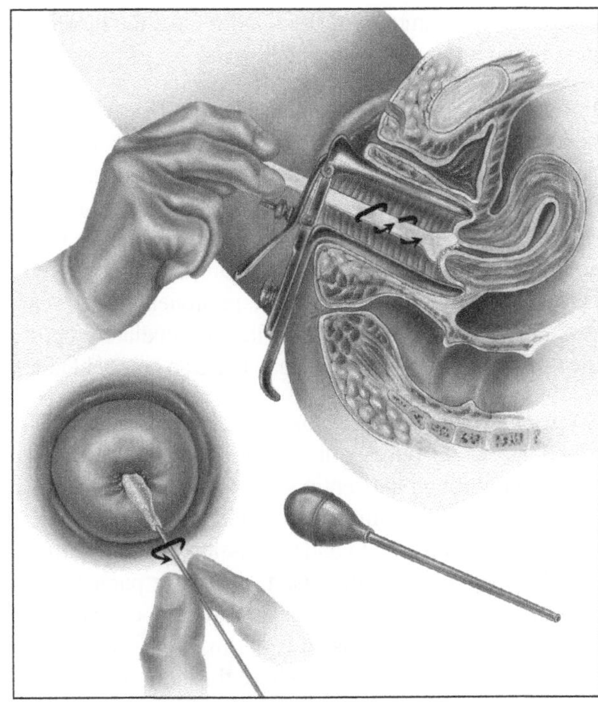

Obtaining a Pap smear. (iStock)

or at age twenty-one, whichever comes first. Until age thirty, women should have annual testing. After age thirty, if the woman is in a monogamous sexual relationship and has had three consecutive normal Pap tests, testing can be done every three years. For women over the age of sixty-five with three normal tests and no abnormal tests for the prior ten years, testing may be discontinued. Women who have had a hysterectomy may stop having Pap tests, unless the hysterectomy was performed because of cancer. These are general guidelines for testing; individual situations must be considered by the health care provider.

Patient preparation: The patient must not be menstruating at the time of testing. It is recommended that the patient avoid sexual intercourse, tampons, douching, and vaginal medications, creams, or sprays for two days before the test. The patient should empty her bladder immediately before the procedure and then undress from the waist down. A patient gown or drape will be provided.

Steps of the procedure: The test is usually done in a health care provider's office during a gynecological examination, which includes a breast and pelvic examination. The patient is placed in lithotomy position on the examination table. In this position, the patient is lying on her back with feet in stirrups at the end of the table and is draped with a sheet.

The examiner will push the patient's knees apart to inspect the external genital area. A plastic or metal speculum is lubricated with water or a water-based gel and is inserted into the vagina. The curved blades of the speculum are opened and the cervix is located. A thin plastic brush with an end that looks like a broom is inserted into the opening of the cervix and is rotated 360 degrees to collect endocervical cells. The patient may feel a slight pinching sensation. The collection device and the speculum are removed. The broom end is placed into a small container with preservative chemicals and is sent to the laboratory for evaluation of the cervical cells. In the past, samples of cells were obtained with a small wire brush and smeared on a glass slide and sent to the laboratory. Newer technology with the broom is more accurate than the older methods.

After the Pap test, the provider will then place lubricant on two fingers and insert them into the vagina while feeling with the other hand on top of the abdomen. This is done to feel the uterus, cervix, and ovaries for any abnormalities, tenderness, or masses. Then, a rectal examination may be done in some patients. The rectal wall lies against the back of the vaginal wall. A tilted uterus may be examined during a rectal examination.

After the procedure: The patient may need to remove lubricant if it is used during the test. The patient is allowed to go home immediately after the examination and resume previous levels of activity.

Risks: Brief mild discomfort may occur in some patients during a Pap test. Some may experience a small amount of vaginal bleeding or spotting during or after the test. Some women may experience embarrassment during the examination. These risks are minor given the benefits of early detection of cervical cancer with the likelihood of successful treatment.

Results: The results are generally available within one week. A normal or negative Pap test will have no abnormal cells or infectious agents present. An abnormal Pap test may show abnormal noncancerous cells, abnormal cancer cells, or infection. If a patient has an abnormal Pap test, then further evaluation is needed. A repeat Pap test may be performed in approximately three months. This time lapse is to allow possible infections to be resolved that may be the cause of the abnormal test. Other patients may have a more detailed test or a biopsy. If cancer is detected, then surgery is generally performed. Rarely, the test may give a false negative result when the test is actually abnormal. This may occur from a poor sample or from laboratory error.

Amy Bull, D.S.N., A.P.N.

For Further Information

Carlson, Karen J., Stephanie A. Eisenstat, and Terra Ziporyn. *The New Harvard Guide to Women's Health.* Cambridge, Mass.: Harvard University Press, 2004.

Minkin, Mary Jane, and Carol V. Wright. *A Woman's Guide to Sexual Health.* New Haven, Conn.: Yale University Press, 2004.

Rosenthal, M. Sara. *The Gynecological Sourcebook.* 4th ed. New York: McGraw-Hill, 2003.

Other Resources

National Cervical Cancer Coalition
http://www.nccc-online.org

National Women's Health Information Center
http://www.4women.gov/faq/pap.htm

See also: Antiviral therapies; Cervical cancer; Colposcopy; Conization; Diethylstilbestrol (DES); Endometrial cancer; Fertility drugs and cancer; Gynecologic cancers; Human Papillomavirus (HPV); Hysterectomy; Hystero-oophorectomy; Loop Electrosurgical Excisional Procedure (LEEP); Pelvic examination; Pregnancy and cancer; Vaccines, preventive; Virus-related cancers

▶ Paracentesis

Category: Procedures
Also known as: Abdominal tap, abdominal paracentesis, peritoneal tap

Definition: Paracentesis is the insertion of a needle or catheter through the peritoneum, the membrane that lines the abdominal cavity, to sample or drain excess fluid.

Cancers diagnosed or treated: Most metastatic cancers, especially liver cancer, mesothelioma, and ovarian cancer

Why performed: Primarily a diagnostic but sometimes a therapeutic procedure, paracentesis is performed to identify new cancer cells that have metastasized to the abdomen, or to analyze the extent of an existing cancer that is causing fluid buildup (ascites) in the peritoneal space. In the latter case, physicians may perform paracentesis to remove a large amount of fluid and relieve the patient of pain in the lungs, kidneys, and bowels.

Patient preparation: The physician will discuss risks, benefits, and alternatives with the patient and ask him or her to sign an informed consent form. A few days before the procedure, the patient undergoes blood tests to confirm that there are no clotting or bleeding problems in the abdomen. On the day of the procedure, a radiologist will perform an ultrasound scan of the peritoneal space to assess the size and area of the ascites. Immediately before the test, the patient must urinate to leave an empty bladder.

Steps of the procedure: Non-emergency paracentesis is scheduled in an outpatient setting. The abdominal area is cleaned with an antiseptic soap, and a local anesthetic such as lidocaine is injected into the patient's abdomen. Based on the ultrasound and percussion of the abdomen, the physician chooses the insertion site for paracentesis. Typically, the patient sits in a semi-recumbent position, so a site just below the navel is optimal for insertion and fluid aspiration. A nurse will shave this area of the abdomen if needed. When enough fluid has been removed (10 to 50 milliliters in diagnostic paracentesis and up to 10 liters in therapeutic paracentesis), the physician withdraws the needle from the abdomen and applies direct pressure to the puncture site with a sterile dressing. Large accumulations of fluid require the insertion of a vacuum-pressurized catheter through which the fluid can drain into a container. Results are sent to the laboratory for analysis right away. The entire procedure takes ten to thirty minutes.

After the procedure: The patient rests for one to four hours while vital signs, incision site, and fluid drainage are monitored. If large amounts of fluid are drained, then nurses will actively monitor the patient's blood pressure for hypotension and shock. An intravenous (IV) line may be inserted to avoid fluid shifts in the body and prevent kidney failure. Slight fluid drainage from the puncture site may continue for one to two days. Normally, the patient does not require an overnight stay.

Risks: Paracentesis is a relatively safe procedure. Although the incidence of any particular complication is rare, a range of intraprocedure complications may occur. The paracentesis needle may perforate the bladder, bowels, or blood vessels in the abdomen, causing internal bleeding or hemorrhage. Infection of the peritoneal fluid or the spread of cancer inside the abdomen are also risks associated with the paracentesis needle. The risk of external infection around the puncture site is increased if there is persistent leakage from the puncture site.

Results: Patients undergo paracentesis only if they have ascites, an abnormal condition, in the abdomen. Several laboratory tests are performed on the peritoneal fluid to assess the abnormality. A high white blood cell count may indicate inflammation, bacterial perotinitis, infection, or cancer in the abdomen. High albumin protein content in the fluid, as compared to the content in the patient's blood serum, may indicate tuberculosis, kidney disorder, pancreatitis, or cancer. Lower protein content may indicate liver cirrhosis or portal hypertension. A high level of the enzyme lactate dehydrogenase in the fluid may indicate infection or cancer. A high level of the enzyme amylase may indicate pancreatitis. A low level of glucose may indicate infection. To confirm the type of infection or cancer, cells from the fluid will undergo culture and pathology in the laboratory. A biopsy may also be performed.

Bharat Burman, B.A.

For Further Information

Aziz, K., and G. Y. Wu. *Cancer Screening: A Practical Guide for Physicians*. Totowa, N.J.: Humana Press, 2002.

Foley, K. M., et al. *When the Focus Is on Care: Palliative Care and Cancer*. Atlanta: American Cancer Society, 2005.

Waller, A., and N. L. Caroline. *Handbook of Palliative Care in Cancer*. Boston: Butterworth-Heinemann, 2000.

Other Resources

American Cancer Society

Treatment of Mesothelioma by Stage
http://www.cancer.org/docroot/CRI/content/CRI_2_4_4X_Treatment_Options_by_stage_29.asp?sitearea=

National Cancer Institute

Screening and Testing to Detect Cancer
http://www.cancer.gov/cancertopics/screening

See also: Ascites; Mesothelioma

▶ Pelvic examination

Category: Procedures
Also known as: Female gynecologic examination, reproductive health examination

Definition: A pelvic examination is a visual inspection of external female genitalia, followed by insertion of a speculum into the vagina to visualize the cervix and a bimanual examination of the uterus and adnexa (ovaries, Fallopian tubes, and uterine ligaments) for masses, tenderness, and overall impression.

Cancers diagnosed: If a collection of cells for a Pap (Papanicolaou) test is done as part of the pelvic examination, then screening for cervical cancer and precursor cellular changes (precancerous conditions) is included; visual inspection of the external genitalia may reveal abnormal tissue to be biopsied for the detection of vulvar or vaginal cancer.

Why performed: A pelvic examination allows for examination of internal and external genitalia as well as the collection of specimens. Some pelvic examinations include laboratory specimen collection for Pap testing (with the collection of cervical and endocervical samples either by fixed slides or the newer liquid cytologic methodology); examination of vaginal discharge for bacterial vaginosis, trichomonas, or yeast vaginitis; and testing for common infections such as gonorrhea and chlamydia. Any particular pelvic examination, however, may include only some or none of these tests. It is important for patients to be aware that not all pelvic examinations include Pap testing. Exams may be performed for routine screening, including a Pap smear, or for symptomatic gynecologic problems.

Patient preparation: The patient should empty her bladder prior to the exam and should have a chance to express any concerns or apprehensions. She should not douche prior to the exam. It is preferable for patients not to be menstruating when examined, although this may not be possible depending on the reason for the visit. Having

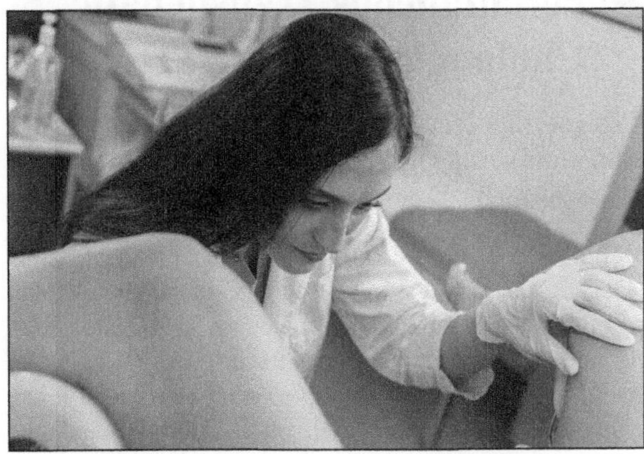

Pelvic examinations allow doctors to check for several types of cancer. (iStock)

the patient move down to the far end of the table relieves some pressure from the speculum.

Steps of the procedure: A pelvic exam involves the external examination and palpation of the genitalia, followed by insertion of a vaginal speculum, collection of specimens, and a bimanual examination with palpation of uterine and adnexal size, mobility, position, contours, presence of masses, and tenderness with palpation.

After the procedure: The physician will help the patient sit up slowly when the exam is completed. Bleeding is possible following a pelvic examination but is not a cause for alarm unless excessive or prolonged.

Risks: Pelvic examinations may be embarrassing and emotionally and physically uncomfortable for some patients, but they carry no known risks.

Results: The results of a pelvic examination depend on visual examination and any clinical or laboratory findings.

Clair Kaplan, R.N., M.S.N., A.P.R.N. (WHNP), M.H.S., M.T. (ASCP)

See also: Antiviral therapies; Cervical cancer; Colposcopy; Conization; Diethylstilbestrol (DES); Endometrial cancer; Fertility drugs and cancer; Gynecologic cancers; Human Papillomavirus (HPV); Hysterectomy; Hystero-oophorectomy; Loop Electrosurgical Excisional Procedure (LEEP); Pap test; Pregnancy and cancer; Transvaginal ultrasound; Uterine cancer; Vaccines, preventive; Vaginal cancer; Virus-related cancers; Vulvar cancer

▶ Percutaneous Transhepatic Cholangiography (PTHC)

Category: Procedures
Also known as: Operative cholangiography, T-tube cholangiography, cystic duct cholangiography

Definition: Percutaneous transhepatic cholangiography (PTHC) is a diagnostic test used to visualize the the liver or bile ducts. Although this procedure is frequently performed in the operating room at the time of exploration of the biliary tract for nonpalpable stones or tumors, it can also be performed postoperatively in the radiology suite to assess catheter patency and drainage and to evaluate for the presence of residual stones or residual narrowing or obstruction of the biliary tract.

Cancers diagnosed: Bile duct carcinoma, pancreatic cancer

Why performed: The main application of PTHC is to avoid common bile duct surgical exploration and to identify calculi that have escaped palpation, as well as to evaluate for the presence of biliary tract tumors or pancreatic tumors. The intrapancreatic segment of the common bile duct is often altered by pancreatic cancer, and PTHC can be used for its evaluation. Postoperative cholangiography is usually performed in the X-ray suite prior to removal of the T tube placed at the time of surgery to demonstrate the patency of the common duct, the absence of retained stones, and the free passage of bile into the duodenum.

Patient preparation: This procedure is frequently performed in the operating room at the time of exploration of the biliary tract for nonpalpable stones or tumor. Therefore, patient preparation is determined by the surgeon prior to the procedure and commonly involves the usual preadmission testing performed before any surgical procedure, as well as instructions such as nothing by mouth after midnight the night before the procedure.

Steps of the procedure: Radiopaque material is injected by the surgeon into the cystic duct while the patient is still in the operating room. Alternatively, after surgery, radiopaque material may be injected into the T tube by a radiologist in the radiology suite. This tube was placed in the common duct intraoperatively using sterile technique under fluoroscopic guidance. In both situations, X-ray films are then taken. In some cases, a trained interventional radiologist, under fluoroscopic control and using sterile technique, can insert a fine needle directly into the biliary tree and outline the intrahepatic ducts, the common hepatic ducts, and the common bile duct using a contrast medium.

After the procedure: If a T tube was placed in the common duct intraoperatively, then the procedure is performed as an inpatient procedure (during the patient's hospital stay). Patients should consult their health care providers if they have any questions or concerns regarding the use of a T-tube cholangiogram or PTHC.

Risks: Patients will consult with their health care providers regarding the need for the study, its risks, how it will be done, and what the results indicate.

Results: The X-ray films taken during the procedure are read by the radiologist the same day. The patient will need to contact the doctor or health care provider for the radiology report and for follow-up therapy. Results are dependent on the reason for the study, such as exploration of the biliary tract for nonpalpable stones or tumors.

Debra B. Kessler, M.D., Ph.D.

See also: Bile duct cancer; Gallbladder cancer

▶ Pericardiocentesis

Category: Procedures
Also known as: Pericardial tap, percutaneous pericardiocentesis

Definition: Pericardiocentesis is the insertion of a needle or catheter through the pericardium, the membrane that surrounds the heart, to drain excess fluid.

Cancers diagnosed or treated: Mesothelioma, advanced breast cancer

Why performed: Primarily a therapeutic but sometimes a diagnostic procedure, pericardiocentesis is performed to remove from the pericardium excess fluid that is inhibiting the heart's pumping action. If this pericardial effusion has accumulated rapidly, causing a life-threatening condition known as cardiac tamponade, then the procedure is performed on an emergency basis to avoid sudden death. In cases of suspected metastatic cancer, fluid buildup requires both relief and pathology.

Patient preparation: A few days before the procedure, an electrocardiogram (EKG), an echocardiogram, and blood tests confirm that it is safe to perform the operation. Patients must not eat or drink for several hours beforehand.

Steps of the procedure: Nonemergency pericardiocentesis is scheduled in a hospital. An intravenous (IV) line is inserted in the patient's arm or hand for medications. The puncture site is sterilized and a local anesthetic given. With the patient's head elevated 30 to 60 degrees, the physician, guided by an image on a video monitor, inserts a needle beneath the breastbone and into the pericardium. When enough fluid has been removed, the needle is withdrawn and direct pressure is applied. Large accumulations of fluid require the insertion of a catheter through which the fluid can drain into a bag. Extreme cases require general anesthesia and open surgery.

After the procedure: The patient stays in an intensive care unit while vital signs, the incision site, and fluid drainage are monitored. Nurses especially watch for bulging of the jugular vein in the neck, which suggests problems with blood flow. The length of the hospital stay may be as short as overnight or as long as a few days.

Risks: With guided imaging, pericardiocentesis is relatively safe, with a 5 percent risk of these side effects: air embolism (air in a blood vessel, blocking blood flow); infection of the pericardial membranes (pericarditis) or at the incision site; irregular heartbeat (arrhythmia); heart attack (myocardial infarction); pneumopericardium (introduction of air into the pericardial sac); and puncture of the heart muscle (myocardium), stomach, lungs, liver, or a coronary artery.

Results: Normal pericardial fluid is clear, straw-colored, and low in viscosity. High viscosity, low clarity, and the presence of blood, bacteria, abnormal cells, high levels of protein, or an excessive number of white blood cells indicate an abnormal result. The latter three conditions particularly suggest the spread of cancer to the pericardium, which is confirmed with biopsy and pathology.

Christina J. Moose, M.A.

See also: Acupuncture and acupressure for cancer patients; Bronchoalveolar lung cancer; Mediastinoscopy; Mesothelioma; Pericardial effusion; Thoracoscopy; Thymomas

▶ Peritoneovenous shunts

Category: Procedures
Also known as: Peritoneovenous ascites shunts

Definition: Peritoneovenous shunts are surgically implanted devices used to relieve intractable cases of ascites. This condition, characterized by excess buildup of fluids in the peritoneal (abdominal) cavity, generally results from chronic liver disease but also from malignancy in one out of ten cases. The shunt—a plastic or silicone rubber tube—serves to drain fluid from the abdominal cavity into the jugular vein in the neck.

Cancers treated: Ovarian, endometrial, colon, gastric, breast, and pancreatic cancers

Why performed: Tumor-induced ascites is difficult to manage and is usually a manifestation of late-stage cancer. It causes abdominal swelling, nausea, loss of appetite, and shortness of breath as a result of fluid accumulation in the chest cavity. Peritoneovenous shunting carries potential risks but may be recommended to ease discomfort when medical therapy consisting of salt restriction, diuretics, repeated fluid aspirations, chemotherapy, or immunotherapy fails to reduce ascites.

Patient preparation: Before surgery, the patient undergoes routine laboratory tests, including a coagulation profile and liver panel, and imaging tests, such as computed tomography (CT) scan and ultrasonography, to assess the extent of ascites and the condition of the veins selected for shunting. The operation is contraindicated if an additional test shows that the ascitic fluid is infected.

Steps of the procedure: The patient is given a sedative and undergoes either local or general anesthesia at the hospital. The surgeon makes a small incision and inserts a shunting tube under the skin of the chest that will run from the abdominal cavity to the jugular vein. The tube is then passed down to the superior vena cava, a large vein that returns blood to the heart. With a pump chamber and a one-way valve that prevents backflow, the shunt drains ascitic fluid into the systemic circulation.

After the procedure: After surgery, the patient's vital signs are monitored by a nursing staff, and for up to forty-eight hours the shunt is checked to make sure that it functions properly. Antibiotics and pain medication are prescribed as needed. Patients are instructed to pump the shunt daily to remove fluid from the abdomen, to take their prescribed medication, and to restrict sodium intake.

Risks: Complications are common and include shunt malfunction, infection, blood clots, edema, leakage of ascitic fluid, and heart failure.

Results: The procedure is deemed successful when fluid in the abdomen gradually ceases to accumulate after surgery, but frequently a blood clot or scar tissue will form around the shunt and block the valve or tube.

Anna Binda, Ph.D.

See also: Ascites; Cytology; Gallbladder cancer; Gastrointestinal cancers; Krukenberg tumors; Mesothelioma; Pancreatic cancers; Paracentesis

▶ Pheresis

Category: Procedures
Also known as: Apheresis, automated blood collection

Definition: Pheresis is a process in which the patient's blood is withdrawn from the body, various cells or proteins are removed from the blood, and then the blood is infused back into the patient. There are different types of therapeutic pheresis that can occur: Leukapheresis (removal of white blood cells), Platelet pheresis (removal of platelets), and Plasmapheresis (removal of plasma). Pheresis can be used to collect donor platelets from healthy people and give them to cancer patients who have no platelets Pheresis is also used for patients who are undergoing a peripheral blood stem cell transplant.

Cancers treated: Hematological (blood) cancers

Why performed: Blood cancers can cause the bone marrow to malfunction and produce too many platelets or white blood cells, creating a life-threatening situation if the levels of these cells are not decreased. Oral medications can be given if levels are only slightly elevated, but for more acute cases, pheresis may be used. Specialized pheresis treatments are also performed, including: 1) photopheresis to treat graft-versus-host disease as well as lymphoma, 2) pheresis to harvest peripheral stem cells for bone marrow transplantation, and 3) therapeutic plasma exchange, which removes large-molecular-weight substances such as harmful antibodies from the plasma to in order to treat the side effects of such diseases as lung cancer, breast cancer, colon cancer, thymomas, and Hodgkin disease.

Patient preparation: Patients who have low levels of calcium may need to take a calcium supplement prior to undergoing pheresis. Patients may also receive calcium tablets during the procedure to help with the side effects associated with low calcium counts.

Steps of the procedure: The procedure can take place in a variety of settings including the bedside, in a clinic, or even in a mobile pheresis lab. First, the patient is positioned for comfort, usually in a recliner or a bed. Intravenous (IV) lines are placed in both arms, usually the antecubital area as it has larger veins. Blood is drawn from one site, travels from the IV through a tube, and then circulates through the pheresis machine to pull out the cells. Finally, the blood is then returned into the other arm. The procedure can take two to three hours to perform.

After the procedure: After pheresis, the patient is monitored for bleeding from the IV site. Pressure may need to be applied directly to the insertion site for five to ten minutes, especially for patients who have altered coagulation times related to their disease and its treatment. Patients are monitored for tingling of the face and arms (which indicates low calcium levels), as well as dizziness. Cancer patients with an elevated platelet count or white blood cell count have their counts lowered to a safe level. They then are placed on an oral agent or receive chemotherapy to maintain the safe levels.

Risks: Bleeding and infection may occur. Rare episodes of an air embolus have occurred with the removal of access lines.

Results: The patient will have the blood count lowered to a safe level in order to receive chemotherapy for the underlying cancer diagnosis. If a patient is given pheresis because the count is too high and does not follow up with additional medications, then the count will again rise to an unsafe level and the patient will need to receive pheresis therapy again.

Katrina Green MSN, RN, OCN

For Further Information

Aqui, N., & O'Doherty, U. (2015). Leukocytapheresis for the treatment of hyperleukocytosis secondary to acute leukemia. *Hematology,* 2014(1): 457-460.

Krejci, M., Janikova, A., Folber, F., Kral, Z., & Mayer, J. (2015). Outcomes of 167 healthy sibling donors after peripheral blood stem cell mobilization with G-CSF 16µg/kg/day: Efficacy and safety. *Neoplasma,* 5(62): 787-792

Pham, H. P., & Schwartz, J. (2015). How we approach a patient with symptoms of leukostasis requiring emergent leukocytapheresis. *Transfusion,* 55(10):2306-2311.

Röllig, C., & Ehninger, G. (2015). How I treat hyperleukocytosis in acute myeloid leukemia. *Blood,* 125(21): 3246-3452.

Other Resources

American Cancer Society
http://www.cancer.org

American Red Cross
http://www.redcross.org

National Cancer Institute
http://www.cancer.gov

See also: Blood cancers; Bone Marrow Transplantation (BMT); Breast cancers; Chronic Myeloid Leukemia (CML); Infection and sepsis; Lambert-Eaton Myasthenic Syndrome (LEMS); Leukapharesis; Lymphomas; Myasthenia gravis; Mycosis fungoides; Myeloproliferative disorders; Side effects; Waldenström Macroglobulinemia (WM)

▶ Pleural biopsy

Category: Procedures

Also known as: Needle biopsy of the pleura, open pleural biopsy, closed pleural biopsy

Definition: A pleural biopsy is the removal of a sample of the pleura (the membrane that surrounds the lungs) so that it can be tested by a pathologist for cancer or other diseases.

Cancers diagnosed: Lung cancer, metastatic pleural tumor, malignant pleural mesothelioma

Why performed: This test may be used to diagnose mesothelioma, a tumor in the pleural membrane, or lung cancer. It is indicated when a pleural fluid sample shows possible cancer or when a chest X ray shows a thickening or mass in the pleura.

Patient preparation: Pleural biopsy may be done in a doctor's office or in the hospital using a local anesthetic. A blood test may be required before the test to ensure that the patient does not have a prolonged bleeding or clotting time.

Steps of the procedure: In a percutaneous biopsy, the doctor uses a large-bore needle. The skin around the site is cleaned and injected with a local anesthetic. The patient sits up and may be asked to hold his or her breath to prevent air from entering the chest during the procedure. The physician makes an incision and inserts the needle through the chest wall and into the pleura. Ultrasound can be used to help view the progress of the needle. When it is in place, a biopsy trocar is inserted through the needle to remove a sample of tissue. The doctor usually removes three samples, places them in fixative, and sends them to the laboratory. The procedure can take less than thirty minutes.

To obtain larger specimens of the pleura, the biopsy can also be performed during a thoracoscopy, using a laparoscope (a tube with a tiny camera on the end) that the doctor inserts through the skin and into the chest, or as an open pleural biopsy, a surgery performed under general anesthesia.

After the procedure: A bandage is placed over the incision. The patient is observed for respiratory distress and bleeding. After returning home, the patient should be aware of any shortness of breath. Light-headedness or an increased pulse rate might indicate internal bleeding.

Risks: Potential complications from this procedure include respiratory distress, pneumothorax (presence of air in the chest outside the lung), injury to the lung, infection, and bleeding.

Results: Preparation of a tissue sample and analysis by a pathologist may take several days. The pathologist can identify the presence or apparent lack of cancer cells in the tissue.

Marcia Pinneau, R.N.

See also: Bronchoalveolar lung cancer; Lung cancers; Mesothelioma; Needle biopsies; Pleural effusion; Pleurodesis; Thoracentesis; Thoracoscopy

▶ Pleurodesis

Category: Procedures

Definition: Pleurodesis is the binding together of the pleural membranes surrounding the lungs to make breathing easier.

Cancers treated: Mesothelioma, lung cancer

Why performed: Pleurodesis is used to help lung cancer patients with malignant pleural effusions breathe more easily. Normally, the membranes of the pleural cavity that surrounds the lungs are coated with fluid that provides surface tension to make them adhere, causing the lungs to inflate when the diaphragm moves during inspiration. Extra fluid in this cavity (pleural effusion) makes it difficult to breathe because pleural surfaces do not stick together and also because the lungs do not have room to expand completely. During pleurodesis, the extra fluid is removed and a sclerosant (chemical irritant) such as sterile talc or an antibiotic is injected into the pleural cavity. The irritation causes inflammation in the membranes, which makes them stick together and also prevents more fluid accumulation. Alternatively, the surfaces can be mechanically irritated (scraped) during a surgical procedure.

Patient preparation: Patients are typically hospitalized, although pleurodesis can also be done on an outpatient basis. Patients should report any allergies to medications or other substances, such as iodine. They may be asked to stop taking medications that can increase the risk of bleeding.

Steps of the procedure: The skin and chest wall are injected with a local anesthetic and a chest tube is inserted into the pleural cavity (a procedure called a thoracotomy). A chest X ray is taken to ensure proper placement. Any fluid in the cavity is drained, in some cases over several days. Before injection of the sclerosant, the patient may receive an analgesic and/or sedative to prevent discomfort. Sometimes the patient is asked to rotate from side to side. Then the excess sclerosant is drained and the doctor removes the chest tube, which may take only a few hours. An occlusive dressing is applied over the opening to prevent air from entering the chest.

After the procedure: Patients are observed for serious complications such as respiratory distress, a collapsed lung, or bleeding. The occlusive dressing is typically left in place for two days; if stitches are used to close the opening, then they may remain in place for a week. Additional pain medication may be needed once the anesthetic has worn off. A low-grade fever is a common response to the inflammation.

Risks: The risks of pleurodesis include respiratory distress, infection, a collapsed lung, and bleeding. Patients may also have a reaction to the irritant.

Results: After a successful pleurodesis, the patient will find breathing is easier. This procedure may be repeated if needed.

Marcia Pinneau, R.N.

See also: Bronchoalveolar lung cancer; Lung cancers; Mesothelioma; Pleural biopsy; Pleural effusion

▶ Pneumonectomy

Category: Procedures
Also known as: Lung removal, extrapleural pneumonectomy

Definition: Pneumonectomy is the surgical removal of the entire lung. Extrapleural pneumonectomy is the surgical removal of the lung, a portion of the membrane covering the heart, the membrane lining the affected side of the chest cavity, and a portion of the diaphragm.

Cancers treated: Lung cancer, mesothelioma

Why performed: Pneumonectomy is a surgical procedure used to treat lung cancer when the tumor cannot be removed by a less extensive procedure. It may also be performed in the presence of severe chest trauma. Rarely, pneumonectomy is used for treatment of bronchiectasis, lung abscesses, or extensive unilateral tuberculosis. Extrapleural pneumonectomy is sometimes a treatment option for those patients with malignant mesothelioma.

Patient preparation: Before planning surgery, a computed tomography (CT) scan of the head and abdomen and a bone scan are typically performed to confirm that the cancer has not spread to other areas of the body. If the cancer has spread, then pneumonectomy may not be a treatment option.

Before surgery, studies are performed to check for abnormalities and establish a baseline for postoperative comparison. These studies include a chest X ray, electrocardiogram (EKG), bleeding time, and blood tests to check kidney function; electrolyte, hemoglobin, and oxygen levels; and white blood cell count. Pulmonary function tests are performed to evaluate lung function and to determine whether the remaining lung is healthy enough to handle the increased workload. A blood sample is also drawn to check the patient's blood type in case a transfusion is needed during surgery.

A week before surgery, aspirin and anti-inflammatory drugs are stopped. The patient is given special instructions about when to stop taking anticoagulants, if prescribed. The patient must not eat or drink for at least eight hours before surgery, and an intravenous (IV) catheter is inserted for the delivery of fluids and medications. An indwelling urinary catheter is also inserted so that urine output can be monitored closely during and after the procedure.

Steps of the procedure: When the patient arrives in the operating suite, an arterial catheter may be inserted to monitor the patient's blood pressure and oxygenation. An

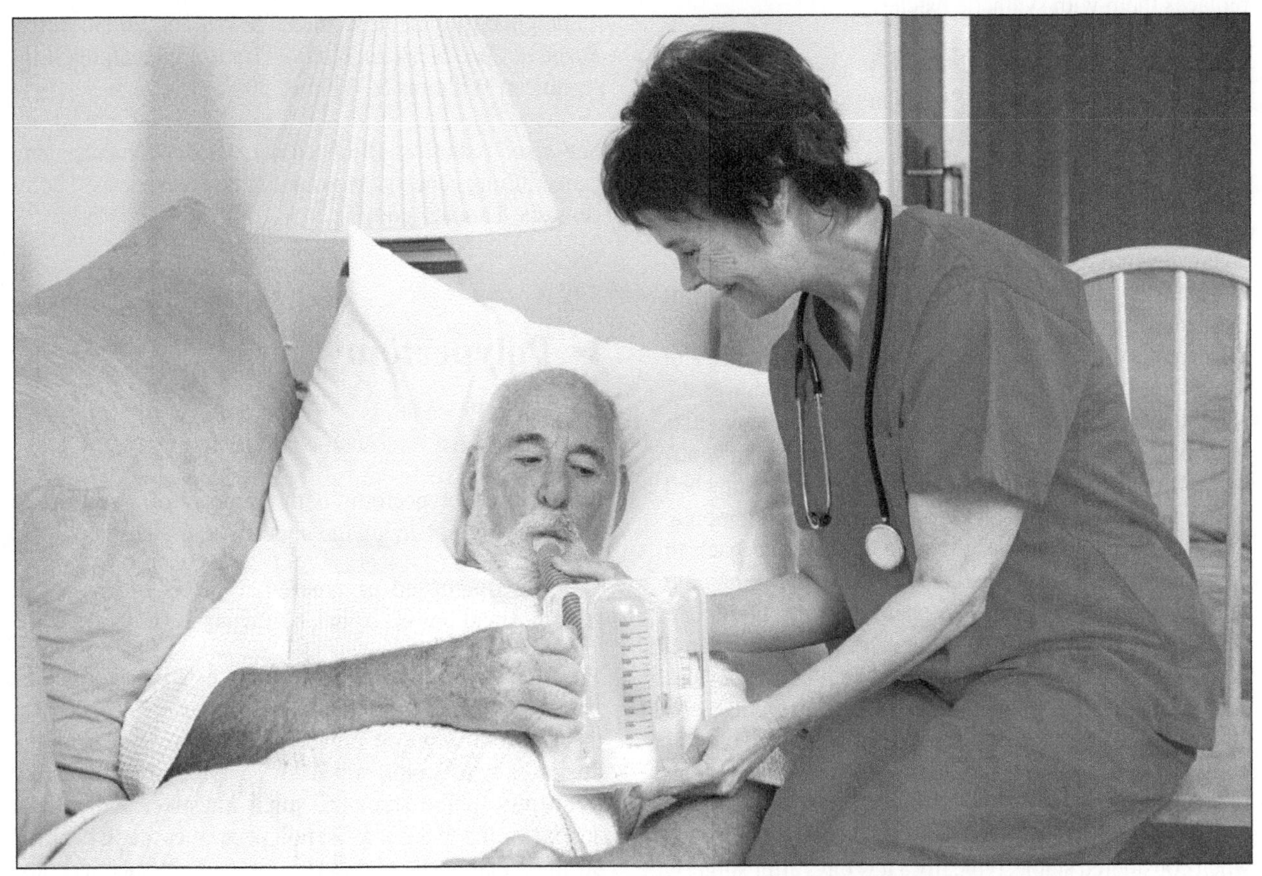

After lung surgery, patients are asked to exercise their lungs by using a spirometer. (iStock)

epidural catheter may also be inserted for postoperative pain control. An endotracheal tube is inserted through the nose or mouth to maintain the patient's airway and provide oxygenation during surgery.

After the patient is anesthetized, the surgeon makes an incision into the chest cavity. When the chest cavity is entered, the lung collapses. The surgeon locates and ties off the pulmonary artery supplying the lung and the pulmonary veins. The ribs are spread, and the lung is exposed for removal. In some cases, it is necessary to remove a rib. The mainstem bronchus is divided, and the affected lung is removed. The surgeon staples or sutures the bronchial stump. Chest tubes typically are not inserted into the chest; instead fluid is permitted to accumulate inside the empty chest cavity, preventing mediastinal shift. Finally, after making sure that the bronchial stump is not leaking air, the surgeon closes the chest cavity and applies a sterile dressing.

When an extrapleural pneumonectomy is necessary, the surgeon removes the lung, a portion of the membrane covering the heart, the membrane lining the affected side of the chest cavity, and a portion of the diaphragm and replaces them with synthetic patches.

After the procedure: The patient is transferred to the surgical intensive care unit (SICU) and attached to a monitor that displays the patient's heart rhythm, blood pressure, and oxygen saturation. These devices help the SICU nurses monitor the patient's condition closely. The patient may have an endotracheal tube in place and require mechanical ventilation to assist breathing. If mechanical ventilation is not necessary, then the patient will receive supplemental oxygen through a nasal cannula or facemask. The patient is encouraged to cough, deep-breathe, and use an incentive spirometer to prevent pneumonia. If the patient requires mechanical ventilation immediately after surgery, then early extubation is the goal to prevent ventilator-associated pneumonia. The head of the patient's bed is elevated at least 30 degrees to help prevent pneumonia. The patient is turned every two hours from the back to the nonoperative side to prevent the heart and remaining lung from shifting toward the operative side. Fluids are administered conservatively through an IV infusion pump to prevent fluid overload. Sequential compression devices are attached to the patient's legs to help prevent blood clot formation. Pain medications are administered continuously either through an epidural catheter or through an IV catheter, as needed.

The patient is transferred to a medical surgical floor when considered stable, typically a few days after surgery, and then discharged to home. The patient is instructed to resume activities of daily living slowly in order to allow the remaining lung to compensate for its increased workload. Recovery commonly takes several months because shortness of breath significantly limits the patient's ability to exercise. Some patients require lifelong supplemental oxygen therapy.

Risks: The risks of pneumonectomy include surgical site infection, pneumonia, empyema (pus in the pleural space), hemorrhage, pulmonary edema, myocardial infarction, cardiac arrhythmia, pulmonary embolism, and ventilator-dependent respiratory failure. Rarely, stump failure results in cardiopulmonary arrest.

Results: Pathologic examination of the lung specimen reveals the type of cancer.

Collette Bishop Hendler, R.N., M.S.

For Further Information

Lorigan, Paul. *Lung Cancer*. Dana-Farber Cancer Institute Handbook. Philadelphia: Mosby, 2007.

Smeltzer, Suzanne C., et al., eds. *Brunner and Suddarth's Textbook of Medical-Surgical Nursing*. 11th ed. Philadelphia: Lippincott Williams & Wilkins, 2008.

Surgical Care Made Incredibly Visual! Philadelphia: Lippincott Williams & Wilkins, 2006.

See also: Asbestos; Bilobectomy; Bronchoalveolar lung cancer; Lung cancers; Mesothelioma; Pleurodesis; Thoracentesis; Thoracoscopy

▶ Polypectomy

Category: Procedures
Also known as: Endoscopic polypectomy

Definition: Polypectomy is the removal of a protruding growth (polyp), leaving the underlying tissue.

Cancers diagnosed or treated: Cancers of the colon, rectum, small bowel, stomach, uterus, and nose

Why performed: Most polypectomies are performed to remove polyps that are or are likely to become cancerous, thereby controlling or preventing the disease. Such polyps arise most frequently in the colon and rectum; less frequently in the stomach, small intestine, and uterus; and rarely in the nose. Most polypectomies are performed during a diagnostic endoscopic procedure (such as colonoscopy, gastroscopy, hysteroscopy, or sigmoidoscopy).

Polyps that cannot be removed with an endoscope, such as polyps that are too large or too numerous, require local excision or major surgery to remove the polyp and underlying tissue completely with a margin of healthy tissue.

Patient preparation: A few days before the procedure, the patient may need to stop certain medications. For gastrointestinal procedures, the patient may need to cleanse the bowel and may not eat or drink after midnight.

Steps of the procedure: Endoscopic procedures are scheduled in an outpatient setting. For the procedure, sensors are placed to monitor the patient's condition. An intravenous (IV) line is started for fluids and medications. The patient lies on the side, and sedation is given. If the patient has an electronic implant, then special precautions are taken. The appropriate endoscope is inserted through the anus (to examine colonic and rectal polyps), mouth (gastric and small intestinal polyps), or vagina (uterine polyps). The physician slowly withdraws the endoscope, carefully viewing the entire lining. When a polyp is found, its location, size, and appearance are documented. The physician may sample (biopsy), destroy (ablate), or remove (excise and retrieve) the polyp. If the polyp was not totally removed, then its location is marked with a small tattoo. All biopsy samples and excised tissues are taken to the laboratory for histopathologic evaluation.

After the procedure: The patient's condition is monitored until he or she awakens and then the patient may leave, transported by a companion. The next day, the patient resumes normal activities.

Risks: Polypectomy is relatively safe, with a small risk of perforation, bleeding, infection, postpolypectomy coagulation syndrome, or reaction to the sedative.

Results: The completeness of removal varies with the polyp's size and shape (such as broad or stalked) and the removal technique (such as type of excision, with or without ablation). Histopathologic evaluation determines whether each polyp is or is not likely to become cancerous and, if so, whether all diseased tissue was removed. Additional treatment, follow-up examinations, or both may be recommended.

Patricia Boone, Ph.D.

See also: Biopsy; Colon polyps; Colonoscopy and virtual colonoscopy; Colorectal cancer; Colorectal cancer screening; *DPC4* gene testing; Hysteroscopy; Infection and sepsis; Juvenile polyposis syndrome; Polyps; Rectal cancer; Sigmoidoscopy; Small intestine cancer; Stomach cancers; Uterine cancer

▶ Positron Emission Tomography (PET)

Category: Procedures
Also known as: PET scan, ^{18}F-FDG PET, ^{18}F-FET PET

Definition: Positron emission tomography (PET) scanning is a procedure in which a small amount of radioactive glucose or amino acid is injected into a vein and a scanner is used to make detailed, computerized pictures of areas inside the body. Since cancer cells often utilize more glucose and amino acids than normal cells, the pictures can be used to find cancer cells in the body by looking for areas with higher uptake of these nutrients.

Cancers diagnosed: A wide range of cancers

Why performed: PET scans are used to screen for tumors in cancer diagnosis and to aid in tumor staging, locating metastases, and assessing treatment response, such as tumor recurrence. In addition to cancers, PET scans are effective for determining the presence of infections, heart disease, brain disorders, abnormal blood flow, and bone disorders.

Patient preparation: Patients should restrict the amount of sugar and caffeine consumed on the day before the scan. On the day of the scan, patients should not ingest anything except water for a minimum of six hours before the scan. Prior to the PET scan, blood glucose levels should be less than 120 milligrams per deciliter in nondiabetics and should fall between 150 and 200 milligrams per deciliter in diabetics. Patients are asked to drink 500 milliliters of water after injection of a radioactive compound approximately 1 hour before the PET scan. For renal or pelvic imaging, 20 to 40 milligrams of furosemide may be given ten to fifteen minutes after the injection of radioactive glucose or amino acid. Patients should also refrain from strenuous exercise for twenty-four hours before PET to minimize uptake of the radioactive compound by the muscles during the test. Just before the scan, patients are asked to remove any dentures, jewelry, or metal objects that may interfere with imaging.

Steps of the procedure: Patients are injected with glucose (FDG) or tyrosine (FET) labeled with radioactive fluorine (^{18}F). The compounds are given about an hour to distribute throughout the body. The patient then empties the bladder and lies still on the scanner bed. The PET scan takes approximately forty-five to sixty minutes, depending on the type of scan taken and the model of scanner used. Commonly, an initial whole-body scan is conducted about an hour after injection of the radioactive compound. This scan typically samples from the angle of the jaw to the level of the mid-thigh. A later scan, known as a delayed scan, is then taken approximately two hours after the injection, focusing on the organ or tissue of interest.

A major complication in interpreting PET data is the presence of multiple primary and metastatic lesions throughout the body. The uptake of radioactive glucose or amino acids into these tumors and into the surrounding normal tissues is a dynamic process that peaks at different times, depending on the specific tissues examined, patient preparation, and other factors. Thus if a patient undergoes serial PET scanning, then the time between injection of the radioactive compound and PET imaging should be the same in the baseline study and in subsequent studies. The National Cancer Institute consensus recommendations for FDG-PET scanning in clinical trials states that serial PET scans should be conducted at the same institution, using the same type of camera, the same dose of radioactive compound, the same imaging times, and the same acquisition and reconstruction parameters.

After the procedure: The patient is asked to drink plenty of fluids for a day after the scan in order to flush the radioactive compound from the body. The PET scans are interpreted by a trained radiologist, who sends the results to the referring physician.

Risks: The procedure is completely painless, with no side effects. The amount of radiation exposure is very small and similar to that from a standard X ray. Like any other procedure involving radiation, however, PET is accompanied by a small risk of tissue damage. Some patients may also experience soreness in the arm where the intravenous (IV) line was placed. Pregnant patients should inform the doctor of their condition, as PET scans may be harmful to the fetus.

Results: PET scans can identify regions in the body with abnormal metabolism of nutrients, which may indicate the presence of cancer cells. These areas can then be examined more closely by computed tomography (CT) or magnetic resonance imaging (MRI) to confirm that tumors are present and, if so, where they are located. PET scans may be useful in determining the extent of spread of certain cancers, assessing how the cancer responds to treatment, and determining if the cancer has recurred. Cancers may use more energy than surrounding tissues and therefore appear brighter on the PET scan.

PET scanning can be used in combination with CT scanning to produce anatomical pictures of organs and tissues that show regions of abnormal metabolism. PET/CT scanning machines are now available at many medical centers. This combination method can be more powerful than either technique used alone. R. A. Kuker and colleagues showed that a combination of delayed-phase FDG-PET and CT could identify liver tumors and metastases that could not be detected by CT alone.

Several important factors must be considered when analyzing PET scans. A crucial factor in analyzing PET data is the time of measurement. For example, whole-body images are composites of static images that are obtained at various predetermined times after the injection of the radioactive compound. These scans must be corrected for signal attenuation over time. Other factors that have an impact on data analysis are the volume of distribution, body weight, lean body mass, body surface area, and normal serum glucose or amino acid concentrations. After correcting for these factors, the standardized uptake value (SUV) is the most common assessment used. When suspected lesions are identified on a PET scan, both maximum and mean SUV are determined for regions in the tumor and in normal tissue in the same organ. The tumor-to-normal-tissue SUV (T/N) ratio can be calculated. A value for the maximum SUV T/N ratio, for example, can be set as a threshold above which a suspected lesion is considered positive.

When using PET to determine tumor response to treatment, experts recommend conducting PET studies six to eight weeks after radiation therapy and two weeks after chemotherapy. The SUVs of the target tumors are determined before and after treatment. The SUVs of normal tissue in the organs in which the tumors occur are also obtained as a reference, and T/N ratios are obtained. This ensures that the SUV changes are attributable to either tumor progression or treatment response, and not to normal changes in the cells over time. The shape and size of tumors frequently change during the course of treatment. These changes should be recorded along with the changes in tumor uptake values. The interpretation of PET data is key to obtaining accurate and reliable results. Many types of cancer do not appear on PET scans and may be detected only by imaging techniques with a higher resolution, such as PET/CT or MRI. Some noncancerous tissues can also appear similar to tumors on a PET scan, resulting in false positives.

Ing-Wei Khor, Ph.D.

For Further Information

Christian, Paul E., and Kristen M. Waterstram-Rich, eds. *Nuclear Medicine and PET: Technology and Techniques*. 6th ed. St. Louis: Mosby/Elsevier, 2007.

Kubota, K. "From Tumor Biology to Clinical PET: A Review of Positron Emission Tomography (PET) in Oncology." *Annals of Nuclear Medicine* 15 (2001): 471-486.

Kuker, R. A., G. Mesoloras, and S. A. Gulec. "Optimization of FDG-PET/CT Imaging Protocol for Evaluation of Patients with Primary and Metastatic Liver Disease." *International Seminars in Surgical Oncology* 4 (2007): 17-21. Also available online at http://www.issoonline.com.

Shankar, L. K., J. M. Hoffman, S. Bacharach, et al. "Consensus Recommendations for the Use of ^{18}F-FDG PET as an Indicator of Therapeutic Response in Patients in National Cancer Institute Trials." *Journal of Nuclear Medicine* 47 (2006): 1059-1066.

Other Resources

Cedars-Sinai Health System
http://www.csmc.edu

Mayo Clinic
Positron Emission Tomography (PET) Scan: Detecting Conditions Early
http://www.mayoclinic.com/health/pet-scan/CA00052

National Cancer Institute
http://www.cancer.gov

PETNET solutions
Patient Preparation
http://www.petscaninfo.com/zportal/portals/pat/my_pet_scan/for_patients

See also: Angiography; Barium enema; Barium swallow; Bone scan; Bronchography; Computed Tomography (CT)-guided biopsy; Computed Tomography (CT) scan; Cystography; Ductogram; Endoscopic Retrograde Cholangiopancreatography (ERCP); Gallium scan; Hysterography; Imaging tests; Lymphangiography; Magnetic Resonance Imaging (MRI); Mammography; Nuclear medicine scan; Radionuclide scan; Thermal imaging; X-ray tests

▶ Progesterone receptor assay

Category: Procedures
Also known as: PgR assay, hormone-response assay

Definition: A progesterone receptor assay is an immunoassay performed on sections from breast tumors removed during surgery or on small samples obtained with core needle biopsy.

Cancers diagnosed: Hormone-responsive breast cancer, ductal carcinoma in situ

Why performed: A progesterone receptor assay is used to determine whether a cancer is likely to respond to hormonal therapy.

Patient preparation: The assay is performed on sections of breast tumors removed during surgery or by needle biopsy. For needle biopsy, patients are usually asked not to use powder, deodorant, or perfume the day of the biopsy.

Steps of the procedure: Tumors that were removed during surgery are fixed and stained and then examined by a pathologist to determine whether the cells of the tumor express receptors for progesterone. For core needle biopsy, the patient is either upright or lying on her stomach. A local anesthetic is used to numb the breast, and a needle, which may be guided by X-ray imaging, is inserted into the breast mass. Samples of the mass are aspirated into the needle and then sent to a pathologist, who will stain the samples for the assay.

After the procedure: After surgery, the patient will be given specific instructions by the physician about activities. Patients can usually resume normal activity immediately after a needle biopsy.

Risks: For needle biopsy, the biopsied breast may occasionally show mild bruising.

Results: The progesterone receptor is a member of the steroid receptor superfamily of nuclear receptors. The steroid hormone progesterone binds to the receptor in the cell and regulates the expression of genes involved in growth and cell division. Expression of progesterone (PgR) or estrogen (ER) receptors in cancer cells indicates that they will respond to signals that inhibit their growth and division, including drugs that block signaling by estrogen and progesterone. The results are presented as positive or negative based on the number of hormone-responsive cells. A positive result, particularly in early-stage cancers that are both ER- and PgR-positive, suggests that a cancer will likely respond to hormonal (endocrine) therapies and generally signals a favorable prognosis. Such therapies may include removing the ovaries in premenopausal women, treating with an antiestrogen drug such as tamoxifen, or treating with an aromatase inhibitor to block the synthesis of estrogen by the body. A negative result on the progesterone receptor assay indicates that other types of treatments should be pursued.

Michele Arduengo, Ph.D., ELS

See also: Adjuvant therapy; Breast cancers; Hormone receptor tests; Immunocytochemistry and immunohistochemistry; Leiomyomas; Meningiomas; Receptor analysis; Tumor markers

▶ Prostate-Specific Antigen (PSA) test

Category: Procedures
Also known as: PSA blood test

Definition: The protein-specific antigen (PSA) test is a simple blood test used to screen for prostate cancer. PSA is a protein produced by both normal and cancerous prostate cells that is released into the blood. High levels of PSA may be indicative of prostate cancer, as well as other noncancerous conditions such as benign prostatic hyperplasia (BPH) or an infection or inflammation in the prostate. The first PSA test determines the baseline level. The PSA levels are compared each year and monitored for any changes.

Cancers diagnosed: Prostate cancer

Why performed: The benefit of this test is that it can detect signs of early-stage prostate cancer when there are no symptoms. When this cancer is treated in the early stages of the disease, there is a high probability of cure.

Prostate cancer is the second most common form of cancer among men in the United States—the most common is skin cancer—and the second leading cause of death behind lung cancer. It is estimated that nearly 235,000 men in the United States were diagnosed with this disease in 2006, and more than 27,000 men died from it.

Certain groups of men are at a greater risk of developing prostate cancer. Age is a risk factor; the older a man gets, the higher the risk of getting prostate cancer. More than 70 percent of all diagnosed prostate cancer is found in men sixty-five years of age or older. Men with a family history of prostate cancer in an immediate relative, such as a father, brother, or son, are two to three times more likely to develop the disease. It is also more common among African American men, with more men in this racial group dying from the disease than in any other ethnic group. It is less common in men who are Hispanic, Asian, Native American, or from the Pacific Islands.

Men who are at high risk for the disease should begin testing with both a digital rectal examination (DRE) and a PSA test at age forty-five. The recommended guidelines suggest testing for all other men beginning at age fifty. The test should be repeated yearly unless a medical provider suggests otherwise.

Patient preparation: No special preparation is needed for this blood test. There are indications that a recent urinary tract infection, a recent urinary catheter, prostate stones, a prostate massage, or a DRE right before the blood test may cause the PSA levels to rise. Therefore, it is recommended to avoid those situations before the blood test in order to avoid a false rise in PSA.

Steps of the procedure: Since this procedure is a blood test, it takes only a few minutes to perform. The blood is then sent to a laboratory for analysis. It may take a few days up to two weeks before the test results are available.

After the procedure: The patient can return to normal activity. It is important to follow up on the results of the blood test to ensure that the PSA levels are within normal limits.

Risks: No risks are associated with this procedure.

Results: There are several ways to interpret PSA results. A more traditional approach considers less than 4 nanograms per milliliter (ng/mL) to be normal, 4 to 10 ng/mL slightly elevated, 10 to 20 ng/mL moderately elevated, and over 20 ng/mL significantly elevated. Other physicians evaluate the PSA level based on age and suggest that the normal ranges vary by age group. For physicians who take that approach, less than 2.5 ng/mL is normal for men forty to forty-nine years old, less than 3.5 ng/ml is normal for men fifty to fifty-nine years old, less than 4.5 ng/mL is normal for men sixty to sixty-nine years of age, and less than 6.5 ng/mL is normal for men seventy or older.

If the initial PSA level is found to be within normal limits, then one of the most important factors in determining whether prostate cancer is present is the change in PSA level from year to year. A dramatic rise in PSA levels from one screening to the next may be indicative of the presence of prostate cancer or other problems with the prostate. When the PSA level is elevated, it is important to have additional testing to determine the cause. Additional tests may include a transrectal ultrasound, in which a small probe is inserted into the rectum to take video images of the prostate, or a biopsy of the prostate, which involves inserting a needle into the prostate to take tissue samples. These samples are then checked for evidence of cancer.

Vonne Sieve, M.A.

For Further Information

American Cancer Society. *Cancer Facts and Figures*. Atlanta: American Cancer Society, 2005.

Bostwick, D. G., et al. "Human Prostate Cancer Risk Factors." *Cancer* 101, suppl. 10 (2004): 2371-2490.

Ellsworth, Pamela, John Heaney, and Cliff Gill. *One Hundred Questions and Answers About Prostate Cancer*. Sudbury, Mass.: Jones & Bartlett, 2003.

U.S. Department of Health and Human Services. *United States Cancer Statistics: 1999-2002 Incidence and Mortality Web-Based Report*. Atlanta: Centers for Disease Control and Prevention and National Cancer Institute, 2005. Also available online at http://www.cdc.gov.

Other Resources

Centers for Disease Control and Prevention
Cancer Prevention and Control
http://www.cdc.gov/cancer

Prostate Cancer Foundation
http://www.prostatecancerfoundation.org

See also: Benign Prostatic Hyperplasia (BPH); Carcinomas; Digital Rectal Exam (DRE); Immunocytochemistry and immunohistochemistry; Pathology; Prevention; Prostate cancer; Prostatectomy; Prostitis; Proteomics and cancer research; Screening for cancer; Transrectal ultra sound; Tumor markers; Watchful waiting; Wine and cancer

▶ Prostatectomy

Category: Procedures
Also known as: Radical prostatectomy, transurethral resection of the prostate (TURP)

Definition: Prostatectomy is the surgical removal of part or all of the prostate gland. A radical prostatectomy refers to removal of the prostate gland and surrounding tissue. A transurethral resection (TURP) refers to removal of part of the prostate.

Cancers treated: Prostate cancer

Why performed: A radical prostatectomy is performed to remove cancer that is confined to the prostate gland and surrounding area. This procedure is not usually done when cancer has spread beyond the prostate gland to distant tissues or organs.

A TURP is commonly done to relieve symptoms associated with benign prostatic hyperplasia (BPH). With BPH, the prostate gland is enlarged and squeezes the urethra, creating problems with urination. Removal of part of the prostate gland can usually alleviate those symptoms.

Patient preparation: Generally, no food or drink is consumed after midnight on the day before undergoing general anesthesia. The evening before a radical prostatectomy, a bowel preparation is usually taken to cleanse the colon.

Steps of the procedure: For a radical prostatectomy, the procedure varies depending on which method the surgeon uses: open, laparoscopic, or laparoscopically assisted prostatectomy. Typically, general anesthesia is used with all these procedures.

Open surgery involves an incision in the lower abdomen if the retropubic approach is done or in the groin between the anus and the penis for the perineal approach. The retropubic approach is most common and allows the surgeon to remove the prostate gland and the lymph nodes, if necessary, to be checked for cancer spread beyond the prostate. This approach allows the surgeon to attempt preservation of the nerves that help control bladder and sexual function. Lymph node removal can be done with the perineal approach, but a separate incision must be made, and preservation of sexual function is not possible. The open procedure can take from one and a half to four hours to complete.

With the laparoscopic and laparoscopically assisted approach, several small incisions are made in the lower abdomen. The laparoscope allows the surgeon to see inside the abdominal cavity and remove the prostate and surrounding tissue. With the robot-assisted procedure, the surgeon performs the procedure remotely with the use of a robot. Occasionally, a laparoscopic procedure may need to be converted to an open procedure if difficulty is encountered. This procedure may take four hours or more to perform.

No abdominal incision is needed for a TURP. A cutting instrument or a heated wire loop is inserted through the penis to the prostate gland to remove or destroy prostate tissue. The bladder is then flushed with sterile solution to remove the destroyed tissue from the body.

With all these procedures, a small flexible tube called a urinary catheter is inserted into the bladder and left in place to drain urine during the healing process.

After the procedure: An open prostatectomy is considered major abdominal surgery. Patients typically remain in the hospital from two to four days. Recovery time can be as long as twelve weeks. A laparoscopic procedure is less invasive. The hospital stay is usually two days, and recovery time averages two to four weeks. The urinary catheter is typically removed one to three weeks after the procedure.

With a TURP, the hospital stay is generally two to four days. The urinary catheter is generally left in place for one to three days after the procedure.

Risks: General complications from undergoing a major surgical procedure may include bleeding, blood clots, heart problems, infection, allergic reaction to anesthesia, and, in rare cases, death.

Short-term complications from a radical prostatectomy may include urinary incontinence, which is the inability to control the bladder. This condition generally improves, and full bladder control is regained over time. Long-term complications may include erectile dysfunction and urinary incontinence.

The risks from a TURP may include excessive bleeding, a urinary tract infection, or pain with urination. Some men temporarily develop problems as a result of the large amounts of irrigating fluid used to flush out the bladder. A more permanent condition that can develop is a stricture, a permanent narrowing of the urethra that can occur if the urethra is damaged during the procedure.

Results: When prostate cancer is confined to the prostate gland, the cure rate is very high. Five-year survival approaches 100 percent. Overall, prostatectomy success rates are about 76 to 98 percent for men with low-risk disease, 60 to 76 percent for men with moderate-risk disease, and 30 to 76 percent for men with high-risk disease. These rates vary depending on the surgeon's technique and experience with the procedure.

Erectile dysfunction is a common side effect. The nerves that control erections are located on both sides of the prostate gland and are easily damaged, or may be removed, during the procedure. Age and erectile function before surgery can affect the likelihood of problems after the procedure.

Urinary incontinence is another common problem with this procedure and includes occasional urine leakage to complete inability to control urine flow. In some cases, additional surgery may be necessary to correct the problem.

With a TURP, urination problems generally stop after the swelling has subsided.

After the surgical procedure, it is important for the patient to discuss monitoring his condition with additional testing to ensure that the problems have not returned.

Vonne Sieve, M.A.

For Further Information

Ellsworth, Pamela, John Heaney, and Cliff Gill. *One Hundred Questions and Answers About Prostate Cancer*. Sudbury, Mass.: Jones & Bartlett, 2003.

Marks, Sheldon. *Prostate Cancer: A Family Guide to Diagnosis, Treatment, and Survival.* Cambridge, Mass.: Fisher Books, 2000.

Wainrib, Barbara, et al. *Men, Women, and Prostate Cancer: A Medical and Psychological Guide for Women and the Men They Love*. Oakland, Calif.: New Harbinger, 2000.

See also: Benign Prostatic Hyperplasia (BPH); Carcinomas; Exenteration; Infection and sepsis; Obesity-associated cancers; Prostate cancer; Psychosocial aspects of cancer; Sexuality and cancer; Urinary system cancers; Urologic oncology

▶ Protein electrophoresis

Category: Procedures
Also known as: Serum protein electrophoresis (SPEP)

Definition: Protein electrophoresis is a laboratory test used to measure the amounts of major proteins in a patient's blood serum, urine, or cerebrospinal fluid.

Cancers diagnosed: Most metastatic cancers, especially multiple myeloma

Why performed: Serum protein electrophoresis is used to screen for cancer or evaluate the extent of an existing cancer, particularly multiple myeloma. It can also be used to identify other diseases, including kidney, liver, intestinal, and immune disorders, as well as malnutrition. These disorders are associated with abnormal levels of different blood proteins, which can be detected by electrophoresis.

Patient preparation: There is no special preparation for this procedure. Patients undergo a normal blood test and should tell their physicians which prescription medications they are taking.

Steps of the procedure: A physician or nurse will draw blood from a vein in the patient's arm in an outpatient setting. The blood sample is transferred to the laboratory, where it is centrifuged to separate serum, the plasma without clotting factors, from the blood cells. Blood proteins are retained in the serum. A small amount of serum is then transferred to an electrophoretic paper or gel such as cellular acetate or agarose, respectively. Since proteins are charged molecules and vary in size, they will migrate differentially when a current is applied to the electrophoretic field. A fluorescent agent that binds to proteins is added to the serum for illumination. The result is a gradient of separated bands, or fractions, of proteins. A laboratory specialist studies an image of the gel to determine the relative concentrations of different proteins in the blood serum.

After the procedure: A bandage is applied to the patient's arm at the puncture site, and the patient can go home.

Risks: No risks are associated with protein electrophoresis. A blood draw, however, may cause minor bleeding or bruising at the puncture site. The patient may also feel light-headed, and there is a possibility of fainting after the blood draw.

Results: The major blood proteins consist of albumin and globulins. There are four types of globulin proteins: alpha-1 globulins, alpha-2 globulins, beta globulins, and gamma globulins. Normally, albumin makes up more than half of the proteins in the blood serum and is important for normal tissue growth. High levels of albumin proteins are a result of dehydration, while low levels suggest inflammatory disease, liver disease, malnutrition, or a kidney disorder. High levels of alpha-1 globulins (alpha-1 antitrypsin, thyroid-binding globulin, and transcortin) may indicate acute inflammatory disease and malignancies, while a low level can indicate liver disease. The levels of certain alpha-2 globulins (ceruloplasmin, alpha-2 macroglobulin, and haptoglobulin) can aid in cancer diagnosis. For example, a low level of haptoglobin may indicate tumor metastasis or liver disease. Variations in other alpha-2 globulin levels may indicate inflammation, nephrotic syndrome, or hemolysis, which is the loss of hemoglobin from red blood cells. High levels of beta globulin (transferrin and beta lipoprotein) can indicate biliary cirrhosis, hyperthyroidism, diabetes mellitus, and carcinoma in some cases, while decreased levels indicate malnutrition. High levels of gamma globulins (various antibodies) are the most indicative of cancers such as multiple myeloma, lymphocytic leukemia, or malignant lymphoma. In addition, high levels can indicate Hodgkin disease, connective tissue disorders, and chronic or acute infections. A patient whose serum protein electrophoresis yields abnormal results will be referred to a hematologist-oncologist.

Bharat Burman, B.A.

For Further Information

Aziz, Khalid, and George Y. Wu. *Cancer Screening: A Practical Guide for Physicians*. Totowa, N.J.: Humana Press, 2002.

Hoffman, Ronald, et al. *Hematology: Basic Principles and Practice*. 4th ed. Philadelphia: Churchill Livingstone, 2005.

Keren, David F. *High-Resolution Electrophoresis and Immunofixation: Techniques and Interpretation*. 2d ed. Boston: Butterworth-Heinemann, 1994.

O'Connell, T. X., et al. "Understanding and Interpreting Serum Protein Electrophoresis." *American Family Physician* 71, no. 1 (January 1, 2005): 105-112.

Wallach, Jacques. *Interpretation of Diagnostic Tests*. 8th ed. Philadelphia: Wolters Kluwer Health/Lippincott Williams & Wilkins, 2007.

Other Resources

American Cancer Society
How Is Multiple Myeloma Diagnosed?
http://www.cancer.org/cancer/multiplemyeloma/

National Cancer Institute
Screening and Testing to Detect Cancer
http://www.cancer.gov/cancertopics/screening

See also: Immunoelectrophoresis (IEP); Lactate Dehydrogenase (LDH) test; Multiple myeloma; Myeloma

▶ Proton beam therapy

Category: Procedures

Definition: Proton beam therapy is a procedure for delivering targeted radiation therapy using protons instead of the electrons used by traditional radiation therapies.

Cancers treated: Primarily cancers of the prostate, lung, head, neck, and brain

Why performed: Proton beam therapy, like traditional radiation therapy, is performed to kill cancer cells. It may be performed as a primary treatment for a tumor, to kill any cancer cells that remain after surgical cancer treatment, or in addition to other cancer treatment options. Proton beam therapy is only offered at a few locations in the United States, and for many cancers it is still considered an experimental treatment.

Proton beam therapy is a site-specific therapy, so it is designed to treat cancers that have not spread to large areas or throughout the body. It is mainly used to treat cancers occurring in the prostate, lung, head, neck, and brain, although it is being tested in clinical trials for use on cancers occurring in many other areas as well.

Patient preparation: The patient should discuss with the cancer care team any necessary preparation for the specific procedure that he or she is undergoing. Necessary preparation may vary depending on the type of cancer being treated and the patient's previous response to any radiation therapy.

Steps of the procedure: Proton beam therapy uses high-speed protons to kill cancer cells, instead of the electrons used by most radiation therapy techniques. Atoms are made up of a nucleus of protons and neutrons surrounded by orbiting electrons. Protons have a positive charge, neutrons have no charge, and electrons have a negative charge. When free protons come very close to an atom, the electrons orbiting the nucleus are attracted to the positive charge of the protons. The electrons are then pulled out of their orbits. This is called ionization of the atom. Atoms that have been ionized are not as stable as normal atoms. This change to the atom means that changes also occur to the molecule of which the atom is part, and eventually to the cell of which the molecule is part. If the cell cannot repair the damage caused, then it eventually dies.

Proton beam therapy begins with protons traveling around a synchrotron, a machine that makes the protons go very fast and energizes them. The protons are then sent through vacuum tubes to the machine that actually aims them at the area of the patient that will receive the radiation. The patient is positioned and held still so that the proton beam can be aimed as accurately as possible. Complex computer technology helps the doctors and technicians aim the proton beam very accurately so that it hits as little healthy tissue as possible.

The protons are released in a directed stream toward the cancer cells. The protons are traveling very quickly at first, but they slow down as they get closer to the cancer. When they are traveling fast, they do not have a very strong effect on the atoms they are passing. When they are slower, however, they have an extremely strong effect. This is one reason that proton beam therapy causes less damage to healthy cells than does traditional radiation therapy. Traditional radiation therapy uses X rays, which strongly affect all the cells with which they come into contact, which makes it hard to deliver enough radiation to the cancer cells without also killing healthy cells. With proton beam therapy, doctors aided by computers can determine the right way to release the protons so that they have the maximum impact just as they come into contact with the cancer cells. Proton beam therapy may need to be repeated one or more times depending on the size and type of the cancer and other factors.

After the procedure: After proton beam therapy, many individuals experience no negative side effects. Some individuals, however, may experience pain, fatigue, nausea, or diarrhea.

Risks: The risks associated with proton beam therapy are believed to be somewhat lower than those associated with traditional radiation therapy for most people. This is the case because proton beam therapy causes less damage to surrounding healthy cells, so healthy tissue is less likely to be significantly damaged. Some of the risks of proton beam therapy include nausea, diarrhea, and fatigue. Damage to healthy tissue is still a possible risk of proton beam therapy.

Results: The goal of proton beam therapy is generally to destroy a tumor, to reduce the size of a tumor, to reduce related symptoms, or to kill any residual cancer cells left after a tumor has been surgically removed. Success rates for proton beam therapy can vary drastically depending on the type of cancer, its size, and how far it has spread. It is generally found to be successful at reducing the side effects usually associated with traditional radiation therapy. If the procedure is done to completely destroy a tumor or residual cancer, then the procedure is generally considered to have been successful if the cancer does not return for five years or more. If the procedure was done to reduce tumor size, then it is considered successful if quality of life is improved.

Helen Davidson, B.A.

For Further Information

Barton-Burkey, Margaret, and Gail M. Wilkes. *Cancer Therapies*. Sudbury, Mass.: Jones and Bartlett, 2006.

Chan, Helen S. L. *Understanding Cancer Therapies*. Jackson: University of Mississippi Press, 2007.

DeLaney, Thomas F., and Hanne M. Kooy, eds. *Proton and Charged Particle Radiotherapy*. Philadelphia: Lippincott Williams & Wilkins, 2008.

Haas, Marilyn L., et al. *Radiation Therapy: A Guide to Patient Care*. St. Louis: Mosby/Elsevier, 2007.

Other Resources

The National Association for Proton Therapy
http://www.proton-therapy.org

See also: Afterloading radiation therapy; Brain scan; Cancer care team; External Beam Radiation Therapy (EBRT); Gastrointestinal complications of cancer treatment; Meningiomas; Nausea and vomiting; Neurologic oncology; Radiation oncology; Radiation therapies; Virus-related cancers

▶ Radiation therapies

Category: Procedures
Also known as: Radiotherapy, external beam radiation therapy (EBRT), internal beam radiation therapy (IBRT), systemic radiation therapy, stereotactic radiosurgery, afterloading radiation, implants, brachytherapy, tomotherapy, proton therapy, intensity-modulated radiation therapy (IMRT), image-guided radiation therapy (IGRT), Mammosite therapy, radioimmunotherapy

Definition: Radiation therapy uses high doses of radiation to kill cancer cells and prevent metastasis (the spread of disease). Most cancers may be treated with one or more of the three types of radiation therapy. About 50 to 60 percent of all cancers may be treated by radiation therapy during the initial treatment phases, and an additional 12.5 percent of patients may need a second course of treatment later in their disease to manage symptoms caused by the growth of their tumor. The radiation oncologist, with other physicians involved in the care of the patient, will determine if the patient's cancer is appropriately treated with radiation.

Cancers treated: Most, such as breast, prostate, thyroid, and gynecological cancers

Why performed: Radiation therapies are performed to kill, stop, or slow the growth of cancer cells in the body. Cancer is usually treated with surgery, chemotherapy, and radiation, which is called multimodal therapy. Radiation, as a component of this combined approach to care, may be used before, during, or after surgery; in combination with chemotherapy; or alone. Some patients who are not able to tolerate aggressive surgeries or chemotherapies may benefit, to some degree, from radiation therapy. Many patients develop side effects from their cancers that may be treated with radiation. Spinal cord compression or bony metastases may be treated to reduce paralysis or pain.

There are three ways to administer radiation to a patient. When a machine outside the body delivers radiation to a tumor inside the body, the process is called external beam radiation therapy (EBRT). Internal beam radiation therapy (IBRT) uses sources, applicators, or a high-dose remote afterloader to place radioactive material in the body near the cancer site. Systemic radiation therapy uses a radioactive substance that is injected or swallowed and then travels to cancer cells in tissues of the body.

EBRT uses X-ray beams that may be given by a linear accelerator, a machine that generates high-energy radiation beams; by a machine with a radioactive source, cobalt 60; by a tomotherapy unit, which is a linear accelerator coupled with a computed tomography (CT) scanner that delivers radiation in spirals around the body; or by a robotically controlled accelerator that delivers radiation while tracking and controlling for patient movement or organ movement during the treatment. Proton beam therapy, one of the newer of the external beam radiation therapies, uses a machine that generates protons to damage the deoxyribonucleic acid (DNA) of cancer cells. With proton therapy, the radiation beam of protons enters the body with a low dose of radiation, deposits its highest dose at the site being treated, and then stops without traveling through the body.

Advances in external beam therapy, based on the ability to better plan therapies, continue to develop rapidly. Conformal radiation therapy (3D-CRT) develops a three-dimensional model of the tumor and then uses shaped beams to treat the cancer from several directions. Intensity-modulated radiation therapy (IMRT) uses sophisticated treatment planning to vary the strength of the radiation beam in an attempt to lessen damage to the normal tissues surrounding the tumor. Tomotherapy is considered a type of IMRT and image-guided radiation therapy (IGRT), as the beams spiral around the body, allowing for precise and focused radiation beams based on data from a CT scan. IGRT is used to visualize the tumor location prior to treatment, as tumor movement occurs daily, and to control for tumor movement with respiration (respiratory gating). In addition to a CT scan, ultrasound may be used.

Stereotactic radiosurgery is a type of radiation therapy that delivers a large, precise dose to a defined tumor site. It is most commonly used for brain tumors, but applications in the abdomen and other sites are being explored. A cobalt 60 source machine is used with a head frame for brain tumors, and a robotically control linear accelerator may be used for both brain tumors and tumors outside the head (extracranial tumors). It is called radiosurgery because of its accuracy. The radiation beam is considered as accurate as a knife (or scalpel) and may treat tumors that surgeons cannot reach using traditional surgical techniques.

Intraoperative radiation therapy is used at the time of surgery to deliver external beam radiation directly to the tumor during the surgical procedure. The surgeon locates the cancer and moves normal tissues and organs out of the way, and then an accelerator delivers radiation directly to the tumor. The patient is asleep (under anesthesia) during the procedure, which is done in a special lead-lined operating room.

IBRT is delivered by several methods and is often referred to as brachytherapy. IBRT using a remote-controlled machine called a high-dose remote afterloader (HDR) unit sends high-dose radioactive material through catheters or needles placed in the patient for a period of minutes, and then the sources are withdrawn, so that the patient is not radioactive. When patients are exposed to radiation sources for a period of hours or days, the process is called low-dose-rate brachytherapy. Applicators or cases that house radioactive sources are placed in the patient and left for a prescribed period of time. The area around the patient is considered radioactive until the source is removed. Therefore, staff must limit their exposure to the patient, and visitors are not allowed. Permanent brachytherapy is a type of low-dose therapy in which radioactive seeds are placed in the patient and remain while giving off low doses of radiation for weeks or months. The patient gives off some radioactivity in very small doses. The primary safety consideration is to keep children away from the area of the implant. For example, a man undergoing permanent brachytherapy for prostate cancer must not allow children to sit on his lap.

Systemic radiation therapy is given as a capsule or liquid swallowed by the patient, or it may be given in a vein (injected intravenously). The radioactive liquid then moves throughout the body. The patient may stay in a special room in the hospital, and body fluids are handled carefully, as the radiation materials are eliminated from the body through urine, saliva, and sweat. When the radioactivity has dipped to safe levels, the patient may be discharged from the hospital. In some cases, the patient may be able to go home after treatment with special instructions about handling wastes.

Breast cancer is one of the most commonly treated cancers using external beam radiation therapy. Use of an HDR unit decreases the treatment time of several weeks to just five days. This procedure is often referred to as Mammosite therapy, named for the company that initially developed the procedure for commercial use. Prostate cancer may also use external beam radiation, an HDR unit, or implantable seeds (low-dose brachytherapy) to kill cancer cells. Thyroid cancer is often treated with radioactive iodine, a systemic radiation therapy in a liquid form that is swallowed by the patient. Gynecological cancers may be treated with an HDR unit or low-dose brachytherapy with an applicator that is left in for a period of time.

Patient preparation: The radiation oncologist, a physician with specialized training in radiation therapy care, will see the patient in a consult visit to determine if radiation therapy is appropriate for his or her cancer. Patients are generally referred to the radiation oncologist by the patient's surgeon or medical oncologist. The physicians treating the patient will discuss whether external, internal, or systemic radiation is most appropriate. Prior to receiving treatment, patients have a simulation using a CT scanner or fluoroscopic simulator to allow the physician to visualize the area to be treated. A simulation may take up to two hours. To assist in positioning the patient for treatment, small marks may be placed on the skin. Later in the treatment room, the marks will be used with wall-mounted positioning lasers to place the patient in the correct position to receive the treatment. The simulation data are used to plan the radiation dose amounts to be given by the linear accelerator, the HDR unit, or any other source of radiation, such as implantable seeds. The simulation information is given to the physicist and dosimetrist, who load the data into a sophisticated treatment-planning computer. The physician then verifies the treatment site, the treatment plan, and the radiation dose to be given.

Steps of the procedure: The steps of the radiation treatment will depend on the type of radiation therapy that the patient receives. Regardless of whether external, internal, or systemic therapy is used, treatment planning is still the key to accurate radiation placement and dosing. For external beam therapy, the treatment plan will outline the patient position on the treatment table, determine the shape of the beam, define the number of treatments to be given, and prescribe the daily and cumulative doses the patient is to receive. The patient has four to six weeks of treatment depending on the treatment plan, five days a week, with two days a week off for normal cells to rest and recover. If an HDR unit is to be used, then catheters may be implanted at the time of surgery, or hollow needles may be placed just before the treatment. HDR treatments usually take place once or twice a day for approximately five days.

For patients receiving internal radiation, a simulation and treatment plan are still necessary. For low-dose brachytherapy, such as prostate seed implants, additional imaging studies may be needed. Seeds are implanted during a surgical procedure with the patient under general anesthesia. Low-dose brachytherapy, such as used in gynecological cancers, may use applicators that are placed in a treatment room and then loaded with the radioactive source. Patients receiving systemic radiation also need treatment planning to determine the amount of radioactive liquid needed to treat the cancer.

After the procedure: Most external beam treatments are done on an outpatient basis, and the patient may leave immediately after the daily treatment. Patients are not radioactive during treatments. A few external beam treatments, such as intraoperative radiation therapy and select stereotactic radiosurgery, may require hospitalization. Internal beam radiation treatments may be done on either an inpatient or an outpatient basis, depending on the method used to deliver the radiation therapy. If an HDR unit is used to deliver high-dose radiation, then the patient may be able to go home between treatments. If the internal beam radiation therapy requires that the radioactive source stay in the patient for a period of hours or days, then the patient is usually hospitalized, as the bodily fluids are emitting radioactive waste. Systemic radiotherapy may be either inpatient or outpatient in nature.

Risks: The risks from radiation depend on the site being treated and the type of radiation therapy being used. EBRT is a local treatment, so risks involve the area around the site being treated. For example, if abdominal radiation is used, then bowel and bladder problems may develop. Skin reactions, similar to sunburn, may occur. Hair loss, called alopecia, may occur if radiation is given to the head or other body areas with hair follicles. Xerostomia, or dry mouth, may occur with radiation of the head and neck areas, and dental problems may also occur with this radiation site. Fatigue is often associated with any radiation procedure. Side effects usually go away within two to three months after therapy is completed. Late side effects, those developing six or more months after therapy is completed, may include infertility, lymphedema, joint pain, or other problems, as well as a risk of a second cancer due to the radiation. There is always a risk that not all cancer cells will be killed by the radiation.

Results: Cancer cell kill is expected after any method of radiation treatment.

Patricia Stanfill Edens, R.N., Ph.D., FACHE

For Further Information

Penson, D. F., M. S. Litwin, J. L. Gore, et al. "Quality of Life After Surgery, External Beam Irradiation, or Brachytherapy for Early Stage Prostate Cancer." *Urologic Oncology* 25, no. 5 (September/October, 2007): 442-443.

Tao, Y., D. Lefkopoulos, D. Ibrahima, et al. "Comparison of Dose Contribution to Normal Pelvic Tissues Among Conventional, Conformal, and Intensity-Modulated Radiotherapy Techniques in Prostate Cancer." *Acta Oncologica*, September 28, 2007, 1-9.

Other Resources

American Cancer Society
http://www.acs.org

American Society for Therapeutic Radiology Oncology
http://www.astro.org

Medline Plus
Radiation Therapy
http://www.nlm.nih.gov/medlineplus/radiationtherapy.html

National Cancer Institute
Radiation Therapy and You
http://www.cancer.gov

See also: Accelerated Partial Breast Irradiation (APBI); Afterloading radiation therapy; Angiography; Barium enema; Barium swallow; Bone scan; Boron Neutron Capture Therapy (BNCT); Brachytherapy; Brain scan; Bronchography; Cobalt 60 radiation; Computed Tomography (CT)-guided biopsy; Computed Tomography (CT) scan; Cystography; Ductogram; Endoscopic Retrograde Cholangiopancreatography (ERCP); External Beam Radiation Therapy (EBRT); Gallium scan; Gamma Knife; Hysterography; Imaging tests; Intensity-modulated Radiation Therapy (IMRT); Iridium seeds; Linear accelerator; Lymphangiography; Magnetic Resonance Imaging (MRI); Mammography; Microwave hyperthermia therapy; Nuclear medicine scan; Positron Emission Tomography (PET); Proton beam therapy; Radiation therapies; Radiofrequency ablation; Radionuclide scan;

Radiopharmaceuticals; Stereotactic needle biopsy; Stereotactic Radiosurgery (SRS); Thermal imaging; Thyroid nuclear medicine scan; Wire localization; X-ray tests

▶ Radical neck dissection

Category: Procedures
Also known as: Classical radical neck dissection

Definition: A radical neck dissection is a surgical procedure that involves the excision of a primary malignant cancer and several adjacent head and neck structures (salivary glands, sternocleidomastoid muscle, cervical lymph nodes, fatty tissue, jugular vein, and spinal accessory nerve).

Cancers treated: Squamous and basal cell carcinomas of the head and neck, lymphoma, thyroid carcinoma, metastatic cancer

Why performed: On gross examination of the neck, masses that preserve the outer tissue can suggest a benign tumor but cannot eliminate the possibility of cancer. Microscopically, benign tumor cells have an increased, orderly growth while malignant cells have an increased, disorderly growth and large nuclei relative to the surrounding cytoplasm. Cervical lymph node samples possessing cancerous cells strongly suggest microscopic spread outside the neck.

Extensive infiltration of the neck by a tumor can affect breathing, speech, and movement as well as blood circulation to the head. Surgery may be necessary to restore the function of the affected structures. The procedure is performed when malignant cancer has spread to adjacent facial and neck structures. Introduced in 1906 by George W. Crile, it remains the standard surgical treatment for metastasis.

Patient preparation: Surgical risk assessment, tissue biopsy, and computed tomography (CT) and/or magnetic resonance imaging (MRI) are done.

Steps of the procedure: A hockey-stick-shaped incision is made over the anterolateral neck. The superficial neck muscle (platysma) is cut and retracted. The submandibular gland and duct, lymph nodes, a segment of the facial artery, and the tail of the parotid gland are removed or ligated. The sternocleidomastoid muscle is cut above the clavicle and retracted. The posterior omohyoid, anterior trapezius, spinal accessory nerve, jugular vein, surrounding lymph nodes, and the upper border of the sternocleidomastoid are ligated, cut, and removed.

After the procedure: The patient is monitored until stable. A breathing tube may be put in place to protect the airway until the wound heals. Food intake may be withheld for at least twenty-four hours after the operation. The patient may be discharged if stable after a few days.

Risks: Bleeding is the most common complication because of the dense capillary network around the head and neck. Breathing problems, infections, formation of an abnormal connection between the esophagus and the trachea, shoulder muscle paralysis, and significant disfigurement can also occur.

Results: Although neck dissection has veered toward preserving function, radical neck dissection remains a sound surgical option for advanced stages of cancer.

Aldo C. Dumlao, M.D.

For Further Information

Brockstein, Bruce, and Gregory Masters, eds. *Head and Neck Cancer*. Boston: Kluwer Academic, 2003.

Kelloff, Gary, Ernest T. Hawk, and Caroline C. Sigman. *Cancer Chemoprevention*. Totowa, N.J.: Humana Press, 2004.

Thaller, Seth R., and W. Scott McDonald. *Facial Trauma*. Miami: Informa Health Care, 2004.

See also: Basal cell carcinomas; Benign tumors; Carcinomas; Computed Tomography (CT) scan; Imaging tests; Infection and sepsis; Lymphomas; Magnetic Resonance Imaging (MRI); Metastasis; Metastatic squamous neck cancer with occult primary; Oral and maxillofacial surgery; Salivary gland cancer; Thyroid cancer

▶ Radiofrequency ablation

Category: Procedures
Also known as: RFA, thermal ablation

Definition: Radiofrequency ablation is the application of high-energy radio waves (radiofrequency thermal energy) through a catheter probe to heat and destroy abnormal tissues. As a cancer treatment, radiofrequency ablation is used to ablate (destroy) cancerous tumors by directing the radiofrequency heat directly to the tumor, causing the cancerous cells to die.

According to the Society of Interventional Radiology, radiofrequency energy is safer than many cancer therapies because it is absorbed by living tissues as simple heat, and the heat generated by radiofrequency does not alter the basic chemical structure of cells.

Radiofrequency ablation technology was originally developed for the treatment of cardiac arrhythmias in the early 1990's and has since been used as a cancer treatment after clinical studies proved its efficacy. The technology is approved by the Food and Drug Administration (FDA).

Radiofrequency applications vary, depending on the type of catheter used and the dose of energy applied. Newer RFA applications involve ablation with multiple electrodes to treat large or multiple tumors and ablation with liposomal therapy, a method of delivering heat-activated chemotherapy drugs via synthetic capsules called liposomes. The coating on the liposome capsules allows the medication to remain in the circulation for a longer period of time, so the drugs selectively target cancer cells and decrease the side effects for healthy tissue.

Cancers treated: Primary and metastatic liver cancer, early-stage breast cancer, lung cancer, bone cancer, prostate cancer, and kidney and adrenal gland cancers; RFA is also being investigated as a treatment option for many other cancers

Why performed: Radiofrequency ablation is a minimally invasive, percutaneous procedure that offers an alternative treatment option for some patients with tumors that cannot be surgically removed, for patients who are not surgical candidates because of comorbid conditions or other risk factors, or for those who desire a less invasive treatment. In some cases, radiofrequency ablation can be used to ease certain side effects of cancer treatment, such as chronic pain caused by some cancers. Radiofrequency ablation may be used in combination with chemotherapy or other cancer treatments to improve a patient's quality of life and survival.

The recommendation for radiofrequency ablation is dependent on the type of cancer, the patient's overall medical condition, the number of tumors, and the tumor size and location.

Patient preparation: Tests performed before the procedure include positron emission tomography (PET) testing and computed tomography (CT) scanning. Radiofrequency ablation does not interfere with most standard cancer therapies and can be performed for some patients who are actively receiving chemotherapy.

A few days before the procedure, patients must stop taking aspirin and products containing aspirin, ibuprofen, and anticoagulants, as directed by the physician. Other anticoagulant medications may be prescribed if necessary before the procedure. Antiarrhythmic medications may also need to be discontinued. Patients with diabetes may need to adjust their diabetes medications, insulin dosages, or meal plan, as directed by the physician. Patients must not eat or drink for eight hours beforehand.

Patients should remove all makeup and nail polish. The patient will change into a hospital gown before the procedure.

Steps of the procedure: An intravenous (IV) line is inserted into a vein in the patient's arm to deliver medications. A sedative is usually given before the procedure so that the patient will be in a form of light sleep during the procedure. General anesthesia is used in some cases. An interventional radiologist usually performs the procedure, although a surgeon can also do so.

If general anesthesia is not used, then a local anesthetic is injected into the procedure site to numb the area. A thin, needlelike probe is placed through a puncture or small incision in the skin and is guided by ultrasound or CT into the core of the tumor. Once it is in place, thin, hook-shaped wires (tines) on the end of the probe extend upon deployment to an area beyond the diameter of the tumor. Localized radiofrequency energy is transmitted through the probe, which is attached to a radiofrequency generator. Energy is applied for ten to fifteen minutes to each targeted area, thereby heating and destroying the tissue. The temperature of the applied energy is carefully controlled; beyond 60 degrees Celsius, cells begin to die, resulting in an area of tissue death surrounding the probe. The probe may be deployed more than once for tumors larger than 3 centimeters.

Multiple tumors may be treated during the ablation procedure. A small region of normal cells around the tumor (margin) is also heated and destroyed with the goal of eradicating cancer in surrounding tissues. The procedure lasts from two to four hours.

After the procedure: The RFA probe is removed and pressure is applied to the insertion site to prevent bleeding. No stitches are needed unless a small incision was made. A small sterile dressing (bandage) will cover the insertion site. The patient may need to stay in bed from one to six hours after the procedure to prevent bleeding.

Most patients stay in the hospital overnight for observation after the procedure, but some patients go home the same day of the procedure. The patient may experience discomfort for two to three days afterward. Pain medication may be prescribed, or the patient may take acetaminophen (Tylenol) to relieve discomfort as needed.

The patient should not drive or operate machinery for eight hours after the procedure. Within twenty-four hours, the patient is usually able to return to light activity but should avoid vigorous physical activity and heavy lifting after the procedure, as directed by the physician. The average recovery time is from three to seven days, after which the patient may resume regular activities. The recovery time for radiofrequency ablation is much faster than that for surgical treatment, which can take from two to three months for full recovery.

Patients usually have a follow-up CT or magnetic resonance imaging (MRI) scan one week after the procedure to evaluate the effectiveness of the treatment. Thereafter, follow-up CT scans and blood tests are performed every three months or more frequently, based on the patient's condition.

Risks: The risks of radiofrequency ablation vary in relation to the type of cancer being treated and the area that is being ablated. For example, the risks of RFA applications for lung cancer include pleural effusion and pneumothorax. The risks of RFA applications for liver cancer include portal vein thrombosis, liver abscess, or acute renal insufficiency. The physician performing the procedure will discuss the potential risks of the procedure with the patient, depending on the type of cancer that is being treated.

The rate of overall complications is 1 to 4 percent, according to the Society of Interventional Radiology, depending on the disease treated and the patient's overall health. Most complications are minor and are often relieved on their own without further treatment or intervention. The risk of infection is rare, since there is no open wound associated with the procedure.

Results: Radiofrequency ablation is a safe and effective treatment option. Tumors from 1 to 10 centimeters in size can be successfully treated with radiofrequency ablation. A tumor or lesion that is successfully ablated should be reduced in size, or disappear altogether, and show no blood flow on follow-up CT scans. In addition to other cancer treatments, radiofrequency ablation can reduce the size of an inoperable tumor. RFA also can ease tumor-related symptoms, such as flushing, diarrhea, or hypertension, that are associated with some hormone-secreting tumors.

Long-term outcomes following radiofrequency ablation are promising. Based on literature reviews, complete tumor ablation with low recurrence rates can be achieved, particularly for smaller cancers. Research is ongoing to evaluate the long-term outcomes of the procedure. For example, RFA in combination with standard radiation therapy has shown two-year and five-year survival rates of 50 and 39 percent, respectively, for the treatment of Stage I and Stage II non-small-cell lung cancer. Research shows the local recurrence rate after RFA of colorectal cancer liver metastases averages less than 10 percent. Recurrence rates are related to the lesion size.

Repeat radiofrequency ablations can be performed for patients who develop new or recurrent tumors. Radiofrequency ablation does not preclude patients from undergoing other cancer treatments if necessary.

Angela M. Costello, B.S.

For Further Information

Ellis, Lee M., et al. *Radiofrequency Ablation for Cancer: Current Indication, Techniques, and Outcomes.* New York: Springer, 2003.

Patti, Jay W., et al. "Radiofrequency Ablation for Cancer-Associated Pain." *The Journal of Pain* 3, no. 6 (2002): 471-473.

Phillips, Carmen. *Radiofrequency Ablation Making Inroads as Cancer Treatment.* Bethesda, Md.: National Cancer Institute, 2005. Also available online at http://www.cancer.gov.

Wood, B. J., et al. "Percutaneous Tumor Ablation with Radiofrequency." *Cancer* 94, no. 2 (2002): 443-451.

Other Resources

American Cancer Ablation Centers
http:///www.cancerablation.com

American Society of Clinical Oncology
http://www.asco.org

Society of Interventional Radiology
http://www.sirweb.org

See also: Adenoid Cystic Carcinoma (ACC); Adrenal gland cancers; Bone cancers; Bone scan; Breast cancers; Carcinoid tumors and carcinoid syndrome; Computed Tomography (CT) scan; Hyperthermia therapy; Liver cancers; Lung cancers; Prostate cancer; Virus-related cancers

▶ Radionuclide scan

Category: Procedures
Also known as: Nuclear medicine scan

Definition: A radionuclide scan is the detection of electromagnetic radiation, usually gamma rays, emitted from an injected radioactive tracer that has been taken up by an organ in the body to be studied, with the goal of producing an image. The most common radioisotope used is technetium 99m, whose gamma rays are absorbed by a sodium iodide crystal detector. The radiation absorbed by this detector is used to generate an image that is interpreted by a radiologist or nuclear medicine physician. The exceptions are positron emission tomography (PET) scanning, which uses positron emission; gallium scanning, which uses gallium as the radionuclide; and some thyroid imaging, which uses iodine.

Cancers diagnosed: Virtually all types of cancer, especially metastases

Why performed: A radionuclide scan is used to diagnose primary and secondary cancer (bone scan, iodine scan, PET scan) and to diagnose various ailments, including but not limited to the following: hypothyroidism or hyperthyroidism (thyroid scan), bone fractures and bone infection (bone scan), kidney obstruction (renal scan), inflammatory disorders such as sarcoid and fever of unknown origin (gallium scan), cardiomyopathy multiple uptake gated acquisition (MUGA scan), coronary artery disease (cardiac single photon emission computed tomography, or SPECT) pulmonary embolus (lung scan), and Alzheimer's disease (brain SPECT).

Patient preparation: The preparation for a radionuclide scan is minimal to none; the scan is usually performed as an outpatient procedure. For some procedures, the patient may be asked to fast several hours prior to the scan.

Steps of the procedure: The radioisotope is prepared by the technologist and injected into a peripheral vein by the radiologist or nuclear medicine physician. The patient is then placed supine on a table under a gamma camera that houses the detectors. The scan time is usually about one hour.

After the procedure: The scan is generated by the computer attached to the camera and read by the radiologist the same day. The patient will need to contact his or her doctor for the radiologist's report and any follow-up therapy.

Risks: The risks of this type of scan include minor pain or bruising at the injection site. If the patient is pregnant, then the scan should be avoided if possible, since the radiation dose, although small in most cases, is not negligible. Radioactive iodine should not be administered to a pregnant patient because of risk to the fetus.

Results: The scan results are dependent on the type of scan performed and the reason for the study.

Debra B. Kessler, M.D., Ph.D.

See also: Appendix cancer; Bone scan; Electromagnetic radiation; Gallium scan; Imaging tests; Ionizing radiation; Nuclear medicine scan; Positron Emission Tomography (PET); Thyroid cancer

▶ Receptor analysis

Category: Procedures
Also known as: Receptor status test

Definition: Receptor analysis refers to diagnostic testing procedures carried out on cells or tissues to determine the abundance or functional integrity of specific receptors.

Cancers diagnosed: Breast cancer, colorectal cancer, prostate cancer, lung cancer, leukemia

Why performed: Many factors that stimulate cell growth start the mitogenic cascade by binding to specific cellular receptors, and one of the hallmarks of cancer is cell growth in the absence of these factors. This observation points to the critical role that receptors play in tumor cell growth and provides the basis for selecting among drug regimens that target receptor-signaling pathways. Breast cancer is the most prominent tumor type in which receptor analysis plays a role, but abnormal growth factor receptors may also be a feature of other solid tumors (colorectal, prostate, lung) and some hematologic (blood) malignancies.

Patient preparation: Tissue samples are required and are obtained as part of tumor resection surgery or biopsy. Procedures done under general anesthetic require an overnight fast. Receptor analysis is performed on tumor tissue that is removed, and the patient requires no special or additional postoperative care. Sample collection in leukemia and lymphoma patients is by a simple blood draw, which requires no fasting or special postvenipuncture care.

Steps of the procedure: After the appropriate tumor tissue samples are collected by the surgeon or phlebotomist, receptor analysis proceeds by fixing and processing the tissue for immunohistochemistry (IHC) or deoxyribonucleic acid (DNA) sequence analysis. IHC involves placing a very thin slice of tumor on a microscope slide and incubation with antibody preparations that react with the receptors of interest. After a washing step, other reagents are added that bind to the antireceptor antibodies and lead to chemical reactions that produce a visible color in cells that have the receptors. Pathologists then examine the tissue to determine the percentage of tumor cells that express the receptor. In breast cancer, receptors for estrogen and progesterone are routinely determined by IHC, as is the orphan receptor HER2/neu (Erb B2). IHC is also used to determine androgen receptor expression in prostate cancer. In lung and colorectal cancer, DNA sequence analysis is done to characterize mutations in the epidermal growth factor receptor (EGFR). In suspected lymphoproliferative disorders, analysis of the T-cell receptor gene by polymerase chain reaction can be used to determine monoclonal expansion (a sign of malignancy).

After the procedure: The operative or biopsy site is kept clean and dry to avoid infection. No special instructions regarding receptor analysis are required.

Risks: The risks and side effects of the sample acquisition procedure may be significant; however, receptor analysis itself carries no additional risk to the patient. Some assays for the estrogen receptor have large interlaboratory variability and high false negative rates for tumors with low receptor expression.

Results: In general, retention of normal receptor status by malignant cells is a favorable prognostic sign and forms the basis for a range of endocrine-based therapeutic options. In breast cancer patients, 25 to 35 percent of patients are expected to have amplified HER2/neu receptors, and a humanized monoclonal antibody to HER2 overexpressing breast cancer cells inhibits growth of the cells. The antibody trastuzumab (marketed as Herceptin) increases the clinical benefit of first-line chemotherapy in metastatic breast cancer that overexpresses HER2. Breast cancers that express estrogen and progesterone receptors may grow in response to these hormones, and patients may therefore benefit from antiestrogen drugs such as tamoxifen.

In prostate cancer cells, androgen receptors (ARs) are often overexpressed, and loss of the receptors is an unfavorable sign. AR-positive prostate cancer patients can be treated with leuprolide, which acts at the pituitary to decrease the secretion of gonadotropins. Lower gonadotropin levels result in lower androgen levels, which slows the growth of AR-positive tumor cells.

Tumors that are found to overexpress the EGFR may be treated with cetuximab, a monoclonal antibody that competitively inhibits the receptor, or with small molecules that inhibit the kinase activity of the receptor.

Tumors can express a wide variety of other growth factor receptors, notably those for insulin-like growth factor I (IGF-I) and for vascular endothelial growth factor (VEGF). Inhibiting these receptors with specific compounds is a promising area of cancer research.

John B. Welsh, M.D., Ph.D.

For Further Information

Carpenter, G., ed. *The EGF Receptor Family: Biologic Mechanisms and Role in Cancer*. Amsterdam: Elsevier Academic Press, 2004

Chang, J., et al. "Prediction of Clinical Outcome from Primary Tamoxifen by Expression of Biologic Markers in Breast Cancer Patients." *Clinical Cancer Research* 6 (2000): 616-621.

Chen, W. Y., and G. A. Colditz. "Risk Factors and Hormone-Receptor Status: Epidemiology, Risk-Prediction Models and Treatment Implications for Breast Cancer." *Nature Clinical Practice Oncology* 4 (2007): 415-423.

Schally, A. V., and A. M. Comaru-Schally. "Hypothalamic and Other Peptide Hormones." In *Holland-Frei Cancer Medicine 7*, edited by D. W. Kufe et al. Hamilton, Ont.: BC Decker, 2006.

Sequist, L. V., et al. "Molecular Predictors of Response to Epidermal Growth Factor Receptor Antagonists in Non-Small-Cell Lung Cancer." *Journal of Clinical Oncology* 25 (2007): 587.

Slamon, D., et al. "Use of Chemotherapy Plus a Monoclonal Antibody Against HER2 for Metastatic Breast Cancer That Overexpresses HER2." *New England Journal of Medicine* 344 (2001): 783-792.

Taube, S. E., et al. "Cancer Diagnostics: Decision Criteria for Marker Utilization in the Clinic." *American Journal of Pharmacogenomics* 5 (2005): 357-364.

Wang, Y., et al. "Inhibition of the IGF-I Receptor for Treatment of Cancer: Kinase Inhibitors and Monoclonal Antibodies as Alternative Approaches." *Recent Results in Cancer Research* 172 (2007): 59-76.

See also: Androgen drugs; Antiestrogens; Biopsy; Breast cancer in children and adolescents; Breast cancer in men; Breast cancer in pregnant women; Breast cancers;

Bronchial adenomas; Colorectal cancer; Colorectal cancer screening; Epidemiology of cancer; HER2/neu protein; Hormone receptor tests; Leukemias; Lung cancers; Lymphomas; Medical oncology; Monoclonal antibodies; Oncology; Progesterone receptor assay; Prostate cancer; Rectal cancer; Risks for cancer

▶ Reconstructive surgery

Category: Procedures
Also known as: Plastic surgery, cosmetic surgery

Definition: Reconstructive surgery is surgery to rebuild areas lost as a result of cancer or cancer treatment, as well as injury.

Cancers treated: Many different types of cancers, especially breast and skin cancers

Why performed: Reconstructive surgery may be performed to correct problems caused by cancer or cancer treatment. It is often performed to restore better functioning to the affected area. It can also be performed for cosmetic reasons. When it is done for cosmetic reasons, it is usually performed to restore a more symmetrical appearance, to reduce the signs left by cancer and cancer treatment, and to improve self-esteem.

Patient preparation: Patient preparation depends in large part on the procedure that is being done. Preparation before surgery generally includes not eating or drinking any fluids for a certain number of hours before the surgery, stopping certain medications such as blood thinners, or beginning to take medications such as antibiotics to help prevent infection. The surgeon and the surgeon's health care team will provide the patient with the necessary information about what to do, and what not to do, in the hours, days, and weeks before the surgery. In some cases, mental health support may be suggested for before the surgery, as well as afterward, if the surgery is going to make a great change in the individual's appearance.

Steps of the procedure: The steps of reconstructive surgery will vary depending on the type of surgery. For many types of surgery, there will be more than one option, and the surgeon will decide which one to use based on the desires of the patient, the patient's health level, body type, and other factors.

Most reconstructive surgery involves using skin, fat, muscle, or tissue from one area of the body and moving it to another location to reconstruct the desired area. Sometimes prosthetics are used in addition to the material from another area of the patient's body. For example, one possible method of breast reconstruction involves using some tissue from the patient in addition to an implant made of saline.

Five main types of procedures are used during cancer treatment and afterward. The first type is a simple closure of the wound area, in which the wound created by the removal of cancerous tissue is closed using sutures. This generally allows for healing with minimal scarring and a coloration that matches the surrounding skin.

If the area removed is too large to be closed using sutures, then a skin graft might be used. In this procedure, skin is removed from another site on the patient's body and is placed over the area that needs to be closed. A donor site will usually be selected for the best possible match of coloration to the recipient area, and minimal visibility.

When more than just skin is desired, a local flap may be used. The surgeon will take skin and tissue from an area next to the site of the wound and move it over the wound. The flap remains connected to its original surroundings by veins and arteries.

If a local flap is not available or appropriate for some reason, then the surgeon may decide to use a pedicle flap, a section of tissue that is removed from one area but left attached to the blood supply in that area. The flap is anchored to the recipient site with its original source of blood still intact.

The other alternative is to use a free flap. A free flap is completely removed from the donor site, including the severing of all arteries and veins. The flap is then moved to the recipient site and connected. This is generally a longer and more complex surgery than a local or pedicle flap, because the surgery team must use microsurgery to connect the flap to the adjacent area so that blood can flow in and out of the tissue, keeping it alive.

After the procedure: The aftercare for reconstructive surgery will vary depending on the type of procedure and the area of the surgery. Usually there will be a hospital stay of short to moderate duration after the procedure, although some more minor procedures may be performed on an outpatient basis. Healing will take varying lengths of time depending on the type of procedure used and the location on the body of the surgery. For most reconstructive surgeries, as with most surgeries, it will take a few weeks or longer for the patient to return to their normal level of activity.

Some reconstructive surgeries can be followed up at a later time, generally after the wound has mostly or completely healed, with additional cosmetic procedures. For example, after breast reconstruction, the nipple can be reconstructed at a later time, after the breast itself has healed. Additionally, tattooing of the nipple and areole can be done at a later time to try to match the existing breast as nearly as possible.

Risks: There are risks associated with any kind of surgical procedure. The risks of reconstructive surgery are generally low when the procedure is performed by a certified reconstructive surgeon who is experienced in the procedure. A patient who has questions about the surgeon's training, qualifications, or experience with the type of procedure being considered should never hesitate to ask.

The risks associated with reconstructive surgery are generally the same as those associated with any other type of surgery, including excessive bleeding, infection, pooling of blood beneath the skin, bruising, and problems with wound healing. Procedures that are done under general anesthesia have the risks associated with general anesthesia, including changes in blood pressure or heart rhythm. Complications from general anesthesia are generally rare, although certain diseases and conditions can increase these risks.

Reconstructive surgery is generally considered to be relatively low risk for individuals who are otherwise in reasonably good health. Certain diseases and conditions can interfere with the healing process or can cause an increased risk of complications. Individuals who have high blood pressure, diabetes, or immune system problems or who have conditions that affect the blood's ability to clot may be at increased risk of complications. Individuals who smoke may be required to quit smoking for a few months before the surgery to decrease the likelihood of side effects or complications and to increase the body's ability to heal effectively. This kind of requirement generally depends on the specific surgeon who is doing the procedure. In general, individuals who smoke have a more difficult time healing completely after surgery and may have increased visibility of scars.

In addition to the risks associated with any type of surgery, each reconstructive procedure may have its own associated risks. For example, there is a small risk of breast implant rupture associated with breast reconstruction. Individuals should talk carefully with their surgeons and any other health care providers to discuss all the possible risks associated with the specific procedure that they are considering before making a final decision.

Results: Reconstructive surgery is often very successful. It is important, however, for the individual to talk to his or her surgeon about what realistic expectations for the procedure should be, as the results of reconstructive surgery can vary. Nearly all procedures will result in some scarring, which will usually fade with time but never disappears completely. Reconstructive surgeries often cannot change some things with which the individual was unhappy before the cancer. In many cases, the procedure is a large improvement, but the reconstruction is not a 100 percent perfect match because of a number of factors. In cases of skin grafts, the area from which the skin is taken is usually not a perfect match in terms of pigmentation and tone for the area to which it is moved. For breast reconstruction, the reconstructed breast is often a close match, but not a perfect match, of the other breast. The more realistic the expectations of the reconstructive procedure, the more likely the individual is to be satisfied with the results.

Helen Davidson, B.A.

For Further Information

Berry, Daniel J., and Scott P. Steinmann. *Adult Reconstruction*. Philadelphia: Lippincott Williams & Wilkins, 2007.

Kryger, Zol B., and Mark Sisco, eds. *Practical Plastic Surgery*. Austin: Landes Bioscience, 2007.

Park, Stephen S. *Facial Plastic Surgery: The Essential Guide*. New York: Thieme, 2005.

Sarwer, David B., and Thomas Pruzinsky, eds. *Psychological Aspects of Reconstructive and Cosmetic Plastic Surgery: Clinical, Empirical, and Ethical Perspectives*. Philadelphia: Lippincott Williams & Wilkins, 2006.

Other Resources

American Society of Plastic Surgeons
http://www.plasticsurgery.org

See also: Aids and devices for cancer patients; Basal cell carcinomas; Breast reconstruction; Exenteration; Eyelid cancer; Fibrosarcomas, soft-tissue; Gynecologic oncology; Head and neck cancers; Infection and sepsis; Lip cancers; Orthopedic surgery; Otolaryngology; Psychosocial aspects of cancer; Risks for cancer; Sexuality and cancer; Skin cancers

▶ Rehabilitation

Category: Procedures

Definition: Rehabilitation aims to treat the physical, emotional, and psychological limitations often experienced by cancer patients. The goal of rehabilitation is to help the individual with cancer participate as fully and independently as possible in daily life. During rehabilitation, the cancer patient works to regain skills and abilities that were lost through the effects of cancer or cancer treatment.

Cancers treated: All types of cancers beginning before, during, or after cancer treatment

Why performed: The specific goals of rehabilitation are different for each individual. In general, the goal of rehabilitation is to allow the individual to function as fully and independently as possible. The rehabilitation team will include different allied health professionals depending on the goals and needs of the individual. Often the rehabilitation team will include many health professionals, such as a physical therapist, an occupational therapist, a rehabilitation nurse, a psychologist or psychiatrist, a nutritionist or registered dietician, the individual's physician or oncologist, pain management specialists, a case manager, and home health workers.

The rehabilitation team will work together with the patient and the patient's family and loved ones to help the patient regain as high a degree of functioning as possible. The specific activities included in the rehabilitation plan usually comprise dressing, bathing, cooking, eating, and other activities of daily living. Some individuals may receive help recovering the ability to drive, take public transportation, or other aspects of mobility.

For individuals whose job skills were affected by cancer or cancer treatment, regaining the skills necessary to return to a job is usually considered a high priority. An occupational therapist or other member of the rehabilitation team may help the individual determine what skills are required, work to improve those skills, and seek ways to modify the employment environment so that the individual may return to work sooner.

The individual may have goals in addition to those necessary for return to employment or for daily living. Many recreation and leisure activities that were formerly pleasurable may become difficult or impossible because of cancer or cancer treatment. Rehabilitation therapists listen to the patient to address additional goals, such as the ability to go camping or sailing, play sports, or play music.

Patient preparation: Before beginning to meet with a rehabilitation specialist, it may help the patient to consider specific goals for rehabilitation. Making a list of activities or skills on which the patient would like to work can help the rehabilitation therapist look beyond the activities of daily living to other activities important in that individual's life. Goals can be very specific, such as being able to knit or type again, or more general, such as being able to play with children or grandchildren.

The patient preparation required before the individual rehabilitation sessions will vary depending on the type of therapy. The rehabilitation specialist will give the patient specific information about what steps to take before a session, which may include things such as doing gentle stretches to warm up or even mentally preparing to meet the challenges that rehabilitation therapy provides.

Steps of the procedure: The steps of rehabilitation are very individualized. They depend on the type of therapy that is being done and on the specific needs and goals of the patient. Rehabilitation therapy often breaks down the goal activity or skill into smaller parts or steps and then works on one step at a time. For example, an occupational therapist who is helping a cancer patient regain the ability to feed himself may work on the action of bringing the food to the mouth as one activity, the act of using a spoon or fork to scoop food as a separate activity, and the act of cutting food as yet a separate skill. As these different aspects of the skill of feeding oneself are mastered, they can be combined into more complex sequences of actions.

Another way of approaching rehabilitation can be from the standpoint of increasing the day-to-day abilities of the patient in the affected areas. In this case, the rehabilitation therapist might focus on getting food from the plate or bowl and into the mouth using the hands and then slowly add skills, such as beginning to help the patient use a spoon, then a fork, and then working on cutting food.

Rehabilitation also often helps to identify assistive devices that individuals can use to help them accomplish various tasks. In some cases, these devices are only necessary for a short time; in other cases, they will be used by the individual for the rest of his or her life. For instance, a rehabilitation specialist may help an individual regain the ability to walk using a walker, or may help an individual who had a leg amputated master the use of a prosthetic leg.

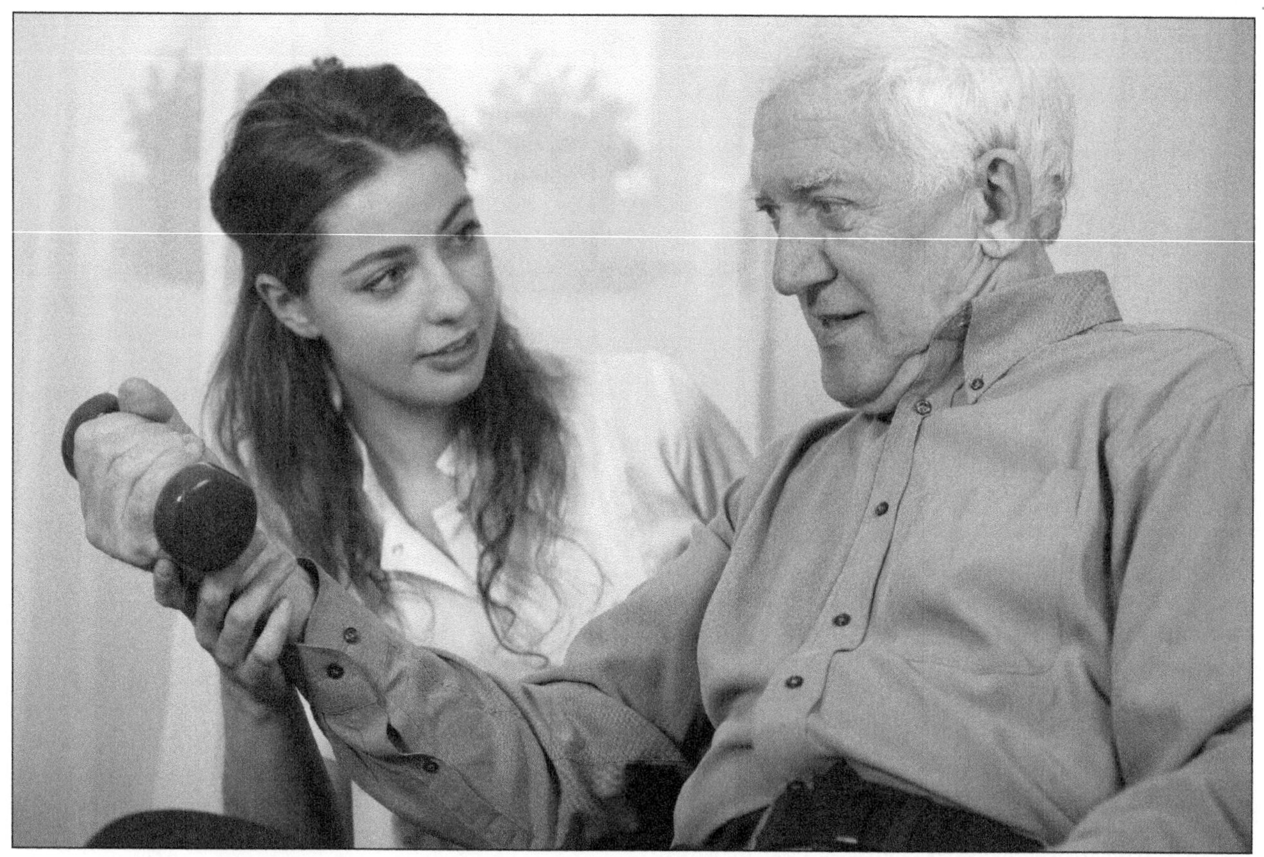

Rehabilitation enables the patient with cancer to participate as fully and independently as possible in daily life. (iStock)

After the procedure: The steps after rehabilitation will vary depending on the type of therapy performed. After therapy that involves physical activity or exercise, a series of stretches and cooldown activities is usually performed. Often the rehabilitation therapist will assign the individual exercises or activities to practice each day, sometimes several times a day, before the next session. This approach can help to ensure that the progress made during the session is maintained until the next session. The patient's family members or caregivers may be shown how to help the individual complete these exercises.

Rehabilitation therapy may be continued for weeks, months, or even longer. When the therapy has ended, the therapist may give the patient a list or set of exercises or activities to continue to do to help keep up the skills that were gained during therapy, or to help the patient continue to make improvements.

Risks: The risks associated with rehabilitation are generally mild but are different for different forms of rehabilitation therapy. There are some risks that during physical therapy individuals may strain or pull muscles, or otherwise overextend or injure themselves, especially if the proper stretching and warmup routine is not followed before the therapy. Risks of occupational therapy and other forms of rehabilitation therapy that involve the patient working to perform certain actions or movements, such as the movements of dressing or bathing, may also result in strain or injury if the individual pushes too hard to accomplish the task before his or her body is ready. An individual working on regaining the ability to walk may fall if not carefully monitored. Generally, these and other physical risks from rehabilitation are very low if the therapy is overseen by a qualified health professional.

There may also be some emotional risks relating to rehabilitation. The issues discussed with a psychologist or psychiatrist can often be painful or upsetting as they help the individual with cancer work through the fear, uncertainty, and feelings of hopelessness that often accompany cancer diagnosis and treatment. Although discussions with a psychologist or therapist can often be very upsetting, they can usually help the patient deal effectively with these new emotions.

Results: The results of rehabilitation are usually very positive. With consistent effort by the patient and the rehabilitation team, many skills and abilities that have been lost can be regained. Many people can return to jobs and activities in which they would not have been able to participate without rehabilitation. Psychological and emotional rehabilitation is usually effective at helping the individual regain a positive outlook and overcome the fear and unhappiness often associated with cancer and cancer treatment. A comprehensive rehabilitation plan that involves many different allied health professionals, as well as family, friends, or other caregivers, is often especially effective.

It is important for the rehabilitation team to help the patient develop a realistic view of the amount of work required by rehabilitation, the length of time that it will take to reach rehabilitation goals, and what rehabilitation goals are likely to be realistic overall. Having realistic expectations can help reduce frustrations and negative feelings that may occur during the rehabilitation process as hurdles are met and overcome.

Helen Davidson, B.A.

For Further Information

Davis, Carol M., ed. *Complementary Therapies in Rehabilitation*. 2d ed. Thorofare, N.J.: Slack, 2004.

Galvin, Jan C., and Scherer Marcia J., eds. *Evaluating, Selecting, and Using Appropriate Assistive Technology*. Austin, Tex.: Pro-Ed, 2004.

Macky, Hazel, and Susan Nancarrow. *Enabling Independence: A Guide for Rehabilitation Workers*. Malden, Mass.: Blackwell, 2006.

Stidwill, Howard. *Exercise Therapy and the Cancer Patient: A Guide for Health Care Professionals and Their Patients*. Belgium, Wisc.: Champion Press, 2005.

Other Resources

National Rehabilitation Information Center
http://www.nairc.com

See also: Aids and devices for cancer patients; Amputation; Cancer care team; Case management; Cognitive effects of cancer and chemotherapy; Cordectomy; Exercise and cancer; Head and neck cancers; Home health services; Limb salvage; Nutrition and cancer treatment; Occupational therapy; Pain management medications; Self-image and body image; Transitional care

▶ Salpingectomy and salpingo-oophorectomy

Category: Procedures
Also known as: Unilateral or bilateral salpingo-oophorectomy

Definition: Salpingectomy is the surgical excision of one or both Fallopian tubes to diagnose suspicious tubo-ovarian masses that are, or may become, cancerous; salpingo-oophorectomy includes surgical excision of one or both ovaries for the same reason.

Cancers diagnosed or treated: Invasive cervical, uterine, and ovarian cancers; hydatidiform mole; rarely, Fallopian tube cancer

Why performed: Salpingectomy is performed in order to remove and examine tubal or tubo-ovarian masses suspicious for cancer and to determine the extent of malignant disease spread. These masses may be fluid-filled (cystic), solid, or mixed and can also be hormone-secreting or hormone receptive. A salpingo-oophorectomy is often performed alongside a hysterectomy in women who are postmenopausal and are suspected of having an endometrial, tubal, and/or ovarian mass at risk for encroaching on other pelvic organs. It is also performed in women of childbearing age who have a suspected malignancy and have completed their families. Women with localized, unilateral disease who still wish to bear children may have only the diseased Fallopian tube and ovary removed, although this is not recommended in the light of the more common occurrence of disease in both tubes and ovaries. Salpingo-oophorectomy may also be done to remove masses of an infectious origin (for example, tubo-ovarian abscess caused by pelvic inflammatory disease) or endometriosis that has irreversibly damaged these organs. A bilateral salpingo-oophorectomy is performed prophylactically when patients are at high risk for developing gynecologic cancers associated with *BRCA1* and *BRCA2* gene mutations, particularly ovarian and breast cancers.

Patient preparation: The patient undergoes preoperative evaluation for any contraindications to the procedure (such as a pregnancy test) and evaluation of coexisting diseases to determine her fitness to undergo surgery and general anesthesia. Patients are instructed to take nothing per mouth the night before the procedure.

Steps of the procedure: After the patient is anesthetized, placed in the lithotomy position, and the vagina, external genitalia, pubic area, and inner thighs have been surgically prepped and draped, a transverse or vertical incision is made above the pubic bone. An incision extended up to the level of the umbilicus is preferred, as it provides a wider surgical field and provides a wider incision through which a large mass can be removed. The incision is taken down to the pelvic cavity. The uterine and ovarian vessels are identified, dissected, and separated from the ureters. The supporting broad, round, and suspensory ovarian ligaments of the Fallopian tubes and ovaries with their vessels are then dissected, isolated, cut, and ligated. In a simultaneous hysterectomy, the uterus and uterine vessels are also dissected away from other pelvic structures, cut, and ligated. When disease extending outside the reproductive tract is suspected, biopsies of suspicious lesions, sampling of lymph nodes around the pelvis and abdominal aorta, and abdominal cavity washings are done.

Laparoscopic removal of the Fallopian tubes and ovaries is done in conjunction with a hysterectomy. It is done through two small abdominal incisions through which sleeved trochars accommodating a scope and any of several instruments for probing, grasping, cutting, and cauterizing are inserted. The uterus, Fallopian tubes and ovaries, vessels, and ligaments are dissected, cut, and ligated. The organs are removed vaginally, and the remaining vaginal cuff is closed off.

After the procedure: The patient is monitored in the postanesthesia care unit until she is fully awake and her vital signs are stable. Once the patient is stable in unit, she may be discharged to the gynecologic ward for postoperative monitoring. Once the patient is stable, ambulatory, urinating, and eating, she may be discharged home after a few days.

Risks: The most significant risk of a salpingectomy is an ectopic pregnancy. Other risks include deep vein thrombosis, pulmonary embolism, perforation of the bladder or bowel, and intractable bleeding.

Results: Cross-sectional examination of both grossly normal and diseased Fallopian tubes should be done, documenting size, depth of penetration, and location along the length of the specimen, although primary tubal cancers account for only 0.1 to 1.8 percent of all female reproductive tract cancers. When a mass encompassing both Fallopian tube and ovary is encountered intraoperatively, it is presumed to be of ovarian origin until proven otherwise during pathological examination, where tubal tissue is recognized within the mass. A gross and microscopic examination of tubal or ovarian masses may reveal whether they are cancerous by evaluating individual cells and the tissue architecture for signs of cancerous changes. On gross examination, masses that preserve the outer tissue surrounding the ovaries can suggest no malignancy but cannot eliminate the possibility of early invasive cancer. Central necrosis and hemorrhage may be present in large tumors as they outgrow their blood supply but do not necessarily imply malignancy, as they can occur in both benign and malignant masses. Microscopic changes pointing to a nonmalignant origin of the tumor include increased but orderly growth of ovarian cells but no elements of disordered growth of abnormal cells and distortion of the tissue architecture. Microscopic examinations that reveal disordered growth and abnormal cells of tubal or ovarian origin are suggestive of Fallopian tube cancer or ovarian cancer. An invasive hydatidiform mole that has spread from the uterus can exhibit characteristic cells and tissues of placental and fetal origin. Lymph node samples and washings from the abdominal cavity possessing cancerous cells strongly suggest microscopic spread outside the reproductive tract.

Aldo C. Dumlao, M.D.

For Further Information

Haas, Adelaide, and Susan L. Puretz. *The Woman's Guide to Hysterectomy: Expectations and Options*. Berkeley, Calif.: Celestial Arts, 2002.

Memorial Sloan-Kettering Cancer Center. "Cancer-Reducing Benefits of Preventive Surgery May Be Specific to Gene Mutation." *Science Daily*, June 5, 2006. Also available at http://www.science daily.com.

Rosenthal, Sara M. *The Gynecological Sourcebook*. 4th ed. New York: McGraw-Hill, 2003.

See also: *BRCA1* and *BRCA2* genes; Cervical cancer; Fallopian tube cancer; Gynecologic cancers; Hydatidiform mole; Hysterectomy; Hystero-oophorectomy; Laparoscopy and laparoscopic surgery; Oophorectomy; Ovarian cancers; Pregnancy and cancer; Risks for cancer; Uterine cancer

▶ Sentinel Lymph Node (SLN) biopsy and mapping

Category: Procedures

Definition: A sentinel lymph node (SLN) biopsy is a procedure in which the first lymph nodes to which cancer is likely to spread from the primary tumor are removed and examined to determine whether cancer cells are present.

The process of identification of the SLNs is called SLN mapping.

Cancers diagnosed or treated: Mainly breast cancer and malignant melanoma; SLN is being studied for use with other cancer types

Why performed: Cancer cells spread first to one or several lymph nodes, called the sentinel lymph nodes (SLNs), before spreading to more distal lymph nodes and other sites in the body. Determining whether a SLN contains cancer cells provides the doctor with valuable information about whether the cancer has spread from its primary location.

Patient preparation: A small dose of a radioactive tracer compound and a blue dye are injected near the patient's tumor several hours before surgery to allow these chemicals time to travel from the tumor region to any SLNs.

Steps of the procedure: Once the radioactive tracer compound and dye have reached the lymph nodes, the surgeon scans the area with a small Geiger counter and removes the radioactive lymph nodes through a small incision, using the presence of the blue dye for additional visual confirmation. A pathologist performs a preliminary examination of the nodes under a microscope, and if cancerous cells are seen while the patient is still in surgery, additional lymph nodes may be removed at that time.

After the procedure: Pain or bruising at the biopsy site and temporary discoloration of urine or skin may occur. Some patients report postoperative nerve damage or swelling caused by lymph fluid accumulation in the area of the surgery. Rarely, a patient may be allergic to the blue dye used for sentinel node identification. Patients undergoing the procedure typically spend one day or less in the hospital.

Risks: A low percentage of SNL biopsies for breast cancer can turn out to be negative when other lymph nodes in the area do contain cancer.

Results: Doctors use SLN biopsy results to help determine the stage of cancer. A negative result implies that the cancer has not spread to the lymph nodes, and a positive result indicates that cancer is present in the SLN and therefore may be present in other lymph nodes. In this case, removal of other lymph nodes in the area may be performed.

Jill Ferguson, Ph.D.

See also: Axillary dissection; Biopsy; Breast cancer in children and adolescents; Breast cancer in men; Breast cancer in pregnant women; Breast cancers; Lymphadenectomy; Lymphangiography; Lymphedema; Mastectomy; Melanomas; Merkel Cell Carcinomas (MCC); Penile cancer

▶ Sigmoidoscopy

Category: Procedures
Also known as: Proctosigmoidoscopy

Definition: Sigmoidoscopy is the insertion of a slender, lighted tube (sigmoidoscope) through the anus to examine the lining of the rectum and lower colon. Sigmoidoscopes vary in insertion tube design (such as size, flexibility, and viewing angle), viewing technology (lens, fiber-optic, or electronic), and procedural capabilities (sample, destroy, remove, or treat abnormalities).

Cancers diagnosed: Sigmoid colon cancer, rectal cancer

Why performed: For cancer, sigmoidoscopy may be performed as a screening procedure to detect abnormalities in the rectum and lower colon; as a diagnostic procedure to determine the cause of symptoms, confirm other findings, or plan treatment; or as a follow-up procedure to verify that tissues healed properly after surgery.

Patient preparation: A few days before the procedure, the patient may need to stop certain medications (such as aspirin products and blood thinners). The day of the procedure, the patient cleans his or her rectum and lower colon (such as with an enema).

Steps of the procedure: Sigmoidoscopy is scheduled in a physician's office or other outpatient setting. The patient wears a gown and lies on the side, awake; if needed, sedation or local anesthetic may be given. First, the physician performs a digital rectal exam. The sigmoidoscope (.25 to .5 inch wide, 10 to 26 inches long) is lubricated and carefully inserted through the anus. Puffs of air gently expand the rectum and lower colon as the physician advances the sigmoidoscope, steering around bends until the sigmoidoscope is fully inserted. The physician slowly withdraws the sigmoidoscope, carefully viewing the lining for abnormalities. When an abnormality is found, its location and characteristics are recorded. Depending on the abnormality, it may be sampled (biopsied), destroyed (ablated), removed (excised and retrieved), or otherwise treated. All biopsy samples and excised tissues are taken to the laboratory for histopathologic evaluation.

After the procedure: The patient leaves and resumes normal activities, unless sedation or anesthetic was needed. The patient may feel bloated and have cramps until the extra air passes.

Risks: Sigmoidoscopy is relatively safe, with a small risk for these side effects: perforation, bleeding, infection, irritation, and discharge.

Results: A normal bowel has smooth folds lining the muscular wall, with an even distribution of blood vessels. Abnormalities include inflammation, stricture, vascular changes, anatomic distortions, and abnormal growths, such as mucosal growths, polypoid lesions (polyps), and cancer. Histopathologic evaluation determines whether an abnormal growth is or is not likely to become cancerous and, if the abnormal growth was removed, whether the diseased tissue was completely removed. Additional treatment, follow-up examinations, or both may be recommended.

Patricia Boone, Ph.D.

See also: Adenomatous polyps; Anal cancer; Colon polyps; Colorectal cancer; Colorectal cancer screening; Diarrhea; Digital Rectal Exam (DRE); Endoscopy; Enterostomal therapy; Fecal Occult Blood Test (FOBT); Gastrointestinal complications of cancer treatment; Hemorrhoids; Hereditary polyposis syndromes; Medicare and cancer; Peutz-Jeghers Syndrome (PJS); Polypectomy; Polyps; Premalignancies; Primary care physician; Rectal cancer; Screening for cancer

▶ Splenectomy

Category: Procedures
Also known as: Spleen removal

Definition: A splenectomy is the surgical removal of the spleen. The spleen is located in the upper-left portion of the abdominal cavity. The function of the spleen is to filter the blood, removing old or damaged blood cells from the circulation and eliminating bacteria, parasites, and other organisms that can cause infection. The spleen also produces and stores blood.

Cancers diagnosed or treated: Hodgkin disease (staging), non-Hodgkin lymphoma, chronic myelogenous leukemia, chronic B-cell leukemias (hairy cell leukemia and prolymphocytic leukemia)

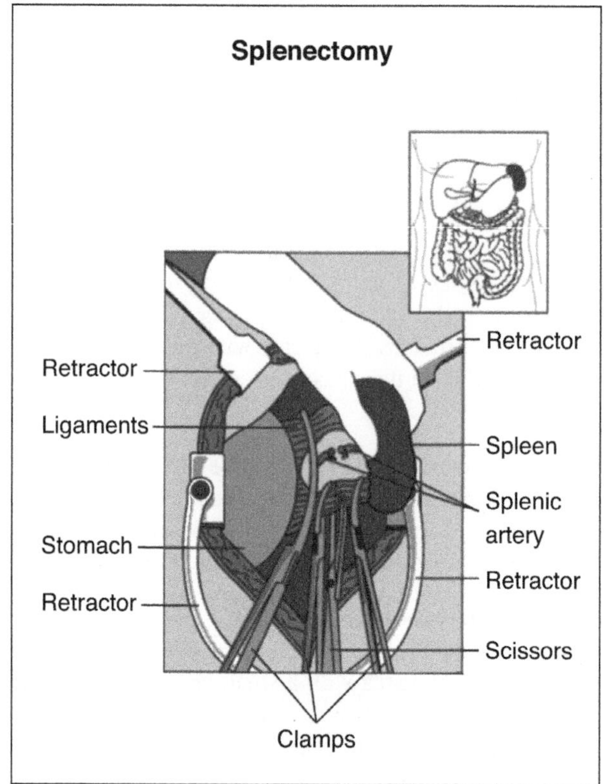

Why performed: A splenectomy is most commonly performed on a ruptured spleen, which, if not immediately treated, can cause life-threatening bleeding into the abdominal cavity. Splenectomies are also performed in patients with Hodgkin disease for staging the extent of disease; with non-Hodgkin lymphoma, leukemias, and splenomegaly for symptom control; or for correction of cytopenias (low blood cell counts) in patients with immune-mediated destruction of one or more blood elements.

Patient preparation: A few days before the procedure, blood and urine tests and X rays of the abdomen are performed. Immunizations against pneumococcal and meningococcal infections are administered, preferably a couple of weeks before the procedure (frequently this is not possible, particularly in the case of a ruptured spleen as a result of trauma or injury). If blood counts (red blood cells or platelets) are low, then a transfusion may be necessary before the procedure can be performed.

Steps of the procedure: A splenectomy may be performed by the classic, open incision method or by laparoscopy. Before the procedure, anesthesia is administered and an airway tube is placed in the windpipe.

In the classic surgery method, one incision is made in the abdomen over the spleen, and the blood vessels to and around the spleen are cut and tied off. This detaches the spleen from the rest of the body, and no further exchange of blood between the spleen and the rest of the body can occur. The spleen is then removed. If bleeding occurs, then it may be controlled with a cautery, which burns the tissue, or by tying the blood vessels. The incision is cleaned and closed with stitches or staples, which are generally removed approximately one week after surgery.

During a laparoscopy, three to four small incisions are made in the abdomen. A laparoscope (a lighted tube with a small camera that projects a view of the internal structures to a video monitor) is inserted through one of these incisions. Specialized instruments are inserted through the two to three additional incisions for the doctor to perform the procedure. To provide more room for the doctor to work, carbon dioxide gas is pumped into the abdomen to inflate the abdomen. As with the classic surgery, blood vessels to the spleen are cut and tied off and the spleen is removed. The incisions are closed with stitches and covered with surgical tape.

After the procedure: Blood tests and a pathology exam of the removed spleen may be performed. If necessary, a blood transfusion may be administered.

Risks: Factors that may increase the risk for complications during the procedure include obesity, smoking, poor nutrition, recent or chronic illness, diabetes, advanced age, or a preexisting heart or lung disease. Complications that may be associated with a splenectomy include an increased risk for infection and, though rare, injury to surrounding organs (pancreas, stomach, or colon). Possible complications of any surgery include infection and excess bleeding. Additional complications that may occur with any surgery involving anesthesia include a collapsed lung, deep-vein blood clots, or thromboembolism (blockage of a blood vessel caused by a blood clot), especially in older adults.

Results: Recovery time can vary depending on the underlying disease or condition. In general, however, complete healing from the procedure occurs in about four to six weeks. The results of splenectomy also vary according to the reason for the procedure:

- Ruptured spleen: Once a ruptured spleen is removed, the risk of life-threatening bleeding is eliminated.
- Splenomegaly: Pain and discomfort are effectively reduced if the patient was experiencing symptoms attributable to splenomegaly.
- Chronic myelogenous leukemia: A splenectomy significantly improves symptoms and simplifies management (by reducing transfusion requirements) in patients with chronic myelogenous leukemia.
- Chronic B cell leukemia: A splenectomy may also be an effective secondary treatment for hairy cell leukemia and prolymphocytic leukemia, significantly reducing the tumor.
- Cytopenias: Splenectomy has been shown to correct cytopenias in a large proportion of patients with immune-mediated destruction of one or more cellular blood elements.

Anita P. Kuan, Ph.D.

For Further Information

Bridget, S. Wilkins, and Dennis H. Wright. *Illustrated Pathology of the Spleen*. New York: Cambridge University Press, 2000.

"Guidelines for the Prevention and Treatment of Infection in Patients with an Absent or Dysfunctional Spleen." *BMJ* 312 (1996): 430-434. Also available at http://www.bmj.com.

Hiatt, Jonathan R., Edward H. Phillips, and Leon Morgenstern, eds. *Surgical Diseases of the Spleen*. New York: Springer, 1997.

Townsend, Courtney M., Jr., et al., eds. *Sabiston Textbook of Surgery*. 17th ed. Philadelphia: Elsevier Saunders, 2005.

"Updated Guidelines: The Prevention and Treatment of Infection in Patients with an Absent or Dysfunctional Spleen." British Committee for Standards in Haematology. *BMJ*, June 2, 2001. Also available at http://www .bmj.com.

Uranus, S. *Current Spleen Surgery*. Munich: Zuckschwerdt, 1995.

Other Resources

Cleveland Clinic
http://www.clevelandclinic.org

Familydoctor.org
Splenectomy
http://familydoctor.org/online/famdocen/home/articles/655.html

Lymphoma Research Foundation
http://www.lymphoma.org

National Institutes of Health
http://www.nih.gov

See also: Chronic Lymphocytic Leukemia (CLL); Hairy cell leukemia; Hodgkin disease; Laparoscopy and laparoscopic surgery; Leukemias; Lymphomas; Myelofibrosis; Myeloproliferative disorders; Non-Hodgkin lymphoma

▶ Sputum cytology

Category: Procedures

Definition: Sputum cytology is a screening for the presence of abnormal cells in sputum (saliva).

Cancers diagnosed: Lung cancer

Why performed: If a tumor is centrally located and has invaded the airways, then this procedure may allow visualization of tumor cells for diagnosis. It is a risk-free and inexpensive procedure.

Patient preparation: A sputum sample may be collected from coughed-up mucus (sometimes induced by an inhaled saline mist) or by bronchoscopy, which uses a bronchoscope to examine the throat and airways.

No special preparation is required if the sputum sample is to be collected by coughing with or without a saline mist at home or in the doctor's office. If a sputum sample is to be obtained by bronchoscopy, then the patient may not eat or drink for eight to ten hours before the procedure. The patient may be given medications to dry the secretions in the mouth and airways. A chest X ray may also be done before bronchoscopy.

Steps of the procedure: For simple coughing procedures, three sputum samples are usually collected over three days in a container with fixative to preserve the sample.

Bronchoscopy is performed with a flexible or a rigid bronchoscope. Rigid bronchoscopy requires general anesthesia. In either case, the patient must sign a consent form.

After the procedure: There are no requirements following sputum collection by coughing. A second chest X ray is taken after bronchoscopy, and the patient should be driven home. Patients should call immediately if they cough up more than two tablespoons of blood, have difficulty breathing, or have a fever for more than twenty-four hours.

Risks: There is no risk in collecting sputum samples by coughing procedures. Bronchoscopy is usually a safe procedure, and complications are rare. Complications that may occur include spasms of the bronchial tubes, irregular heart rhythms, infections, hoarseness, and bubbles under the skin.

Results: The most common screening tests for lung cancer are a chest X ray and sputum cytology. According to a 2007 report by the United States National Cancer Institute, the results of many studies have shown no evidence that screening for lung cancer using sputum cytology or chest X ray reduces lung cancer mortality. The institute also concludes that screening could lead to false positive tests and unnecessary, invasive diagnostic procedures and treatments. Hence, these tests are not used for routine screening of healthy individuals but only when symptons indicate their use.

Bernard Jacobson, Ph.D.

See also: Bronchial adenomas; Bronchoalveolar lung cancer; Carcinoid tumors and carcinoid syndrome; Coughing; Head and neck cancers; Hemoptysis; Infection and sepsis; Lung cancers; Mesothelioma; Pneumonia; Radon; Screening for cancer

▶ Staging of cancer

Category: Procedures
Also known as: Clinical staging, pathological staging, restaging

Definition: Staging is the process in which the location, extent, and degree of metastasis (spread) of a primary, or original, cancerous tumor is determined.

Cancers diagnosed or treated: Essentially all solid tumor cancer diagnoses are staged similarly. Nonlocalized leukemias are staged in unique ways according to the specific diagnosis. The diagnostic processes used to stage a specific case vary somewhat according to cancer type and location.

Why performed: Cancer staging plays an integral role in determining overall disease prognosis as well as influencing treatment modality choices. Stage assessment also plays an important role in assuring effective communication among the patient's medical team and accurate disease surveillance and epidemiology efforts.

Patient preparation: Patient preparation will vary according to the technique, or supporting procedures, used to help stage the cancer. These procedures range from physical examination and imaging—X rays, ultra sounds, computed tomography (CT), magnetic resonance imaging (MRI) scans—to laboratory tests, biopsies, and surgical excisions with subsequent pathological examination of the tumor. Any preparation normally required of these supporting procedures will apply to the process.

Steps of the procedure: Cancer staging is composed of three distinct phases: clinical staging, pathological staging, and restaging. Clinical staging is accomplished by nonpathologic means based on physical examination and imaging technology such as X ray, MRI, and CT, as well as immunologic and molecular blood tests to detect and measure cancer markers where applicable.

Pathological staging is accomplished following tissue removal by biopsy in which surgical tumor excision is assessed as a sound treatment option. The biopsied tissue and/or removed tumor, surrounding tissue, and nearby lymph nodes are examined microscopically and histologically to determine the type and extent of the cancer from a pathologic perspective. Because treatment considerations and survival statistics are based on the stage of a patient's cancer, the initial stage assessment remains static throughout the course of the disease regardless of progression and/or response to treatment.

Should a cancer patient enter remission but subsequently present with a recurrence, restaging may be accomplished if additional treatment is planned. The restaging process is identical to the original one, including both clinical and pathological staging, but is now designated with a lowercase *r*. For example, a restaged Stage IV grouping would be recorded as Stage rIV.

In order to maintain terminology consistency, a limited number of classification systems are utilized, and efforts toward additional interpretive continuity are ongoing. Although the type of cancer dictates which specific categorization is applied, common elements include tumor location, size and number, lymph node involvement, and degree of metastasis (spread). The most prevalent systems used include tumor-node-metastasis (TNM) and overall group staging.

The tumor-node-metastasis (TNM) classification is adapted by the American Joint Committee on Cancer (AJCC) and the Union Internationale Contre le Cancer/International Union Against Cancer (UICC).

The category T, for tumor, provides information about the original tumor such as measurement (in millimeters, centimeters) at the site of origin and its degree of invasion into nearby tissues and organs.

- TX: Cannot be measured/evaluated
- T0: No evidence of primary tumor
- Tis: In situ tumor (tumor limited to cell layers of the original site)

Beyond Tis, numerical tumor categorization offers a relative degree of severity, with higher numbers reflecting a larger tumor and/or more aggressive invasion.

- T1: Smaller tumor, least aggressive
- T2
- T3
- T4: Larger tumor, most aggressive

The tumor grade is the degree of abnormality (amount of differentiation from normal cells) and is determined pathologically—by microscopic analysis. Typically, well-differentiated, or low-grade, tumors are considered the least aggressive and are associated with the best outcomes overall.

- GX: Cannot be determined
- G1: Tumor cells well differentiated from surrounding tissue
- G2: Tumor cells moderately well differentiated from surrounding tissue
- G3: Tumor cells poorly differentiated from surrounding tissue
- G4: Tumor cells undifferentiated from surrounding tissue

Special cases are prostate cancer and central nervous system (CNS) cancers. The most common approach to classification of prostate cancer is the Gleason system, which is based on the degree of glandular change, including size, shape, and pathologic differentiation. The Gleason Score or Sum (GS) represents the sum of the primary and secondary grade of the prostate tumor. Based on a ranking from G2 (least aggressive, best prognosis) to G10 (most aggressive, poorest prognosis), the higher the sum is, the more severe is the disease. There are several, similar classification systems used to grade CNS/brain cancers: World Health Organization (WHO), Kernohan, or Ringertz. Rather than tumor size, grading is based on tissue differentiation and degree of vascularity and necrosis. Classification is made based on a three- or four-grade system, with the higher number associated with more aggressive cancer.

The category N, for node, describes the degree that lymph nodes have been affected by cancer. This is typically accomplished by a process termed "sentinal node biopsy." The (nearby) sentinal node or nodes are detected by injection of a radioactive or colored dye solution at the tumor site. The indicator solution will travel a path within the lymph system that circulating cancer cells would be expected to follow. The area is then scanned to detect the presence of the indicator solution in nearby, or sentinal, lymph nodes. One or more lymph nodes are then removed and examined pathologically for the presence of cancer cells. Positive findings will typically result in further removal and testing of nearby lymph nodes to determine extent.

- NX: Cannot be measured/evaluated
- N0: Nearby lymph nodes are clear of cancer

Beyond N0, numerical categorization describes the size, location, and number of lymph nodes affected. The higher the number, the more lymph nodes are involved.

- N1: Fewer lymph nodes affected
- N2
- N3: More lymph nodes affected

The M category, for metastasis, describes the degree to which the primary tumor has spread (metastasized) into surrounding tissues and/or organs.

- MX: Cannot be measured/evaluated
- M0: No cancer metastasis detected
- M1: Cancer metastasis detected

Although the TNM metrics are relatively universal, each cancer type has a customized version of this classification system. In some instances, there may be many additional subcategories to refine tumor classification and offer additional prognostic information to the provider. In other cases, the staging classification may be simplified by means of truncated categorization.

Based on the established TNM categories, an overall cancer group stage is determined. Although criteria for stage assignment varies somewhat according to cancer type, the following provides a top-level overview of stage groupings:

- Stage 0: Carcinoma in situ (cancer is limited to the site of origin)

Stages I through III classify cancer where higher numbers indicate more extensive and aggressive disease. Some cancers types utilize subcategories in staging to provide more specific information about type, behavior, and prognosis.

- Stage IV: Distant metastatic cancer (cancer has spread to another, distant organ)

Special cases are female reproductive cancers, Hodgkin disease/lymphoma, colorectal cancer, and leukemia. Female reproductive cancers are stage according to the International Federation of Gynecologists and Obstetricians (FIGO). Although FIGO staging classification guidelines generally follow the general TNM/group staging approach, many of the female reproductive cancers, including those of the breast, cervix, and uterus, are subclassified in great detail.

Hodgkin disease and other cancers of the lymphoid system are staged using the Ann Arbor classification system. Stages I through IV are defined by the anatomical location of affected lymph nodes. The higher the stage number, the more lymph nodes are affected and the more aggressive is the disease. Each stage assignment is then subclassified as either "A" (asymptomatic) or "B" (symptomatic).

Colorectal cancer uses the Dukes' staging classification, an older system that corresponds closely to group staging. Dukes' A through D colorectal cancer stages effectively translate to group Stages I through IV.

Because leukemia involves the bone marrow and has often affected many organs, including the liver, spleen, and lymph nodes, staging is based primarily on the patient's survival outlook according to disease progression. Although not all forms of leukemia utilize a formal staging system, each form that does has a dedicated staging classification system. For example, chronic myelogenous leukemia (CML) is classified into three phases (as opposed to stages):

- Chronic: Fewer than 5 percent immature cells in circulation/bone marrow; mildly symptomatic, readily responsive to treatment
- Accelerated: 5 to 30 percent immature cells in circulation/bone marrow; more symptomatic, less responsive to treatment
- Acute/blast phase: Less than 30 percent immature cells in circulation/bone marrow; very aggressive, acute disease

Additional staging classifications, such as Rai (Stages 0-IV; U.S. predominant) and Binet (Stages A, B, and C; European predominant), are used for chronic lymphocytic leukemia (CLL). Still other systems are applied to different leukemia types such as the Stage 1 through Stage 3 classification based on level of anemia and spleen size for hairy cell leukemia (HCL).

In addition to providing information on the size, extent, and prognostic status of each cancer case, staging plays a vital role in epidemiology and treatment studies. The National Cancer Institute Surveillance, Epidemiology, and End Results (SEER) program and other cancer registries such as the National Program of Cancer Registries (NPCR) use summary staging classification in their surveillance and epidemiology efforts. For these purposes, all cancers are grouped into one of the following five summary categories:

- In situ: Early-stage cancer, present only in the cell layers where first detected
- Localized: Cancer localized to tissue/organ where first detected; no evidence of metastasis
- Regional: Cancer metastasized to nearby lymph nodes, tissues, organs
- Distant: Cancer metastasized to distant lymph nodes, tissues, organs
- Unknown: Insufficient data available to classify

Data collected are made available to clinical and research professionals so that they may better understand and address the cancer burden according to a variety of demographics and metrics, including cancer stage.

Results: Cancer staging is a vital component of the diagnostic process. Accurate stage assessment will guide the medical team in making optimal treatment recommendations for patient care according to prognostic expectations. Because the epidemiologic value of the original stage is significant, the classification remains constant throughout the course of disease. Restaging occurs only if treatment is planned following a recurrence.

Pam Conboy, B.S.

For Further Information

Benedet, J. L., et al. "FIGO Staging Classifications and Clinical Practice Guidelines in the Management of Gynecologic Cancers." *International Journal of Gynecology and Obstetrics* 70 (2000): 209-262.

Greene, F. L. "Updates to Staging System Reflect Advances in Imaging, Understanding." *Journal of the National Cancer Institute* 22 (2002): 1664-1666.

_______. "Updating the Strategies in Cancer Staging." *American College of Surgeons Bulletin* 87 (2002): 13-15.

Greene, F. L., et al., eds. *American Joint Committee on Cancer Staging Manual*. 6th ed. New York: Springer, 2002.

O'Dowd, G. J., et al. "The Gleason Score: A Significant Biologic Manifestation of Prostate Cancer Aggressiveness on Biopsy." *PCRI Insights* 4, no. 1 (January, 2001).

Wittekind, C., et al. "TNM Residual Tumor Classification Revisited." *Cancer* 94 (2002): 2511-2516.

Other Resources

American Cancer Society
http://www.cancer.org

American Joint Committee on Cancer (AJCC)
http://www.cancerstaging.org/

CancerCare
http://www.cancercare.org

Centers for Disease Control and Prevention (CDC) National Program of Cancer Registries (NPCR)
http://www.cdc.gov/cancer/npcr/

CureSearch
http://www.curesearch.org

International Federation of Gynecologists and Obstetricians (FIGO)
http://www.figo.org

International Union Against Cancer
http://www.uicc.org/

Lung Cancer Online Foundation
http://www.lungcanceronline.org

National Cancer Institute
http://www.cancer.gov

See also: Biopsy; Cancer care team; Carcinomas; Chemotherapy; Childhood cancers; Dukes' classification; Epidemiology of cancer; Gleason grading system; Leukemias; Lymphomas; Medical oncology; Metastasis; National Cancer Institute (NCI); Oncology; Sentinel Lymph Node (SLN) biopsy and mapping; Statistics of cancer; TNM staging

▶ Stent therapy

Category: Procedures

Definition: Stent therapy is the placement of a rigid plastic or expandable metal tube to open a blocked airway, a stenosed blood vessel, the colon, or the esophagus.

Cancers treated: Lung cancer, esophageal cancer, colon cancer, gastric carcinoma, vena cava syndrome

Why performed: When cancerous growth constricts or occludes an airway or major blood vessel, a stent can be an important option if removal of tissue alone is not effective. Stents can be used to strengthen a weakened airway or blood vessel.

Stents made by the Schneider company are used as an entro-endo prosthesis for colonic stenting and also for gastroduodenal stenting. Such stents are used for two purposes: preoperative relief of obstruction and palliative treatment. Stricture formation can be a major problem among patients who have an anastomosis between the esophagus and stomach or jejunum following subtotal or total gastrectomy.

Although first used as a simple adjunct to radiotherapy, stenting of the superior vena cava can be an effective first-line procedure for immediate relief in patients with malignancy. Growth of malignant lesions surrounding the vena cava often causes stenosis or obstruction of the vena cava and symptoms of venous congestion result, the so-called vena cava syndrome. Stent therapy can be effective to treat such cases and to improve quality of life for patients with advanced malignant disease.

Patient preparation: Patients diagnosed with superior vena cava (SVC) syndrome caused by severe stenosis secondary to mediastinal malignancy may be referred for stent insertion. Most cases of SVC syndrome are attributable to an underlying primary thoracic malignancy, lymphoma, or metastatic tumor. Symptoms include venous congestion and edema in the upper half of the body. These symptoms are associated with dyspnea, dysphagia, and cognitive dysfunction as a result of cerebral venous hypertension. In these cases, patients must decide along with their doctors whether to undergo stent therapy or instead proceed with radiotherapy and chemotherapy.

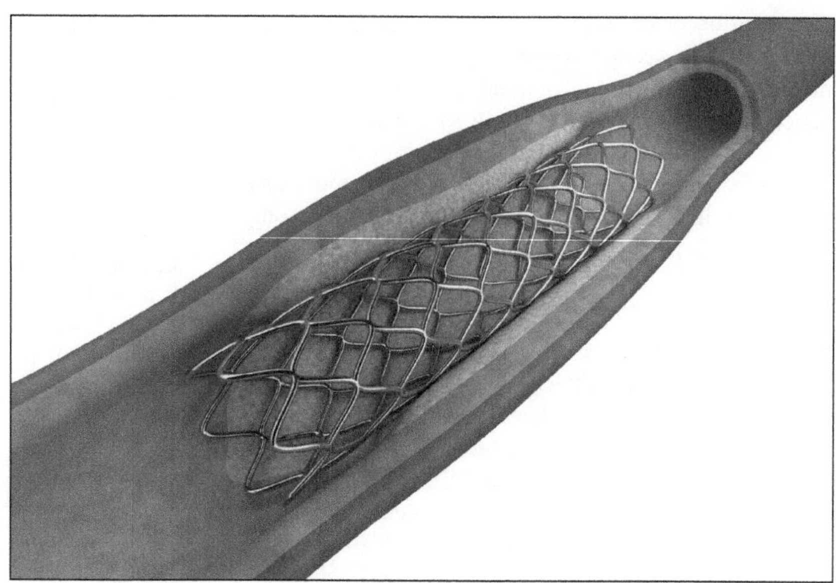

This metallic mesh stent holds open the duodenum of a woman with a pancreatic carcinoma. (iStock)

Prior to SVC stent therapy, patients undergo a bilateral arm venography to determine the site and degree of stenosis. Patients in which the SVC is severely stenosed and the obstruction involves confluence of the brachiocephalic veins may be candidates for stent therapy. Patients with very extensive total occlusions involving both SVC and subclavin veins may be referred to other therapy. Short occlusions can also be treated with thrombolysis and then stented.

Steps of the procedure: For preoperative relief of colon obstruction, the stent is placed across the acute obstruction, with the intent of decompressing and cleaning the colon, which may allow a single-stage procedure. In studies of stent treatment of colon cancer, successful stent placement is usually achieved in lesions of the sigmoidal colon, descending colon, and transverse colon. The stent delivery system is quite flexible and can be maneuvered into the transverse colon if necessary.

Effective symptom relief can be achieved with an expandable stent. The rigid plastic tube stent, on the other hand, is shoved through the distal tumor with the use of a pusher-tube device. The newest type of stent treatment is the self-expanding metal stent, which was first modified for esophageal use in 1991. One example is the Schneider Wallstent, which can be mounted onto a delivery catheter where it is held in check with a sheath.

Percutaneous access can be achieved via the right common femoral vein for SVC stent insertion. An angled guidewire is inserted, dilatation is achieved with a small balloon, and a self-expanding stent (such as produced by Boston Scientific) is inserted.

After the procedure: The duration of palliative stent therapy, when placed properly, averages seventeen weeks and can extend as long as sixty-four weeks. Stent insertion is successful for most patients receiving treatment for SVC syndrome, with patients experiencing symptomatic relief within a few hours of the procedure. Few major complications are reported, and most patients are able to start radiotherapy the next day after stenting. During the procedure, heparin is administered to prevent clotting.

Risks: Insertion of a self-expanding metallic stent into an esophagojejunal anastomotic stricture can be a successful and uncomplicated therapy. The risks of palliative stent therapy for treatment of colon cancer include migration in the colon with colonic motility. Especially when the stent is placed at an anatomical curve such as the splenic flexure, these stents are much more likely to migrate. Migration in the treatment of colon cancer occurs in about 20 percent of cases. Perforation can occur, although this outcome is often the result of balloon dilation performed before the stent is placed.

Results: Stent therapy to treat SVC syndrome usually results in patients being able to undertake an ideal radiotherapy course, which maximizes the quality and length of their lives.

Michael R. King, Ph.D.

For Further Information

Altman, Arnold J., ed. *Supportive Care of Children with Cancer: Current Therapy and Guidelines from the Children's Oncology Group*. Boston: Johns Hopkins University Press, 2004.

Boyiadzis, Michael, et al. *Hematology-Oncology Therapy*. New York: McGraw-Hill, 2006.

Talamonti, Mark S., and Sam G. Pappas, eds. *Liver-Directed Therapy for Primary and Metastatic Liver Tumors*. New York: Springer, 2001.

Other Resources

Library of the National Medical Society
http://www.medical-library.org

See also: Colorectal cancer; Esophageal cancer; Gastrointestinal cancers; Lung cancers; Palliative treatment; Superior vena cava syndrome

▶ Stereotactic needle biopsy

Category: Procedures
Also known as: Breast biopsy, image-guided biopsy

Definition: Stereotactic needle biopsy is an outpatient procedure, usually performed by a radiologist or breast surgeon, in which a biopsy is obtained following imaging of a breast lesion using X rays. A stereo pair of the breast to be biopsied is generated using an X-ray tube at two slightly different positions and the images are combined with a computer, much the way the eyes capture the same object with two slightly different images that the brain then unites to form the final three-dimensional image.

Cancer diagnosed: Breast cancer

Why performed: Stereotactic needle biopsy is used to determine whether a suspicious lesion is cancer.

Patient preparation: Before stereotactic needle biopsy, sterile technique is observed, and a topical anesthetic is administered.

Steps of the procedure: The doctor obtains the informed consent of the patient and verifies the correct breast to be biopsied. A stereotable is used, whereby the patient is prone with the affected breast hanging down through an opening in the table. A stereo pair of the breast is generated and the relative shift in the lesion's position between the two X-ray pictures, called parallax shift, allows the computer to determine the exact location of the lesion in three dimensions.

The skin surface of the breast to be biopsied is cleaned with antiseptic and local anesthetic is given. The needle is inserted into the breast lesion through a tiny nick in the skin under computer guidance. Several samples of the lesion are then obtained. Adhesive skin closures (Steri-Strips) are applied to close the nick in the skin, and a sterile dressing is then applied. The samples are labeled and sent to pathology.

After the procedure: The patient is given discharge instructions, including to avoid the use of aspirin or ibuprofen and to instead take acetaminophen (Tylenol) for pain, to apply cold compresses over the biopsy site that evening to reduce swelling, to avoid exercise for seventy-two hours, and to monitor for any sign of fever or infection.

Risks: The risks of this procedure, although minimal, include infection, bleeding at the biopsy site, and bruising and/or scarring.

Results: The pathology results are usually available within forty-eight hours postprocedure, and if the lesion is benign, then no further workup is usually necessary. If the lesion is cancer, however, an open surgical biopsy may then be necessary to ensure complete removal.

Debra B. Kessler, M.D., Ph.D.

See also: Acoustic neuromas; Astrocytomas; Biopsy; Cordotomy; Core needle biopsy; Craniopharyngiomas; Gamma Knife; Medulloblastomas; Microcalcifications; Needle biopsies; Needle localization; Radiation oncology; Stereotactic Radiosurgery (SRS); Surgical biopsies

▶ Stereotactic Radiosurgery (SRS)

Category: Procedures
Also known as: Fractionated stereotactic radiosurgery

Definition: Stereotactic radiosurgery (SRS) is a noninvasive procedure that uses multiple beams of radiation to treat a selected target, such as a brain tumor or a difficult-to-reach tumor in the chest or abdomen. The radiation comes from either cobalt or a linear accelerator.

Cancers treated: Benign and malignant brain tumors, acoustic neuroma, metastases, head and neck cancers, lung cancer, pancreatic cancer, gynecological cancers, liver cancer, spinal cancer, other cancers that are difficult to reach

Why performed: SRS is the most precise in tumor targeting of the radiation therapy interventions. While stereotactic radiosurgery is noninvasive and similar to radiation therapy, it is so accurate that it is considered surgical in nature. Most often, SRS is used to reach tumors that are not candidates for surgery or near structures that could be damaged by a surgical approach. SRS provides the option for an outpatient procedure rather than a traditional surgery that may require several days or weeks of hospitalization. In some instances, SRS may be used when patients have had previous radiation.

Patient preparation: Stereotactic radiosurgery preparation depends on the site of the tumor and the type of equipment used. The traditional approach to SRS in the head uses a lightweight halo frame attached to the skull with four small screws and cobalt radiation beams for treatment. Another option for SRS is a robotically controlled linear accelerator that delivers multiple beams and uses a variety of techniques to hold the patient still. A facial mask or a body frame is fitted for each patient when the robotically controlled linear accelerator is used. Since treatments may last thirty minutes to two hours, positioning devices help the patient lie still during the treatment.

A computed tomography (CT) scan with contrast dye, a magnetic resonance imaging (MRI) scan, or an angiogram, all very accurate radiology procedures, may be done to determine the size and location of the tumor or blood vessels to be treated. If treatment is in the head, then a neurosurgeon will work with a radiation oncologist to review the images and other patient data to determine the site to be treated. Other physician specialists may be involved in planning the SRS treatment for other body sites along with the radiation oncologist. Information is loaded into a treatment-planning computer that calculates how much radiation the patient is to receive and precisely where to direct the beams. The patient may receive a mild drug to be more comfortable during the treatment.

Steps of the procedure: For a stereotactic radiosurgery treatment of the head using a cobalt radiation source, the patient lies down on the treatment table and the halo head frame is attached to the equipment, securing the position of the head to prevent movement that might cause the radiation beams to stray onto normal tissue. Up to 201 separate beams may be used to shape the treatment area. The treatment may last two to forty-five minutes during the session. There is no pain during the treatment.

For a stereotactic radiosurgery treatment using a robotically controlled linear accelerator, the patient lies down on the treatment table and the premade positioning devices are adjusted to hold the patient in one position for the treatment. One beam of radiation is used as the linear accelerator moves around the patient in a circle to shape the treatment area. A single treatment or a daily treatment of one or two sessions for five or more days may be used.

Regardless of equipment, the patient is awake and can talk with the radiation therapy staff using an intercom. The staff watches the patient on closed-circuit television. The patient may hear noises from the equipment as adjustments of the beam are made to move around the tumor.

After the procedure: If a head frame was used, then it is removed. Depending on the procedure and the site treated, the patient may be able to go home in just a few hours or may stay overnight in the hospital. The patient may need to lie still for a while after the procedure. The doctor will provide information about when the patient may resume normal activities, but it is usually in just a few days. It is safe for patients to be around others, including children and pregnant women, because no radiation is in the body.

Risks: Side effects depend on the site treated but may include headache, swelling as the tumor cells die, minor swelling where the head frame was attached to the skin, nausea, skin irritation, diarrhea, or bladder problems. There is a slight chance of paralysis or other deficits, such as weakness or difficulty with speech or hearing, when the brain or spine receives radiation.

Results: Stereotactic radiosurgery does not work immediately but causes cell death over time. The tumor decreases in size over time based on the type of tumor and its growth rate before treatment. Malignant tumors and metastatic tumors usually respond more rapidly because their growth rate is faster. The patient sees the physician frequently to monitor the tumor destruction and to be sure that side effects are not developing as the cells die.

Patricia Stanfill Edens, R.N., Ph.D., FACHE

For Further Information

Le, Q. T., B. W. Loo, A. Ho, et al. "Results of a Phase I Dose-Escalation Study Using Single-Fraction Stereotactic Radiotherapy for Lung Tumors." *Journal of Thoracic Oncology* 1, no. 8 (October, 2006): 802-809.

National Cancer Institute. *Radiation Therapy and You: A Guide to Self-Help During Cancer Treatment.* NIH Publication 01-2227. Bethesda, Md.: National Institutes of Health, 2001. Also available at http://www.cancer.gov.

Slotman, B. J., T. D. Solberg, and D. Verellen. *Extracranial Stereotactic Radiotherapy and Radiosurgery.* New York: Taylor and Francis, 2006.

Other Resources

American Cancer Society
http://www.cancer.org

International Radiosurgery Association
http://www.irsa.org

See also: Acoustic neuromas; Afterloading radiation therapy; Astrocytomas; Cobalt 60 radiation; Craniopharyngiomas; Gamma Knife; Linear accelerator; Medulloblastomas; Radiation oncology; Radiation therapies; Stereotactic needle biopsy

▶ Surgical biopsies

Category: Procedures
Also known as: Tissue sampling, incisional biopsy, excisional biopsy, endoscopic or laparoscopic biopsy, open biopsy, transvenous biopsy

Definition: A surgical biopsy is the removal of tissue through an incision during an open or laparoscopic surgical procedure. A pathologist examines the tissue sample in the laboratory to detect the presence of cancer cells and determine the grade of the tumor.

There are several types of surgical biopsy procedures. The one performed is dependent on the type of suspected cancer and the area of the body being examined.

In incisional biopsy, a scalpel or similar instrument is used to remove a portion of the suspected cancerous tissue through an incision made in the skin. Incisional biopsies are most commonly used to remove soft tissue, such as skin, connective tissue, breast tissue, muscle, and fat. For skin lesions, an incisional biopsy may be performed with a hollow, circular-shaped instrument (punch biopsy), or a razor may be used (shave biopsy). Depending on the type of procedure, general or local anesthesia may be used.

In excisional biopsy, a whole lump, tumor, or organ and a margin of normal tissue around it are removed. Some open surgical biopsy procedures include laparotomy, thoracotomy, or mediastinotomy. General anesthesia is used for excisional and open biopsy procedures.

In endoscopic or laparoscopic biopsy, an endoscope (small camera on a thin tube) is used to view an internal area and identify the tissue for removal. The endoscope transmits magnified images of the area onto a video monitor to guide the physician during the procedure. The endoscope can be inserted through a natural body opening (endoscopy), such as the throat to remove esophageal tissue, or through a small abdominal incision (laparoscopy). When the laparoscope is used to view the inside of the chest cavity, the procedure is called a thoracoscopy and the scope is called a thoracoscope. When the laparoscope is used to view the mediastinum (space between and in front of the lungs), the procedure is called a mediastinoscopy, and the scope is called a mediastinoscope.

Surgical instruments attached to the endoscope or inserted through other small incisions are used to remove the tissue. Laparoscopic biopsy procedures are the most common type of biopsies and are often used when a tissue sample is needed from more than one area or when a larger tissue sample is needed. Depending on the biopsy site, the patient may be under general or local anesthesia.

Cancers diagnosed or treated: Various, including breast cancer, bone cancer, carcinoid tumors, germ-cell tumors, liver cancer, lung cancer, sarcoidosis, Hodgkin disease, myasthenia gravis, neurogenic tumors, thymic cancer and thymomas, malignant mesothelioma, mediastinal tumors, pericardial tumors, lymphoma, skin cancer, and thyroid cancer

Why performed: Surgical biopsies are performed to diagnose a variety of conditions and to assess the degree of organ damage (disease staging). Surgical biopsies may be performed when abnormalities are found during other tests such as an ultrasound, computed tomography (CT) scan, magnetic resonance imaging (MRI), or a nuclear scan. Surgical biopsies also may be performed to determine the cause of unexplained symptoms or to match organ tissue before a transplant.

An excisional biopsy may be used to remove some types of tumors or suspected cancers that need to be entirely removed for an accurate diagnosis, such as the removal of lymph nodes to accurately diagnose lymphoma. A surgical biopsy procedure also may be recommended when other, less invasive biopsy procedures do not provide conclusive results for an accurate diagnosis to be made.

Patient preparation: Preprocedure tests may include a chest X ray, electrocardiogram (EKG), CT, MRI, and other imaging tests. Urine tests and blood tests are performed before the procedure to evaluate the patient's blood count, platelet count, and blood clotting ability. Depending on the type of surgical biopsy procedure to be performed, additional tests may be required.

The patient preparation for a biopsy procedure varies, depending on the type of procedure and biopsy location. One week before the procedure, patients must stop taking aspirin and products containing aspirin, ibuprofen, and anticoagulants, as directed by the physician. Other anticoagulant medications may be prescribed as needed. In most cases, the patient must not eat or drink for eight to twelve hours beforehand. The patient will receive specific preparation instructions from the health care team.

Patients at most health care facilities must sign a form stating their willingness to permit diagnosis and medical treatment, a process called informed consent.

Steps of the procedure: An intravenous (IV) line is inserted into a vein in the patient's arm to deliver medications. For some surgical biopsy procedures, such as liver biopsy and some laparoscopic procedures, the patient is given a sedative and the procedure is performed under conscious sedation. With conscious sedation, the patient is awake but relaxed and able to respond to the physician's instructions during the procedure. The majority of surgical biopsy procedures, however, are performed while the patient is under general anesthesia.

The biopsy site is cleansed, and sterile drapes may be placed around the area. A local anesthetic is injected into the area. In some cases, such as with sentinel node biopsy, a radioactive substance or dye is injected into the tumor, and a scanner is used to locate the lymph node or tissue containing the radioactive substance or stained with the dye.

During a laparoscopic biopsy, a laparoscope is inserted into a small abdominal incision. The laparoscope transmits magnified images onto a video monitor to guide the physician as laparoscopic instruments are inserted through additional small abdominal incisions to remove tissue samples. Ultrasound or CT guidance may be used to aid the surgeon during the procedure.

Transvenous biopsy is a technique used to remove a tissue sample via a catheter inserted into a vein in the neck. This technique is not common, but it may be used for certain high-risk patients, including those who have a blood-clotting disorder, fluid in the abdomen, or liver failure or who are morbidly obese.

During an incisional biopsy, the surgeon uses a scalpel to remove a sample of tissue from the area. During an excisional biopsy, the lesion and surrounding margin of normal tissue are removed. During an open surgical biopsy, an incision is made in the abdomen (laparotomy), upper chest (thoracotomy or mediastinoscopy), or breast, allowing visualization of the area. The location and size of the tumor are identified, and a tissue sample or lymph nodes can be removed for analysis. Ultrasound or CT guidance may be used to aid the surgeon during the procedure.

After the tissue has been removed, a pathologist sends it to a laboratory for microscopic analysis to determine how much the tissue sample differs from normal tissue. A variety of methods can be used to process tissue samples. Histologic sections involve preparing stained, thin "slices" of tissue mounted on slides. The histologic method may take up to forty-eight hours to produce results. With this method, the tissue sample is placed in a machine that replaces all water in the sample with paraffin wax. The sample is embedded into a larger block of paraffin and is then sliced into very thin sections and stained with dye to aid microscopic analysis. Frozen tissue analysis involves freezing the tissue, slicing it into thin sections, and staining the sections to aid analysis. Smears are tissue samples that are spread onto a slide for examination. The results of smears can usually be obtained very quickly, although the smear technique cannot be used on all types of biopsy samples.

After the procedure: The length of a patient's recovery and the steps for recovery vary depending on the type of biopsy procedure, biopsy location, and type of anesthesia. The patient may stay in an intensive care unit (ICU) or recovery room for a certain amount of time after the procedure. The incision is closed with sutures, and the biopsy site is usually covered with a bandage or dressing. A catheter may remain after surgery to drain urine. Drains or chest tubes may remain in place at the incision site to remove fluid or air that may have accumulated during the procedure. Pain medication is prescribed as needed for relief of pain, which may include discomfort at the biopsy site or muscle pain. The patient usually stays in the hospital overnight but may need to recover in the hospital three to four days, depending on the biopsy site, type of procedure, and type of anesthesia given during the procedure.

Specific instructions for driving, activity, incision care, medications, nutrition, and managing emergencies and a follow-up care schedule are provided to the patient, as applicable. In most cases, the patient is not permitted to drive home after the procedure, and driving or operating machinery may be limited for a certain amount of time. Depending on the physician's instructions, the patient may be required to stay on bed rest at home for a certain amount of time after the procedure.

The patient should avoid vigorous physical activity and heavy lifting after the procedure, as directed by the physician. For one week after the procedure, the patient should avoid aspirin and products containing aspirin, ibuprofen, and anticoagulants, as these medications decrease blood clotting, which is necessary for healing. Other anticoagulant medications may be prescribed if necessary after the procedure. The patient may take acetaminophen (Tylenol) to relieve pain as needed.

Risks: The risks of biopsy procedures are dependent on the type of procedure performed and the biopsy location. Possible risks of all surgical biopsy procedures include allergic reaction to the anesthetic, bleeding, infection, and scarring, and these risks are greater with open surgical biopsy procedures.

The risk of death associated with biopsy procedures is generally very low. The physician can discuss specific mortality rates and risks with the patient, depending on the type of procedure performed.

Results: Biopsy results are available either right away or within twenty-four to forty-eight hours after the tissue removal, depending on the type of biopsy analysis that is being performed. The tissue sample removed during the procedure is either normal, which means it is benign or noncancerous, or abnormal, which means it has unusual characteristics and may be malignant or cancerous. The grade of tumor may also be determined from the biopsy sample, indicating how quickly the tumor is likely to grow and spread. Surgical biopsy procedures remove a larger tissue sample than other biopsy methods, increasing the accuracy of a diagnosis. The type of cancerous cells and extent of disease will help guide the patient's treatment.

Angela M. Costello, B.S.

For Further Information

DeVita, Vincent, Jr., Samuel Hellman, Steven A. Rosenberg, et al., eds. *Cancer: Principles and Practice of Oncology*. 7th ed. Philadelphia: Lippincott Williams & Wilkins, 2005.

McPhee, Stephen J., Maxine A. Papadakis, and Lawrence M. Tierney, eds. *Current Medical Diagnosis and Treatment 2008*. New York: McGraw-Hill Medical, 2007.

Ota, D. M. "What's New in General Surgery: Surgical Oncology." *Journal of the American College of Surgeons* 196, no. 6 (2003): 926-932.

Skandalakis, John E., Panajiotis N. Skandalakis, and Lee John Skandalakis. *Surgical Anatomy and Technique: A Pocket Manual*. 2d ed. New York: Springer, 2000.

Other Resources

American Cancer Society
http://www.cancer.org

American Pathology Foundation
http://www.apfconnect.org

College of American Pathologists
http://www.cap.org

National Cancer Institute
http://www.cancer.gov

Radiology Info, provided by the American College of Radiology and the Radiological Society of North America
http://www.radiologyinfo.org

Society of Interventional Radiology
http://www.sirweb.org

Society for Hematopathology
http://socforheme.org

See also: Biopsy; Liver biopsy; Needle biopsies; Needle localization; Stereotactic needle biopsy

▶ Technetium isotopes

Category: Procedures
Related: CT Scans, MRI, X-rays

Definition: Technetium is a man-made radioactive element extensively used in nuclear medicine for diagnostic procedures. Technetium generators in a hospital transform molybdenum-99 into technetium-99m shortly before injection into a patient. Technetium-99m is a metastable isotope that decays with a half-life of about 6 hours into technetium-99, which itself is radioactive with a half-life of over 200,000 years.

Cancers Diagnosed: Cancers of the internal organs, bone cancers, and blood cancers.

Why performed: Most noninvasive scans of the body (X-rays, CT, and MRI) detect density differences in the body. However, some cancers do not manifest themselves as easily detected tumors. Rather, these cancers manifest themselves more as organ dysfunctions. Scans using technetium radioactive tracers can be used to pinpoint these types of organ dysfunctions. As the most commonly used radioisotope tracer diagnostic tool, tens of millions of technetium scans are performed each year, though only some of them are for cancer diagnosis, as many other conditions can also lead to organ dysfunction. Because the technetium is bound to chemicals in the body, technetium scans generate images based upon body chemistry rather than structural differences like most other scans.

Patient preparation: The technetium-99m is produced and attached to a chemical or nutrient used by a specific organ of interest. This acts as a radioactive tracer. A few hours before the scan, the radioactive tracer is introduced into the patient's body, typically intravenously.

Steps of the procedure: During the scan, the patient lies still on a table. When the technetium-99m decays it emits characteristic gamma rays. A gamma-ray detector, often looking much like an X-ray camera, moves around the patient and measures the radiation emitted by the technetium 99-m decay. Triangulation of regions emitting excess radiation shows where the tracer is being concentrated and used in the body. Depending upon the test being performed, the imaging can take 30 minutes to an hour.

After the procedure: With a half-life of only six hours, close to 94% of the initial technetium-99m decays into the far less radioactive technetium-99 within 24 hours. The less radioactive technetium-99 is normally eliminated from the body relatively quickly, often with 75% being removed within only a couple days.

Risks: As with any radioactive material, radiation exposure is a potential health issue with technetium scans. However, the radiation exposure is rather low, being comparable to that of a CT scan. The rapid decay and removal of technetium from the body also means that the patient poses little radiation risk to others.

Results: Images produced by technetium scans show where the body either concentrates or depletes the radioactive tracer. Since the technetium is attached to chemicals and nutrients normally used by specific organs in the body, the scan can determine whether the organs are working as they should. Together with other diagnostic procedures, technetium scans can help determine the location and extent of various types of cancer or other organ dysfunctions.

Raymond D. Benge, Jr., MS

For Further Information

Raloff, J. (2009). Desperately seeking moly. *Science News,* 176(7): 16-20.

Scerri, E. (2013). *A tale of 7 elements.* New York: Oxford.

Other Resources

American Cancer Society
Nuclear Medicine Scans
http://www.cancer.org/treatment/understandingyourdiagnosis/examsandtestdescriptions/imagingradiologytests/imaging-radiology-tests-nuc-scan

Mayo Clinic
Nuclear Medicine
http://mayoclinichealthsystem.org/locations/barron/medical-services/radiology-and-imaging/nuclear-medicine

See also: Radiation oncology

▶ Testicular Self-Examination (TSE)

Category: Procedures

Definition: Testicular self-examination (TSE) is a procedure done by the patient as a screening tool for early diagnosis of any testicular disorders. The exam is performed by manually examining the scrotum and testes.

Cancers diagnosed: Testicular cancer

Why performed: A self-exam of the testicles is an effective way of becoming familiar with this area of the body and thus enabling the early detection of abnormalities that can lead to testicular cancer. It can be the first line of defense against cancer because testicular cancer comes with virtually no obvious symptoms or pain. Testicular cancer primarily develops in younger men, and it is the most common form of cancer developed by men between the ages of twenty and thirty-five. Therefore, monthly performance of the testicular self-exam is recommended for men over age fourteen.

Patient preparation: Because heat relaxes the scrotum, a TSE is best performed after a warm bath or shower.

Steps of the procedure: The first step in TSE is to stand in front of a mirror and observe any possible swelling on the scrotal skin. Next, the patient should elevate one leg for better access and examine each testicle with both hands. With the index and middle fingers under the testicle and the thumbs placed on top, the testicle should be rolled gently between the thumbs and fingers. This process should not be painful, but if pain or tenderness is experienced, the patient should notify a physician. The testicles should feel firm and round, but not hard, and it is normal for one testicle to be slightly larger than the other. It is important to feel for any lumps on the testicle, which can range in size from a pea to a golf ball and are frequently very hard. If any lumps are detected, then it is critical for the patient to see a physician as soon as possible to determine if the lumps are benign (noncancerous) or malignant (cancerous).

The next step in the TSE is to locate the epididymis, a soft, tubelike structure behind the testicle that collects and carries sperm. It is important to become familiar with this structure to avoid mistaking it for a lump or mass.

After the procedure: No aftercare is required.

Risks: There are no risks with this procedure if the patient performs the exam without inflicting pain.

Results: If any abnormalities (swelling, change in color, lumps, hardness, pain) are detected during the testicular self-exam, a physician (urologist) should be consulted. Generally any suspicions can be confirmed or ruled out by the physician with an exam and/or ultrasound.

Robert J. Amato, D.O.

For Further Information

Johanson, Paula. *Frequently Asked Questions About Testicular Cancer*. New York: Rosen, 2007.

Kurth, Karl H., Gerald H. J. Mickisch, and Fritz H. Schröder. *Renal, Bladder, Prostate, and Testicular Cancer*: An Update. New York: Parthenon, 2001.

Parker, James N., and Philip M. Parker, eds. *The Official Patient's Sourcebook on Testicular Cancer: A Revised and Updated Directory for the Internet Age*. San Diego, Calif.: Icon Health, 2002.

See also: Embryonal cell cancer; Lumps; Risks for cancer; Symptoms and cancer; Testicular cancer; Ultrasound tests

▶ Thermal imaging

Category: Procedures
Also known as: Digital infrared thermal imaging (DITI)

Definition: Thermal imaging is a procedure to measure the skin surface temperature by detecting infrared radiation emitted from the circulation. Since tumors have higher metabolic rates than normal tissues, they tend to recruit and/or create more surrounding blood vessels than normal tissues. This process provides nutrients and oxygen for tumor cell survival and increases surface temperature.

Cancers diagnosed: Primarily breast cancer

Why performed: Thermal imaging is an extremely sensitive test performed to detect and monitor cancers. It is an alternative to other screening options that carry the risk of radiation exposure. Additionally, multiple images over time may aid in analyzing responses to treatment.

Patient preparation: Because thermal imaging measures temperature changes, patients should maintain normal circulation and body temperature prior to the imaging, including the avoidance of excessive sun exposure one week prior to testing. Also, patients should avoid hot water exposure and the use of topical analgesics two hours prior to testing, as well as nicotine, caffeine, alcohol, strenuous physical exercise, and hot or cold beverages four hours prior to testing. Medications affecting the sympathetic nervous system may need to be withheld twelve to twenty-four hours prior to the evaluation as well.

Steps of the procedure: Patients will wear a hospital gown and lay on an examination table in a temperature-controlled room (68 degrees Fahrenheit) for approximately ten minutes to equilibrate the patient to the room temperature. Both sides of the body will be scanned with a thermal camera, also called an imaging radiometer, and the scans will be used as a thermal reference because of the body's natural thermal symmetry.

After the procedure: After thermal images are taken, no more action is required by the patient. The emitted infrared radiation will be detected and converted into a monochrome or multicolored image, known as a thermogram, and displayed on a monitor screen.

Risks: The risks of this procedure are negligible, since it is noninvasive and does not use tracer dyes, radiation, or chemicals.

Results: The thermal images are analyzed with the assistance of software programs, where shades or colors represent thermal patterns. The test result would be normal if the sides of the body are mirror images, indicating a symmetrical thermal pattern. Areas of increased heat, however, would indicate a potentially cancerous mass as a result of increased local blood vessels emitting more infrared radiation. Because thermal imagers cannot pinpoint specific tumor sites, an abnormal result would likely be followed up with other imaging or clinical laboratory tests.

Elizabeth A. Manning, Ph.D.

See also: Breast cancer in children and adolescents; Breast cancer in men; Breast cancer in pregnant women; Breast cancers; Imaging tests; Risks for cancer

▶ Thoracentesis

Category: Procedures
Also known as: Thoracocentesis, pleural tap

Definition: Thoracentesis is the removal of pleural fluid from the layers of the pleura, the membranes lining the lungs and chest cavity. The pleural fluid is removed through a needle inserted through the chest wall, between the ribs, and is analyzed in a laboratory to determine the underlying cause of the fluid accumulation.

Cancers diagnosed or treated: Lung cancer, breast cancer, lymphoma, leukemia

Why performed: A thoracentesis is performed as a diagnostic procedure to determine the cause of a pleural effusion, the abnormal collection of excess fluid between the layers of the pleura. Normally, only a small amount of fluid is present in the pleural cavity to lubricate the pleural surfaces. This procedure is also performed as a therapeutic procedure to remove excess fluid and help reduce pressure on the lungs when an effusion is large and causing symptoms, such as shortness of breath or other breathing problems. A thoracentesis may be used as a palliative treatment to relieve symptoms of advanced cancers.

Patient preparation: Tests performed before the procedure include a chest X ray to confirm the presence of the pleural effusion and identify its location, ultrasound of the chest, and blood tests, such as a complete blood count, to exclude any blood-clotting abnormalities. One week before the procedure, patients must stop taking aspirin and products containing aspirin, ibuprofen, and anticoagulants, as directed by the physician. Other anticoagulant medications may be prescribed if necessary before the procedure. There are no specific eating or drinking guidelines in preparation for a thoracentesis.

Steps of the procedure: The patient usually sits upright on the edge of a chair or bed with the head and arms resting on a table. Sedating medications are not usually given for this procedure. The skin around the procedure site between the ribs and back of the chest is cleansed, and sterile drapes are placed around the area. A local anesthetic is injected into the skin to numb the area. The thoracentesis needle is inserted into the pleural space. Ultrasound guidance may be used to direct the biopsy needle into the effusion. Fluid is withdrawn through a syringe attached to the biopsy needle and collected for analysis in the laboratory.

Sclerosing agents such as talc, doxycycline, bleomycin, and quinacrine may be inserted through a chest tube during thoracentesis to prevent recurring, symptomatic malignant effusions.

The patient may experience mild pain or discomfort at the puncture site. The patient should not cough or breathe deeply during the procedure and must remain as still as possible to prevent injury to the lung. If the patient develops a cough or chest pain during the procedure, then the procedure should be stopped immediately.

After the procedure: Pressure is applied at the site where the needle was inserted. A dressing or adhesive bandage is placed over the site to help prevent infection. Supplemental oxygen may be given to the patient. The patient's breathing will be monitored after the procedure. A chest X ray is performed to ensure that the lung was not injured during the procedure. The patient should immediately report chest pain, shortness of breath, or difficulty breathing to the nurse. After the patient goes home within a few hours of the procedure, he or she should seek emergency treatment if these symptoms occur. A follow-up chest X ray may be scheduled within two to four weeks.

Risks: The risks of a thoracentesis are decreased when the procedure is performed with ultrasound guidance. In most cases, there are few complications. The risks, however, include reaccumulation of fluid in the pleural space or fluid in the lungs (pulmonary edema), bleeding, infection, respiratory distress, or collapse of the lung (pneumothorax). Pneumothorax occurs when air has built up in the pleural space because of a leak in the lung. Pneumothorax often does not require treatment, but in some cases it may require placement of a chest tube thoracostomy, a procedure to drain air from the space around the lungs to allow the lung to reexpand. Rarely, damage to the spleen or liver may occur as a result of a puncture from the thoracentesis needle.

Results: The fluid sample that was removed during the procedure is first examined for color and consistency by the physician and is then analyzed in a laboratory. The fluid may be exudative (protein-rich) or transudative (watery, protein-poor). Pleural fluid analysis is useful in determining the cause of the effusion such as infection, pneumonia, blood in the pleural space (hemothorax), cancer, heart failure, cirrhosis, or kidney disease. It may also help identify other conditions such as pancreatitis, pulmonary embolism, or thyroid disease. The goals of therapeutic thoracentesis include draining excess fluid, treating infection, fully reexpanding the lung, and relieving symptoms such as shortness of breath, chest pain, or dry cough. If a large amount of fluid was removed, then the patient will experience a relief of symptoms soon after the procedure.

A repeat thoracentesis procedure may be needed if the effusion reaccumulates, which often occurs when the underlying cause is a malignancy.

Angela M. Costello, B.S.

For Further Information

Colice, Gene L., et al. "Medical and Surgical Treatment of Parapneumonic Effusions: An Evidence-Based Guideline." *Chest* 118 (2000): 1158-1171.

Ferrer, Jaume. "Predictors of Pleural Malignancy in Patients with Pleural Effusion Undergoing Thoracoscopy." *Chest* 127 (2005): 1017-1022.

Other Resources

American College of Chest Physicians
http://www.chestnet.org

American Thoracic Society
http://www.thoracic.org

Society of Thoracic Surgeons
http://www.sts.org/sections/patientinformation

See also: Bronchoalveolar lung cancer; Lung cancers; Mesothelioma; Needle biopsies; Pleural biopsy; Pleural effusion; Pleurodesis; Radiofrequency ablation; Thoracentesis; Thoracoscopy; Ultrasound tests

▶ Thoracoscopy

Category: Procedures
Also known as: Pleuroscopy, minimally invasive or video-assisted thoracic surgery

Definition: Thoracoscopy is an endoscopic procedure used to view inside the chest cavity with a thoracoscope (small videoscope). The thoracoscope transmits images of the surgical area onto a computer screen to guide surgeons during the procedure. Compared to open-chest surgery that requires one 6- to 8-inch incision, thoracoscopy uses several small, 1-inch incisions to access the chest, thereby minimizing trauma, decreasing postoperative pain, and promoting a shorter hospital stay and a quicker recovery.

Cancers diagnosed or treated: Pleural effusion, malignant mesothelioma, lung cancer, thymomas, and mediastinal and pericardial tumors

Why performed: Thoracoscopy may be used as a diagnostic procedure to determine the cause of a pleural effusion, perform a lung biopsy, or evaluate tumors. Thoracoscopy may be used to perform therapeutic procedures including thoracoscopic pneumonectomy, lobectomy, or wedge resection for lung cancer treatment; thoracentesis to drain excess pleural fluid; and removal of tumors in the esophagus, mediastinum, pericardium, or thymus.

Patient preparation: Preprocedure tests may include a chest X ray and ultrasound, pulmonary function test, computed tomography (CT) scan, electrocardiogram (EKG), and blood tests. In general, patients must not eat or drink for eight hours before the procedure. Depending on the type of procedure to be performed, additional tests or patient preparations may be required.

Steps of the procedure: General anesthesia is used in most cases. The thoracoscope and surgical instruments are inserted through three or four small chest incisions between the ribs. The thoracoscope is manipulated to view the area, and the surgical instruments may be used to remove tissue.

After the procedure: A chest tube drains fluid and removes air that may have accumulated during the procedure. Cardiac function and blood oxygen levels are monitored, and daily chest X rays evaluate lung reexpansion and chest tube placement. The hospital recovery is about three to four days. The chest tube is removed. and the patient receives a follow-up schedule and homegoing instructions. The patient can generally return to normal activities three to four weeks after discharge.

Risks: The risks of thoracoscopy include accumulation of fluid in the pleural space, fluid in the lungs (pulmonary edema), bleeding, infection, respiratory distress, or collapse of the lung (pneumothorax). The risk of death is rare and occurs in about 0.24 percent of patients.

Results: Pleural fluid removed during the procedure is analyzed in the laboratory, and the biopsy tissue is examined for malignancy. The type and extent of disease will help guide the patient's treatment.

Angela M. Costello, B.S.

See also: Bronchoalveolar lung cancer; Endoscopy; Gastrointestinal oncology; Hematologic oncology; Lung cancers; Medical oncology; Mesothelioma; Pediatric oncology and hematology; Pleural effusion; Pleurodesis; Surgical biopsies; Thoracentesis; Thymomas

▶ Thoracotomy

Category: Procedures
Also known as: Lung surgery

Definition: A thoracotomy is the surgical opening of the chest wall so that the lungs, esophagus, or heart may be accessed. It can be performed on the right or left side or the midline of the chest.

Cancers diagnosed or treated: Lung cancer, esophageal cancer, cancer of the heart

Why performed: A thoracotomy is performed to biopsy and/or remove a tumor, to close a bleb (blister) in the external wall of the lung, or to drain an abscess.

Patient preparation: Several days before the thoracotomy, the patient will require blood work and an electrocardiogram (EKG). The patient will have to fast after midnight the day of the procedure.

Steps of the procedure: Before the thoracotomy, the patient will have an intravenous (IV) line inserted and be hooked up to a heart monitor. After the patient is sedated, an endotracheal tube is placed through the patient's nose or mouth into the trachea and attached to a ventilator, which breathes for the patient.

A midline thoracotomy is performed for surgery on the heart or esophagus. The patient lies on the back, and the surgeon splits the sternum to gain access to the chest. A right or left thoracotomy is used for surgery on the lungs. The patient lies on the opposite side with the arm over the head, and the surgeon makes an incision over the fifth intercostal (between the ribs) space.

After the surgery and before the chest wall is closed, one or two chest tubes are placed through the chest wall into the pleural space. They are necessary to reestablish the negative pressure in the chest. The chest tubes are attached to a drainage unit, which has a water seal to keep air from entering the pleural space.

After the procedure: The patient is sent to an intensive care unit (ICU) for close monitoring of vital signs, breathing, heart rhythm, and chest drainage. The patient will remain in the hospital for five or ten days. Usually the chest tubes can be removed after three to five days.

Risks: The risks of a thoracotomy are pneumothorax (collapse of the lung), air leaks, infection, bleeding, local nerve damage, and respiratory failure. After a thoracotomy, the patient may have severe pain with breathing.

Results: The lungs should be fully inflated. The tumor should be removed and the local lymph nodes evaluated.

Christine M. Carroll, R.N., B.S.N., M.B.A.

See also: Bilobectomy; Biopsy; Bronchial adenomas; Bronchoalveolar lung cancer; Esophageal cancer; Esophagectomy; Lung cancers; Pleural effusion; Pleurodesis; Pneumonectomy; Surgical biopsies

▶ Thyroid nuclear medicine scan

Category: Procedures
Also known as: Thyroid scintiscan, technetium thyroid scan

Definition: The thyroid nuclear medicine scan is an imaging technique using a gamma camera to help assess the health and anatomy of the thyroid gland following the administration of a radioisotope, a radiation-emitting form of an element. The radioisotopes most commonly used are iodine 123, iodine 131, and technetium pertechnetate. Other isotopes, such as gallium 67 and thallium 201, are also in use for their characteristic correlation in malignancy profiling. Still others are being scrutinized for better visualization of specific thyroid cancers.

When radiation is given off during the procedure, it is recorded by the scanner on radiographic film or on a screen, which allows direct viewing or photographing of the thyroid image. The radioactive substance used often gives name to the procedure, such as a technetium thyroid scan or a radioactive iodine uptake scan (RAIU test). These studies are possible because of the thyroid's special affinity for radioactive substances and its normal uptake of iodine in the production of thyroid hormones.

Cancers diagnosed: Thyroid cancers (papillary, follicular, medullary, or anaplastic)

Why performed: Thyroid scans are helpful in evaluating masses in the neck area, in defining specific types of hyperthyroidism, and in assessing thyroid nodules, metastatic tumors, and thyroid cancer. They are an important tool in determining the position, size, and structure of the thyroid gland and, together with other tests, help assess thyroid function. Scans are especially helpful in evaluating patients with suspected thyroid nodules. Thyroid nodules are either functioning (hot or warm) or nonfunctioning (cold), and this has important implications in assessing malignancy.

The butterfly-shaped thyroid is an endocrine gland consisting of two lobes located on either side of the trachea connected by bridging tissue called an isthmus. Assessing thyroid health is critical because of its central role to basic human physiology. The iodine-laden hormone produced in the thyroid gland regulates oxygen consumption, body temperature, heart function, skeletal growth, skin function, and carbohydrate, lipid, and fat metabolism.

Patient preparation: The scintiscan may be performed either in an outpatient X-ray center or a hospital radiology department. The patient is instructed to discontinue iodine-containing medications such as thyroid drugs, corticosteroids, phenothiazines, salicylates, anticoagulants, and antihistamines for several weeks to twenty-four hours prior to the scan, depending on the amount of time that the substance takes to clear from the body. If the radioisotope is to be administered orally, then the patient should fast after the midnight preceding the test. Fasting is not required for intravenous (IV) injection.

Steps of the procedure: The patient will receive the radioisotope either intravenously or orally. The patient takes the oral medication (iodine 123 or iodine 131) as either a tasteless liquid or a capsule twenty-four hours prior to imaging or receives an IV injection (pertechnetate) twenty to thirty minutes before imaging. During the scan, the patient will be lying down with the face up. The camera is then positioned over the thyroid area in the neck, and the radioactive response is displayed on a monitor and recorded on X-ray film. The procedure is usually complete in less than thirty minutes.

When evaluating thyroid function, the radioisotope iodine 123 or iodine 131 is measured at six hours and again at twenty-four hours after dosing.

After the procedure: This is a noninvasive procedure, and there are no special precautions or instructions. Regular eating can continue two hours after imaging.

Risks: The radioactive dose is very small and is generally considered harmless, but pregnant or lactating women, as well as patients allergic to iodine, shellfish, or the tracers used in the imaging, should not undergo the procedure.

Results: Many types of thyroid pathology may be revealed through imaging, and fortunately most are not cancerous. One of the ways in which the scintiscan makes this distinction is through the assessment of thyroid nodules. A thyroid nodule is a nonspecific term for a swelling in the thyroid gland. It might be no more than an accumulation of thyroid cells or a cyst. Even though they are common, they might grow large enough to interfere with swallowing or breathing, or they can produce so much hormone that hyperthyroidism results. They can also become cancerous about 5 percent of the time.

On scintiscan, the nodules are seen as hot, warm, or cold. An area of increased radionuclide uptake may be called a hot nodule, signifying that a benign growth has become overactive. An area of decreased radionuclide uptake, representing low thyroid activity, is a cold nodule. A variety of conditions, including cysts, nonfunctioning benign growths, localized inflammation, or cancer, may produce a cold spot. Hot or warm nodules are rarely malignant, while almost all cancerous nodules are cold. A cold nodule is not exclusive to malignancy, however, as most benign nodules, cysts, and localized areas of inflammation are cold as well.

Neoplasms are graded according to cell abnormality and for their potential for invasiveness and growth as a guide to treatment options and prognosis. The minimally invasive, encapsulated, and well-circumscribed growth is a grade I neoplasm. As the neoplasm becomes more aggressive and infiltrates the surrounding gland and the cells become more irregular and mitotic, the neoplasm is considered grade II. Grade III describes even more extensive growth, with possible invasiveness beyond the gland and increased cellular irregularity and mitosis. Further classification is done by anatomic staging, which defines the extent of the disease process.

The results of a thyroid nuclear medicine scan serve as a guide and are almost always used in conjunction with other tests to establish a diagnosis.

Richard S. Spira, D.V.M.

For Further Information

Beers, Mark H., et al., eds. *The Merck Manual of Medical Information, Second Home Edition*. Whitehouse Station, N.J.: Merck Research Laboratories, 2003.

Feld, Stanley. *AACE Clinical Practice Guidelines for the Diagnosis and Management of Thyroid Nodules*. New York: American Association of Clinical Endocrinologists, 1996.

Other Resources

American Thyroid Association
http://www.thyroid.org

MedlinePlus
http://www.nlm.nih.gov

Thyroid Foundation of America
http://www.allthyroid.org

See also: Cobalt 60 radiation; Cold nodule; Corticosteroids; Endocrine cancers; Imaging tests; Nuclear medicine scan; Pathology; Pregnancy and cancer; Radionuclide scan; Risks for cancer; Staging of cancer; Thyroid cancer; X-ray tests

▶ TNM staging

Category: Procedures
Also known as: Tumor/nodes/metastases staging

Definition: TNM (an abbreviation for tumor, node, and metastasis) staging is a system used to describe the extent and severity of solid malignant tumors and how much they have spread.

Cancers diagnosed or treated: Solid tumors such as breast, colorectal, kidney, larynx, lung, and prostate cancers and melanoma

Why performed: Staging of cancer is important because the stage at diagnosis is the most powerful predictor of survival. Doctors use staging information to help plan a patient's treatment, to estimate a patient's prognosis, to select changes in treatment, and to identify appropriate clinical trials for patients.

TNM staging provides a common language with which oncologists and all other members of the health care team can communicate when discussing cancer patients, as well as evaluate and compare the results of clinical trials. Staging data, when collected over time, can be valuable to epidemiologists for analysis of similar types of cancer or for use in special studies.

Patient preparation: Tissue samples are taken from a variety of tumors; patient preparation depends on the type of tumor and its location. Often, samples are taken as part of the surgical process to remove the tumor.

Steps of the procedure: Staging is based on an understanding of the way in which cancer develops. A tumor is formed at the primary site as cancer cells grow and divide in an uncontrolled fashion. As a tumor grows, its cells can invade neighboring tissues or leave the tumor to migrate through the bloodstream or lymph system to new sites in the body, a process called metastasis.

Staging systems for cancer have evolved over time and continue to be upgraded as cancer becomes better understood. The American Joint Committee on Cancer, established in 1988 to address the inadequacies of the traditional method of staging cancer using I-IV, created the TNM system for staging solid tumors throughout the body. Most types of solid tumors have TNM designations, although some do not (for example, cancers of the brain and spinal cord). As of 2008, the TNM system was in its sixth edition. In the TNM system, each factor is evaluated separately and given a number. For instance, a T1N1M0 cancer means that the patient has a T1 tumor, N1 lymph node involvement, and no metastases.

The precise definitions of T, N, and M are specific to each type of cancer, but general definitions of each element are tumor, node, and metastasis. Tumor (T) describes the extent of the primary tumor and carries a number of 0 to 4, with 0 being a tumor that is entirely contained at the local site and 4 being a large primary tumor that has probably invaded other organs. Node (N) describes regional lymph node metastasis and can also be ranked from 0 to 4, with 0 being no lymph node involvement and 4 being extensive involvement. Metastasis (M) describes the presence or absence of distant metastases;

it is 1 if distant metastases are present and 0 if not. For example, breast cancer T3N2M1 describes a large tumor that has spread outside the breast to nearby lymph nodes and to other parts of the body, whereas prostate cancer T2N0M0 describes a tumor located only in the prostate that has not spread to the lymph nodes or any other part of the body.

The category X is used in each element where no assessment of that characteristic was made. For example, NX indicates that the status of lymph nodes was not assessed. It is important not to confuse this category with N0, which indicates that no lymph node involvement was found by the diagnostic tools used.

The types of tests that are used for staging depend on the type of cancer but can include physical examination; imaging studies such as X rays, computed tomography (CT) scans, magnetic resonance imaging (MRI), or positron emission tomography (PET) scans; laboratory values such as tests for liver function or tumor markers; pathology reports; and surgical reports. The TNM system has evolved as advances have been made in diagnosis and treatment of different types of cancer. For instance, endoscopic ultrasound imaging of esophageal and rectal tumors has improved the accuracy of the clinical T, N, and M classifications. Advances in treatment have necessitated more detail in some T4 categories.

Clinical TNM staging and pathological TNM staging are distinct evaluations. Clinical staging is based on all available information obtained before pathology results are available. It may include information obtained by physical examination, radiologic examination, and endoscopy, for example. Pathologic staging includes information gained by microscopic examination of the primary tumor and regional lymph nodes. These two categories of staging are denoted by a small *c* or *p* before the stage, such as cT2N2M0 or pT3N4M1. It is also possible to stage a case at recurrence after a disease-free interval, at which time an *r* precedes the TNM designation.

After the procedure: Aftercare depends on the type of biopsy taken and whether the patient was placed under anesthesia. For most types of biopsy for which a patient is not already hospitalized, patients will arrange transportation to and from the health care facility and will have a family member or friend's supervision afterward. Often, a postsurgical hospital stay is required.

Risks: The risks to patients are related to the type of sample taken and the disease involved.

Results: Staging is an important aspect of understanding a patient's cancer. It guides treatment decisions and provides insight into the patient's prognosis.

Jill Ferguson, Ph.D.

For Further Information

Bernick, P. E., and W. D. Wong. "Staging: What Makes Sense? Can the Pathologist Help?" *Surgical Oncology Clinics of North America* 9 (2000): 703-720.

Kehoe, J., and V. P. Khatri. "Staging and Prognosis of Colon Cancer." *Surgical Oncology Clinics of North America* 15 (2006): 129-146.

Sobin, L. H. "TNM: Evolution and Relation to Other Prognostic Factors." *Seminars in Surgical Oncology* 21 (2003): 3-7.

Other Resources

American Joint Committee for Cancer
General Guidelines for TNM Staging
http://training.seer.cancer.gov/module_staging_cancer/unit03_sec03_part04_ajcc_guidelines.html

National Cancer Institute
Staging: Questions and Answers
http://www.cancer.gov/cancertopics/factsheet/Detection/staging

See also: Biopsy; Blood cancers; Breast cancers; Epidermoid cancers of mucous membranes; Head and neck cancers; Imaging tests; Kidney cancer; Lung cancers; Melanomas; Metastasis; Risks for cancer; Staging of cancer; Surgical oncology; Thyroid cancer; Tumor markers; Ultrasound tests

▶ Tracheostomy

Category: Procedures
Also known as: Tracheotomy, trach tube

Definition: Tracheostomy is a surgical procedure performed to aid breathing. An incision is made in the neck, just below the larynx (voice box), to directly access the trachea (windpipe). A tracheostomy tube is inserted through the opening, called a stoma, to keep the airway open. The tracheostomy tube may be connected to oxygen or mechanical ventilation.

Cancers treated: Neck, laryngeal, thyroid, and some congenital cancers

Why performed: A tracheostomy is performed for patients who have an upper airway obstruction, difficulty breathing, or excess secretions in the airway. It is also performed for patients recovering after tracheal or laryngeal surgery and for patients who are having difficulty being weaned from mechanical ventilation.

Patient preparation: With a planned tracheostomy, patients must stop taking aspirin and products containing aspirin, ibuprofen, and anticoagulants, as directed by the physician, one week before the procedure. Patients must not eat or drink for eight hours beforehand.

Steps of the procedure: The procedure is usually performed by a surgeon in an operating room while the patient is under general anesthesia. In emergent cases, the procedure may be performed at the patient's bedside in an emergency room or an intensive care unit (ICU). If the procedure is emergent, then the patient lies on the back with a rolled-up towel between the shoulders. A local anesthetic is injected and the procedure is performed.

In nonemergent cases, an intravenous (IV) line is inserted into the patient's arm to deliver medications. A small clip placed on the patient's finger is attached to an oximeter monitor to check the patient's blood oxygen level during the procedure. Electrodes, placed on the patient's chest, are attached via wires to an electrocardiograph (EKG) machine to monitor the patient's heart rhythm. The patient receives general anesthesia through the IV. The neck is cleaned, and sterile drapes are placed around the surgical area. Incisions are made in the neck and through the second and third tracheal rings to create an opening in the trachea. The tracheostomy tube is inserted into the opening. Tape or stitches hold the tube in place.

A newer technique, called tube-free tracheostomy, may be performed when a long-term tracheostomy is anticipated. A permanent opening in the trachea is created with skin and muscle flaps. After a one-month recovery period, the patient is usually able to talk efficiently by contracting the neck muscles, without the use of valves or devices.

After the procedure: The patient will not be able to talk or eat by mouth immediately after the procedure and while remaining on mechanical ventilation. Most patients will need several days to adjust to breathing through the trach tube. Nutrition is given directly into the stomach through a percutaneous endoscopic gastrostomy tube until the tracheostomy tube is removed. The patient will communicate with others by writing and nonverbal communication in response to questions. With training and an adaptive valve on the tracheostomy, patients are able to resume speaking as they adjust to the tracheostomy. A speech therapist can help the patient learn to speak with the tube in place.

Antibiotics may be given to reduce the risk of infection. A nurse or respiratory therapist will remove secretions from the trach tube using a suction device to clear the breathing passages.

A tracheostomy is not necessarily permanent. The patient's condition and the purpose of the tracheostomy will determine when and if the tube can be removed. If the tube is eventually removed, then the area heals quickly, leaving a small scar.

The patient and caregiver will learn how to care for the tracheostomy before leaving the hospital. The patient is usually able to go home in three to five days after the procedure, depending on his or her medical condition and rate of recovery. Some patients go home with mechanical ventilation, depending on their condition. A nurse will teach the patient and caregiver how to care for the equipment; suction, clean, and change the tube; and manage emergencies. Routine tracheostomy care must be performed at least once daily at home. A loose covering or tracheostomy cover is recommended to prevent foreign particles from entering the stoma. The patient must take precautions to avoid getting water in the opening.

The patient will feel some pain and discomfort in the neck area for about one week after the procedure, and pain medication will be prescribed as needed. It may take up to one month for the patient to heal completely. Most activities can eventually be resumed within six weeks after the procedure.

Risks: Like all surgeries, the tracheostomy procedure has risks. Complications are rare but may include bleeding, damage to the larynx or airway with a permanent change to the voice, need for further surgery, infection, scarring of the airway or neck, or impaired swallowing function. The health care team will discuss the potential risks of the procedure with the patient and his or her family or caregiver beforehand if the tracheostomy is not being performed as an emergent procedure.

Results: A tracheostomy can help the patient breathe more easily and allows the health care provider to clear secretions from the patient's breathing passages. In many cases, the tracheostomy is temporary and is removed when the patient is able to breathe without the help of a ventilator.

Angela M. Costello, B.S.

For Further Information

Cooper, Sue, ed. *Tracheostomy Care*. Hoboken, N.J.: John Wiley & Sons, 2006.

Lewarski, Joseph. "Management of the Tracheostomy Patient in the Home." *RT for Decision Makers in Respiratory Care*, August, 2006. Available online at http://www.rtmagazine.com.

Pierson, D. J., S. K. Epstein, C. G. Durbin, Jr., et al. "Twentieth Annual New Horizons Symposium: Tracheostomy from A to Z." *Respiratory Care* 50 (2005): 473-549.

See also: Infection and sepsis; Laryngeal cancer; Laryngeal nerve palsy; Laryngectomy

▶ Transfusion therapy

Category: Procedures

Also known as: Blood transfusion, red cell transfusion, platelet transfusion, plasma transfusion, cryoprecipitate transfusion, granulocyte transfusion

Definition: Transfusion therapy is the infusion of blood components.

Cancers treated: All

Why performed: Cancer patients may need transfusion of blood components because of the disease itself or as a result of cancer treatments. Some cancers, such as those of the digestive system, may cause loss of blood through internal bleeding. Patients with cancers affecting the production or storage of blood cells may need transfusion if blood counts become too low. Treatments such as chemotherapy and radiation may destroy enough cells that patients need transfusion. Patients having surgery for cancer may need blood to replace blood loss during the procedure.

Patient preparation: The physician admits the patient to an inpatient or outpatient facility. The physician discusses benefits and risks of transfusion with the patient or legal guardian and asks him or her to sign an informed consent for transfusion. Patients experiencing previous allergic reactions to blood components are given a pretransfusion medication such as diphendydramine (Benedryl).

Steps of the procedure: A phlebotomist collects a sample of blood. In some facilities, a special transfusion armband is placed on the patient's arm at the time that the blood sample is collected. Other facilities use the standard hospital patient armband for identification. The sample is sent to transfusion services.

Transfusion services staff test the sample to determine the patient's blood type. An antibody screening is also done to detect any unusual antibodies, proteins that may cause adverse reactions if the corresponding antigen is present on the donor cells. These antibodies may be naturally occurring, formed from exposure to a blood cell antigen during previous blood transfusions, or, in females, during childbirth. If unusual antibodies are present, then donor units that lack the corresponding antigen are used for transfusion. Transfusion services staff select appropriate components from storage. If the component is red cells, then a crossmatch is performed to ensure compatibility between the patient's serum and the donor red cells. Platelets, fresh frozen plasma, or cryoprecipitate do not need to be crossmatched. The selected components are tagged with the patient's name and identification number, the component unit number, blood type of the patient and the donor, results of antibody screening, and any special needs.

Special needs that the physician may order are leukoreduction and/or irradiation of cellular components (red cells and platelets). Leukoreduction is the removal of white cells, which decreases exposure to leukocyte antigens and cytomegalovirus (CMV). Irradiation is done to prevent graft-versus-host disease.

A nurse inserts an intravenous (IV) line into the patient's arm. Two nurses verify identification of the patient and that information on the component tag matches the patient and donor information. Before starting the transfusion, the nurse checks and records the patient's temperature, pulse, and blood pressure. During the first fifteen minutes of the transfusion, the nurse stays at the bedside and observes the patient for any signs of adverse reaction. At the end of fifteen minutes, the nurse again checks and records pulse, temperature, and blood pressure. Transfusion of blood components takes as little as fifteen minutes to as long as four hours, depending on the component and the rate of transfusion that the physician orders. At the end of the transfusion, the nurse again checks and records the pulse, temperature, and blood pressure, comparing them with the beginning rates. Changes that are greater than established standards at any time or adverse patient symptoms may result in stopping the transfusion. The physician reviews the information and may order a reaction workup.

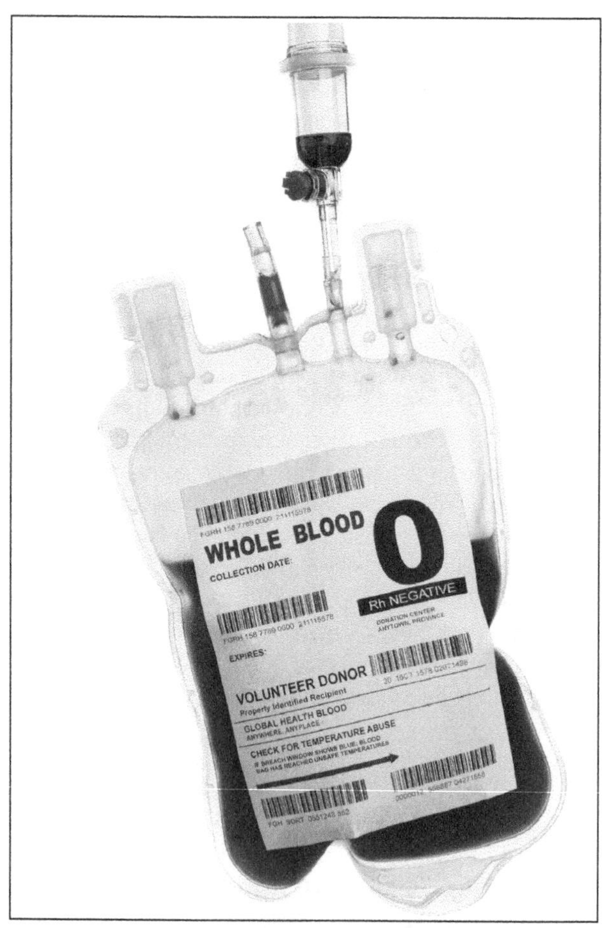

Cancer patients may require blood transfusions because of either the disease itself or cancer treatments. (iStock)

In the event of a reaction workup, any remaining component and the transfusion tubing are sent to transfusion services. A phlebotomist collects a new sample of blood and sends it to transfusion services. Nursing staff and transfusion services staff review all patient identification, paperwork, and donor information. Repeat testing is performed on pretransfusion and posttransfusion blood samples and the donor sample. Additional tests such as a culture for bacteria or other blood and chemistry tests may be done. A pathologist reviews the results of the transfusion reaction workup and determines the cause. The patient will not be transfused with additional components until the completion of the workup.

After the procedure: The IV line is removed. The nurse advises the patient about signs and symptoms to watch for and report. Blood samples may be collected to test for hemoglobin, platelet count, or clotting factors. If transfusion is done on an outpatient basis, then the patient may be discharged shortly after completion of the transfusion.

Risks: The risks of transfusion are allergic reactions, transmission of viruses or infectious diseases, fever iron overload, lung injury, acute hemolytic reaction, delayed hemolytic reaction, and graft-versus-host disease.

Results: Red cells are given to replace blood loss or correct anemia. Platelet transfusions are given to replace platelets to prevent bleeding. Plasma and cryoprecipitate are given to correct coagulation factors. Rarely, granulocytes are given to increase the white blood cell count.

Wanda E. Clark, M.T. (ASCP)

For Further Information

Abeloff, Martin D., et al. *Clinical Oncology*. 3d ed. Philadelphia: Churchill Livingstone Elsevier, 2004.

Klein, Harvey G., and David J. Anstee. *Mollison's Blood Transfusion in Clinical Medicine*. 11th ed. Malden, Mass.: Blackwell, 2005.

Other Resources

American Association of Blood Banks, America's Blood Centers, and the American Red Cross

Circular of Information for the Use of Human Blood and Blood Components

http://www.fda.gov/cber/gdlns/crclr.pdf

American Cancer Society

Why Cancer Patients Might Need Blood Product Transfusions

http://www.cancer.org/docroot/ETO/content/ETO_1_4x_Why_Cancer_Patients_Might_Need_Blood_Product_Transfusions.asp?sitearea=ETO

National Heart and Lung and Blood Institute Diseases and Conditions Index

What Is a Blood Transfusion?

http://www.nhlbi.nih.gov/health/dci/Diseases/bt/bt_whatis.html

See also: Anemia; Aplastic anemia; Autologous blood transfusion; Biological therapy; Blood cancers; Bone marrow aspiration and biopsy; Fanconi anemia; Hematemesis; Hematologic oncology; Hemochromatosis; Hemolytic anemia; Hepatitis B virus (HBV); Hepatitis C virus (HCV); Infusion therapies; Pathology; Risks for cancer

▶ Transrectal ultrasound

Category: Procedures
Also known as: Prostate sonography

Definition: Transrectal ultrasound is a procedure that uses ultrasonic waves to evaluate the prostate gland, primarily by acting as a guide for prostate biopsies.

Cancers diagnosed: Prostate cancer

Why performed: Since the sensitivity of transrectal ultrasound is only 60 to 70 percent for the detection of prostate cancer, it is not a screening test. Therefore, the primary role of transrectal ultrasound is to guide prostate biopsies. The sonographic appearance of prostate cancer is variable, with approximately 70 percent of cancer appearing hypoechoic (lower in density) compared to the peripheral zone. The remainder of prostate cancer can appear hyperechoic (higher in density) or a mixture of both and can be either nodular or infiltrative. Cystic cancer is rare. Although classically cancer of the prostate presents as a hypoechoic nodule in the peripheral zone, only 20 to 30 percent of such nodules actually represent cancer. Benign conditions that can be visualized on transrectal ultrasound include prostatitis, atrophy, fibrosis, infarct, and benign prostatic hyperplasia (BPH).

Patient preparation: The scan is usually performed as an outpatient procedure, and patients are not asked to perform any special preparation.

Steps of the procedure: The patient is placed on his side on a table, and the technologist or the radiologist applies a water-based conducting gel to the probe in order to study the organ or body part of interest, in this case the prostate gland. The transducer is designed to be inserted inside the rectum, and it may feel uncomfortable. The sonographer then rubs the handheld probe or transducer across the surface of the the prostate gland. There will be some discomfort from pressure, but the ultrasound waves themselves are painless.

After the procedure: The scan is generated by the computer attached to the ultrasound probe and read by the radiologist the same day. The patient will need to contact his doctor or health care provider for the radiology report and for any follow-up therapy,

Risks: The study is painless and relatively harmless, as no radiation is involved. Use of the transrectal probe is a decision made by the health care provider, not the sonographer or radiologist. The patient should consult his health care provider if he has any questions or concerns regarding use of the transrectal probe and talk to his health professional about any concerns regarding the need for the ultrasound, its risks, how it will be done, and what the results indicate.

Results: The results are dependent on the type of scan performed and the reason for the study. If evidence of cancer is found, additional tests will be ordered to confirm the diagnosis and suggest a course of treatment.

Debra B. Kessler, M.D., Ph.D.

See also: Benign Prostatic Hyperplasia (BPH); Endorectal ultrasound; Prostate cancer; Prostate-Ppecific Antigen (PSA) test; Prostatitis; Screening for cancer; Ultrasound tests

▶ Transvaginal ultrasound

Category: Procedures
Also known as: Transvaginal sonogram

Definition: Transvaginal ultrasound is a diagnostic procedure that uses an internal probe or transducer to enter the vagina.

Cancers diagnosed: Uterine, ovarian, and endometrial cancers; noncancerous fibroids

Why performed: Transvaginal ultrasound is a diagnostic procedure used to evaluate women with dysfunctional uterine bleeding to detect pelvic masses, ectopic pregnancy, and pelvic inflammatory disease. In postmenopausal women, the thickness of the endometrium is evaluated to check for overgrowth (hyperplasia) or cancer. Since the ovaries shrink after menopause, a gynecologist cannot feel them during a routine pelvic examination. The ovaries can be examined by transvaginal ultrasound.

Patient preparation: Little preparation is needed for the transvaginal ultrasound. The patient undresses from the waist down and lies face-up on the examination table. Either the patient will place her feet in stirrups or a bolster is placed under the hips to tilt the pelvis upward for insertion of the probe as well as the examination. The bladder is empty.

Steps of the procedure: Often the woman inserts the probe herself (similar to inserting a tampon). Warm gel is used to lubricate the probe. There may be slight pressure when the transducer is inserted. A transducer is used to transmit high-frequency sound waves, which bounce back to produce images that can be seen on a video monitor or recorded on X-ray film. There is no radiation exposure during transvaginal ultrasound, and the results are available immediately. The procedure is performed by a radiological technician or physician radiologist and read by a physician radiologist.

After the procedure: The patient can resume normal activities immediately. There may be a small amount of leakage from the gel used, which can be absorbed by using a sanitary pad.

Risks: No risks are associated with this procedure.

Results: The results of a transvaginal ultrasound may be normal or abnormal. Normal results mean that no abnormal areas are found in the uterus. It is normal in shape and size with no abnormal thickness, masses, or growths. Abnormal results include growths (masses or cysts) and unanticipated thickness. Because there is a risk of false positive results, abnormal findings should be evaluated and confirmed by magnetic resonance imaging (MRI) or biopsy.

Marcia J. Weiss, J.D.

See also: Endometrial cancer; Gynecologic cancers; Hereditary Leiomyomatosis and Renal Cell Cancer (HLRCC); Imaging tests; Pelvic examination; Ultrasound tests; Uterine cancer

▶ Tumor markers

Category: Procedures

Also known as: Biomarkers, cancer markers, tumor-associated antigens, tumor-specific antigens

Definition: Tumor markers are molecules whose presence or abnormal concentration in body fluids or tissue samples is associated with malignancy. They are most often individual, well-characterized proteins or nucleic acids. Increasingly, multiple tumor markers are interpreted in combination.

Cancers identified: Many, notably prostate, ovarian, and gastrointestinal cancers

How tumor markers are used: Tumor markers have been sought for every type of cancer, and tumor-marker determinations can be used in several contexts. In risk assessment, mutations in the *BRCA1* and *BRCA2* genes confer an increased risk of breast and ovarian cancer, and mutations in the *APC* gene are associated with increased colorectal cancer risk. Knowledge of increased risk can motivate more frequent screening procedures or more aggressive treatment decisions if cancer is eventually diagnosed.

In early detection efforts, three serum tumor markers are widely used:

- Cancer antigen 125 (CA 125) for ovarian cancer
- Carcinoembryonic antigen (CEA) for gastrointestinal cancer
- Prostate-specific antigen (PSA) for prostate cancer

Because of the need for very high specificity, only one tumor marker (PSA) is recommended for screening of asymptomatic individuals; most early detection efforts focus on clinical and radiological findings. In diagnostic confirmation procedures, markers such as alpha-methylacyl-CoA racemase (AMACR) can be interrogated on biopsy specimens; the presence of AMACR in prostate tissue helps rule out benign mimickers of prostate cancer. In molecular classification efforts, tumor markers can resolve different types of cancer that might otherwise be misdiagnosed. Four malignancies appearing histologically as small round blue cell tumors—neuroblastoma, non-Hodgkin lymphoma, rhabdomyosarcoma, and Ewing sarcoma—fall into this category; tumor markers are needed to distinguish among them.

Therapy selection can also be guided by tumor markers, such as the ABCB1 (more commonly known as MDR1) protein and the estrogen and progesterone receptors (ER/PR). Low levels of MDR1 correlate with better response to treatment in ovary and lung cancer patients, whereas presence of the ER/PR tumor marker in advanced breast cancer patients correlates with a high response rate to endocrine ablation. Breast cancer patients whose tumors overexpress the HER2/neu (also known as ERBB2, c-erb-B2) protein are another important subgroup identified by tumor-marker analysis, since these patients are uniquely appropriate for therapy with anti-HER2-based therapies such as trastuzumab. Tumor-marker concentrations often correlate with tumor burden or activity, providing information on the effectiveness of treatment. Rapid normalization of serum CA 125 levels following ovarian cancer treatment, for example, has favorable prognostic significance.

The next important application of tumor markers is in long-term follow-up of patients with previously diagnosed and treated cancer, because early detection of recurrent or metastatic disease can hasten intervention and improve outcome. The tumor markers CA 15-3 (breast), CEA (colorectal), CA 125 (ovary), and PSA (prostate) are used in this context.

Finally, scientists performing cancer research are seeking improved diagnostic assays and clues to novel therapies; tumor markers are an integral part of these efforts. Overexpression of fatty acid synthase, for example, was noted in several types of tumors; subsequent efforts to inhibit the enzyme demonstrated this to be a promising therapeutic modality.

Significant barriers exist to more extensive use of tumor markers in oncology. Primarily, the clinical value of the marker must be proven; that is, the result should trigger or remand a treatment decision that benefits patients, this benefit must be demonstrated in a large and rigorous trial, and the benefits must outweigh the costs of implementation and follow-up. After this is accomplished, oncologists must be convinced of the need to change their established practices by incorporating the marker.

Data analysis: After the appropriate material is obtained from the patient, several options exist for tumor-marker determination and data analysis. The method for tumor-marker quantification depends both on the marker and on the specimen; the method of analysis depends largely on the form and amount of data present.

Serum protein markers are typically measured with specific antibody-based assays. A popular immunoassay format is the enzyme-linked immunosorbent assay (ELISA), which provides a numerical readout of the marker's concentration. Protein markers can also be determined in tissue biopsy slices or individual cells by immunohistochemistry (IHC) or immunocytochemistry (ICC). In contrast to the ELISA, samples analyzed by IHC or ICC must be assessed visually for an estimate of tumor-marker abundance. However, IHC and ICC allow precise localization of the tumor marker within the cell. IHC and ICC are appropriate for tumor markers that are not shed into the extracellular space. Enzymes such as lactate dehydrogenase are sometimes employed as tumor markers; their concentration is inferred from their catalytic activity. Highly complex protein mixtures present in body fluids such as serum or urine can be analyzed by protein chips coupled with surface-enhanced laser desorption ionization/time-of-flight mass spectrometry (SELDI/TOF-MS). In this case, the relative abundance of hundreds to thousands of proteins in a sample is determined in a single run.

Tumor markers that are products expressed by genes (messenger ribonucleic acid, or mRNA, molecules) can be measured by the reverse transcriptase polymerase chain reaction (RT-PCR) or on a larger scale by oligonucleotide microarrays. In reverse transcriptase polymerase chain reaction, the mRNA sample is first reverse-transcribed into deoxyribonucleic acid (DNA), then amplified by standard polymerase chain reaction. Relative quantification is achieved by monitoring the abundance of the polymerase chain reaction products spectrophotometrically during the thermal cycling process. Messenger RNA-based tumor-marker assays can estimate the risk of breast cancer recurrence in women who are diagnosed with Stage I or II hormone-responsive cancer that has not spread to the surrounding lymph nodes. In this setting, the abundance of multiple different transcripts in breast tumor tissue is determined by reverse transcriptase polymerase chain reaction.

Tumor markers that exist as mutated or disrupted genes can be analyzed by several methods. Chromosomes can be inspected microscopically to confirm changes in genomic DNA. For example, abnormal amplification of *MYCB* (also known as *N-myc*) in neuroblastoma can be visualized as a homogenous staining region on chromosome 2p. Other tumor risk markers, such as mutated *APC*, can be detected through DNA sequencing or single-strand conformational polymorphism.

Tumor markers that exist as small organic compounds such as 5-hydroxyindoleacetic acid (carcinoid tumors) are measured with chemical techniques such as high-performance liquid chromatography.

Results: Numerical results (concentrations) for single tumor markers can be interpreted only with knowledge of the marker's normal concentration range and its sensitivity, specificity, and positive and negative predictive value for the tumor type in question. Also essential are knowledge of the tumor's prevalence and the patient's clinical history. Serial tumor-marker determinations offer additional information by demonstrating the rate of the tumor marker's increase or decrease. In the case of PSA, a short time to doubling may prompt more concern than higher levels that remain steady. No single tumor marker reaches the ideal standards of 100 percent sensitivity and specificity. Many proposed tumor markers are ultimately rejected by practitioners because of unacceptably low sensitivity or specificity.

Results from multiplexed assays consist of patterns of individual data points that can yield more biologically relevant and clinically useful information than single markers. Analysis requires sophisticated and sometimes proprietary pattern-matching algorithms. Protein chips coupled with SELDI/TOF-MS, for example, have identified tumor-marker patterns that correctly classified individuals with and without early-stage ovarian cancer with high sensitivity and specificity. Gene expression chips (oligonucleotide microarrays) have also shown remarkable accuracy in identifying the primary sites of poorly differentiated metastatic lesions. Test results are highly reproducible and provide information to aid the physician and patient in making treatment decisions.

John B. Welsh, M.D., Ph.D.

For Further Information

Bigbee W., and R. B. Herberman. "Tumor Markers and Immunodiagnosis." In *Cancer Medicine*, edited by James F. Holland and Emil Frei. 6th ed. Hamilton, Ont.: BC Decker, 2003.

Diamandis, E. P., et al., eds. *Tumor Markers: Physiology, Pathobiology, Technology, and Clinical Applications*. Washington, D.C.: AACC Press, 2002.

Hartwell, L., et al. "Cancer Biomarkers: A Systems Approach." *Nature Biotechnology* 24 (2006): 905-908.

Nakamura, R. M., et al., eds. *Cancer Diagnostics: Current and Future Trends*. Totowa, N.J.: Humana Press, 2004.

Perkins, G. L., et al. "Serum Tumor Markers." *American Family Physician* 68 (2003): 1075-1082.

Petricoin, E. F., et al. "Use of Proteomic Patterns in Serum to Identify Ovarian Cancer." *Lancet* 359 (2002): 572-577.

Taube, S. E., et al. "Cancer Diagnostics: Decision Criteria for Marker Utilization in the Clinic." *American Journal of Pharmacogenomics* 5 (2005): 357-364.

Other Resources

Lab Tests Online

Tumor Markers

http://www.labtestsonline.org/understanding/analytes/tumor_markers/glance.html

National Cancer Institute

Tumor Markers: Questions and Answers

http://www.cancer.gov/cancertopics/factsheet/Detection/tumor-markers

See also: Alpha-Fetoprotein (AFP) levels; Bone cancers; CA 15-3 test; CA 19-9 test; CA 27-29 test; CA 125 test; Carcinoembryonic Antigen antibody (CEA) test; Carcinomas; Embryonal cell cancer; Endocrine cancers; Germ-cell tumors; Gynecologic oncology; Lactate Dehydrogenase (LDH) test; Liver cancers; Malignant tumors; Neuroendocrine tumors; Placental Alkaline Phosphatase (PALP); Proteomics and cancer research; Testicular cancer; TNM staging

▶ Ultrasound tests

Category: Procedures
Also known as: Sonogram, echogram

Definition: An ultrasound test is a type of radiologic study that utilizes sound waves to detect an abnormality in an organ of the body under evaluation using a principle similar to sonar used in ship navigation. Ultrasound waves are mechanical pressure waves that occur at a higher frequency compared to audible sound waves, hence the name ultrasound. These high-frequency sound waves reflect off body surfaces and structures. Different tissues in the body have different acoustic velocities or speeds of sound propagating through them. The time that it takes for a pulsed sound wave to travel from a transducer to a reflector and back again can be measured and then, along with the known acoustic velocity of a tissue, can be used to calculate their separation and thus the depth from the skin surface of the organ or organ part under study. Bone, for example, has a higher acoustic velocity than soft tissue. One would expect higher-amplitude echoes from soft tissue-bone interfaces and lower-amplitude reflection or echoes from soft tissue-soft tissue interfaces because of the almost matched acoustic velocities among the latter.

The ultrasound transducer converts the amplitude of the mechanical energy received from the organ under study into an electrical signal and vice versa. The emitting and receiving element of an ultrasound transducer is a piezoelectric crystal. The electrical signals from the transducer are fed into a computer, and an image is produced that can be stored on compact disc (CD), printed on film, or viewed on a computer monitor by the sonographer and the radiologist, who is ultimately responsible for the quality and interpretation of the study.

Cancers diagnosed: Breast, thyroid, testicular, uterine, ovarian, prostate, renal (kidney), bladder, gallbladder, liver, spleen, and pancreatic cancers; cancers associated with pregnancy, such as gestational trophoblastic disease; unsuspected adenopathy often detected as an incidental finding during ultrasound examination, especially during examination of the thyroid, breast, and abdomen

Why performed: Ultrasound is used to diagnose primary cancers, both benign and malignant, as well as secondary cancers (also known as metastases). It is also used to diagnose ailments depending on the patient's symptoms, including but not limited to the following: right-upper-quadrant abdominal pain caused by acute and chronic cholecystitis (both calculus and acalculus) and postoperative leaks following cholecystectomy (gallbladder and right-upper-quadrant ultrasound); goiter, Hashimoto's thyroiditis, and ectopic parathyroid (thyroid ultrasound); mastitis and Paget disease of the breast (breast ultrasound); pain in the right lower quadrant of the abdomen caused by appendicitis (ultrasound of the appendix); scrotal pain caused by testicular torsion, testicular trauma, orchitis, epididymitis, and hydrocele, as well as undescended testes (testicular ultrasound); pain in the back caused by kidney stones, kidney obstruction, or infection (renal ultrasound); pain and swelling in the legs caused by deep venous thrombosis (DVT study); pain in the epigastric area caused by pancreatitis (abdominal ultrasound); pain in the left upper abdomen caused by splenic infarct or splenic trauma (abdominal ultrasound); pain in the right upper quadrant caused by liver trauma, liver infection, or liver cysts and evaluation for the presence of ascites (abdominal ultrasound); valvular heart disease (cardiac ultrasound or echocardiography); atherosclerosis of the lower-extremity arteries, abdominal aortic aneurysm, and carotid artery atherosclerosis (vascular or arterial Doppler ultrasound); and polycystic ovarian syndrome or pelvic pain and/or bleeding caused by ovarian torsion, uterine polyps, uterine fibroids, and retained products of conception (pelvic and transvaginal ultrasound).

In addition, pregnancy in all three trimesters is evaluated by ultrasound. Ultrasound is also useful in guiding amniocentesis for evaluation of possible fetal anomalies such as Down syndrome (trisomy 21) involving sampling of fluid surrounding the fetus; sampling and removal of fluid from various body cavities in the adult, such as the lung (pleural effusion tap) and abdominal cavity (ascites); and guiding biopsy of various organs in the adult, such as liver, breast, thyroid, and kidney.

Patient preparation: Patients are asked to fast at least four to eight hours prior to gallbladder ultrasound, as food causes the gallbladder to contract and minimizes the area visible for the ultrasound evaluation. Patients are asked to drink at least four glasses of water at least one half hour prior to pelvic ultrasound in order to distend the bladder, which acts as an acoustic window for the study (sound travels well through water). This enables the sonographer, usually a technologist, to evaluate the baby and the womb during pregnancy and to evaluate the state of the uterus, cervix, and ovaries in both the pregnant and the nonpregnant state.

Steps of the procedure: The patient is placed on the back on a table, and the technologist and/or the radiologist applies a clear, water-based conducting gel to the skin over the organ or body part of interest. The gel helps in the transmission of sound waves and may feel wet and cold. The sonographer then rubs a handheld probe or transducer across the surface of the organ of interest. There will be some discomfort from pressure on a full bladder, but the ultrasound waves themselves are painless. Some transducers are designed to be inserted inside a body cavity, such as a transvaginal probe or transrectal probe, which may feel uncomfortable.

After the procedure: The scan is generated by the computer attached to the ultrasound probe and read by the radiologist the same day. The patient will need to contact his or her doctor or health care provider for the radiology report and for follow-up therapy.

Risks: The study is painless and relatively harmless, as no radiation is involved; transvaginal ultrasound is generally done early in a pregnancy to determine fetal age or to detect a suspected ectopic pregnancy. Use of the transvaginal probe late in pregnancy is a decision made by the health care provider, not the sonographer or radiologist.

Results: The results are dependent on the type of scan performed and the reason for the study. Some ultrasound tests are screening tests and may be normal, while others are ordered by a health care provider when an abnormality is suspected.

Debra B. Kessler, M.D., Ph.D.

For Further Information

Bushong, Stewart C. *Diagnostic Ultrasound.* New York: McGraw-Hill, 1999.

Curry, Thomas S., III, James E. Dowdey, and Robert C. Murry, Jr. *Christensen's Physics of Diagnostic Radiology.* 4th ed. Philadelphia: Lea & Febiger, 1990.

Rumak, Carole M., S. R. Wilson, and J. W. Charboneau. *Diagnostic Ultrasound.* St. Louis: Mosby-Year Book, 1991.

See also: Breast ultrasound; Endorectal ultrasound; Pregnancy and cancer; Screening for cancer; Transrectal ultrasound; Transvaginal ultrasound

▶ Umbilical cord blood transplantation

Category: Procedures
Also known as: Cord blood transplantation

Definition: Umbilical cord blood is the blood that remains in the umbilical cord and placenta soon after an infant is born. Instead of discarding the umbilical cord as medical waste, the cord blood can be collected as a rich source of hematopoietic (blood-forming) stem cells and stored in a private or public blood bank for future use. Umbilical cord blood transplantation is the infusion of the cord blood stem cells into a recipient for the treatment of a malignant or non-malignant hematologic (blood-based) disease.

Cancers treated: Acute and Chronic Leukemias, Non-Hodgkin and Hodgkin Lymphoma, Myeloma, Neuroblastoma, Other Diseases Treated: Sickle Cell Disease, Bone Marrow Failure Syndromes, Metabolic Disorders, Immunodeficiency Syndromes

Why performed: Under circumstances in which the hematopoietic stem cells of the bone marrow are malfunctioning, due to a malignant disease or non-malignant condition, properly functioning stem cells from a healthy donor can be administered to replace these malfunctioning cells. The healthy hematopoietic stem cells can be transplanted into the recipient after obliterating the malfunctioning cells from the recipient's bone marrow and body, using chemotherapy and/or radiation. While stem cells from adult bone marrow or peripheral blood can be used to replace malfunctioning cells, umbilical cord blood stem cells have become increasingly utilized as an alternative stem cell source for transplantation.

Umbilical cord blood transplantation may be chosen for treatment due to the accessibility and availability of cord blood grafts. For patients with an urgent need of a stem cell transplant, cryopreserved cord blood (frozen in liquid nitrogen) is quickly accessible for treatment. Additionally, a greater degree of genetic mismatch between the donor and recipient can be tolerated in umbilical cord blood transplantation, rather than in bone marrow or peripheral blood transplantation, due to the immunologically naïve nature of the lymphocytes present in an infant's cord blood. Thus, suitable cord blood donors are widely available for all patients, including those who may have difficulty finding a related or unrelated adult stem cell donor. For example, some ethnic or racial minorities may only have a 16-19% probability of finding a matched adult donor due to the presence of specific genetic polymorphisms (natural variations in genes). However, the same patients have an 88-99% chance of finding a suitable cord blood donor, making umbilical cord blood transplantation a desirable treatment option.

Patient preparation: Patient Preparation: Prior to umbilical cord blood transplantation, the patient undergoes a preparative myeloablative or non-myeloablative conditioning regimen to rid the bone marrow and body of the malfunctioning cells. Myeloablative conditioning utilizes a more toxic chemotherapy cocktail and total body irradiation (TBI) regimen used to destroy all of the stem cells in the bone marrow and lymphocytes circulating throughout the body. Myeloablative conditioning may be too toxic for older patients (>55 years old) or patients with multiple health problems. In such cases, the patient may undergo non-myeloablative (reduced-intensity) conditioning to only suppress the bone marrow and immune system, rather than destroy it, prior to umbilical cord blood transplantation.

Before transplantation, confirmatory human leukocyte antigen (HLA)-typing is also performed at three to eight genetic loci on the recipient and potential cord blood donor units to find a suitably matched graft. Human leukocyte antigens are the genetic fingerprints of an individual's cells that recognize and initiate an immune response against foreign cells. Cord blood donors with a minimum 4/6 or 5/8 HLA-match to the recipient are typically chosen for umbilical cord blood transplantation.

Another important aspect to consider prior to umbilical cord blood transplantation is the total nucleated cell (TNC) dose of the potential donor units. A cord blood unit usually contains approximately 10% of the number of stem cells found in a bone marrow or peripheral blood transplant. Therefore, a single cord blood unit is often insufficient for larger adolescents or adults. However, under circumstances in which a single cord blood unit does not contain a sufficient TNC dose, two cord blood units from completely different donors can be transplanted into a single patient in a procedure known as "double cord blood transplantation."

Steps of Procedure: After suitable cord blood units have been selected and the patient has undergone an appropriate conditioning regimen, the patient is prepared for the umbilical cord blood transplantation procedure. "Day 0" of the process is defined as the day the patient actually receives the infusion of cord blood stem cells. After being thawed, the stem cells are administered to the patient using a peripherally inserted central venous catheter (PICC). Patients often receive blood transfusions in conjunction with the cord blood transplant because their red blood cell count will remain depleted until engraftment occurs.

After Procedure: After the umbilical cord blood transplant, the patient is monitored for engraftment; i.e., when the donor stem cells migrate to the bone marrow and begin differentiating into erythrocytes, leukocytes, and platelets. In the clinical setting, engraftment is denoted by an absolute neutrophil count (ANC) of 500/µl or greater for three consecutive days and a platelet count of 20,000-50,000/µl. Routine complete blood count (CBC) tests are performed on the patient's blood during the post-transplant period to track the patient's progress. It takes an average of 21 to 35 days for neutrophil engraftment to occur and as long as 8 weeks post-transplant for platelet engraftment. For double cord blood transplant recipients, chimerism will also be studied because one of the two cord blood grafts usually becomes the dominant unit that repopulates the patient's bone marrow.

Risks: Prior to engraftment, patients are at high risk for life-threatening nosocomial (hospital-derived) infections due to the immunosuppression caused by the conditioning regimen. Until platelet engraftment occurs, the patient is also at risk for hemorrhages in mucus membranes, such as the lungs or eyes. After transplantation, graft-vs.-host disease (GVHD) is another potentially life-threatening risk. GVHD occurs when the donor stem cells recognize the transplant recipient's cells as foreign and initiate an immune response against the recipient's tissues. Umbilical cord blood transplant patients may experience GVHD in the form of skin rashes, gastrointestinal irritation, and/or abnormal liver function. Although, the engraftment period is extended for cord blood transplant recipients, several studies have shown that umbilical cord blood transplantation has a lower incidence of GVHD than bone marrow or peripheral blood stem cell transplantation.

Results: The desired result of umbilical cord blood transplantation is remission of cancer or cure of the non-malignant condition. For double cord blood transplant recipients, another potential outcome is mixed chimerism in which a dominant cord blood donor is not established, but both donors engraft and are expressed in the patient's new immune system. In some circumstances, a patient may experience graft-failure in which the donor stem cells never migrate to the bone marrow and begin differentiating. Unfortunately, patients may relapse after umbilical cord blood transplantation and require additional therapy.

Wanda Todd Bradshaw
Updated by: Paige E. Albert, B.S.

For Further Information

Cornetta K., Lauglin M., Carter S., Wall D., Weinthal, J., Delaney, C., ... Chao, N. (2005). Umbilical cord blood transplantation in adults: Results of the prospective cord blood transplantation (COBLT). *Biology of Blood and Marrow Transplantation,* 11(2), 149-160.

Diaconescu R., Flowers C., Storer B., Sorror, M. L., Maris, M. B., Maloney, D. G. ... Storb, R. (2004). Morbidity and mortality with nonmyeloablative compared with myeloablative conditioning before hematopoietic cell transplantation from HLA-matched related donors. *Blood,* 104(5), 1550-1558.

Eapen M., Klein J., Ruggeri A., Spellman S., Lee, S. J., Anasetti, C., ... Center for International Blood and Marrow Transplant Research, Netcord, Eurocord, and the European Group for Blood and Marrow Transplantation. (2014). Impact of allele-level HLA matching on outcomes after myeloablative single unit umbilical cord Blood transplantation for hematologic malignancy. *Blood,* 123(1), 133-140.

Gragert, L., Eapen, M., Williams, E., Freeman, J., Spellman, S., Baitty, R., ... Maiers, M. (2014). HLA match likelihoods for hematopoietic stem-cell grafts in U.S. registry. *The New England Journal of Medicine,* 371(4), 339-348.

Stavropoulos-Giokas C. & Papassavas, A. (2012). The role of HLA in cord blood transplantation. *Bone Marrow Research,* 2012, doi:10.1155/2012/485160.

Van Deerlin V. & Reshef R. (2016). Chimerism testing in allogeneic hematopoietic stem cell transplantation. In Debra G.B. Leonard (Ed.), *Molecular Pathology in Clinical Practice* (pp. 823-848). New York, NY: Springer.

Yap Y.S., Karapetis C., Lerose S., Iyer S., & Koczwara B. (2006). Reducing the risk of peripherally inserted central catheter line complications in the oncology setting. *European Journal of Cancer,* 15, 342-347.

Other Resources

UW Health – Blood and Bone Marrow Transplant: Double Cord Blood Transplantation
http://www.uwhealth.org/blood-and-bone-marrow-transplant/double-cord-blood-transplantation/31899

Seattle Cancer Care Alliance - Improving Cord Blood Transplants
http://www.seattlecca.org/diseases/improving-cord-blood-transplants.cfm

See also: Acute Lymphocytic leukemia (ALL); Bone marrow aspiration and biopsy; Bone Marrow Transplantation (BMT); Chemotherapy; Chronic Lymphocytic Leukemia (CLL); Chronic Myeloid Leukemia (CML); Graft-Versus-Host Disease (GVHD); Leukemias; Lymphomas; Myeloma; Stem cell transplantation

▶ Upper Gastrointestinal (GI) endoscopy

Category: Procedures
Also known as: Esophagogastroduodenoscopy (EGD)

Definition: An upper gastrointestinal (GI) endoscopy is a diagnostic procedure in which a thin tube with a light and camera is inserted into the throat to evaluate the inside of the esophagus, stomach, and first part of the small intestine (duodenum).

Cancers treated: Esophageal cancer, gastric (stomach) cancer, duodenal cancer

Why performed: An upper endoscopy helps identify the cause of unexplained abdominal or chest pain, nausea and vomiting, heartburn, bleeding, and swallowing disorders. It can evaluate tumors, ulcers, and areas of inflammation.

Patient preparation: Patients who have heart valve disease, rheumatic heart disease, and some other cardiovascular conditions may need to take an antibiotic before the procedure to reduce the risk of infection. Patients must not eat solid foods for eight hours before the procedure, but clear liquids may be allowed until a few hours before the procedure, depending on the specific guidelines of the testing center. Before the procedure, an assessment of the patient's health history is conducted, and the potential risks of the procedure will be discussed.

Steps of the procedure: The patient will change into a hospital gown. An intravenous (IV) line is inserted into a vein in the patient's arm to deliver medications. A blood pressure cuff is placed on the patient's arm to monitor blood pressure, a small clip placed on the patient's finger is attached to an oximeter monitor to check the patient's blood oxygen level, and the patient's pulse is monitored during the procedure.

The patient lies on the left side during the procedure. A sedative is given (conscious or moderate sedation), so the patient is awake but relaxed and able to respond to the physician's instructions during the procedure. A pain-relieving medication is infused in the IV, and a local anesthetic is applied via a spray at the back of the patient's throat to numb it and reduce the natural gag reflex. A mouthpiece is placed in the patient's mouth through which the endoscope is passed. The physician may ask the patient to swallow several times to help pass the endoscope down the throat to the stomach. An endoscope is a long, thin, lighted flexible instrument with a camera on the end that transmits images of the esophagus, stomach, and duodenum onto a video monitor to guide the physician during the procedure. The procedure lasts from twenty to thirty minutes.

If an abnormality such as a polyp or lesion is found during the procedure, then instruments can be inserted through the endoscope to remove it. Tissue samples (biopsy) can be removed through the endoscope. If bleeding is found during the procedure, then a sclerosing agent can be injected or another instrument can be inserted through the endoscope to stop the bleeding.

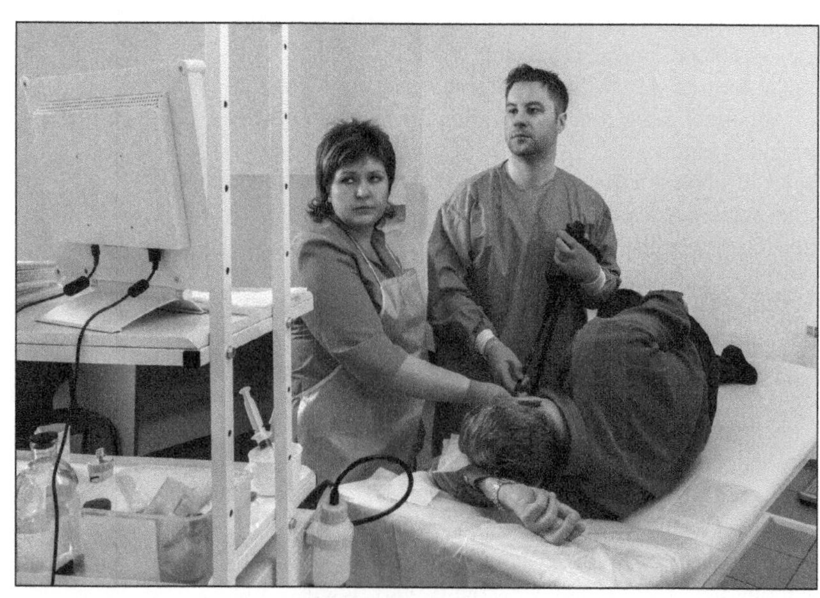

A physician performs an upper gastrointestinal endoscopy. (iStock)

After the procedure: The patient is observed in a recovery room for one to two hours as he or she recovers from the effects of the sedation. The patient will receive home-going instructions from the nurse, including diet restrictions and medication and activity guidelines. The patient should not drive or operate machinery for eight hours after the procedure and should avoid vigorous physical activity after the procedure, as directed by the physician. The patient may have temporary throat soreness for a few days after the procedure, which can be relieved with throat lozenges. If a polyp or tissue sample was removed, then the patient may need to avoid aspirin and products containing aspirin, ibuprofen, and anticoagulants for one week. The physician will provide specific guidelines. Within seventy-two hours after the procedure, the patient should call the physician if he or she experiences severe abdominal pain, black or bloody stools, a continuous cough, fever, chills, chest pain, nausea, or vomiting.

Risks: Complications associated with an upper endoscopy procedure are rare but may include bleeding and puncture of the stomach lining. The risk of complications associated with the sedation given during the procedure is also rare, occurring in less than 1 in every 10,000 people, according to the American College of Gastroenterology. In general, most patients experience only a mild sore throat after the procedure.

Results: If the results of the test indicate that prompt treatment is needed, then the physician will discuss the treatment options with the patient and his or her family and the necessary arrangements will be made. The abnormal tissue or biopsy sample is sent for analysis in the laboratory to determine if there is a malignancy. If bleeding in the stomach lining or duodenum is found, then a peptic or duodenal ulcer may be diagnosed and a proton pump inhibitor or H_2 antagonist medication may be prescribed. Barrett esophagus (a condition that increases the risk of esophageal cancer) is revealed by upper endoscopy in up to 5 percent of high-risk patients with gastroesophageal reflux disease (GERD), according to the American College of Gastroenterology.

When the laboratory results are available within two to three days, the physician will notify the patient with the results. If another physician referred the patient for the procedure, then he or she will also receive a copy of the results.

Angela M. Costello, B.S.

For Further Information

Cohen, J., et al. "Quality Indicators for Esophagogastroduodenoscopy." *American Journal of Gastroenterology* 101 (2006): 886-891.

Faigel, D. O., et al. "Quality Indicators for Gastrointestinal Endoscopic Procedures: An Introduction." *American Journal of Gastroenterology* 101 (2006): 866-872.

Other Resources

American College of Gastroenterology
http://www.acg.gi.org

American Gastroenterological Association
http://gastro.org

American Society for Gastrointestinal Endoscopy
http://www.askasge.org

International Foundation for Functional Gastrointestinal Disorders
http://www.iffgd.org

National Digestive Diseases Clearinghouse, National Institute of Diabetes and Digestive and Kidney Diseases
http://digestive.niddk.nih.gov/index.htm

See also: Barrett esophagus; Duodenal carcinomas; Endoscopy; Esophageal cancer; Gastrointestinal complications of cancer treatment; Gastrointestinal oncology; *Helicobacter pylori*; Infection and sepsis; Nausea and vomiting; Small intestine cancer

▶ Upper Gastrointestinal (GI) series

Category: Procedures
Also known as: Barium swallow, upper GI and small bowel series

Definition: An upper gastrointestinal (GI) series is a radiographic examination of the upper digestive tract, including the esophagus, stomach, and small intestine. Moving X-ray images of the digestive tract are produced with a fluoroscopy machine.

Cancers diagnosed: Esophageal, gastric, duodenal, and laryngeal cancers

Why performed: An upper GI series helps identify structural or functional abnormalities of the upper digestive tract, including a tumor in these organs, hiatal hernia, narrowing of the esophagus, esophageal muscle disorders, esophageal varices (enlarged veins), gastroesophageal reflux disease (GERD), achalasia, ulcers, strictures, polyps, diverticula, some causes of intestinal inflammation, and certain swallowing disorders. It also may be performed to determine the cause of frequent heartburn or unexplained abdominal pain.

Patient preparation: Specific dietary restrictions may be given to be followed for a few days before the procedure. A laxative may need to be taken the day before the procedure to clear the digestive tract. Patients must not eat or drink anything or smoke after midnight the night before the procedure. In most cases, the patient can continue taking regularly scheduled medications, but they must be taken with small sips of water. Patients with diabetes should ask how to adjust their meal plans, insulin, or other diabetes medications in preparation for the test. Patients should tell the physician if they are allergic or sensitive to contrast dyes, certain medications, iodine, shellfish, or latex. Female patients should tell the physician if they are pregnant or think they might be pregnant; this test is not advised for pregnant women, so another test may be recommended.

Steps of the procedure: The patient will change into a hospital gown. The X-ray technician will first take a regular X ray of the stomach and abdomen. A medication may be injected into a vein in the patient's arm to temporarily slow bowel movement. The patient is asked to drink 16 to 20 ounces of a barium solution that coats the lining of the esophagus, stomach, and duodenum to allow these organs to be seen on the X rays. Using a fluoroscope, a radiologist passes a continuous X-ray beam through the part of the digestive system being examined, and detailed pictures of the organ and its motion are transmitted on a monitor as the barium moves through the digestive system. The patient will be asked to hold his or her breath as each picture is taken so that the movement of breathing does not interfere with the images. The patient may be lying on a table or standing during the test and will be asked to turn in different positions as the barium moves through the digestive system. In some cases, the table may move to tilt the patient in different positions. The patient may be asked to swallow a "fizzy" tablet that produces air bubbles in the stomach. After the fluoroscopy part of the test, another regular X ray is taken of the stomach and abdomen. The procedure lasts about one to two hours, including the barium preparation time.

After the procedure: The patient will receive homegoing instructions from the nurse, including diet restrictions and medication and activity guidelines. The patient can go home right after the procedure and resume regular activities and diet, unless otherwise instructed by the physician. The patient should increase the intake of fluids and high-fiber foods to help flush the barium. The patient will pass what remains of the barium during the next few days after the procedure, and the stool may be light-colored or white. If constipation occurs after the procedure, then the patient should ask his or her doctor about taking a laxative. The patient should call the physician if he or she experiences abdominal pain within twenty-four hours after the procedure or constipation for more than two days after the procedure.

Risks: There are no significant risks of the upper GI series. There is a low exposure of radiation during the test, but the amount of radiation is minimal and not likely to cause any health problems. The patient may find the taste of the barium solution unpleasant and may experience constipation after the procedure.

Results: Normal values indicate that there are no structural abnormalities found on the upper GI examination. The physician will notify the patient within two to three days about the test results after the radiologist has reviewed the fluoroscopy films. If a structural or functional problem was identified during the procedure, then the physician will discuss the appropriate treatment options with the patient. If another physician referred the patient for the procedure, then he or she will receive a copy of the test results.

Angela M. Costello, B.S.

For Further Information

Allen, J. I., et al. "Best Practices: Community-Based Gastroenterology Practices." *Clinical Gastroenterology and Hepatology* 4 (2006): 292-295.

McPhee, Stephen J., Maxine A. Papadakis, and Lawrence M. Tierney, eds. *Current Medical Diagnosis and Treatment*, 2008. New York: McGraw-Hill Medical, 2007.

Other Resources

American College of Gastroenterology
http://www.acg.gi.org

American Gastroenterological Association
http://gastro.org

American Society for Gastrointestinal Endoscopy
http://www.askasge.org

International Foundation for Functional Gastrointestinal Disorders
http://www.iffgd.org

National Digestive Diseases Clearinghouse, National Institute of Diabetes and Digestive and Kidney Diseases
http://digestive.niddk.nih.gov/index.htm

See also: Barium swallow; Cobalt 60 radiation; Colon polyps; Duodenal carcinomas; Endoscopy; Fiber; Gastrointestinal oncology; Imaging tests; Laryngeal cancer; Laryngeal nerve palsy; Laxatives; Polyps; Pregnancy and cancer; Risks for cancer; Small intestine cancer; X-ray tests

▶ Urinalysis

Category: Procedures
Also known as: UA, routine urinalysis, complete urinalysis

Definition: A routine complete urinalysis is the physical, chemical, and microscopic examination of the urine and a comprehensive overview of kidney function.

Cancers diagnosed: While urinalysis is the most cost effective and least invasive evaluation of kidney and urinary tract function, it is not a screening method for the detection of cancer. Suspicious cells may be seen, however, upon microscopic review of the urine sediment and forwarded for cytological examination and further pathology review to rule out cancer of the bladder or kidney.

Why performed: Urinalysis is the single most important evaluation of kidney function. It may detect urinary tract infections, systemic diseases such as diabetes mellitus, glomerulonephritis, and malignancy.

Patient preparation: First morning voided urine of a minimum of 10 milliliters is the preferred specimen for a urinalysis. A random urine sample taken at any time during the day is acceptable. The patient collects the urine sample at midstream while urinating.

The source of the urine sample may also be through the catherization of the bladder through the urethra or, rarely, through a suprapubic transabdominal needle aspirate of the bladder.

If the physician suspects a urinary tract infection, then the urine must be a clean-catch sample in which contaminating bacteria are absent. For more detailed studies, a twenty-four-hour urine specimen may be required. A sample contaminated by vaginal discharge or hemorrhage will be rejected for analysis.

Steps of the procedure: After the patient voids the urine sample into a cup or other container, it is labeled and sent to the clinical laboratory. A sample might have to be collected again if the transport to the clinical laboratory has been delayed, the quantity is insufficient, or there is bacterial overgrowth.

The clinical laboratory completes three evaluations of the urine. The physical characterization of the urine includes a description of the color (pale yellow, yellow, red orange, or brown), appearance or transparency (clear to cloudy to opaque), odor if abnormal, and specific gravity. The chemical evaluation includes the pH, protein, glucose, occult blood, ketones, leukocyte esterase, nitrite, bilirubin, and urobilinogen. These chemistry detection systems are each impregnated on a series of reagent pads

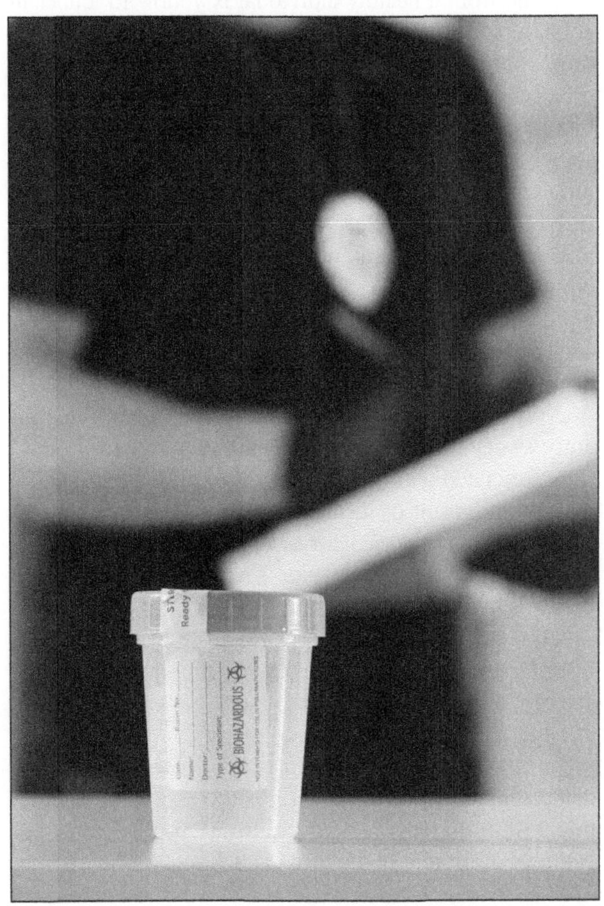

Urinalysis is invaluable for evaluating kidney function. (iStock)

on a dipstick that are activated when dipped into the urine and can be read manually or with an instrument. The microscopic examination of the urine sediment looks for bacteria, cells, and other formed elements such as casts, squamous epithelial cells, and crystals.

After the procedure: The urine sample is analyzed as soon as possible after voiding, ideally in less than two hours after collection. The results are sent to the physician who ordered the test.

Risks: There are no risks to collecting a routine urine sample other than inconvenience.

Results: Fresh normal urine is sterile, pale to dark yellow or amber in color, clear, and faintly aromatic, with a specific gravity between 1.003 and 1.035 grams per milliliter and a pH of 4.5 to 8.0. The dipstick chemistries are negative, and the microscopic observation is absent of cells or other elements. The normal twenty-four-hour urine volume is 750 to 2,000 milliliters.

Urine from a healthy individual is yellow to amber in color. A pale urine may suggest diabetes insipidus. A milky urine may be caused by fat globules or by white cells in a urinary tract infection. A red urine may be the result of red blood cells, medications, or certain foods. A greenish urine suggests the presence of bile associated with jaundice. A brown/black urine suggests hemorrhage or poisoning.

Normal urine is clear, through which newsprint can be read. Cloudy to turbid urine may be the result of precipitation of mucin or calcium phosphates, neither of which merits pathological significance. Milky urine may suggest the pathological presence of fat globules. Turbid urine can point to a urinary tract infection.

Normally urine presents a faintly acrid odor. A pleasantly sweet-smelling urine may suggest ketone production associated with diabetes mellitus. Strong acrid odors may be the result of medications or ingestion of certain foods, such as an acrid odor associated with asparagus.

The urinary specific gravity is a reliable indicator of a person's hydration status.

The body maintains a narrow acid-to-base ratio (pH) in order to sustain life. The kidney monitors metabolic activity, and excess acid or base ions are excreted in the urine to maintain that balance.

In healthy persons, protein is not present in urine in detectable amounts. Proteinuria is the excretion of more that 150 milligrams per day or 10 to 20 milligrams per deciliter of protein in the urine and is a classic symptom of renal disease. The proteinuria may be transient or persistent. If the proteinuria is persistent, then additional studies will determine if the cause is glomerular, tubular, or the result of overflow in which low-molecular-weight proteins overwhelm the ability of the system to reabsorb filtered proteins.

In healthy persons, glucose is filtered by the glomerulus and reabsorbed in the proximal tubule. Glucose appears in the urine when the amount of glucose overwhelms the ability of the tubule to reabsorb it. Further evaluation determines the source of the glycosuria: diabetes mellitus, Cushing syndrome, liver and pancreatic diseases, or Fanconi syndrome.

A positive test for occult blood indicates the presence of hemoglobin or myoglobin. A finding of blood in the urine chemistry and the presence of red blood cells in the microscopic examination of urinary sediment (hematuria) requires the clinician to determine the source of the bleeding. The hematuria may be caused by an infection; glomerular, tubular, renovascular, or metabolic disorders; tumors; or calculi (stones). The hematuria may be induced by exercise, such as long-distance running.

Ketones are the end products of the body's fat metabolism and are not usually detected in the urine. The clinician determines the cause of the presence of ketones (ketonuria): carbohydrate-free dieting, uncontrolled diabetes, or starvation.

Normally, fresh voided urine is sterile. In the case of urinary tract infections and subsequent pyuria, the white blood cells produce leukocyte esterase, which is detected on the dipstick reagent strip.

A healthy person does not have nitrites in the urine. In the case of a urinary tract infection, gram-negative and some gram-positive microorganisms reduce the nitrates in the urine to nitrites, which can be detected.

Normally, unconjugated bilirubin is water insoluble and cannot pass through the glomerulus. Conjugated bilirubin is water soluble, however, and appears in the urine, suggesting liver disease or biliary obstruction.

The urine is also tested for urobilinogen, a colorless derivative of bilirubin formed by the action of intestinal bacteria.

Urinalysis also checks for microscopic formed elements. Except for an occasional epithelial, white, or red cell, the microscopic examination of normal healthy urine sediment is without comment. Any of the following may or may not suggest pathology and require clinical interpretation in context of patient history: white blood cells (leukocytes), red blood cells (erythrocytes), casts, crystals, and bacteria.

Casts are cylindrical bodies with a protein matrix, formed in the lumen of the renal tubules. They may demonstrate a homogenous or cellular matix and include any of the following types: hyaline, waxy, erythrocyte, leukocyte, epithelia, bacteria, granular, fatty, or broad. Crystals result from the precipitation of urinary solute out of the urine. They are not normally present in fresh voided urine, and many are not clinically significant. Examples include calcium oxalate, uric acid, triple phosphate (struvite), and cystine.

Five bacterial organisms per high-power field from a clean-catch urine sample is the classic diagnostic criteria for bacteriuria and a diagnosis of a urinary tract infection. Typically five organisms per high-power field represents 100,000 colony-forming units when the urine is cultured.

Jane Adrian, M.P.H., Ed.M., M.T. (ASCP)

For Further Information

Brunzel, Nancy A. *Fundamentals of Urine and Body Fluid Analysis*. 2d ed. Philadelphia: W. B. Saunders, 2004.

Ringsrud, Karen Munson, and Jean Jorgenson Linne. *Urinalysis and Body Fluids: A Colortext and Atlas*. Philadelphia: Elsevier, 1994.

Simerville, Jeff A., William C. Maxted, and John J. Pahira. "Urinalysis: A Comprehensive Review." *American Family Physician*, March 15, 2005, 1153.

Strasinger, Susan King, and Marjorie Schaub Di Lorenzo. *Urinalysis and Body Fluids*. 5th ed. Philadelphia: F. A. Davis, 2008.

Other Resources

American Urological Association
http://www.auanet.org

Lab Tests Online
http://www.labtestsonline.org

Onco Link
http://www.oncolink.com

See also: Calcium; Cushing syndrome and cancer; Exercise and cancer; Fanconi anemia; Hematuria; Pathology; Risks for cancer; Tubular carcinomas; Urethral cancer

▶ Urography

Category: Procedures

Also known as: Intravenous pyelography (IVP), oral urography, retrograde urography, magnetic resonance urography, computed tomography urography

Definition: Urography allows an assessment of the health and functioning of the urinary system by injecting a contrast material (dye) into the bloodstream. When this contrast material reaches the urinary tract, its soft-tissue structures become visible on imaging scans, so that abnormalities can be detected.

Cancers diagnosed: Cancers of the kidney (renal cell carcinoma), ureters, and bladder

Why performed: The urinary system is composed of the kidneys, ureters, bladder, and urethra. The kidneys are two bean-shaped organs located in the lower back below the rib cage. Their function is to filter blood, remove waste products, and help maintain the proper balance of fluid in the body. The ureters carry excess water and waste materials from the kidney to the bladder, where these waste materials are stored. The urethra removes this urine from the body. Urography allows these structures to be examined for cancer and other abnormalities in a noninvasive way.

Most often, urography is done for reasons unrelated to cancer. Kidney stones, for example, can cause obstruction in the urinary system accompanied by extreme pain. In this case, urography is done on an emergency basis to locate the obstruction. Cancer tumors can also cause obstruction or blood in the urine. Urography to detect cancer is done on a nonemergency basis in a radiology center or other outpatient setting.

Urography can be done in several different ways using various imaging techniques. Sometimes it is necessary to use more than one method in order to acquire precise information about the location of tumors. In intravenous pyelography (IVP), a dye containing iodine is injected into a vein in the hand or arm. When the dye reaches the urinary tract, the tissues become visible on conventional X rays. The only difference between oral urography and IVP is that the individual drinks the dye instead of having it injected. Retrograde pyelography is similar to an IVP, only the dye is placed directly in the urinary tract by way of a catheter (thin tube) inserted into the urethra. In computed tomography (CT) urography, contrast material is injected into the bloodstream, but instead of using conventional X rays to visualize the kidneys, ureters, and bladder, a CT scanner takes multiple cross-sectional images of the body and uses a computer to compile a three-dimensional image. In magnetic resonance imaging (MRI) urography, contrast material is injected, and then the individual is placed in a special tube while a three-dimensional picture is obtained through MRI. This type of urography is used most often to locate bladder cancer that has spread into the pelvic region.

Patient preparation: For nonemergency urography, the physician will review the patient's medications to make sure that they do not interact with the contrast material. Patients should tell their physicians if they are allergic to seafood or iodine, as this increases the likelihood that they may have an allergic reaction to the contrast dye. Women who are or think they might be pregnant should not have urographic tests that expose them to X rays.

The night before the test, the patient takes a laxative to empty the bowel and should not eat or drink on the day of the test. During the test, the patient will wear a hospital gown.

Steps of the procedure: The contrast material is injected into a vein (most commonly), injected into the urethra, or given by mouth. The patient may briefly feel a warm, tingling sensation. In rare cases, the patient can develop breathing problems or experiences swelling in the throat or elsewhere. This is a sign of an allergic reaction, and the physician should be notified immediately.

The patient is placed on the X-ray table, and a series of X rays are taken at timed intervals, usually at zero, five, ten, twenty, and sometimes forty minutes. While each X ray is being taken, the patient must remain still. Between X rays, the patient may move. For the final X ray, the patient is asked to urinate, and an X ray is taken of the bladder. CT and MRI urography are very similar. MRI urography takes about one hour and requires the patient to remain still during that time.

After the procedure: After the procedure, the patient may eat, drink, and resume normal activities. The patient may have a mild headache or slight nausea from the contrast material. Urine will appear normal; the contrast material does not change its color.

Risks: This is a minimally invasive procedure with few risks. Rarely does a patient have a serious allergic reaction to the contrast material. Although X rays are very safe, pregnant women should not have them because of potential damage to the developing fetus. These women can have MRI or CT urography, neither of which uses X rays.

Results: In a healthy kidney, the dye will show up on the X rays soon after it is injected. In people with kidney damage, the dye takes longer to appear in the X rays.

Martiscia Davidson, A.M.

For Further Information

Anderson, E. M., et al. "Multidetector Computed Tomography Urography (MDCTU) for Diagnosing Urothelial Malignancy." *Clinical Radiology* 62, no. 4 (April, 2007): 324-332.

Guermazi, A., ed. *Imaging of Kidney Cancer*. New York: Springer, 2006.

Strum, Stephen, and Donna L. Pogliano. *A Primer on Prostate Cancer: The Empowered Patient's Guide*. Hollywood, Fla.: Life Extension Media, 2002.

Other Resources

eMedicinehealth.com

Intravenous Pyelogram

http://www.emedicinehealth.com/intravenous_pyelogram/article_em.htm

See also: Bladder cancer; Gastrointestinal complications of cancer treatment; Hematuria; Imaging tests; Kidney cancer; Nephrostomy; Prostate cancer; Urethral cancer; Urinary system cancers; X-ray tests

▶ Urostomy

Category: Procedures
Also known as: Urinary diversion

Definition: A urostomy is a surgical opening (stoma) through the abdominal wall that allows urine to drain from the diseased bladder into an artificial pouch, to be emptied intermittently, when long-term drainage from the bladder is not possible. A urostomy can be conventional or standard, with an ileal conduit, or feature a continent urinary reservoir.

Cancers treated: Bladder cancer

Why performed: When a bladder is diseased, the body must have a way to excrete urine, liquid human waste. A surgeon creates a urostomy to drain urine from the kidney.

Patient preparation: The surgeon discusses the risks and benefits of the urostomy with the patient and examines the patient's abdomen to locate the best place for the stoma. Some patients try flat pouches at the predetermined place to see if the location allows maximum comfort and minimal interference in activities of daily living. Patients should tell the surgeon if their work or hobbies need special consideration.

Steps of the procedure: The steps of the procedure depend on the type of surgery performed. In a conventional urostomy, a small pouch or urine reservoir is created surgically from a small bowel segment. A passage is created from the kidney and ureters to the ileal segment that bypasses the bladder (which may or may not be removed). The far end of the ileal segment is brought through the abdominal wall to make a stoma.

After the procedure: Education regarding how to care for a pouch after surgery is provided by an ostomy specialist. After surgery, the stoma may swell but will decrease in size over six to eight weeks. Most health care facilities have ostomy visitors who have experienced a urostomy and understand concerns about body image. They can answer questions that the patient may have after surgery. Support groups are also useful.

Risks: Typical risks include urinary crystals, infection, and skin irritation. A pouch that fits well along with adequate fluid intake and appropriate skin care with a protectant barrier can minimize problems. The patient should notify the health care provider if bleeding occurs from the stoma, if ulcers form on the skin around the stoma, or if fever or a strong odor in the urine (a sign of a kidney infection) occurs.

Results: The urostomy can improve quality of life for the bladder cancer patient, who can return to most normal activities. Managing the urostomy will become routine with practice.

Marylane Wade Koch, M.S.N., R.N.

See also: Bladder cancer; Enterostomal therapy; Exenteration; Nephrostomy; Self-image and body image

▶ Vascular access tubes

Category: Procedures
Also known as: Peripherally inserted central catheters (PICC), subcutaneous ports, Hickman catheters, Groshong catheters, Broviac catheters

Definition: A vascular access tube is a catheter inserted into the veins of the arm, neck, or just beneath the collarbone for long-term intravenous access (greater than seven to ten days). The catheter can also be used to draw blood for lab tests. Patients receiving long-term chemotherapy, pain medications, nutrition, or antibiotics will have vascular access.

Cancers treated: All requiring long-term therapy

Why performed: Many patients have poor veins or are unable to receive treatment without access.

Patient preparation: Vascular access lines can be placed at the bedside, in the operating room (OR), or in vascular radiology. Procedures at the bedside have no preprocedure preparation. Patients going to the OR or vascular radiology are not allowed to eat or drink for at least eight hours before line placement as a result of the anesthesia.

Steps of the procedure: All lines are placed using sterile technique. For peripherally inserted central catheters (PICC), a catheter is inserted through the antecube to be threaded up the arm and to end in the superior vena cava. PICC lines are flushed at least once a day and their dressings are changed once a week.

For ports, a small titanium or plastic reservoir is inserted and stitched into place in the upper chest. The catheter is attached to the reservoir and inserted into the vein and then threaded into the superior vena cava. The reservoir is accessed through the patient's chest wall with special needles. Ports must have a needle inserted and flushed at least once a month to prevent clotting. This line can be placed in the OR or vascular radiology.

Hickman, Broviac, or Groshong catheters are also placed in the upper chest wall. The line is inserted through a small incision and into the vein and follows until the end rests in the superior vena cava. It is held into place by a small cuff located under the skin; typically stitches are not used. The patient or caregiver will be responsible for flushing the access and changing the dressing every seven days.

After the procedure: Line placement is verified by a chest X ray. Once the line has been verified, it can be used to infuse therapy or for lab sampling. The patient or caregiver is responsible for home care, including flushing the access and changing the dressing.

Risks: The risks associated with vascular access lines are pneumothorax (collapsed lung), bleeding, and infection.

Results: The result of this procedure is reliable venous access to receive therapy and for blood draws.

Katrina Green, R.N., B.S.N., O.C.N.

See also: Caregivers and caregiving; Chemotherapy; Infection and sepsis; Nutrition and cancer treatment; Pain management medications; Superior vena cava syndrome

▶ Vasectomy and cancer

Category: Procedures
Also known as: Sterilization, permanent birth control

Related cancers: None

Definition: Vasectomy, a form of permanent birth control for men, is a commonly performed procedure that results in sterilization and is more than 99 percent effective in preventing pregnancy. No link has been established between having this procedure and developing cancer.

Vasectomy facts: More than 13 million vasectomies have been performed in the United States. Of the men who had vasectomies, 91 percent were married or cohabiting, 87 percent were white, and 81 percent were educated beyond high school. Although vasectomy is effective at preventing pregnancy, it does not prevent or protect from sexually transmitted diseases.

History: In 2004, prostate cancer was the most commonly identified new cancer in American men and the second highest cause of cancer mortality in men. Some questions were raised about a possible association between vasectomy and cancer, with the greatest concern being an association with prostate cancer. The cause of prostate cancer is unknown, and therefore there was concern that an association might be found between cancer and vasectomy.

Several studies have been conducted in an effort to determine if there is a causal relationship between the two. The major studies done in 1993 found that it was not possible to show a correlation. There were too many other factors that introduced bias into the ability to draw the conclusion. Similarly, it has been impossible to identify a correlation between vasectomy and testicular cancer. Testicular cancer is a cancer of young men (ages fifteen to thirty-four), while prostate cancer is seen in older men.

A 2002 study looked at vasectomy and the risk of prostate cancer and concluded that the association was small and could be explained by bias. This means that there were too many factors that interfered with the ability to scientifically make an association. The researchers concluded that studies should continue because of the popularity of vasectomy. Men should discuss any cancer concerns with their physician prior to having a vasectomy, but there is no evidence to show that a man should not have a vasectomy because of concerns about cancer.

Janet R. Green, M.S.P.H.

See also: Birth control pills and cancer; Fertility issues; Pregnancy and cancer; Prostate cancer; Relationships; Sterility; Testicular cancer

▶ Wire localization

Category: Procedures
Also known as: Needle localization

Definition: Wire localization is the insertion of a fine wire under radiologic guidance to mark for biopsy areas of breast density or calcifications that can be seen on mammograms but are not detectable by touch.

Cancers diagnosed: Breast cancers

Why performed: Certain types of images seen on mammograms may indicate precancer or developing cancer. Some of these lesions cannot be seen with the naked eye or felt by touch. Wire localization enables the surgeon to accurately target areas for biopsy. A follow-up radiologic image after the biopsy assures that the suspect tissue was removed.

Conditions of concern that require wire localization include microcalcifications and certain types of breast densities. Microcalcifications are tiny calcium deposits in the breast tissue, which show up on mammograms as white specks. Microcalcifications are generally only of concern when they appear in irregular patterns or are concentrated in one area of the breast. In these patterns or concentrations, they may indicate the rapid cell growth associated with precancer.

Patient preparation: Patients usually get a local anesthetic to numb feeling in the area of the breast where the wire will be inserted.

Steps of the procedure: To locate the area for biopsy, the surgeon uses radiologic images in which the wire site is marked. X ray is the preferred method used for wire localization. Ultrasound can also be used, but conditions requiring wire localization are often not visible by ultrasound. Guided by radiologic images of the breast, a radiologist locates the area in question, first inserts a thin, hollow needle into the area and then, through the needle, a fine wire with a hook. The hook keeps the wire in place in the breast and marks the specific area for biopsy. The wire in the breast provides a guide for where the incision is made. The wire is removed along with the breast tissue.

After the procedure: After the biopsy, the patient remains in the operating room until a repeat radiologic image confirms that the suspect area was removed. If the target area was missed, then another biopsy can be done immediately.

Risks: The risks of wire localization are minimal and include minor pain, possible bruising, and limited radiation exposure.

Results: Wire localization and follow-up radiologic images assure accurate targeting of the area for biopsy.

Charlotte Crowder, M.P.H., ELS

See also: Biopsy; Breast cancers; Calcifications of the breast; Calcium; Mammography; Microcalcifications; Needle localization; Ultrasound tests

▶ X-ray tests

Category: Procedures
Also known as: Radiology, medical imaging, radiologic procedures, radiographic imaging

Definition: An X-ray test uses a machine to produce radiation that is passed through a particular body part. The size and density of the part show up as light and dark tones in the image on radiographic film, which helps the doctor diagnose the patient. Radiology encompasses many diagnostic types of imaging. Body parts, regions, and systems that can be seen by radiography include the chest, abdomen, skeletal system (skull, pelvis, spine, facial bones, extremities), brain, sinus, circulatory system (veins, arteries), lymphatic system, glands, muscles, urinary system, digestive system, reproductive system, cysts and tumors, and any soft tissues or organ in the body.

Radiologic exams may include routine X rays; computed tomography (CT) scans, previously known as a computed axial tomography (CAT) scans; angiography to study the veins and arteries; intravenous urography (IVU), previously known as intravenous pyelogram (IVP), which uses tomography imaging to view the kidneys, ureters, and bladder; upper gastrointestinal (UGI) series, also known as barium swallow, to show the esophagus, stomach, and small intestines; colon imaging, also known as barium enema or lower GI, to demonstrate the large intestine, colon, rectum, and appendix; dental radiography and panoramic tomography, also known as Panorex imaging, to view the teeth, jaw, and tempromandibular joint; sinus radiography to view the paranasal sinus; bone densitometry scans to evaluate bone porosity; digital subtraction angiography (DSA) to illustrate the blood vessels; ER, also known as emergency room, portables, and trauma, to take radiographic images during emergency situations in surgery and in the emergency room; fluoroscopy, which shows an actively moving video image of the part being evaluated; mammography, which takes medical images of the breasts; single photon emission computerized tomography (SPECT) scans which shows an increase in blood flow; and nuclear medicine and positron emission tomography (PET) which use radioactive tracer materials or radiopharmaceuticals that are injected, inhaled, or swallowed by the patient to create images of the whole body and show areas of increased radioactive uptake according to the organ's functioning ability.

Other imaging technologies that fall outside the scope of X-ray technologies include magnetic resonance imaging (MRI), ultrasound, and endoscopy, which do not use radiation to produce an image. MRI uses a powerful magnet to produce images on film, ultrasound uses sound waves to create its images, and an endoscope is a flexible viewing camera inserted orally or rectally to take internal pictures.

Cancers diagnosed: Medical imaging using X rays is designed to help diagnose cancers, metastases, diseases, fractures, or abnormalities. These diagnostic tests are not to be confused with radiation therapy, which is used to destroy cancers. Most cancers can be seen with the use of radiographic imaging; however, all cancers vary widely in their visibility. Some cancers hide until late in the disease process and then metastasize (grow and spread) quickly.

X-ray tests help diagnose bone cancers, bone marrow cancers, soft-tissue cancers, cancers of vital organs, blood-related cancers, lung cancers, lymph node and lymphoma cancers, spinal cord cancers, abdominal and pelvic cancers, head and neck cancers, liver and gallbladder cancers, reproductive organ cancers, breast cancers, leukemia, esophageal and colon cancers, Hodgkin and non-Hodgkin diseases, advanced skin cancers, brain cancers, and metastases.

Why performed: Diagnostic X rays are used to identify fractures, pneumonias, cancers, sinus infections, bowel obstructions, foreign objects, and anatomical abnormalities, or to confirm that there are no abnormalities. CT, MRI, nuclear medicine scans, and angiography are extremely helpful in locating diseases and cancers that are hard to find. Clinical observation and laboratory tests,

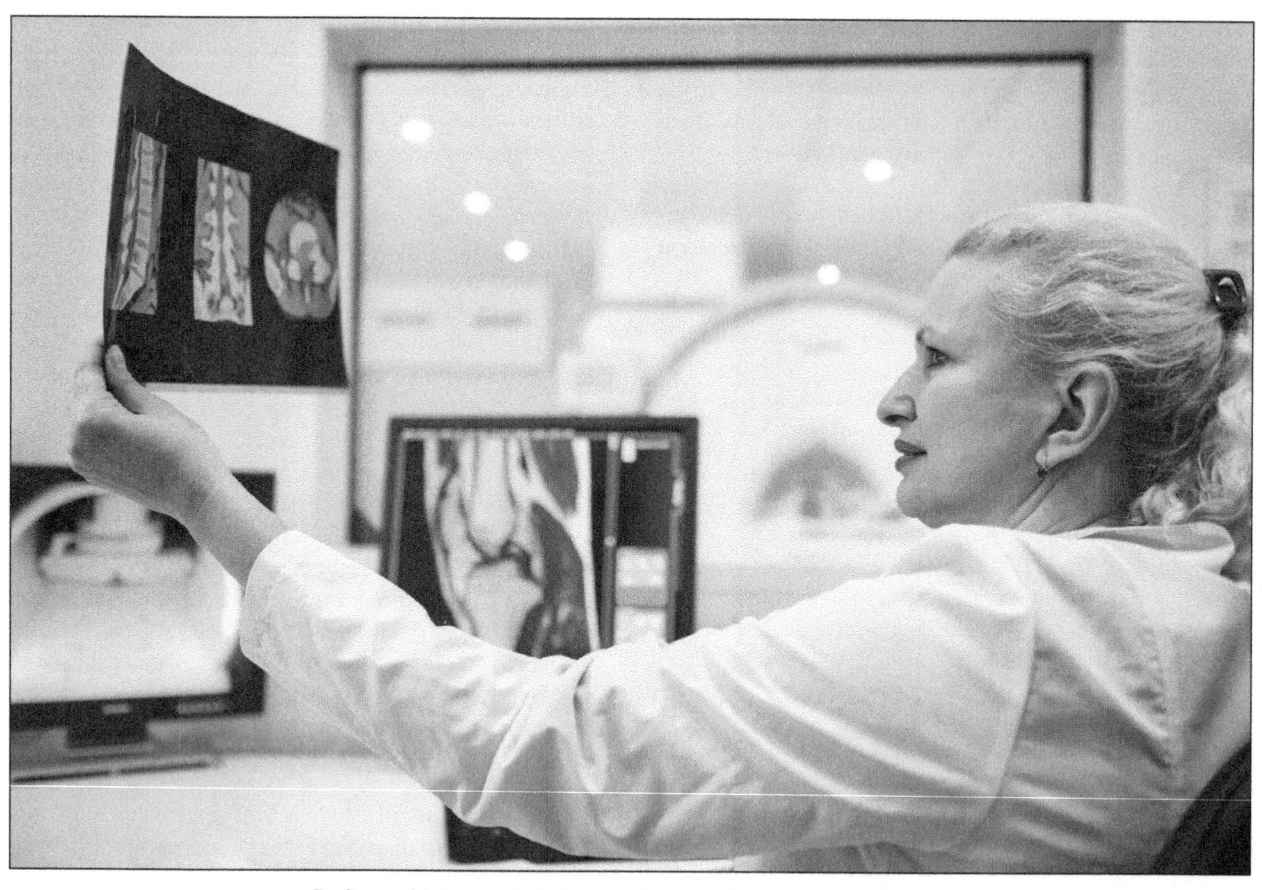

Radiographic images help doctors detect and treat cancers. (iStock)

combined with X-ray imaging, give the physician a more complete view of the extent of a particular disease. The combination of all tests and exams helps the doctor form a treatment plan for the patient. Any of these imaging devices may also be used to assist with guiding a biopsy, in needle placement, or to verify the location of wires and instruments during surgical procedures.

Patient preparation: Because there is such a wide variety of exams and a vast range of reasons for a radiology exam, it is best for the patient to consult with the medical doctor or discuss the preparation with the technologist three days prior to the exam. Some of the tests are routine, involving no preparation. Others may require eating or drinking restrictions, an increase in the amount of fluids in the bladder, or ingestion of contrast preparations for enhanced viewing in certain areas.

Steps of the procedure: The patient should tell the X-ray technician if there is any chance of pregnancy. If pregnancy is not a factor, then the patient is positioned between the X-ray tube and the radiographic film. Depending on the procedure and part being radiographed, the patient may be sitting, standing, or lying on a table for the exam. A lead shield (radiation protection device) is placed on the area surrounding, but not on, the region to be radiographed. Technique is set according to the size and density of the part. The length of time for procedures varies from five minutes to two hours depending on the test. Often, several images using different angles are needed. Some X-ray exams require the use of a contrast medium (dye). It may be taken orally or injected into the patient prior to or during the imaging process. Contrast materials are used when specific parts need to be enhanced or defined on film.

Contrast materials include barium sulfate (for upper GI and colon studies), iodine-based media (for IVP, CT, and angiography), gadolinium (for MRI), radioactive pharmaceutical materials and radioactive isotopes (for nuclear medicine scans), and xenon gas (for lung scans).

After the procedure: A radiologist will view the X-ray images and document the findings. The report will be given to the patient's doctor. At a follow-up appointment, the results will be discussed. If the imaging used a contrast material, then it is often suggested that the patient drink plenty of fluids to flush the contrast from the body. Over the next several days, the contrast will be eliminated through the body's waste products. Depending on the type of contrast and amount used, an unpleasant taste can linger in the mouth for a few weeks.

Risks: The physician will evaluate the patient's medical situation and determine if the diagnosis and treatment from the radiographic knowledge outweigh the potential risk from the X rays. If the patient is pregnant, then the procedure may be canceled or rescheduled or the patient may be double-shielded to protect the fetus. With the use of high-speed film, fast and accurate imaging equipment, collimation, and lead shielding, radiation is kept to a minimum for the patient. Diagnostic X-ray procedures carry no obvious short-term effects; however, any amount of radiation has the potential to harm cell structure. High doses of radiation that produce ill effects are seen in radiotherapy for cancer treatments. Long-term or high-dose effects of radiation can cause fetal or genetic defects, mutations or cancers, nausea, diarrhea, vomiting, or death.

In addition to medical and dental X rays, the general population is exposed to background radiation that increases their total body exposure when they live in a brick house, walk by a brick building, fly in an airplane, smoke or breathe secondhand smoke, live at higher elevation levels, heat their home with natural gas, breathe air pollution, work with natural elements or radiation in their profession, watch television, and work or play on a computer. One can calculate the radiation dose from many potential sources at http://www.epa.gov/radiation/students/calculate.html.

Other risks of X rays include claustrophobia in CT or MRI scanners and allergic reactions to contrast materials. Allergic reactions can include rash, itching, hives, nausea, vomiting, coma, or death.

Results: The radiographic image is developed and viewed by the radiology technician, who gives the film to the physician or radiologist. Depending on the procedure, the patient may receive a preliminary diagnosis or may have to wait until the final report from the radiologist, which may be several days later. The patient's current health status and extent of disease help determine a treatment plan.

Suzette Buhr, R.T.R., C.D.A.

For Further Information

Frank, Eugene D., Bruce W. Long, and Barbara J. Smith. *Merrill's Atlas of Radiographic Positions and Radiologic Procedures*. 11th ed. St. Louis: Mosby/Elsevier, 2007.

Goldmann, David R., and David A. Horowitz, eds. *American College of Physicians Complete Home Medical Guide*. New York: DK, 2003.

Putman, Charles E., and Carl E. Ravin. *Textbook of Diagnostic Imaging*. 2d ed. Philadelphia: W. B. Saunders, 1994.

Other Resources

American Cancer Society

http://www.cancer.org

University of Iowa Hospital and Clinics

Radiation Exposure: The Facts vs. Fiction

http://www.uihealthcare.com/topics/medicaldepartments/cancercenter/prevention/preventionradiation.html

See also: Barium enema; Barium swallow; Brain and central nervous system cancers; Breast cancers; Computed Tomography (CT) scan; Endoscopy; Imaging tests; Lymphomas; Mammography; Radiation therapies; Upper Gastrointestinal (GI) series; Urography

Appendixes

▶ Drugs Classified by Drug Classes/Trade Names

1. Antibiotics

a. Antibacterial Agents

Trade Name	*Generic Name*	*Indicated For*
Abbott-56268	Clarithromycin	*H. pylori* infection; various bacterial infections
Augmentin	Amoxicillin – Clavulanate potassium	Various bacterial infections
Avelox	Moxifloxacin	Various bacterial infections
Bactrim	Trimethoprim - Sulfamethoxazole	*Pneumocystis jiroveci* pneumonia; various bacterial infections
Biaxin	Clarithromycin	*H. pylori* infection; various bacterial infections
Cipro	Ciprofloxacin	Inhaled anthrax; postexposure; susceptible disease
Cotrim, Septa	Trimethoprim - Sulfamethoxazole	*Pneumocystis jiroveci* pneumonia; various bacterial infections
Maxipime	Cefepime hydrochloride	Upper respiratory tract and urinary tract infections, febrile neutropenic conditions
Mycobutin	Rifabutin	Prevention and treatment of *Mycobacterium avium* complex (MAC) and tuberculosis in patients with HIV infection
Viagmox	Moxifloxicin hydrochloride	Various bacterial infections

b. Antifungal Agents

Trade Name	*Generic Name*	*Indicated For*
Abelcet	Amphotericin B lipid complex	Invasive, systemic fungal infections
Amphotec, Amphocil	Amphotericin B cholesteryl sulfate complex	
AmBisome	Amphotericin B liposomal	
Ancoba	Flucytosine	Candidiasis; cryptococcosis; chromomycosis; common used in combination with Amphotericin B or fluconazole
Cancidas	Caspofungin	Candidiasis
Cresemba	Isavuconazole	Invasive aspergillosis; invasive mucormycosis
Diflucan	Fluconazole	Antifungal, prophylaxis in allogeneic bone marrow transplantation; candidiasis; cryptococcal meningitis

Trade Name	*Generic Name*	*Indicated For*
Eraxis	Anidulafungin	Candidemia
Fungarest	Ketoconazole	Seborrheic dermatitis; prostate cancer
Fungoral	Ketoconazole	Seborrheic dermatitis; prostate cancer
Mycamine	Micafungin	Systemic fungal infections caused by *Aspergillus*, Cryptococcus, or *Candida* species
Nizoral	Ketoconazole	Seborrheic dermatitis; prostate cancer
Noxafil	Posaconazole	Fungal infection prevention for immunocompromised host
Orifungal M	Ketoconazole	Seborrheic dermatitis, Prostate cancer
Panfungol		
R-41400		
Sporanox	Itraconazole	Fungal infections
Vfend	Voriconazole	Invasive, systemic fungal infections; invasive candidiasis, invasive aspergillosis, and emerging fungal infections in immunocompromised patients
Xolegel	Ketoconazole	Seborrheic dermatitis, Prostate cancer

c. Antiviral Agents

Trade Name	*Generic Name*	*Indicated For*
3TC	Lamivudine	Anti-HIV (nucleoside reverse transcriptase inhibitor)
ABC	Abacavir	Anti-HIV (nucleoside reverse transcriptase inhibitor)
Acyclovir	Acyclovir	Chicken pox, shingles, and oral and genital herpes
Agenerase	Aprenavir	Anti-HIV (protease inhibitor)
Alferon N	Recombinant interferon alfa	Used as antiviral and antitumor agent
Atripla	Emtricitabine – Tenofovir disoproxil – Efavirenz combination	AIDS-related complex HIV infection; HIV transmission; prevention
Aztec	Zidovudine (azidothymidine; AZT)	AIDS-related complex; HIV infection; HIV transmission, prevention (nucleoside reverse transcriptase inhibitor)
Combivir	Amivudine & Zidovudine combination	AIDS-related complex HIV infection; HIV transmission; prevention

Trade Name	*Generic Name*	*Indicated For*
Complera	Emtricitabine – Rilpivirine – Tenofovir disoproxil combination	AIDS-related complex HIV infection; HIV transmission; prevention
Crixivan	Idinavir	Anti-HIV (protease inhibitor)
Cymevan	Ganciclovir	Cytomegalovirus (CMV) infections in immunocompromised patients
Denvir	Penciclovir	Herpes cold sores (topical only)
DHPG	Ganciclovir	CMV infections in immunosuppressed patients
Dutrebis	Lamivudine – Raltegravir	AIDS-related complex HIV infection; HIV transmission; prevention
Emtriva	Emtricitabine	Anti-HIV (nucleoside reverse transcriptase inhibitor)
Endurant	Rilpivirine	Anti-HIV (non-nucleoside reverse transcriptase inhibitor)
Epivir	Lamivudine	chronic hepatitis B; HIV infection
Epzicom	Abacavir – Lamivudine	AIDS-related complex HIV infection; HIV transmission; prevention
Evotaz	Atazanavir – Cobicistat	AIDS-related complex HIV infection; HIV transmission; prevention
Famvir	Famciclovir	Shingles, oral and genital herpes
Foscarnet	Foscanet	CMV and Herpes simplex virus infections in immuno-suppressed patients
Fuzeon	Enfuvirtide	Anti-HIV (entry inhibitor)
Genvoya	Elvitegravir – Cobicistat – Emtricitabine – Tenofovir alafenamide combination	AIDS-related complex HIV infection; HIV transmission; prevention
Harvoni	Ledipasvir – Sofosbuvir combination	Hepatitis C infections
Hepsera	Adefovir dipivoxil	Chronic hepatitis B
Intelence	Etravirine	Anti-HIV (non-nucleoside reverse transcriptase inhibitor)
Isentress	Reltegravir	Anti-HIV (integrase inhibitor)
Kaletra	Lopinavir – Ritonavir combination	Anti-HIV (protease inhibitor)
Laroferon	Recombinant interferon alfa	Used as antiviral and antitumor agents
Nordeoxyguanosine	Ganciclovir	CMV infections in immunocompromised patients

Trade Name	*Generic Name*	*Indicated For*
Norvir	Ritonavir	Anti-HIV (protease inhibitor) and hepatitis C infections
Prezcobix	Darunavir – Cobicistat	AIDS-related complex HIV infection; HIV transmission; prevention
Prezista	Darunavir	Anti-HIV ((protease inhibitor)
Rebetol	Ribavirin	Hepatitis C and severe respiratory syncytial virus (RSV) infections
Retrovir	Zidovudine (Azidothymidine)	AIDS-related complex HIV infection; HIV transmission; prevention (nucleoside reverse transcriptase inhibitor)
Roceron; Roceron-A	Recombinant intergferon alfa	Used as antiviral and anticancer agents
Roferon-A	Interferon alfa-2a; recombinant interferon alfa	treating chronic hepatitis C and certain types of leukemia; used as antiviral and antitumor agents
Seizentry	Maraviroc	Anti-HIV (entry inhibitor)
Sovaldi	Sofosbuvir	Hepatitis C infections
Stribild	Elvitegravir – Cobicistat – Emtricitabine – Tenofovir disoproxil combination	AIDS-related complex HIV infection; HIV transmission; prevention
Sustiva	Efavirenz	Anti-HIV (non-nucleoside reverse transcriptase inhibitor)
Technivie	Ombitasavir, paritaprevir, and Ritonavir combination	Hepatitis C infections
Triumeq	Abacavir – Dolutegravir – Lamivudine combination	AIDS-related complex HIV infection; HIV transmission; prevention
Tivicay	Dolutigravir	Anti-HIV (integrase inhibitor)
Trivizir	Abacavir – lamivudine – zidovudine combination	AIDS-related complex HIV infection; HIV transmission; prevention
Truvada	Tenofovir disoproxil – Emtricitabine combination	AIDS-related complex HIV infection; HIV transmission; prevention
Valcyte	Valganciclovir	CMV retinitis
Valtrex	Valacyclovir	Chicken pox, shingles, oral and genital herpes infections
Vidarabine	Vidarabine	Chicken pox, shingles, herpes simplex infections of the eye
Viekira Pak	Ombitasavir, paritapravir, ritonavir, dasasbuvir combination	Hepatitis C infections

Trade Name	*Generic Name*	*Indicated For*
Viracept	Nelfinavir	Anti-HIV (protease inhibitor)
Viramune	Nevirapine	Anti-HIV (non-nucleoside reverse transcriptase inhibitor)
Viread	Tenofovir disproxil	Anti-HIV (nucleotide reverse transcriptase inhibitor)
Virgan	Ganciclovir	CMV infections in immunocompromised patients
Zovirax	Acyclovir	Chicken pox, shingles, oral and genital herpes

d. Viral and Bacterial vaccines

Trade Name	*Generic Name*	*Indicated For*
Ceravix	Bivalent human papillomavirus (HPV) vaccine	Genital warts prophylaxis and cervical cancer prevention; protects against infection by HPV types 16 and 18.
Gardasil	Quadrivalent HPV vaccine	Genital warts prophylaxis and cervical cancer prevention; protects against infection by HPV types 6, 11, 16, and 18.
Gardasil 9	Nonavalent HPV vaccine	Genital and anal warts prophylaxis and cervical and anal cancer prevention; protects against infection by HPV types 6, 11, 16, 18, 31, 33, 45, 52, and 58.
Flumist	Trivalent influenza vaccine	Influenza prophylaxis
Flushield	Trivalent influenza vaccine	Influenza prophylaxis
Fluvirin	Trivalent influenza vaccine	Influenza prophylaxis
Fluzone	Trivalent influenza vaccine	Influenza prophylaxis
Hib TITER vaccine	*Haemophilus influenzae B* vaccine	*Haemophilus influenzae B* prophylaxis
Varivax	Varicella-Zoster vaccine	Chicken pox and shingles prophylaxis
PedvaxHIB	*Haemophilus influenzae* B vaccine	*Haemophilus influenzae* B prophylaxis
Proquad	Varicella-Zoster vaccine	Chicken pox and shingles prophylaxis
Zostavax	Varicella-Zoster vaccine	Chicken pox and shingles prophylaxis

2. Anticoagulants

Trade Name	*Generic Name*	*Indicated For*
Athrombin-K	Warfarin	Pulmonary embolism and thromboembolic disorders, treatment and prophylaxis; venous thrombosis, prophylaxis and treatment
Clexane	Enoxaparin	Deep vein thrombosis, prophylaxis; ischemic complications in unstable angina and non-Q wave myocardial infarction, prophylaxis
Co-Rax, Compound-42, Coumadin	Warfarin	Pulmonary embolism and thromboembolic disorders, treatment and prophylaxis; venous thrombosis, prophylaxis and treatment
Eliquis	Apixaban	Stroke prophylaxis with atrial fibrillation; postoperative prophylaxis of deep vein thrombosis and pulmonary embolism and treatment
Fragmin	Dalteparin (Low molecular weight heparin)	Deep vein thrombosis, prophylaxis; ischemic complications in unstable angina and non-Q wave myocardial infarction, prophylaxis
Innohep	Tinzaparin sodium (Low molecular weight heparin)	Treatment of acute symptomatic deep venous thrombosis (DVT) with or without a pulmonary embolism (PE), in conjunction with warfarin
Lovenox	Enoxaparin (Low molecular weight heparin)	Deep vein thrombosis, prophylaxis; ischemic complications in unstable angina and non-Q wave myocardial infarction, prophylaxis
Panwarfarin, Rodex, WARF Compound 42	Warfarin	Pulmonary embolism and thromboembolic disorders, treatment and prophylaxis; venous thrombosis, prophylaxis and treatment
Pradaxa	Dabigatran	Stroke prophylaxis in those with atrial fibrillation
Savaysa	Edoxaban	Deep vein thrombosis; pulmonary embolism
Xarelto	Rivaroxaban	Nonvalvular atrial fibrillation; deep vein thrombosis and pulmonary embolism treatment
Xaparin	Enoxaparin	Deep vein thrombosis, prophylaxis; ischemic complications in unstable angina and non-Q wave myocardial infarction, prophylaxis

3. Antiplatelet Drugs

Trade Name	*Generic Name*	*Indicated For*
Cyclooxygenase inhibitors		
Aspergum, Ecotrin, Empirin, Entericin, Extren, Measurin	acetylsalicylic acid; aspirin	mild to moderate pain; fever; prevention of arterial and venous thrombosis
GPIIb/IIIa inhibitors		
Aggrastat	Tirofiban	Acute Coronary Syndrome
Integrilin	Eptifibatide	Acute Coronary Syndrome or PCI
ReoPro	abciximab	Percutaneous coronary intervention (PCI)
$P2Y_{12}$ inhibitors		
Brilinta	Ticagrelor	Acute Coronary Syndrome; unstable angina; non-ST elevation; myocardial infarction; ST elevation myocardial infarction; percutaneous coronary intervention
Effient	Prasugrel	Unstable angina; non-ST elevation; myocardial infarction; ST elevation myocardial infarction; percutaneous coronary intervention
Plavix	Clopidogrel bisulfate	Thromboembolic disorders
Phosphodiesterase inhibitors		
Aggrenox	Dipyridamole and aspirin	Stroke prophylaxis, MI prophylaxis in patients with atrial fibrillation
Persantine	Dipyridamole	Stroke prophylaxs
Pletal	Cilostazol	Intermittent claudication
Thrombin receptor antagonists		
Zontivity	Vorapaxar	myocardial infarction; peripheral arterial disease.

ZONTIVITY

4. Steroids

Trade Name	*Generic Name*	*Indicated For*
Aeroseb-Dex, Alba-Dex	Dexamethasone; desamethasone; dexamethasonum; DXM; hexadecadrol; methylfluorprednisolone	Antiemetic (prevents vomiting)

Trade Name	*Generic Name*	*Indicated For*
Andro LA 200, Andro-Cyp 100	Testosterone	Breast cancer in women, palliative
Android	Methyltestosterone	Breast cancer, palliative
Android-F, Androxy	Fluoxymesterone; androfluorene	Certain types of breast cancer
Clinagen LA40	Estradiol	Breast cancer, palliative
Colprosterone	Therapeutic progesterone	Amenorrhea; functional uterine bleeding; infertility; maintenance of pregnancy
Cortalone	Prednisolone	Inflammatory conditions; allergic conditions; hematologic conditions; neoplastic conditions; autoimmune conditions; replacement therapy in adrenal insufficiency
Curretab	Medroxyprogesterone; medroxyprogesterone acetate	Breast carcinoma; endometrial carcinoma; renal cell carcinoma
Cyprostat	Cyproterone acetate	Prostate cancer
Decaderm, Decadrol, Decadrone	Dexamethasone	Antiemetic
Deca-Durabolin	Nandrolone decanoate	Anabolic steroid; anemia of renal insufficiency; metastatic breast cancer
Decasone R.p., Decaspray, Deenar	Dexamethasone	Antiemetic
Delatest	Testosterone	Breast cancer in women, palliative
Delatestryl	Therapeutic testosterone; testosterone; testosterone enanthate; trans-testosterone	delayed puberty, male; hypogonadism; metastatic mammary cancer; breast cancer in women, palliative
Delta-Cortef	Prednisolone	Inflammatory conditions; allergic conditions; hematologic conditions; neoplastic conditions; autoimmune conditions; replacement therapy in adrenal insufficiency
Delta-Dome, Deltasone	prednisone; delta(1)-cortisone; deltacortisone; deltadehydrocortisone; metacortandracin; PRD; prednisonum	Inflammatory conditions; allergic conditions; hematologic conditions; neoplastic conditions; autoimmune conditions; replacement therapy in adrenal insufficiency
Depandro 100	Testosterone	Breast cancer in women, palliative
Depo-Provera	Medroxyprogesterone; medroxyprogesterone acetate	Breast carcinoma; endometrial carcinoma; renal cell carcinoma
Depotest, Depotestosterone	Testosterone	Breast cancer in women, palliative
Deronil, Dex-4, Dexace. Dexameth, Dezone	Dexamethasone	Antiemetic (prevents vomiting)

Trade Name	*Generic Name*	*Indicated For*
Duratest, Durathate 200	Testosterone	Breast cancer in women, palliative
Emcyt	Estramustine phosphate sodium; estramustine phosphate	Prostate cancer
Estinyl	Ethinyl estradiol	Advanced androgen-dependent prostate cancer, palliative; breast cancer, palliative; estrogen replacement; menopausal symptoms; postmenopausal osteoporosis
Estrace, Estradiol Patch, Estragyn LA 5	Estradiol	Breast cancer, palliative
Estratab	Esterified estrogens	Breast cancer
Estro-Cyp, Estrogen patches	Estradiol	Breast cancer, palliative
Ethinoral, Eticylol	Ethinyl estradiol	Advanced androgen-dependent prostate cancer, palliative; breast cancer, palliative; estrogen replacement; menopausal symptoms; postmenopausal osteoporosis
Everone	Testosterone	Breast cancer in women, palliative
Femest	Conjugated estrogens	Advanced androgen-dependent prostate cancer, palliative; breast cancer, palliative
Feminone	Ethinyl estradiol	Advanced androgen-dependent prostate cancer, palliative; breast cancer, palliative; estrogen replacement; menopausal symptoms; postmenopausal osteoporosis
Fempatch	Estradiol	Breast cancer, palliative
Fidelin	Therapeutic dehydroepiandrosterone	Adrenal insufficiency, replacement; systemic lupus erythematosus, treatment and steroid treatment reduction
FIRST-Testosterone, FIRST-Testosterone MC	Testosterone	Breast cancer in women, palliative
Florinef	Fludrocortisone	Breast cancer; adrenal cortical cancer
Gammacorten	Dexamethasone	Antiemetic
Gesterol 100	Therapeutic progesterone	Amenorrhea; functional uterine bleeding; infertility; maintenance of pregnancy
Gynodiol, Gynogen LA 20	Estradiol	Breast cancer, palliative
Halodrin, Halotestrin	Fluoxymesterone; androfluorene	Certain types of breast cancer
Hexadrol	Dexamethasone	Antiemetic
Histerone	Testosterone	Breast cancer in women, palliative
Hydeltra, Hydeltrasol	Prednisolone	Inflammatory conditions; allergic conditions; hematologic conditions; neoplastic conditions; autoimmune conditions; replacement therapy in adrenal insufficiency
Inestra	Ethinyl estradiol	Advanced androgen-dependent prostate cancer, palliative; breast cancer, palliative; estrogen replacement; menopausal symptoms; postmenopausal osteoporosis

Trade Name	*Generic Name*	*Indicated For*
Lipo-Lutin	Therapeutic progesterone	Amenorrhea; functional uterine bleeding; infertility; maintenance of pregnancy
Liquid Pred, Lisacort	prednisone; delta(1)-cortisone; deltacortisone; deltadehydrocortisone; metacortandracin; PRD; prednisonum	Inflammatory conditions; allergic conditions; hematologic conditions; neoplastic conditions; autoimmune conditions; replacement therapy in adrenal insufficiency
Luteohormone	Therapeutic progesterone	Amenorrhea; functional uterine bleeding; infertility; maintenance of pregnancy
Lynoral	Ethinyl estradiol	Advanced androgen-dependent prostate cancer, palliative; breast cancer, palliative; estrogen replacement; menopausal symptoms; postmenopausal osteoporosis
Maxidex	Dexamethasone	Antiemetic (prevents vomiting)
Meditest	Testosterone	Breast cancer in women, palliative
Megace; Megace ES	Megestrol acetate	Appetite enhancement, AIDS patients; breast cancer, palliative; endometrial carcinoma, palliative treatment
Menaval-20	Estradiol	Breast cancer, palliative
Menest	Esterified estrogens	Breast cancer
Meticorten	Prednisone; delta(1)-cortisone; deltacortisone; deltadehydrocortisone; metacortandracin; PRD; prednisonum	Inflammatory conditions; allergic conditions; hematologic conditions; neoplastic conditions; autoimmune conditions; replacement therapy in adrenal insufficiency
Meti-derm	Prednisolone	
Microlut, Neogest	Norgestrel	Oral contraception
Orasone	Prednisone; delta(1)-cortisone; deltacortisone; deltadehydrocortisone; metacortandracin; PRD; prednisonum	Inflammatory conditions; allergic conditions; hematologic conditions; neoplastic conditions; autoimmune conditions; replacement therapy in adrenal insufficiency
Ora-Testryl	Fluoxymesterone; androfluorene; androsterolo	Anabolic steroid; certain types of breast cancer, male hypogonadism, delayed puberty in males
Orestralyn	Ethinyl estradiol	Advanced androgen-dependent prostate cancer, palliative; breast cancer, palliative; estrogen replacement; menopausal symptoms; postmenopausal osteoporosis
Ovaban	Megestrol acetate	Appetite enhancement, AIDS patients; breast cancer, palliative; endometrial carcinoma, palliative treatment
Ovrette	Norgestrel	Oral contraception
Pallace	Megestrol acetate	Appetite enhancement, AIDS patients; breast cancer, palliative; endometrial carcinoma, palliative treatment

Trade Name	*Generic Name*	*Indicated For*
Prednicen-M	Prednisone; delta(1)-cortisone; deltacortisone; deltadehydrocortisone; metacortandracin; PRD; prednisonum	Inflammatory conditions; allergic conditions; hematologic conditions; neoplastic conditions; autoimmune conditions; replacement therapy in adrenal insufficiency
Prednilen	Methylprednisone	Adrenocortical insufficiency; conditions requiring immunosuppression; inflammatory conditions; multiple sclerosis; nephrotic syndrome
Prelone	Prednisone; delta(1)-cortisone; deltacortisone; deltadehydrocortisone; metacortandracin; PRD; prednisonum	Inflammatory conditions; allergic conditions; hematologic conditions; neoplastic conditions; autoimmune conditions; replacement therapy in adrenal insufficiency
Premarin	Conjugated estrogens	Advanced androgen-dependent prostate cancer, palliative; breast cancer, palliative
Progestin	Therapeutic progesterone	Amenorrhea; functional uterine bleeding; infertility; maintenance of pregnancy
Provera. Provera Dosepak	Medroxyprogesterone; medroxyprogesterone acetate	Breast carcinoma; endometrial carcinoma; renal cell carcinoma
Sk-Dexamethasone	Dexamethasone	Antiemetic (prevents vomiting)
Sk-Prednisone Sterapred	Prednisone; delta(1)-cortisone; deltacortisone; deltadehydrocortisone; metacortandracin; PRD; prednisonum	Inflammatory conditions; allergic conditions; hematologic conditions; neoplastic conditions; autoimmune conditions; replacement therapy in adrenal insufficiency
Testamone-100	Testosterone	Breast cancer in women, palliative
Testoderm Testolin	Therapeutic testosterone; testosterone; testosterone enanthate; trans-testosterone	delayed puberty, male; hypogonadism; metastatic mammary cancer; breast cancer in women, palliative
Testopel, Testosterone Enanthate	Testosterone	Breast cancer in women, palliative
Testostroval, Testostroval-PA, Testro, Testro AQ	Therapeutic testosterone, testosterone; testosterone enanthate; trans-testosterone	Delayed puberty, male; hypogonadism; metastatic mammary cancer
Testred	Testosterone	Breast cancer in women, palliative
Virilon	Methyltestosterone	Breast cancer, palliative
Wyacort	Methylprednisone	Adrenocortical insufficiency; conditions requiring immunosuppression; inflammatory conditions; multiple sclerosis; nephrotic syndrome
Zytiga	Abiraterone acetate	Castration-resistant prostate cancer

5. Non-steroidal Anti-inflammatory Drugs (NSAIDs)

Trade Name	*Generic Name*	*Indicated For*
Advil, Midol, NeoProfen, Caldolor, Motrin, Select, Ibu, & Profen	Ibuprofen	Arthritis; inflammatory conditions, pain
Aflodac	Sulindac	Arthritis; inflammatory conditions
Aleve, Anaprox	Naproxen sodium	Fever, inflammatory conditions, pain
Ansaid	Flurbiprofen	Osteoarthritis; rheumatoid arthritis
Aspirin, Empirin	Acetylsalicylic acid	Stroke and myocardial infarction prophylaxis (low dose), fever, inflammatory conditions (high dose); mild to moderate pain
Cambia, Cataflam	Diclofenac	Mild to moderate pain, fever, and inflammation
Clinoril	Sulindac	Arthritis; inflammatory conditions
Celebrex	Celecoxib (Cox-2 specific inhibitor)	Familial adenomatous polyposis (inherited colorectal cancer syndrome)
Daypro	Oxaprozin	Osteoarthritis; rheumatoid arthritis
Disalcid	Sodium salicylate	Fever, inflammatory conditions, pain
Extren	Acetylsalicylic acid; aspirin	Mild to moderate pain; fever; prevention of arterial and venous thrombosis
Feldene	Piroxicam	Rheumatoid arthritis
Flanax	Naproxen sodium	Fever, inflammatory conditions, pain
Indocin	Indomethacin	Dysmenorrhea; inflammatory disorders; pain
Lodine	Etodolac	Moderate pain; osteoarthritis; rheumatoid arthritis.
Mobic	Meloxicam	Osteoarthritis; rheumatoid arthritis
Naprelan, Naprosyn	Naproxen sodium	Fever, inflammatory conditions, pain
Nalfon	Fenoprofen	Osteoarthritis; rheumatoid arthritis
Orudis, Orudis KT, Oruvail	Ketoprofen	Rheumatoid arthritis; osteoarthritis; menstrual cramps; pain
Relafen	Nabumetone	Mild to moderate pain, fever, and inflammation
Tolectin DS; Tolectin 600	Tolmetin	rheumatoid arthritis; osteoarthritis; juvenile arthritis
Toradol	Ketorolac	Moderate to severe pain
Vivlodex	Meloxicam	Osteoarthritis; rheumatoid arthritis
Vivomo	Esomeprazole and Naproxen	Osteoarthritis; rheumatoid arthritis; ankylosing spondylitis.

Trade Name	*Generic Name*	*Indicated For*
Voltaren-XR, Zipsor, Zorvolex	Diclofenac	Mild to moderate pain, fever, and inflammation
Non-NSAID		

6. Antihypertensives

Trade Name	*Generic Name*	*Indicated For*
ACE inhibitors		
Accupril	Quinapril	Hypertension; heart failure; left ventricular dysfunction; diabetic nephropathy
Aceon	Perinopril	
Altace	Ramapril	
Capoten	Captopril	
Lotensin	benzazepril	
Mavil	Trandolapril	
Monopril	Fosinopril	
Prinivil	Lisinopril	
Univasc	Moexipril	
Vasotec	Enalapril	
Zestril	Lisinopril	
Angiotensin II Receptor Inhibitors		
Atacand	Candesartan	Hypertension; kidney failure prophylaxis in diabetics; heart failure; stroke prophylaxis.
Avapro	Irbesartan	
Benicar	Olmesartan	
Cozaar	Losartan	
Diovan	Valsartan	
Edarbi	Azilsartan	
Micardis	telmisartan	
Teveten	Eprosartan	
Beta Blockers		

a. Cardioselective

Trade Name	*Generic Name*	*Indicated For*
Brevibloc	Esmolol	Angina; arrhythmia; hypertension
Kerlone	Betaxolol	
Lopressor	Metoprolol	
Sectral	Acebutolol	
Tenormin	Atenolol	
Toprol-XL	Metoprolol	
Zebeta	Bisoprolol	
b. Noncardioselective		
Cartrol	Carteolol	
Coreg	Carvedilol	
Corgard	Nadolol	
Inderal, InnoPran XL	Propranolol	
Normodyne, Trandate	Labetalol	
Potassium-Sparing Diuretics		
Aldactone	Spironolactone	Hypertension; congestive heart failure; nephrotic syndrome; cirrhosis
Midamor	Amiloride	Hypertension, congestive heart failure
Thiazide Diuretics		
Aquazide H, HydroDIU-RIL, Microzide	Hydrochlorothiazide	Hypertension; edema
Thalitone	Chlorthalidone	
Zaroxolyn	Metolazone	
Miscellaneous vasodilators		
Apresoline	Hydralazine	Hypertension
Loniten	Minoxidil	Hypertension; topically for alopecia
Nitropress	Nitroprusside	Hypertensive emergencies
Proglycem	Diazoxide	Malignant hypertension

7. Analgesics (pain killers)

Trade Name	*Generic Name*	*Indicated For*
Actamin, Apra, Disprol, Mapap, Q-Pap, Tactinal, Tempra, Tycolene, Tylenol, Vitapap	Acetaminophen (also known as paracetamol)	Pain; fever
Actiq, Fentora, Sublimaze	Fentanyl citrate	Breakthrough pain in cancer patients
Combunox	Ibuprofen/oxycodone	Pain relief
Darvocet	Acetaminophen/ Propoxyphene	
Meprozine	meperidine/promethazine	
Morphine, AVINza, Kadi-an, MS Contin	Morphine	
Norco, Hycet, Lorcet, Lortab, Verdrocet, Xodol, Zolvit	Acetaminophen/ Hydrocodone	
Percocet, Percodan	Acetaminophen/ Oxycodone	
Suboxone, Zubsolv	buprenorphine/naloxone	
Talacen	Acetaminophen/ pentazocine	
Vicoprofen	Hydrocodone/ibuprofen	

8. Hormones/Antineoplastics

Trade Name	*Generic Name*	*Indicated For*
Antiandrogen		
Casodex	Bicalutamide	Prostate cancer
Eulexin	Flutamide	
Nilandron	Nilutamide	
Xtandi	Enzalutamide	
Aromatase inhibitor		
Arimidex	Anastrozole	Breast cancers
Aromasin	Exemestane	
Femara	Letrozole	

Trade Name	*Generic Name*	*Indicated For*
Estrogen Receptor Agonist		
Faslodex	Fulvestrant	Breast cancer
Gonadotropin-releasing hormone antagonists		
Firmagon	Degarelix	Breast cancer
Plenaxis	Abarelix	Prostate cancer, palliative
Gonadotropin-releasing hormone agonists		
Histrelin implant	histrelin acetate	palliative treatment of advanced prostate cancer
Lupron, Viadur	Leuprolide acetate; leuprorelin; leuprorelin acetate	Prostate cancer, uterine fibroid tumors
Trelstar, Decapeptyl	Triptorelin; 6-D-tryptophan-LH- RH; 6-D-tryptophanluteinizing hormone-releasing factor; detryptoreline; D-TRP-6-LHRH	Prostate cancer; palliative treatment
Zoladex	Goserelin	Prostate cancer; endometriosis
Progestins		
Megace	Megestrol	Uterine cancer; breast cancer
Evista, Keoxifene	Raloxifene	Breast cancer; cardiovascular disease prophylaxis; osteoporosis
Fareston	Toremifene	Breast cancer
Nolvadex, Soltamox	Tamoxifen	breast cancer, palliative; adjuvant in breast cancer therapy; endometrial cancer; gynecomastia; melanoma; ovarian cancer
Synthetic estrogens		
Acnestrol, Cyren A, Deladumone, Diastyl, Domestrol, Estrobene, Estrosyn, Fornatol, Makarol, Milestrol, Neo-Oestronol I, Oestrogenine, Oestromenin, Oestromon, Palestrol, Stilbestrol; Stilboestrol, Stilbetin, Stilboestroform, Synestrin, Synthoestrin, Vagestrol	diethylstilbesterol; diethylstilbenediol; diethylstilbestrol dipropionate; diethylstilbestrolum; diethylstilboestrol; sinestrol; stilboestrol dipropionate	Breast cancer; prostate cancer

9. Bisphosphonates

Trade Name	*Generic Name*	*Indicated For*
Actonel	Risedronate sodium	Osteoporosis, treatment and prevention; Paget disease
Aredia	Disodium pamidronate; pamidronate disodium	Myeloma, secondary breast cancer; hypercalcemia of malignancy; osteolytic bone lesions of multiple myeloma; osteolytic bone metastases of breast cancer; Paget disease
Binosto, Fosamax	Alendronate	Osteoporosis, treatment and prevention; Paget disease
Bondronate, Boniva	Ibandronate sodium	Osteoporosis, treatment and prevention
Didronel	Etidronate	Treating adults with Paget disease; preventing and treating abnormal bone growth following hip replacement surgery or spinal cord injury
Reclast, Zometa	Zoledronic acid; NDC-zoledronate; zoledronate	Hypercalcemia of malignancy; multiple myeloma and metastatic bone lesions from solid tumors; Paget disease

10. Nutritional or Mineral Supplements

Trade Name	*Generic Name*	*Indicated For*
Acicontral	Calcium citrate; calcium supplement;	Hypocalcemia; osteoporosis; rickets; tetany
Calglucon	Calcium gluconate	Hyperkalemia; hypocalcemic tetany; magnesium intoxication
Carnitor	Levocarnitine	carnitine deficiency; end-stage renal disease
Citracal	Calcium citrate	Calcium supplement; hypocalcemia; osteoporosis; rickets; tetany
Geritol	Multivitamin	Vitamin supplement
Glutacerebro, Glutaven, L-glutamine, Memoril, Nutrestore, Q. Levoglutamide	Glutamine	Short Bowel
Lumitene	Beta-carotene	chemoprevention for cardiovascular disease and cancer
Nicamid, Nicosedine	Niacinamide	Pellagra, treatment and prophylaxis; various dermatologic conditions
Retinol Acetate	Retinyl acetate	dietary supplement; vitamin A deficiency
Revival	Soy protein isolate	heart disease prevention; hyperlipidemia; menopausal symptoms
Solatene	Beta-carotene	Chemoprevention for cardiovascular disease and cancer

Trade Name	*Generic Name*	*Indicated For*
Ubidecarenone,	Coenzyme Q10	Chronic heart failure; mitochondrial cytopathies
Venofer	Iron sucrose injection	Treatment of iron deficiency for both dialysis and non-dialysis patients with kidney disease, with or without concurrent erythropoietin therapy

11. Retinoids

Trade Name	*Generic Name*	*Indicated For*
Aberel, Aknoten, Aquasol A, Avita, Renova, Retin-A; Retin-A MICRO, Vesanoid	Tretinoin; all-trans retinoic acid; all-trans vitamin A acid; beta- retinoic acid; retinoic acid; TRA; trans retinoic acid; trans vitamin A acid; tretinoinum; vitamin A acid	(oral) acute promyelocytic leukemia (APL), characterized by the t(15;17) translocation or the PML/RARa gene; for patients refractory to or who have relapsed from anthracycline chemotherapy, or for where anthracycline-based chemotherapy is contraindicated; (topical) acne vulgaris; other dermatologic conditions; some skin cancers
Accutane	Isotretinoin	Cutaneous T-cell lymphoma; juvenile metastatic neuroblastoma and leukemia
Aknoten	Tretinoin; all-trans retinoic acid; all-trans vitamin A acid; beta- retinoic acid; retinoic acid; TRA; trans retinoic acid; trans vitamin A acid; tretinoinum; vitamin A acid	(oral) acute promyelocytic leukemia (APL), characterized by the t(15;17) translocation or the PML/RARa gene; for patients refractory to or who have relapsed from anthracycline chemotherapy, or for where anthracycline-based chemotherapy is contraindicated; (topical) acne vulgaris; other dermatologic conditions; some skin cancers
Aquasol A, Del-Vi-A, Pedi-Vit-A	vitamin A compound; all trans- retinol; anti-infective vitamin; antixerophthalmic vitamin; axerophthol; axerophtholum; biosterol; lard-factor; oleovitamin A; ophthalamin; retinol; vitamin A; vitamin A alcohol; vitamin A USP; vitamin A1; vitaminum A	diminishing malignant cell growth; enhancing the immune system
Etretin, Soriatane	acitretin; trimethylmethoxyphenyl-retinoic acid	Cutaneous T-cell lymphoma
Panretin	alitretinoin; 9-cis-retinoic acid; retinoicacid-9-cis	topical treatment of cutaneous lesions in patients with AIDS-related Kaposi sarcoma

Trade Name	*Generic Name*	*Indicated For*
Retisol-A, Vitinoin, Avage	Tazarotene	Topical treatment of facial acne vulgaris; stable plaque psoriasis; mitigation (palliation) of facial fine wrinkling; facial mottled hyper- and hypopigmentation; benign facial lentigines
Targretin	bexarotene; 3-methyl TTNEB	oral or topical treatment of manifestations of cutaneous T-cell lymphoma

12. Psychiatric drugs

Trade Names	*Generic Names*	*Indicated For*
Adderall	Dextroamphetamine-amphetamine	Attention deficit/hyperactivity disorder (ADHD); narcolepsy
Alti-Valproic, Depakene, Ergenyl, Novo-Valproic	Valproic acid	epilepsy; mania; migraine
Aricept	Donepezil hydrochloride	Alzheimer's disease and opioid-induced sedation
Buspar, Wellbutrin, Zyban	Buspirone hydrochloride	Alcohol abuse; anxiety; depression; migraine prophylax-is; smoking cessation; panic disorder
Circadin	Therapeutic melatonin	Sleep disorders in blind people with no light perception
Concerta	Methylphenidate hydrochloride	Attention deficit/hyperactivity disorder (ADHD); narcolepsy
Effexor	Venlafaxine	Anxiety; depression
Epitol, Tegretol	Carbamazepine	Epilepsy
Lamictal	lamotrigine	Lamotrigine
Neurontin	Gabapentin	Management of epilepsy; pain; mania; depression and anxiety disorders
Paxil	Paroxetine hydrochloride	Depression
Provigil	Modafinil	Narcolepsy
Zoloft	sertraline hydrochloride	Major depressive disorder; obsessive-compulsive disorder; panic disorder; posttraumatic stress disorder; premenstrual dysphoric disorder; social phobia

13. Antigout drugs

Trade Name	*Generic Name*	*Indicated For*
Alloprim, Zyloprim	allopurinol	treats high levels of uric acid in the body caused by certain cancer medications, especially for patients with leukemia, lymphoma, and solid-tumor malignancies (xanthine oxidase inhibitor)
Elitek	rasburicase; recombinant urate oxidase; urate oxidase	chemotherapy-induced acute hyperuricemia, treatment and prophylaxis
Probalan	**Probenecid**	Gout; hyperuricemia; increases concentrations of some antibiotics.
Uloric	Febuxostat	Treats high levels of uric acid in the body caused by certain cancer medications, especially for patients with leukemia, lymphoma, and solid-tumor malignancies (xanthine oxidase inhibitor)

14. Antinausea drugs

Trade Name	*Generic Name*	*Indicated For*
Aloxi	palonosetron hydrochloride	antinausea; antiemetic (prevents vomiting)
Compazine	Prochlorperazine	antinausea
Kytril	granisetron hydrochloride	Antinausea
Marinol	dronabinol; cannabinol; delta 9-tetrahydrocannabinol; tetrahydrocannabinol	Antinausea; appetite enhancement
Octamide, Reglan	metoclopramide	antinausea
Phenergan	Promethazine	Allergies; motion sickness; pain; nausea; vomiting

15. Radiochemicals

Trade Name	*Generic Name*	*Indicated For*
Bexxar	iodine I 131 tositumomab; 131-I- anti-B1 antibody; 131-I-anti-B1 monoclonal antibody; iodine I 131 MOAB anti-B1; iodine I 131 monoclonal antibody anti-B1; iodine-131 anti-B1 antibody; iodine-131 anti-CD20 monoclonal antibody; tositumomab; anti-CD20 antibody	CD-20-antigen-expressing, relapsed or refractory, low-grade, follicular, or transformed non-Hodgkin lymphoma; CD20 positive follicular non-Hodgkin lymphoma refractory to rituximab
I-125	iodine I 125	prostate cancer

I-131	iodine I 131	hyperthyroidism
131 I-MIBG	iodine I 131 metaiodobenzylguanidine	diagnostic imaging
Iodotope	sodium iodide I 131; iodine I 131	thyroid cancer; hyperthyroidism
Metastron	strontium chloride Sr 89	palliation of pain in bone metastases
Quadramet	samarium SM 153 lexidronam pentasodium; samarium-153 EDTMP; samarium-153 ethylenediaminetetramethyleneph osphonate; samarium-153 ethylenediaminetetramethyleneph osphonic acid; Sm-153 EDTMP	pain due to bone cancer
Sodium Phosphate P32 Solution	Sodium phosphate P32	Polycythemia vera; chronic myelocytic leukemia and chronic lymphocytic leukemia; multiple areas of skeletal metastases, palliative treatment
TheraSphere	yttrium Y 90 glass microspheres	hepatocellular carcinoma, transarterial internal radiation
Zevalin	yttrium Y 90 ibritumomab tiuxetan; 90Y ibritumomab tiuxetan; ibritumomab (In2B8/ Y2B8 radiolabeling kit); ibritumomab tiuxetan; IDEC- Y2B8 monoclonal antibody; Y90 zevalin; Y90-labeled ibritumomab tiuxetan; yttrium-90 ibritumomab tiuxetan	Relapsed or refractory low-grade, follicular, or transformed B-cell non-Hodgkin lymphoma, including patients with rituximab refractory follicular non-Hodgkin lymphoma

Associations and Agencies

American Association for Cancer Research
http://www.aacr.org
Provides programs and services that promote the exchange of knowledge and new ideas among cancer research scientists; provides training opportunities for upcoming cancer researchers and promotes public education about cancer.

American Cancer Society
http://www.cancer.org
Nonprofit organization providing the largest private source of cancer research funds in the United States. Offers prevention and early detection information in addition to a wide variety of patient services programs.

American Lung Association
http://www.lungusa.org
Provides educational materials on treatments and research related to lung cancer, as well as information on the dangers of smoking and secondhand smoke. Offers smoking-cessation support programs.

American Society of Clinical Oncology (ASCO)
http://www.asco.org; http://www.Cancer.Net
A nonprofit organization consisting of more than twenty-five thousand oncology practitioners who conduct clinical cancer research and treat cancer patients. Primary Web site provides news releases, cancer research articles, and new drug information. ASCO also manages a Web site called Cancer.Net (formerly People Living with Cancer), which provides information on different types of cancer, discusses clinical trials, offers suggestions for managing side effects, and features an oncologist database.

Association of American Cancer Institutes (AACI)
http://www.aaci.org
Comprises ninety-one U.S. cancer research centers; promotes cancer research, prevention, treatment, and patient care; provides research news and a list of member cancer centers.

Blue Faery: The Adrienne Wilson Liver Cancer Association
http://www.bluefaery.org
Dedicated to increasing research, education, and advocacy for the prevention, treatment, and cure of primary liver cancer, specifically hepatocellular carcinoma. Web site provides liver cancer information and latest news updates.

Breast Cancer Action
http://www.bcaction.org
Advocates for policy changes related to breast cancer issues and educates people about breast cancer and related topics. Provides a booklet for newly diagnosed breast cancer patients, monthly e-alerts with important breast cancer news, and a bimonthly newsletter called *The Source*. Web site offers recent breast cancer news and downloadable flyers and fact sheets.

The Breast Cancer Fund
http://www.breastcancerfund.org
Identifies environmental and other preventable contributors to breast cancer and advocates for their elimination. Educates the public about cancer prevention. Web site offers a monthly e-newsletter and fact sheets.

The Breast Cancer Research Foundation
http://www.bcrfcure.org
Raises funds for breast cancer research and increases awareness of good breast health. Provides a biannual newsletter.

Caregiver Action Network
http://caregiveraction.org
The Caregiver Action Network or CAN is the major resource for the more than 90 million Americans who care for loved ones with chronic conditions such as cancer. CAN (formerly the National Family Caregivers Association) is a non-profit organization that helps educate caregivers, provide them with peer support and mentoring and provides resources for caregivers free of charge.

C3: Colorectal Cancer Coalition
http://www.fightcolorectalcancer.org
Advocates to promote colorectal cancer research, policy. and awareness in an effort to improve screening, diagnosis, and treatment of colorectal cancer. Provides a monthly e-newsletter and a quarterly print newsletter called Momentum. Offers information on treatment options and clinical trials.

Canadian Cancer Society
http://www.cancer.ca
A Canadian, community-based organization of volunteers that provides information about cancer, prevention, research, support services, and publications. Web site provides information by province/territory in English and French.

Centers for Disease Control and Prevention (CDC)
http://www.cde.gov
Web site offers information on cancer, provides statistical information on cancer diagnosis in the United States, discusses smoking-cessation programs, and provides educational materials on cancer treatment and awareness. It also hosts a cancer survivorship issues page.

Children's Cause for Cancer Advocacy
http://www.childrenscause.org
Works with leading medical, scientific, and public policy experts to advance cancer research and treatment and to provide services for childhood cancer patients, survivors, and families. Web site offers information on Rise to Action Survivors Program and the opportunity to sign up for their newsletter, *The Next Step*.

CureSearch
http://www.curesearch.org
Unites Children's Oncology Group and National Childhood Cancer Foundation in their efforts to cure and prevent pediatric cancer. Web site provides information about types of pediatric cancers, treatment options available, risks and benefits of different treatment methods, prevention of and preparation for side effects, and ways to maintain a healthy lifestyle after treatment.

Esophageal Cancer Awareness Association (ECAA)
http://www.ecaware.org
Dedicated to helping patients, survivors, and caregivers deal more effectively with the uncertainties and consequences of esophageal cancer. Web site provides information about esophageal cancer and its diagnosis, staging, and treatments, as well as their newsletter, *Swallow Tales*, and contact information for members willing to offer support and advice.

Food and Drug Administration (FDA)
http://www.fd a.gov
Web site provides information on clinical trials, discusses clinical trial regulations, and provides consumer education information. The FDA's Cancer Liaison Program provides answers to questions about therapies asked by cancer patients and patient advocates; its Drug Development Patient Consultant Program allows cancer patient advocates to participate in the FDA drug review regulatory process; and its Cancer Patient Representative Program recruits, assesses, and selects patient representatives to serve as members of advisory committees.

Friends of Cancer Research
http://www.focr.org
Pioneers public-private partnerships in research and clinical trials, organizes public policy forums, educates public about prevention, detection, and treatment of cancers, and collaborates with media and the motion picture industry to promote cancer research and education. Web site offers news and events articles related to Cancer and a monthly newsletter.

Hospice Foundation of America
http://hospicefoundation.org
Professional palliative care for terminally-ill patients in the end stages of their lives. Hospice provides the services of a care team who consist of a hospice physician, nurse, medical social worker, home-health aide and chaplain/spiritual adviser who visit the patient at home, medication for symptom control or pain relief, medical equipment (e.g., wheelchairs or walkers) and medical supplies (e.g., bandages and catheters), physical and occupational therapy, speech-language pathology services, dietary counseling, short-term inpatient care, short-term respite care for caregivers, and grief and loss counseling for patients and loved ones.

Hurricane Voices
http://www.huITicanevoices.org
Organizes public awareness campaigns and educational programs and provides grants and sponsorships in support of breast cancer programs. Web site provides news articles about breast cancer and a list of books suggested for families affected by breast cancer.

Inflammatory Breast Cancer Association
http://www.ibchelp.org .
Educates people about inflammatory breast cancer (IBC). Web site provides information about signs and symptoms, screening methods, and treatments of IBC, news reports and videos about mc, an mc forum and registries, as well as survivors' stories.

Inflammatory Breast Cancer Research Foundation
http://www.ibcresearch.org
Educates people about inflammatory breast cancer. Advocates for advancement of research and raises awareness of the symptoms associated with the disease, to aid in early detection. Web site offers educational materials, e-mail discussion lists, and a newsletter.

Institute of Medicine (IOM)
http://www.iom.edu
Consists of volunteer scientists and laypeople not employed by the U.S. government who provide analysis and guidance on important health issues. Web site provides reports on cancer research, survivorship, and palliative care.

Intercultural Cancer Council
http://iccnetwork.org
Advocates for programs, policies, partnerships, and research aimed at eliminating cancer within racial and ethnic minorities and medically underserved populations in the United States. Sponsors biennial symposia. Web site provides cancer fact sheets and a quarterly newsletter called *The Voice.*

International Agency for Research on Cancer (IARC)
http://www.iarc.fr
Part of the World Health Organization, IARC coordinates and conducts cancer research, including monitoring global cancer occurrence, identifying causes of cancer and the mechanisms of carcinogenesis, and developing scientific strategies for cancer control; also distributes scientific information through publications, meetings, courses, and fellowships.

International Psycho-Oncology Society
http://www.ipos-society.org
A global professional society that seeks to foster multidisciplinary care for cancer patients that pays as close attention to the psychosocial facets of cancer as it does to the medical and clinical aspects of the disease. The organization serves advisory, educational, and advocacy roles and holds conferences, provides grants to researchers studying the psychosocial aspects of cancer and recognizes outstanding health care professionals to champion and model the integration of psychosocial care into their treatments regimens for cancer patients.

International Union Against Cancer
http://www.uicc.org
A global association of cancer-fighting organizations that educates people about cancer prevention and control worldwide. Offers fellowship and training opportunities for scientists. Publishes the *International Journal of Cancer*. Web site provides pres releases, new letters, publications, and a list of suggested books.

Joan Scarangello Foundation to Conquer Lung Cancer
http://www.jo..;slegacy.org
Increases awareness about lung cancer and raises money to provide research grants. The Joanie Award recognizes journalists who focus on the problem of lung cancer. Web site offers information on lung cancer and a list of patient resources.

Kidney Cancer Association
http://kidneycancer.org
Provides information on kidney cancer, treatment options, and clinical trials. Funds research, advocates on behalf of patients, and distributes the *Kidney Cancer Journal*. Web site provides links to a forum, calendar of events, online store, and the Fourth Angel Caregiver Mentoring Program.

Leukemia and Lymphoma Society
http://www.leukemia-Iymphoma.org
Provides information on blood cancers such as leukemia, lymphoma, Hodgkin disease, and myeloma. Funds blood cancer research, education, and patient services. Web site offers information on blood cancers, newsletters, a First Connection (peer-to-peer) program, education programs, calendar of events, and a call center.

Multiple Myeloma Research Foundation (MMRF)
http://www.multiplemyeloma.org
Provides research grants and advocates for myeloma research. Web site offers information about the disease, treatment options, and clinical trials, in addition to news and events.

National Asian Women's Health, Organization (NAWHO)
http://www.nawho.org
Raises awareness about the health issues facing Asian American women, including breast cancer and cervical cancer, and provides a list of Asian-language informational resources.

National Breast Cancer Coalition (NBCC)
http://www.natlbcc.org
Promotes breast cancer research and works toward improving access for all women to high-quality breast cancer screening, diagnosis, treatment, and care; informs and trains breast cancer survivors and others in effective advocacy efforts aimed at eradicating breast cancer. Web site provides breast cancer information, latest news, and sign-up for their e-newsletter.

National Cancer Institute (NCI)
http://www.cancer.gov
Part of the medical research agency of the U.S. government, NCI conducts and supports research, training, and information distribution regarding the cause, diagnosis, prevention and treatment of cancer, rehabilitation from cancer, and me continuing care of cancer

patients. Web site offers fact sheets, a dictionary of cancer terms, a dictionary of drug names, suggestions on coping with cancer, research news, and information on cancer prevention and screening, clinical trials, statistics, research funding, and complementary and alternative medicine.

National Cancer Institute of Canada (NCIC)
http://www.ncic.cancer.ca
Provides support for cancer research and related programs undertaken at Canadian universities, hospitals, and other research institutions. Web site offers video of commonly asked questions about cancer, information about program project grants, and an e-newsletter for cancer researchers.

National Cancer institute of Canada Clinical Trials Group (NCIC CTG)
http://www.etg.queensu.ca
Conducts clinical trials related to cancer therapy and prevention. Web site provides a list of publications and descriptions of clinical trials.

National Cervical Cancer Coalition (NCCC)
http://www.nccc-online.org
Educates people about cervical cancer and the importance of early detection, advocates for quality patient care, and provides support through its Phone Pals and E-Pals programs, which match women with cervical cancer survivors. Web site provides links to many resources related to cervical cancer, the NCCC Store, latest news, and its newsletter *Extraordinary Moments*.

National Comprehensive Cancer Network (NCCN)
http://www.nccn.org
A not-for-profit alliance of leading cancer centers. Web site provides information 00 treatment guidelines and supportive care, clinical trials, and member centers for people looking for physicians, pediatric cancer treatment, and genetic testing or screening.

National Institute of Environmental Health Sciences (NIEHS)
http://www.niehs. nih.gov
Part of the medical research agency of the U.S. government, the institute studies how environmental factors affect a person's chances of developing certain diseases, including cancers. Web site offers a library of resources, such as fact sheets, research reports, and a peer-reviewed journal called *Environmental Health Perspectives*. NIEHS performs a long-term study, called the Sister Study, of women whose sisters had breast cancer in an effort to learn how environment and genes affect a woman's chances of developing breast cancer.

National Library of Medicine
http://www.nlm.nih.gov
World's largest medical library offering a link to *PubMed*, an online searchable database of biomedical journal literature, and a link to MedlinePlus, an online searchable database of health and drug information for patients and loved ones, as well as links to many NLM databases and electronic resources.

National Ovarian Cancer Coalition (NOCC)
http://www.ovarian.org
Raises awareness and promotes education about ovarian cancer. Web site lists state chapters, support groups and services, and clinical trials, in addition to providing latest news, NOCC newsletter, and medical information about ovarian cancer.

Ovarian Cancer National Alliance (OCNA)
http://www.ovariancancer.org
An alliance of seven ovarian cancer groups that advocate for ovarian cancer education, policy, and research issues with national policy makers and women's health care leaders. Web site provides educational resources, support services, latest news, and clinical trials.

Prevent Cancer Foundation
http://www.preventcancer.org
Attempts to prevent cancer by funding research, educating people about prevention, and reaching out to communities through events and partnerships with other organizations.

Sarcoma Foundation of America
http://www.curesarcoma.org
Advocates for increased sarcoma research, raises funds to provide research grants to sarcoma researchers, and works to raise awareness of the treatment needs of sarcoma patients.

Skin Cancer Foundation
http://www.skincancer.org
Provides educational material about skin cancer prevention and detection. Web site provides information about different types of skin cancer, an Ask the Expert feature, a link to the SCF Store, and a Physician Finder database.

Stupid Cancer

http://stupidcancer.org

Founded in 2007 by a young adult brain cancer survivor, named Matthew Zachary, Stupid Cancer focuses on young adult cancer and is the largest advocacy organization dedicated to these cancers. It supports a global network of patients, survivors, caregivers, providers and advocates through deployment of an abundant network of resources.

WebMD

http://www.webmd.comlcancer

An online cancer health center that provides timely reports about medical research and other cancer issues. Web site includes links to top cancer news articles, information about common cancers and treatments, current clinical trials and research, blogs, message boards, Ask the Experts resource, drug information, a database for finding a doctor, WebMD video library, sign-up for WebMD newsletter, a symptom checker, and much more.

▶ Cancer Centers and Hospitals

Abramson Cancer Center of the University of Pennsylvania
http://www.penncancer.org
A National Cancer Institute (NCI)-designated comprehensive cancer center in Philadelphia that is part of a network of hospitals throughout Pennsylvania and New Jersey dedicated to providing state-of-the-art cancer care, research, and education.

Arizona Cancer Center at the University of Arizona
http://www.azcc.arizona.edu
An NCI-designated comprehensive cancer center in Tucson, Arizona. Offers specialized care to each patient through research, outreach, education, and information programs (including a patient education library), and support groups as well as social services and interpreters, and leading-edge clinical care.

Barbara Ann Karmanos Cancer Institute/Meyer L. Prentis Comprehensive Cancer Center of Metropolitan Detroit
http://www.karmanos.org
An NCI-designated comprehensive cancer center based in Detroit, Michigan. Videoconferencing and physician-to-physician communication throughout the Karmanos affiliate network al lows for leading-edge patient care, cancer research, clinical trials, and education statewide.

Cancer Institute of New Jersey (CINJ) at Robert Wood Johnson Medical School
http://www.cinj.org
An NCI-designated comprehensive cancer center based in New Brunswick, New Jersey, consisting of a statewide network of sixteen hospitals. Provides cancer research, clinical trials, patient care, support groups, and education. Produces publications useful to patients and their families, including its quarterly newsletter *Oncolyte*.

Cancer Treatment Centers of America (CTCA)
http://www.cancercenter.com
Uses aggressive research and innovative new techniques to provide personalized medical, nutritional, physical, psychological, and spiritual therapies to fight cancer. Several locations nationwide. Web site offers many survivor stories, CTCA news releases, media coverage, brochures, and treatment diagrams.

Case Comprehensive Cancer Center
http://cancer.case.edu
An NCI-designated comprehensive cancer center based in Cleveland, Ohio, in partnership with University Hospitals of Cleveland and the Cleveland Clinic. Uses coordinated interdisciplinary clinical research to improve cancer diagnosis, treatment, prevention, and control.

Chao Family Comprehensive Cancer Center at the University of California, Irvine
http://www.ucihs.uci.edulcancer
An NCI-designated comprehensive cancer center located in Irvine, California, that integrates research, prevention, diagnostic, treatment, and rehabilitation programs to provide patient-centered care for patients and families coping with cancer.

City of Hope
http://www.cityofhope.org
A biomedical research, treatment, and educational institution in Duarte, California, and an NCI-designated comprehensive cancer center dedicated to the prevention and cure of cancer and other life-threatening diseases. Mission follows a compassionate patient-centered philosophy. Supported by a national foundation of humanitarian philanthropy.

Dana-Farber Cancer Institute, Brigham and Women's Hospital, and Massachusetts General Hospital
http://www.cancercare.harvard.edu
Teaching affiliates of Harvard Medical School and founding members of Dana-Farber/Harvard Cancer Center, an NCI-designated comprehensive cancer center, in Boston. Develops and provides comprehensive, multidisciplinary care plans for cancer patients. A major leader in cancer research.

Duke Comprehensive Cancer Center
http://www.cancer.duke.edu
An NCI-designated comprehensive cancer center in Durham, North Carolina, that strives to provide cutting-edge research and compassionate care. Web site provides a tumor registry detailing cancer incidence seen at Duke.

Fox Chase Cancer Center
http://www.fccc.edu
An NCI-designated comprehensive cancer center in Philadelphia that provides basic, clinical, and prevention

research in addition to programs for detection and treatment of cancer and community outreach services.

Fred Hutchinson Cancer Research Center (Seattle Cancer Care Alliance)
hup://www.fhcrc.org (http://www.seattlecca.org)
An NCI-designated comprehensive cancer center in Seattle, Washington. Has pioneered new diagnostic and treatment techniques. Web site offers a Patient Guide to Clinical Trials and information on its Survivorship Program.

H. Lee Moffitt Cancer Center and Research Institute at the University of South Florida
http://www.moffitt.org
A nonprofit, NCI-designated comprehensive cancer center in Tampa, Florida, that provides rapid translation of scientific research discoveries to patient care, a blood and marrow transplant program, outpatient treatment programs, and a lifetime cancer screening program.

Herbert Irving Comprehensive Cancer Center at Columbia University
http://www.ccc.columbia.edu
An NCI-designated comprehensive cancer center in New York, in partnership with New York Presbyterian Hospital, that provides patient care, clinical trials, research, and education.

Holden Comprehensive Cancer Center at the University of Iowa
http://www.uihealthcare.comldeptslcancercenter
An NCI-designated comprehensive cancer center in Iowa City, Iowa, that provides cancer-related research, clinical trials, education, and patient care throughout many departments in the University of Iowa and its hospitals and clinics.

Huntsman Cancer Institute at the University of Utah
http://www.huntsmancancer.org
An NCI-designated cancer center in Salt Lake City, Utah, that consists of scientists, physicians, and health educators working to prevent, diagnose, and treat cancers. Web site offers a link to the Huntsman Online Patient Education (HOPE) Guide.

Indiana University Melvin and Bren Simon Cancer Center
http://iucc.iu.edu
An NCI-designated cancer center in Indianapolis, Indiana, that consists of a partnership between the Indiana University School of Medicine and Clarian Health. Provides quality patient care, research, clinical trials, and educational programs.

John Wayne Cancer Institute at St. John's Health Center
http://www.jwci.org
A cancer research institute in Santa Monica, California, that conducts multidisciplinary basic, clinical translational research, focusing mainly on melanoma, sarcoma, breast cancer, prostate cancer, and colon cancer.

Johns Hopkins Hospital
http://www.hopkinsmedicine.org/
One of the leading hospitals in the United States, Johns Hopkins Hospital is located in Baltimore, MD, and has a long tradition of medical excellence and innovative clinical research. Johns Hopkins Hospital has the following cancer specialty centers: 1) Blood and Bone Marrow Cancers; 2) Brain and Spinal Tumor Program; 3) Breast Cancer Program; 4) Colon Cancer Center; 5) Gynecologic Oncology Program; 6) Head and Neck Cancer Center; 7) Liver Cancer Center; 8) Lung Cancer Program; 9) Melanoma Program; 10) Pancreatic Cancer Center; 11) Pediatric Oncology; and 12) Prostate Cancer and other Genitourinary Cancers.

Jonsson Comprehensive Cancer Center
http://www.cancer.mednet.ucla.edu
An NCI-designated comprehensive cancer center at the University of California, Los Angeles, that provides interdisciplinary, team-oriented care for cancer patients. Provides information on research advances in the laboratory, clinical trials, Food and Drug Administration approved treatments, and psychosocial and supportive care for cancer patients and their families, including people at high risk of cancer due to family histories or inherited genetic mutations.

Kimmel Cancer Center at Thomas Jefferson University Hospital
http://www.kimmelcancercenter.org
An NCI-designated comprehensive cancer center in Philadelphia. Translates latest research discoveries and clinical trials into high-quality patient care, provides patient education and support programs, and maintains a cancer registry.

Lineberger Comprehensive Cancer Center at University of North Carolina
http://cancer.med.unc.edu
A comprehensive cancer center at Chapel Hill's School of Medicine. A member of the Lance Armstrong Foundation Survivorship Network, the center provides multi-disciplinary teams, patient and family support, research, clinical trials, survivor services, and an NC Cancer Hospital oncology newsletter.

Lombardi Comprehensive Cancer Center, Georgetown University Medical Center
http://lombardi.georgetown.edu
An NCI-designated comprehensive cancer center in Washington, D.C., that provides comprehensive patient care, research, clinical trials, and community outreach. The center also provides the Lombardi Cancerline to answer questions confidentially.

M. D. Anderson Cancer Center
http://www.mdanderson.org
In association with Children's Cancer Hospital, a comprehensive cancer center in Houston, Texas, that provides integrated programs in cancer treatment, clinical trials, education programs and cancer prevention.

Massachusetts General Hospital
www.massgeneral.org
Ranked the top hospital in the nation in 2015-2016, Massachusetts General Hospital is home to a formidable list of innovative clinical trials. Besides being a superb research institution, MGH also specializes in multidisciplinary approaches to cancer treatment and care.

Mayo Clinic Cancer Center
http://mayoresearch.mayo.edu/mayo/research/cancercenter
An NCI-designated comprehensive cancer center with three campuses nationwide. Offers research, clinical trials, patient care, and outreach programs, including Outreach to American Indians and Alaska Natives.

Memorial Sloan-Kettering Cancer Center
http://www.mskcc.org
Close collaboration between scientists and physicians underlines this NCI-designated comprehensive cancer center's commitment to exceptional patient care, research, and educational programs. Located in New York.

Norris Cotton Cancer Center at Dartmouth-Hitchcock Medical Center
http://www.cancer.dartmouth.edu/index.shtml
An NCI-designated comprehensive cancer center in Lebanon, New Hampshire. Multidisciplinary teams work to provide the best treatment, cure, and recovery environment possible for patients through research, clinical trials, support groups, and education.

NYU Cancer Institute
http://www.med.nyu.edu/nyuci
Part of the New York University Medical Center in New York, it provides programs in patient care, research, prevention, and community outreach and education dealing with cancer.

Ohio State University Comprehensive Cancer Center
http://www.OSUCCC.osu.edu
An NCI-designated comprehensive cancer center in Columbus, Ohio, that translates research into high-quality patient care by offering educational programs, individualized treatments and preventive strategies designed to meet unique personal health care needs.

Rebecca and John Moores University of California, San Diego, Cancer Center
http://cancer.ucsd.edu
An NCI-designated comprehensive cancer center in San Diego, California, dedicated to translating research into promising new treatments and to providing community outreach to educate the public, especially underserved populations, about prevention studies and cancer information.

Robert H. Lurie Comprehensive Cancer Center of Northwestern University
http://www.cancer.northwestern.edu
An NCI-designated comprehensive cancer center in Chicago that performs laboratory and clinical cancer research and offers innovative cancer treatments involving clinical trials, cancer prevention and control programs, training and education of health care professionals, cancer information services, and community outreach and education.

Roswell Park Cancer Institute
http://www.roswellpark.org
America's first cancer center, now an NCI-designated comprehensive cancer center in Buffalo, New York, includes a comprehensive diagnostic and treatment center and a medical research complex.

St. Jude Children's Research Hospital
http://www.stjude.org
A comprehensive pediatric cancer center in Memphis, Tennessee, St. Jude is America's third-largest health care charity. Concentrates its efforts on researching and curing childhood cancers and diseases, becoming pioneers in unique procedures and cures.

The Sidney Kimmel Comprehensive Cancer Center at Johns Hopkins
http://www.hopkinskimmelcancercenter.org
An NCI-designated comprehensive cancer center in Baltimore, Maryland, dedicated to finding more effective cancer treatments through programs in clinical and

laboratory research, education, community outreach, and prevention and control. Offers counseling, survivors and palliative care programs, and two residences for out-of-town patients.

Siteman Cancer Center at Barnes-Jewish Hospital and Washington University School of Medicine
http://www.siteman.wustl.edu
An NCI-designated comprehensive cancer center in St. Louis, Missouri, that provides expertise of research scientists and physicians, advanced diagnostic and treatment services, and an active outreach program of cancer screening and education.

Stanford Cancer Center
http://cancer.stanford.edu
An NCI-designated cancer center in Stanford, California, that uses the latest detection, diagnosis, treatment, and prevention discoveries with comprehensive support services to provide the most advanced patient care available.

UC Davis Cancer Center
http://www.ucdmc.ucdavis .edu/cancer
An NCI-designated cancer center in Sacramento, California, that provides multidisciplinary teams for patient care, clinical trials, and support groups and services, including the Triumph Fitness Program and the Writing as Healing Program. Web site provides survivor stories, news releases, and a link to its biannual magazine *Synthesis*.

UCLA Medical Center
www.uclahealth.org
Consistently ranked in the top five hospitals in the nation, UCLA Medical Center is home to the UCLA Daltrey/Townshead Teen and Young Adult Cancer Program that specializes in cancers that afflict young people.

UCSF Helen Diller Family Comprehensive Cancer Center
http://cancer.ucsf.edu
An NCI-designated comprehensive cancer center in San Francisco that combines basic science, clinical research, population science, epidemiology/cancer control, and patient care.

University of Alabama at Birmingham Comprehensive Cancer Center
http://www3.ccc.uab.edu
An NCI-designated comprehensive cancer center in Birmingham, Alabama, that includes a large patient resource library, a preventive care program for women's cancers, many support groups, and its magazine called *Crossroads*.

University of Colorado Cancer Center
http://www.uccc.info
An NCI-designated comprehensive cancer center in Aurora, Colorado, that provides a multidisciplinary team approach to patient care. Web site offers information on support groups, patient programs and classes, spiritual counseling, and palliative care.

University of Michigan Comprehensive Cancer Center
http://www.mcancer.org
An NCI-designated comprehensive cancer center in Ann Arbor, Michigan, that provides research, patient care, a patient education resource center, complementary therapies, nutrition counseling, child and family life services, art therapy, and social work services.

University of Minnesota Cancer Center
http://www.cancer.umn.edu
An NCI-designated comprehensive cancer center in Minneapolis that strives to enhance knowledge of the prevention, causes, detection, and treatment of cancer to improve quality of life for patients and survivors through research, clinical trials, and education. Web site offers access to cancer center stories, news, and publications.

University of Nebraska Medical Center Eppley Cancer Center
http://www.unmc.edu:80/cancercenter
A comprehensive cancer center in Omaha, Nebraska, that performs cancer research and provides patient care and educational programs.

University of New Mexico Cancer Center
http://cancer.unm.edu
An NCI-designated cancer center in Albuquerque, New Mexico, integrates research, clinical trials, patient care, support services, and community outreach to serve its region's multiethnic populations.

University of Pittsburgh Cancer Institute
http://www.upci.upmc.edu
An NCI-designated comprehensive cancer center in Pittsburgh, Pennsylvania. Provides research, clinical trials, patient care, and education. Web site offers links to a variety of cancer-related publications.

University of Tennessee Cancer Institute
http://www.utcancer.com
A partnership between the University of Tennessee Health Science Center and Boston Baskin Cancer Group in Memphis, this institute provides surgical oncology, radiation oncology, gynecologic oncology, genetic

counseling, multidisciplinary clinics, and cancer prevention and supportive care programs.

University of Virginia Health System Cancer Center
http://www.healthsystem.virginia.edu/internet/cancer
An NCI-designated cancer center in Charlottesville, Virginia, that provides cancer care teams, research, clinical trials, and support services.

University of Washington Medical Center/Seattle Cancer Care Alliance
http://www.uwmedicine.org/uw-medical-center
A highly-ranked teaching hospital, cancer research center, and cancer care and treatment center. UW is highly regarded for its commitment to patient safety, and is certified for bone marrow, umbilical cord blood, and tissue transplantation by the Foundation for the Accreditation of Cellular Therapy.

University of Wisconsin Paul P. Carbone Comprehensive Cancer Center
http://www.cancer.wisc.edu
An NCI-designated comprehensive cancer center in Madison, Wisconsin that provides research, clinical trials, patient care, and outreach. Web site provides information on news articles and outreach programs, including tobacco cessation and quality of life/pain and symptom management.

USC/Norris Comprehensive Cancer Center
http://ccnt.hsc.usc.edu
An NCI-designated comprehensive cancer center in Los Angeles that provides inpatient and outpatient care in its affiliated hospitals and outpatient clinics, conducts research and clinical trials, and translates that research into new patient therapies.

Vanderbilt-Ingram Cancer Center
http://www.vicc.org
An NCI-designated comprehensive cancer center in Nashville, Tennessee, that performs research and clinical trials and uses an interdisciplinary team approach to patient care; also provides childhood cancer programs.

Vermont Cancer Center at the University of Vermont
http://www.vermontcancer.org
An NCI-designated comprehensive cancer center in Burlington, Vermont, that provides interdisciplinary approaches to cancer research, prevention, patient care, and community education. Web site provides cancer, information, news, and information about support groups and services.

Wake Forest University Baptist Medical Center
http://wwwl .wfubmc.edu/cancer
An NCI-designated comprehensive cancer center in Winston-Salem, North Carolina, that provides patient care, clinical trials, research, pastoral care, support groups, and education. Web site provides drug interaction information, health encyclopedia, nutrition center, alternative and complementary medicine information, and a physician directory.

Yale Cancer Center at Yale University School of Medicine
http://yalecancercenter.org
An NCI-designated comprehensive cancer center in New Haven, Connecticut, that provides specialized team care, customized treatment plans, many support services, and a weekly informative radio show called *Yale Cancer Center Answers*. Web site offers an alphabetical list of cancer information and information on clinical trials and research.

▶ Cancer Support Groups

4th Angel Mentoring Program
http://www.4thangel.org/
Support group that pairs cancer patients with cancer patients and cancer survivors and who serve as mentors for the patient during their treatment and convalescence.

Adenoid Cystic Carcinoma Organization International
http://www.accoi.org
Provides information about adenoid cystic carcinoma. Offers support services in several different languages. Web site provides information on treatment options, research, clinical trials, the ACC tumor registry, and financial resources.

American Cancer Society
http://www.cancer.org
Educates the public about cancer, raises funds for cancer research, and runs support groups across the country. Web site provides links to a variety of support groups.

American Hospice Foundation
http://www.americanhospice.org
Professional palliative care organization that aids terminally ill with the process of dying, and also provides physical and emotional support for the patient's families.

Association of Cancer Online Resources
http://www.acor.org
Provides links to more than one hundred mailing lists and support resources.

BC Cancer Agency
http://www.bccancer.bc.ca
Educates people of British Columbia and the Yukon about cancer, including prevention, screening, early detection, and treatment options, as well as alternative therapies. Offers one-on-one support services and support groups.

The Brain Tumor Society
http://www.tbts.org
Provides educational material and support services, including a newsletter called *Heads Up,* a monthly e-newsletter called *Head Lines,* and a comprehensive resource guide called *Color Me Hope*. Its COPE (Connection of Personal Experiences) program provides sharing of mutual experiences via e-mail and telephone conversations.

Breast Cancer Network of Strength
http://www.networkofstrength.org
Provides support services and resources for people affected by breast cancer and offers a twenty-four-hour breast cancer hotline with interpreters in 150 languages.

CANCER101
http://cancer101.org/
Provides professional medical advice, emotion support, and advocacy for cancer patients. It also gives financial and legal advice for patients. CANCER101 partners with healthcare providers to empower patients and help them own their own health care decisions.

Cancer.Net
www.cancer.net
A repository of high-quality, medical information for a wide variety of cancers and brings cancer expertise to patients to help them make informed medical decisions. This site is also linked to several high-ranking oncology journals and provides professional counseling for biopsy interpretation through the College of American Pathologists,

Cancer Hope Network
http://www.cancerhopenetwork.org
Provides free, confidential one-on-one support to those affected by cancer by specially trained cancer survivor volunteers.

Cancer Support Community
http://www.cancersupportcommunity.org
Professionally led, nonprofit network of cancer support affiliates that offer emotional and social support for cancer suffers worldwide. Their Research and Training Institute conducts psychosocial, behavioral and emotional, and survivorships research, and their Cancer Policy Institute participates in cancer advocacy.

CancerCare
http://www.cancercare.org
Provides free counseling and support, online and by telephone, in English and Spanish, by trained oncology social workers. Also provides financial assistance to those in need and affected by cancer.

The Carcinoid Cancer Foundation
http://www.carcinoid.org
Provides information on carcinoid cancer, treatment options, and clinical trials. Web site offers a list of doctors

in the United States and Canada who specialize in treating carcinoid cancer, a list of carcinoid cancer support groups, resources for medical professionals, financial assistance resources, and archived articles.

The Childhood Brain Tumor Foundation
http://www.childhoodbraintumor.org
Provides information about brain tumors and cancer research, especially that related to childhood brain tumors. Offers the Childhood Cancer Ombudsman Program, which helps families with health insurance analysis and applications and with employment and educational difficulties that may arise during or after treatment.

Children's Cancer Association
http://www.childrenscancerassociation.org
Provides many resources and support services to help children and their families cope with cancer, including the DreamCatcher Wish program, the CCA Caring Cabin, and the Kids' Cancer Pages.

Colon Cancer Alliance
http://www.ccalliance.org
Provides support and educational resources for newly diagnosed colon cancer patients. Web site lists organizations and programs that may help with the financial issues related to medical treatment.

Colorectal Cancer Network
http://clickonium.com/colorectal-cancer.net/html
Provides a support network, including support groups, listserves, chat rooms, and a system of matching longterm survivors with newly diagnosed patients. Web site provides information about prevention and screening, treatment options, advocacy, and resources for newly diagnosed colon cancer patients.

Corporate Angel Network
http://www.corpangelnetwork.org
Arranges free travel on corporate jets, using empty seats on routine business flights, for cancer patients, bone marrow donors, and bone marrow recipients who are traveling to cancer treatment centers.

Florida Prostate Cancer Network
http://www.charityadvantage.com/www.floridaprostate-cancer.org/HomePage.asp
Educates men of Florida about the risks of developing prostate cancer. Supports research and promotes legislation to increase health insurance coverage of prostate cancer screenings. Web site offers information about early detection, support organizations, clinical trials, and current treatment options.

Gilda's Club Worldwide
http://www.gildasclub.org
Provides lectures, workshops, and support groups for those people whose lives have been touched by cancer, including a support program called *Noogieland* for children and teens. Web site lists Gilda's Clubhouse locations across the United States.

The Gynecologic Cancer Foundation
http://www.thegcf.org
Provides brochures and educational materials about gynecologic cancer. Supports research and training related to gynecologic cancers and organizes annual ovarian cancer survivor's courses.

International Myeloma Foundation
http://www.myeloma.org
Provides comprehensive information on myeloma treatment options, disease management, and programs and services for patients, family members, and health care professionals. Resources are available in fourteen languages. Web site offers educational resources, webcasts, a newsletter, and a toll-free hotline.

Lance Armstrong Foundation
http://www.livestrong.org
Provides survivorship education and resources, national advocacy initiatives, community programs, and scientific and clinical research grants. Web site provides information on LiveStrong SurvivorCare, a LiveStrong blog, a LiveStrong survivorship notebook, many cancer survivor brochures, sign-up for the LiveStrong Newsletter, and a link to the LiveStrong Store, where LiveStrong apparel and accessories can be purchased, the proceeds of which help support LiveStrong programs and services.

Leukemia and Lymphoma Society
http://www.leukemia-lymphoma.org
Provides information on leukemia, lymphoma, myeloma, and other blood cancers and support services for newly diagnosed and long-term survivors. Also supports research on blood cancers and pursues advocacy aimed at governmental decision makers. Web site hosts several discussion boards and offers medical news, event listings, and treatment information. Informational booklets are published in English, Spanish, and French.

Linda Creed Breast Cancer Foundation
http://www.lindacreed.org
Provides educational materials about the detection, treatment, and survivorship of breast cancer; offers access

to detection and treatment resources; provides financial assistance to women in the Philadelphia area receiving breast cancer treatment; and advocates for critical cancer legislation and governmental funding for breast cancer research.

Living Beyond Breast Cancer
http://www.lbbc.org
Provides educational programs and services to women affected by breast cancer, including a toll-free Survivors' Helpline, a quarterly newsletter called *Insight*, publications for African American and Latina women, current information about treatment options, and networking programs for women of color and young survivors.

Lung Cancer Alliance
http://www.lungcanceralliance.org
Provides support and advocacy for people at risk for and those living with lung cancer. Offers a peer-to-peer support network, toll-free information and referral services, and a quarterly newsletter called *Spirit and Breath*.

Lustgarten Foundation for Pancreatic Cancer Research
http://www.lustgarten.org/LUS/CDA/HomePage.jsp
Provides research grants to support pancreatic cancer research, information on clinical trials, and patient and caregiver support services. Web site provides information on selecting a treatment provider, an Ask an Expert series, research news, and information on legal, insurance, and benefits assistance.

Lymphoma Research Foundation
http://www.lymphoma.org
Raises funds for lymphoma research; provides educational materials on Hodgkin disease and non-Hodgkin lymphoma; provides information on diagnostic techniques, treatment options, and clinical trials; offers support for people living with lymphoma; sponsors lectures for scientists who conduct lymphoma research; and matches patients with peer support through its Lymphoma Support Network. Web site provides lymphoma news and features, fact sheets and booklets, and access to webcasts and podcasts.

Marti Nelson Cancer Foundation/ CancerActionNow.org
http://www.canceractionnow.org
Advocates for different options for cancer patients when standard treatments have not helped by providing information on nonstandard cancer treatment options, clinical trials, and experimental drugs.

Mautner Project, the National Lesbian Health Organization
http://www.mautnerproject.org
Offers support, advocacy, and educational information for lesbian, bisexual, and transgender women and their families, especially those living with cancer.

Melanoma International Foundation
http://www.melanomainternational.org
Provides melanoma facts, and tips on coping with a melanoma diagnosis. Web site provides an extensive list of melanoma treatment centers, forums, blogs, message boards, the latest news, and upcoming events.

MyOncofertility.org
http://www.myoncofertility.org/
Supports male and female cancer patients who wish to preserve their fertility despite their need to undergo cancer treatments that can diminish fertility. Provides a network of cryopreservation organizations that can isolate and freeze gametes for use after treatment.

National Brain Tumor Foundation
http://www.braintumor.org
Provides information about types of brain tumors, treatments, treatment centers, financial assistance, support services, and upcoming events as well as survivor stories and the latest news.

National Breast Cancer Coalition
http://www.natlbcc.org
Promotes breast cancer research and works toward improving access for all women to high-quality breast cancer screening, diagnosis, treatment, and care; informs and trains breast cancer survivors and others in effective advocacy efforts aimed at eradicating breast cancer. Web site provides breast cancer information, the latest news, and an e-newsletter.

National Cervical Cancer Coalition
http://www.nccc-online.org
Educates people about cervical cancer and the importance of early detection, advocates for quality patient care, and provides support through its Phone Pals and E-Pals programs. Web site provides links to many resources related to cervical cancer, the NCCC Store, and sign-up for its newsletter *Extraordinary Moments*.

National Coalition for Cancer Survivorship
http://www.canceradvocacy.org
Raises awareness about cancer survivorship issues, self-advocacy, and public advocacy, and provides resources for cancer patients, including information on types

of cancer, treatment issues, side effects, financial advice, and other cancer-related topics. Web site offers sign-up for online newsletter called *InterAction* and a Cancer Survival Toolbox.

National Lymphedema Network
http://www.lymphnet.org
Provides information about lymphedema and news about medical and scientific developments, sponsors a national conference and a patient summit, supports research into causes and possible alternative treatments, and advocates to standardize quality treatment for lymphedema patients. Web site lists treatment centers, health care professionals, and support groups.

National Ovarian Cancer Coalition
http://www.ovarian.org
Raises awareness and promotes education about ovarian cancer. Web site lists state chapters, support groups and services, and clinical trials, and provides the latest news, an NOCC newsletter, and medical information about ovarian cancer.

Native American Cancer Research
http://natamcancer.org
Provides culturally sensitive information and support to Native Americans living with cancer. Web site provides information on clinical trials, treatment, the Native American Cancer Survivors Network, and printable handouts.

Native People's Circle of Hope
http://www.nativepeoplescoh.org
A coalition of Native American cancer support groups in which Native American cancer survivors offer culturally sensitive support and counseling for newly diagnosed Native American cancer patients.

Oklahoma Brain Tumor Foundation
http://www.okbtf.org
Provides education, support groups, advocacy, and financial assistance for people in Oklahoma affected by primary brain or central nervous system tumors. Web site provides information about tumors, treatments, clinical trials, and area oncologists.

Oncolink
http://www.oncolink.com
Online cancer resource Web site operated by the University of Pennsylvania with an Ask the Experts page. Includes links to OncoLife, which offers an individualized survivorship care plan created on the basis of answers provided in a questionnaire; OncoTip of the Day; OncoPilot, a guide for navigating the cancer journey; and *OncoLink eNews*, a monthly newsletter.

Ovarian Cancer Canada
http://www.ovariancancercanada.ca
Provides ovarian cancer education, support, a quarterly newsletter, and other resources to Canadian residents. All services are available in English and French.

Ovarian Cancer Research Fund
http://www.ocrf.org
Promotes and raises funds for ovarian cancer research and its early diagnosis, and provides support and information to patients and loved ones, including an informational hotline mainly staffed by ovarian cancer survivor volunteers.

Pediatric Brain Tumor Foundation
http://www.pbtfus.org
Offers educational materials and support to children with brain tumors and their parents, and raises money for pediatric brain tumor research, awareness, and detection.

The Prostate Net
http://www.prostate-online.org
Provides information, support, and resources to simplify the treatment decision-making process.

Research Advocacy Network
http://www.researchadvocacy.org
Provides education, support, and advocacy by working with all participants in the medical research process to improve patient care.

Sarcoma Alliance
http://www.sarcomaalliance.org
Provides guidance, education, and support to those people whose lives have been affected by sarcoma. Web site provides information on services, programs, survivor and caregiver support groups, and an assistance fund developed to help sarcoma patients obtain second opinions from sarcoma specialists across the country.

SHARE: Self-help for Women with Breast or Ovarian Cancer
http://www.sharecancersupport.org
Trained breast or ovarian cancer survivors staff nationwide hotlines and run support groups and educational programs for women with breast or ovarian cancer in the New York metropolitan area.

Sisters Network
http://www.sistersnetworkinc.org
A national African American breast cancer survivorship organization that provides African American women with educational materials about breast cancer risk, symptoms, and treatment, as well as support services.

Skin Cancer Foundation
http://www.skincancer.org
Provides educational material about skin cancer prevention and detection. Web site provides information about different types of skin cancer, an Ask the Expert feature, and a physician finder database.

Stand Up To Cancer
http://www.standup2cancer.org
Brings together researchers from different scientific disciplines and areas of the world to foster innovation, speed the pace of cancer research, and bring new, science-based cancer treatments to the patients who need them. The organization raises funds to support its research and educates the public through celebrity-hosted awareness campaigns.

Support for People with Oral and Head and Neck Cancer
http://www.spohnc.org
Provides information and support groups for people living with oral cancer and cancers of the head and neck. Web site provides educational resources, information on clinical trials, and news releases.

Susan G. Komen for the Cure
http://www.komen.org
Funds research grants; provides breast cancer education; gives information about screening, treatment options, and community support groups; and provides a national tollfree helpline, which is available in English and Spanish.

ThyCa: Thyroid Cancer Survivors' Association
http://www.thyca.org
Provides information and support services for people living with thyroid cancer and hosts survivor workshops and an annual conference. Web site provides access to a new-patient packet, resource list, low iodine cookbook, and an online newsletter.

The Ulman Cancer Fund for Young Adults
http://www.ulmanfund.org
Provides educational programs and support groups for teens and young adults facing the challenges of cancer, and conducts community outreach programs as well as maintains a scholarship fund for young people who are facing or who have overcome cancer.

Us TOO International
http://www.ustoo.com
Provides prostate cancer education and a support network with hundreds of support groups across the United States, and advocates for increased funding for prostate cancer detection, diagnosis, treatment, and research. Web site provides a list of clinical trials, publications, informational newsletters, and a resource kit for newly diagnosed patients.

The Wellness Community
http://www.thewellnesscommunity.org
Provides online support groups in English and Spanish, as well as an online resource guide with information about various types of cancer, clinical trials, and advice on managing treatment side effects.

Wisconsin Multiple Myeloma Support Group
http://www.madison.com/communities/multiplemyeloma
Hosts monthly support meetings and publishes a monthly newsletter that provides a resource list and notes on new research.

Young Survival Coalition
http://www.youngsurvival.org
Provides educational and support services that are unique to young women and breast cancer. Web site provides information about research, clinical trials, and programs; informational brochures; a quarterly newsletter; and an online bulletin board.

▶ Carcinogens

The following list of carcinogens is based on the National Toxicology Program's *Report on Carcinogens* (RoC, 11th ed.). Human carcinogens that are both "known" and "reasonably anticipated" are listed here, with a summary of each carcinogen along with its status (K for "known" or RA for "reasonably anticipated") according to the *ROC*. The *ROC* can be fully accessed as a PDF file for more in-depth technical description from the home page of the National Toxicology Program, http://ntp.niehs.nih.gov.

acetaldehyde: RA. Primarily used in the production of a variety of chemicals. Also found in tobacco, ripe fruit, wine, and other alcoholic beverages. Produced by plants as part of their normal life cycle. Main source of human exposure is through the metabolism of alcohol. Other sources include food, beverages, and, to a lesser extent, the air. Studies indicate an increased incidence of squamous cell carcinomas and adenocarcinomas in exposed laboratory animals; inadequate evidence to evaluate the carcinogenicity in humans.

2-acetylaminofluorene: RA. Used as a positive control by toxicologists. Potential human exposure includes inhalation and skin contact. Resulting cancers in laboratory animals include carcinomas of the urinary bladder and the liver and subcutaneous carcinomas on the face; no adequate data are available to evaluate the carcinogenicity in humans.

acrylamide: RA. Used in treating municipal drinking water and wastewater. Also found in home appliances, building materials, automotive parts, cosmetics, soaps, and lotions. Can be absorbed through unbroken skin, mucous membranes, lungs, and the gastrointestinal tract. Resulting cancers in laboratory animals; no adequate data are available to evaluate the carcinogenicity in humans.

acrylonitrile: RA. Used extensively in the manufacture of synthetic fibers, resins, plastics, elastomers, and rubber for consumer goods such as textiles, dinnerware, food containers, toys, luggage, automotive parts, small appliances, and telephones. A variety of cancers have developed in laboratory animals. Studies have indicated an increased risk of lung cancer in textile plant workers exposed to acrylonitrile.

Adriamycin (doxorubicin hydrochloride): RA. An antibiotic used in antimitotic chemotherapy to treat various neoplastic diseases; human exposure routes include injection, skin contact, and inhalation. Cancers that developed in laboratory animals include mammary tumors, bladder papillomas, urinary bladder tumors, and local sarcomas near injection sites. Although no adequate data are available to evaluate the carcinogenicity in humans, in a study of cancer patients receiving Adriamycin in combination with alkylating agents and radiotherapy, patients developed leukemia and bone cancer.

aflatoxins: K. Toxins produced by *Aspergillus* fungi that grow naturally on grains and other agricultural crops. Exposure occurs by eating contaminated foods or by inhalation of dust containing aflatoxins. Studies have confirmed carcinogenicity in humans resulting in liver cancer (hepatocellular carcinoma and primary liver-cell cancer).

alcoholic beverage consumption: K. Known or suspected as human carcinogens, include acetaldehyde, nitrosamines, aflatoxins, ethyl carbamate (urethane), asbestos, and arsenic compounds. Studies have indicated an increased risk of cancers of the mouth, pharynx, larynx, and esophagus with increased alcoholic beverage consumption, especially when combined with smoking.

2-aminoanthraquinone: RA. Used in the production of anthraquinone dyes, which are used in automotive paints, high-quality paints and enamels, textile dyes, plastics, rubber, and printing inks. Hepatocellular carcinomas, neoplastic nodules, and lymphomas have resulted in laboratory animals that have ingested 2-aminoanthraquinone; however, potential human exposure is through skin contact, and no adequate data are available to evaluate the carcinogenicity in humans.

***o*-aminoazotoluene: RA.** Used in coloring oils, fats, waxes, and medicine, and in the production of the dyes Solvent Red 24 and Acid Red 115. Cancers of the liver, lungs, and urinary bladder have resulted in laboratory animals that have ingested *o*-aminoazotoluene; potential human exposure is through skin contact and inhalation and no adequate data are available to evaluate the carcinogenicity in humans.

4-aminobiphenyl: K. Previously used commercially as a rubber antioxidant, as a dye intermediate, and in the detection of sulfates; later used only in laboratory research because of sufficient evidence for carcinogenicity in humans.

1-amino-2,4-dibromoanthraquinone: RA. Used in the production of dyes, especially those used in textiles. Tumors in various sites have been reported in laboratory animals in which 1-amino-2,4-dibromoanthraquinone had been orally administered; however, no adequate data are available to evaluate the carcinogenicity in humans. Human exposure is primarily through skin contact.

1-amino-2-methylanthraquinone: RA. Was used in the production of dyes for synthetic fibers, furs, and thermoplastic resins, specifically for the dyes Solvent Blue 13 and Acid Blue 47. No longer commercially produced in the United States. Liver and kidney cancer have occurred in exposed laboratory animals; no adequate data are available to evaluate the carcinogenicity in humans. Human exposure would be primarily through skin contact and inhalation.

amitrole: RA. Widely used as an herbicide on annual and perennial broadleaf and grass-type weeds, on noncrop land prior to sowing, and as control of pondweeds. When administered in the diet of laboratory animals, increased incidence of tumors in the liver and thyroid occurred. No adequate data are available to evaluate the carcinogenicity in humans. Human exposure is through inhalation and skin contact or ingestion of contaminated food or drinking water.

***o*-anisidine hydrochloride: RA.** Used in the production of dyes and pharmaceuticals, as a corrosion inhibitor for steel, and as an antioxidant for polymercaptan resins. Tumors of the urinary bladder, the renal pelvis, and the thyroid occurred in laboratory animals. No adequate data are available to evaluate the carcinogenicity in humans. Human exposure is through inhalation and skin contact; the general population may be exposed to the chemical as an environmental pollutant or through cigarette smoke.

arsenic compounds, inorganic: K. Used in a variety of substances ranging from pesticides to medicines; later more commonly used in pressure-treated wood. Effective December 31, 2003, a voluntary phaseout in wood for residential uses began. Also used in the production of lead alloys. Sufficient evidence confirms that humans exposed to arsenic compounds have increased risks of cancers of the skin, lung, digestive tract, liver, bladder, kidney, and lymphatic and hematopoietic systems. Occupational exposure includes inhalation and skin contact. For the general population, exposure is primarily through the ingestion of foods or by inhalation of contaminated air.

asbestos: K. Has been used in roofing, flooring, thermal and electrical insulation, cement pipe and sheets, friction materials, gaskets, coatings, plastics, textiles, paper, and other products. Banned in general-use garments, but it may be used in firefighting garments. Human exposure is primarily through inhalation and ingestion. Although the potential for exposure is widespread be-cause of its previous extensive use, the potential for exposure continues to decline because of the elimination of asbestos products from the market. Sufficient evidence confirms that asbestos exposure in humans causes respiratory-tract cancer, pleural and peritoneal mesothelioma, lung cancer, laryngeal cancer, cancer of the digestive tract, and other cancers.

azacitidine: RA. Has been used in treatment of acute myeloblastic anemia, acute lymphoblastic leukemia, and myelodysplastic syndromes. Has been used in combination with other antineoplastic agents in cancer treatment trial protocols, as well as in clinical trials for beta thalassemia, acute myeloid leukemia, myelodysplastic syndrome, advanced or metastatic solid tumors, non-Hodgkin lymphoma, multiple myeloma, non-smallcell lung cancer, and prostate cancer. Malignant tumor formation at multiple tissue sites occurred in laboratory animals when administered by injection. No adequate data are available to evaluate the carcinogenicity in humans.

azathioprine: K. Used as an immunosuppressive agent, usually in combination with a corticosteroid, to prevent rejection following transplant surgery and to manage severe cases of rheumatoid arthritis in adults, and as a second-line treatment for some immunological diseases. A high occurrence of cancers in patients and others routinely treated with azathioprine confirms carcinogenicity in humans.

benzene: K. Used primarily as a solvent in the chemical and pharmaceutical industries, in the synthesis of numerous chemicals, and in gasoline. Also used in the production of styrene, phenol, acetone, cyclohexane, nitrobenzene, detergent alkylate, and chlorobenzenes. Benzene is known to cause leukemia.

benzidine and dyes metabolized to benzidine: K. Has been used in the production of azo dyes, fast-color salts, naphthols, sulfur dyes, and other dyeing compounds. Also used in clinical laboratories for detection of blood, as a rubber-compounding agent, in the manufacture of plastic films, for detection of hydrogen peroxide in milk, and for quantitative determination of nicotine. Most of these uses have been discontinued because of concerns about potential carcinogenicity. Although potential for exposure is low, human exposure may occur through inhalation, ingestion, or skin contact. Liver cancer has been reported in association with occupational exposure to benzidine, and limited evidence has associated it with a variety of other cancers.

benzotrichloride: RA. Used as a chemical intermediate to stabilize plastics in the presence of ultraviolet light, in the preparation of specific dyes and pigments, and to make benzotrifluoride, hydroxybenzophenone, antiseptics, and antimicrobial agents. Human exposure is through inhalation, ingestion, and skin contact. A variety of cancers have developed in laboratory animals exposed to benzotrichloride. Increased risk of respiratory cancer has been reported in humans involved in the production of chlorinated toluenes, which involves potential exposure to benzotrichloride and other chemicals; otherwise, no data are available to evaluate the carcinogenicity in humans.

beryllium and beryllium compounds: K. Used as an alloy, metal, and oxide in electrical components and in aerospace and defense applications. Also used in molds for injection-molded plastics, computers, home appliances, telecommunications devices, dental applications, bicycle frames, golf clubs, and many other applications. Inhalation of dusts and fumes is the primary route of human exposure, but it may also be ingested in drinking water or food. Studies showing an increased risk of lung cancer in occupational groups exposed to beryllium or beryllium compounds provide sufficient evidence of carcinogenicity in humans.

bromodichloromethane: RA. Used in the synthesis of organic chemicals and as a reagent in laboratory research. Also has been used to separate minerals and salts, as a flame retardant, and in fire extinguishers. It is also formed as a result of the chlorination treatment of drinking, waste, or cooling water. Human exposure is through the consumption of contaminated drinking water, beverages, and food products, and inhalation of contaminated ambient air. Tumors in the kidney, intestine, and liver have been reported in laboratory animals when administered by stomach tube. Sufficient data are not available to evaluate the carcinogenic effects in humans.

2,2-bis-(bromoethyl)-1,3-propanediol (technical grade): RA. Used as a flame retardant, especially in unsaturated polyester resins, molded products, and rigid polyurethane foam. Tumor formation at multiple tissue sites and leukemia occurred in laboratory animals. No data are available to evaluate the carcinogenicity in humans. Contamination occurs in the environment as dust and through wastewater; therefore, human exposure is through inhalation and skin contact.

1,3-butadiene: K. Used in a variety of rubber products. Also used in a number of industrial chemicals and in the manufacture of fungicides. Also found in gasoline, automobile exhausts, and cigarette smoke. Human exposure is primarily through inhalation; some exposure may occur from ingesting contaminated food or water, or through skin contact. Lymphatic and hematopoietic cancers have been reported in humans who have been exposed to 1,3-butadiene.

1,4-butanediol dimethanesulfonate (Myleran): K. Used in chemotherapeutic treatment by ingestion or intravenous administration to treat some forms of leukemia. Also may be used in combination with cyclophosphamide before bone marrow transplants for chronic myelogenous leukemia. Cancer at different tissue sites has been reported among leukemia patients receiving 1,4-butanediol dimethanesulfonate. Also, leukemia was reported in a follow-up study of bronchial cancer patients treated with 1,4-butanediol dimethanesulfonate.

butylated hydroxyanisole (BHA): RA. Used primarily as an antioxidant and preservative in an extensive list of foods (especially those containing vegetable oils and animal fats), food packaging, animal feed, and cosmetics, and in rubber and petroleum products. Administration in the diet induced tumors in the forestomach of laboratory animals. No data are available to evaluate the carcinogenicity in humans. Human exposure is through ingestion and skin contact.

cadmium and cadmium compounds: K. Used primarily in batteries. Cadmium compounds are used in analytical chemistry, calico printing, dyeing, mirrors, electronbeam-pumped lasers, electroplating, fluorescent screens, lubricants, nuclear reactors, photocopying, photographic emulsions, radiation detectors, smoke detectors, solar cells, thin-film transistors and diodes, phosphors, photomultipliers, and vacuum tubes. Also used as a fungicide, nematocide, or ascaricide; to color glass and porcelain; and in the production of cadmium-containing stabilizers and pigments for paints, glass, ceramics, plastics, textiles, paper, and fireworks.

Human exposure is through ingestion of contaminated food, drinking water, soil, and dust, and inhalation of particles of cadmium from ambient air or cigarette smoke. The largest intake of cadmium is estimated to come from cereal grain products, potatoes, and other vegetables. Studies have confirmed that exposure to various cadmium compounds increases the risk of lung cancer. Evidence also suggests an increased risk of prostate, kidney, and bladder cancer.

carbon tetrachloride: RA. Used primarily in the production of Freon 11 and 12. Human exposure is through inhalation, ingestion, and skin contact. The general population is most likely exposed through air and drinking water. Liver tumors occurred in laboratory animals exposed to carbon tetrachloride. Although no adequate data are available to evaluate the carcinogenicity in humans, liver tumors, respiratory cancers, and leukemia have been reported in humans exposed to carbon tetrachloride.

ceramic fibers (respirable size): RA. Used as insulation materials, primarily for lining furnaces and kilns and as replacement for asbestos. Products produced using ceramic fibers are blankets, boards, bulk fibers, felts, vacuum-formed or cast shapes, paper, and textile products. Human exposure is through inhalation, mainly in the manufacturing environment, during installation, and during removal. Tumors of the lung occurred in laboratory animals. No adequate studies have confirmed carcinogenicity in humans.

chlorambucil: K. Used primarily in the treatment of chronic lymphocytic leukemia and primary (Waldenström) macroglobulinemia. Also used as an immunosuppressive agent in the treatment of systemic lupus erythematosus, acute and chronic glomerular nephritis, nephrotic syndrome, chronic active hepatitis, cold agglutinic disease, psoriasis, and Wegener granulomatosis. Human exposure is through ingestion, inhalation, and skin contact. Increased risk of cancers, especially acute nonlymphocytic leukemia, has been reported with exposure to chlorambucil.

chloramphenicol: RA. An antimicrobial agent used to combat serious infections; has restricted use because it causes blood dyscrasia. Human exposure is primarily by the oral or topical route through its use as a drug; exposure also may occur through inhalation, ingestion, skin contact, or contact with contaminated water or soil. Although no adequate studies have confirmed cancers in laboratory animals exposed to chloramphenicol, many human case reports have implicated chloramphenicol as a cause of aplastic anemia and an increased risk of leukemia.

chlorendic acid: RA. Used primarily as a flame retardant in polyester resins and coatings, epoxy resins, and polyurethane foams. Also used in the manufacture of corrosion-resistant polyester resins, oil-modified paints and coatings, flame-retardant additives, extreme pressure lubricants, and epoxy resins used in printed circuit boards. Human exposure is primarily through skin contact; small exposure may occur through inhalation. Tumors of the liver, pancreas, lung, and preputial gland occurred in laboratory animals in which chlorendic acid was administered in the diet. No data are available to evaluate the carcinogenicity in humans.

chlorinated paraffins (C12, 60 percent chlorine): RA. Used primarily as extreme-pressure lubricant additives in metalworking and in flame retardants and plasticizers for plastics. Also used in rubber, paints, adhesives, caulks, and sealants, and as a plasticizer in inks, paper and textile coatings, and flexible polyvinyl chloride. Tumors of the liver, kidney, and thyroid gland, as well as leukemia, occurred in laboratory animals in which chlorinated paraffins were administered by stomach tube. No data are available to evaluate the carcinogenicity in humans.

1-(2-chloroethyl)-3-cyclohexyl-1-nitrosourea (CCNU): RA. Has limited use in the treatment of Hodgkin disease, brain tumors, colorectal tumors, and specific pulmonary malignancies. Human exposure is through ingestion, inhalation, and skin contact. Tumors of the lung and lymphosarcomas occurred in laboratory animals in which CCNU was administered by injection. No adequate data are available to evaluate the carcinogenicity in humans; however, cases of leukemia have been reported in cancer patients who have received CCNU.

1-(2-chloroethyl)-3-(4-methylcyclohexyl)-1-nitrosourea (methyl-CCNU): K. Used an investigational drug in the treatment of several types of cancers. Clinical trials in which cancer patients were given adjuvant treatment with methyl-CCNU showed an increased risk of developing leukemia and preleukemia.

bis(chloroethyl) nitrosourea (BCNU): RA. Used in the treatment of Hodgkin disease, multiple myeloma, and brain tumors. Human exposure is through injection, inhalation, and skin contact. Tumors of the lung and peritoneal cavity have occurred in laboratory animals administered BCNU by injection. Limited evidence of carcinogenicity in humans is available in that BCNU is associated with acute nonlymphocytic leukemia following its use with other anticancer therapies in the treatment of previously existing cancer.

chloroform: RA. Primarily used to produce hydrochlorofluorocarbon-22; also used as a solvent and in certain medical procedures. Human exposure is through inhalation, skin contact with water, and ingestion, primarily drinking water. Tumors of the kidney and liver occurred in laboratory animals that were exposed to chloroform. There is no adequate evidence of carcinogenicity in humans; however, some studies indicate that there is an association between cancer of the large intestine, rectum, and urinary bladder and the components of chlorinated water.

bis(chloromethyl) ether (BCME) and technical-grade chloromethyl methyl ether (CMME): K. Used primarily as chemical intermediates and alkylating agents. Human exposure is through inhalation and skin contact; however, probability of exposure is very low. Potential for exposure is greatest for chemical plant workers, ion-exchange resin makers, laboratory workers, and polymer makers. Studies have demonstrated that occupational exposure causes lung cancer.

3-chloro-2-methylpropene: RA. Used primarily in the production of carbofuran, an insecticide used mostly on corn. Also used in the production of plastics, pharmaceuticals, herbicides, and other organic chemicals; as a textile additive; and as a perfume additive. Human exposure is through inhalation, ingestion, and skin contact. Tumors of the forestomach occurred in laboratory animals when administered by stomach tube. No data are available to evaluate the carcinogenicity in humans.

4-chloro-*o*-phenylenediamine: RA. Patented as a hair dye component and used in the production of a photographic chemical, as a curing agent for epoxy resins, and as a reagent in gas chromatography. Human exposure is through ingestion, inhalation, and skin contact. Little exposure is expected in the general population due to its limited use in consumer products. Tumors of the urinary bladder and liver occurred in laboratory animals when administered in the diet. No data are available to evaluate the carcinogenicity in humans.

chloroprene: RA. Used in the production of neoprene, a synthetic rubber used in the production of automotive and mechanical rubber goods, adhesives, caulks, construction goods, fiber binding, footwear, flame-resistant cushioning, fabric coatings, roof coatings, and sealants for dams or locks in waterways. Human exposure is through inhalation. Inhalation exposure in laboratory animals induced tumor formation at multiple tissue sites. Limited data demonstrating that occupational exposure to chloroprene increases the risk for various tumors may suggest carcinogenicity in humans.

***p*-chloro-*o*-toluidine and *p*-chloro-*o*-toluidine hydrochloride: RA.** Has been used to produce azo dyes for cotton, silk, acetate, and nylon, and to produce Pigment Red 7 and Pigment Yellow 49, as well as in the manufacture of the pesticide chlordimeform. Human exposure is through inhalation, ingestion, and skin contact. Increased incidences of urinary bladder tumors have been documented in workers exposed to *p*-chloro*o*-toluidine; however, as they were also exposed to numerous other compounds, this provides limited evidence of carcinogenicity in humans. Increased incidence of tumors occurred in laboratory animals exposed to *p*-chloro-*o*-toluidine hydrochloride.

chlorozotocin: RA. Used in the investigational treatment of various cancers. Human exposure is through intravenous administration. An increased incidence of sarcoma and mesothelioma in the peritoneal cavity, and tumors of the nervous system, lungs, and forestomach, occurred in laboratory animals in which chlorozotocin was administered. No adequate data are available to evaluate the carcinogenicity in humans.

chromium hexavalent compounds: K. Used as corrosion inhibitors, in wood preservatives, in leather tanning, in metal finishing and chrome plating, in stainless steel production, and in the manufacture of pigments. Also used in textile dyeing processes, printing inks, drilling muds, pyrotechnics, water treatment, and chemical synthesis. Residential uses as wood preservatives are expected to decrease because of a voluntary phaseout that went into effect December 31, 2003. Exposure for the general population is through inhalation of the ambient air, ingestion of water, or skin contact. Increased risks of lung cancer and a rare cancer of the sinonasal cavity among workers engaged in chromate production, chromate pigment production, and chromium plating have been reported. Other studies suggest that exposure to chromium may also be associated with cancer at other tissue sites, including leukemia and bone cancer.

C.I. Basic Red 9 monohydrochloride: RA. Used primarily in a nutrient agar for bacterium identification; as a biological stain; in a commercial magenta dye used for coloring textiles, china clay products, leather, and printing inks; and as a filter dye in photography. Also used in tinting automobile antifreeze solutions and toilet sanitary preparations. Human exposure is primarily through skin contact. A variety of tumors have occurred in laboratory animals exposed to the compound. An increase in urinary bladder tumors in workers involved in the manufacture of magenta dye has been reported; however, inadequate evidence is available to determine if this is attributable to exposure to the magenta or to other intermediates and impurities.

cisplatin: RA. Used in the treatment of various malignancies, often in combination with other cancer treatments. Human exposure is not only through treatment but also through skin absorption and inhalation. Significant increases in the incidence and number of lung adenomas and skin papillomas, as well as leukemia, occurred in laboratory animals in which cisplatin was administered by injection. No adequate data are available to evaluate the carcinogenicity in humans.

coal tars and coal tar pitches: K. Used primarily for the production of refined chemicals and coal tar products. Have also been used in surface-coating formulations, pesticides, and epoxy-resin surface coatings, and as fuel in open-hearth furnaces and blast furnaces in the steel industry. U.S. pharmacopeia-grade coal tar is used in denatured alcohol and in preparations used to treat various skin conditions. Coal tar pitches are used primarily as the binder for aluminum-smelting electrodes and in roofing materials, refractory brick, and surface coatings; as a binder for foundry cores; and to produce pitch coke. Also used for road paving and construction, as well as in the production of naphthalene, recovery of benzene, production of anthracene paste, briquetting of smokeless solid fuel, impregnation of electrodes and fibers, and manufacture of electrodes and graphite. Human exposure is through inhalation, ingestion, and skin contact. Increased incidences of leukemia and a variety of other cancers have occurred in humans exposed to coal tars or coal tar pitches. Coal tars and coal tar pitches contain known and potential carcinogens, such as benzene, naphthalene, and other polycyclic aromatic hydrocarbons.

cobalt sulfate: RA. Used in the electrochemical and electroplating industries; as a drier in lithographic inks, varnishes, paints, and linoleum; and in storage batteries, ceramics, enamels, glazes, and porcelain. Has been used in animal feeds as a mineral supplement and on pastures to supplement forage with cobalt, as well as in beers and to treat anemia in people not responsive to other treatments. Human exposure is through inhalation of ambient air and ingestion of food or drinking water. Occupational exposure also includes skin contact. Tumors of the lung and adrenal gland occurred in laboratory animals when administered by inhalation. No significant data are available to evaluate the carcinogenicity in humans.

coke oven emissions: K. Used in iron-making blast furnaces, to synthesize calcium carbide, and to manufacture graphite and electrodes. Coke oven gas is used as a fuel. Coke by-products may be refined into commodity chemicals, such as benzene, toluene, naphthalene, sulfur, and ammonium sulfate. Human exposure to coke oven emissions is through inhalation and skin contact. A variety of cancers have been reported in humans exposed to coke oven emissions.

***p*-cresidine: RA.** Used exclusively in the production of azo dyes and pigments—such as Direct Orange 72, FD&C Red 40, and Direct Violet 9—to be used in the textile industry. Human exposure is through inhalation and skin contact. Increased incidences of urinary bladder cancer, liver cancer, and olfactory neuroblastomas occurred in laboratory animals when administered in the diet. No adequate data are available to evaluate the carcinogenicity in humans.

cupferron: RA. Used to separate and precipitate metals such as copper, iron, vanadium, and thorium; also used in analytical laboratories. Human exposure is through ingestion and inhalation of dust from the dry salt, and through skin contact. Hemangiosarcomas and a variety of tumors have occurred in laboratory animals when administered in the diet. No data are available to evaluate the carcinogenicity in humans.

cyclophosphamide: K. Used to treat a variety of cancers; also used as an immunosuppressive agent following organ transplants or to treat autoimmune disorders. Exposure for the general population is through medical treatment; occupational exposure is through skin contact or inhalation of dust. Bladder cancer and leukemia have been reported in patients administered cyclophosphamide.

cyclosporin A: K. Used as an immunosuppressive agent in the prevention and treatment of graft-versus-host reactions in bone marrow transplantation and for the prevention of rejection of organ transplants. Has also been tested for the treatment of a variety of diseases. Human exposure is through intravenous and oral administration. Lymphoma and skin cancer have been reported in transplant recipients, psoriasis patients, and rheumatoid arthritis patients treated with cyclosporin A.

dacarbazine: RA. Used in the treatment of Hodgkin disease, malignant melanomas, neuroblastomas, osteogenic sarcomas, and soft-tissue sarcomas, and occasionally in the therapy for other neoplastic diseases that have become resistant to alternative treatment. Human exposure is through injection, inhalation, and skin contact. A variety of cancers have resulted in laboratory animals when administered dacarbazine. No adequate data are available to evaluate the carcinogenicity in humans.

danthron (1,8-dihydroxyanthraquinone): RA. Used in synthetic lubricants, experimental antitumor agents, a fungicide used to control powdery mildew, and certain dyes. Tumors of the colon, cecum, and liver occurred in laboratory animals when administered in the diet. No adequate data are available to evaluate the carcinogenicity in humans.

2,4-diaminoanisole sulfate: RA. Used primarily in hair and fur dyes; also used in production of C.I. Basic Brown 2, which is used to dye clothing and is also an ingredient in shoe polishes. Human exposure is through skin contact and inhalation. Tumors at various tissue sites occurred in laboratory animals when administered in the diet. No adequate data are available to evaluate the carcinogenicity in humans.

2,4-diaminotoluene: RA. Used primarily in the production of toluene diisocyanate, which is used to produce polyurethane. Also used to produce dyes for biological stains, furs, leathers, textiles, and wood. Human exposure is through skin contact and inhalation. Tumors of the liver and mammary gland and lymphomas occurred in laboratory animals when administered in the diet, and local tumors occurred when injected. No adequate data are available to evaluate the carcinogenicity in humans.

diazoaminobenzene (DAAB): RA. Used in organic synthesis and in the manufacture of insecticides and dyes, particularly D&C Red no. 33, FD&C Yellow no. 5 (tartrazine), and FD&C Yellow no. 6, which are used in drugs and cosmetics; the latter two are allowed in food. Human exposure is through ingestion of products containing those dyes or skin contact with these products. DAAB is metabolized to benzene, a known human carcinogen that causes leukemia; evidence also shows that DAAB causes genetic damage.

1,2-dibromo-3-chloropropane: RA. Before being banned by the Environmental Protection Agency in 1985, 1,2dibromo-3-chloropropane was used as a pesticide; later used only for research purposes. Human exposure is probably minimal; however, ingestion of previously contaminated drinking water and food may occur. A variety of cancers have resulted in laboratory animals when exposed to 1,2-dibromo-3-chloropropane. There is inadequate evidence for the carcinogenicity in humans.

1,2-dibromoethane (ethylene dibromide): RA. Used to make vinyl bromide, a flame retardant in modacrylic fibers. Also used as a nonflammable solvent for resins, gums, and waxes, and used in the preparation of dyes and pharmaceuticals. Formerly used in lead gasoline and as a pesticide, it is still detected in ambient air, soil, groundwater, and food. Major source of human exposure is through the ingestion of contaminated drinking water. A variety of cancers have resulted in laboratory animals when exposed to 1,2-dibromoethane. There is inadequate evidence for the carcinogenicity in humans.

2,3-dibromo-1-propanol (DBP): RA. Used in the production of flame retardants, insecticides, and pharmaceuticals. Human exposure is through inhalation and skin contact. A variety of tumors have occurred in laboratory animals when painted onto the skin for numerous weeks. There is inadequate evidence for the carcinogenicity in humans.

tris(2,3-dibromopropyl) phosphate: RA. Previously used as a flame-retardant additive for textiles and plastics. It was banned in 1977 for use in children's clothing and in any textiles intended for use in clothing and is no longer used in the United States; however, in 1978, the Consumer Product Safety Commission identified twenty-two products containing the compound that were still commercially available. Human exposure is through inhalation, skin contact, and ingestion. A variety of cancers have resulted in laboratory animals exposed to tris(2,3-dibromopropyl) phosphate. There is inadequate evidence for the carcinogenicity in humans.

1,4-dichlorobenzene: RA. Used primarily as a space deodorant and as an insecticide fumigant for moth control. Also used in the production of polyphenylene sulfide and in the production of 1,2,4-trichlorobenzene; yellow, red, and orange pigments; air deodorizers; dyes; pharmaceuticals; and resin-bonded abrasives. Also used as a germicide/disinfectant, soil fumigant, insecticide, pesticide, animal repellent, and an agent to control mold and mildew growth. Human exposure is primarily through inhalation; skin contact and ingestion are also routes of potential exposure. Tumors of the kidney and liver occurred in laboratory animals when administered by stomach tube. No adequate data are available to evaluate the carcinogenicity in humans.

3,3′-dichlorobenzidine and 3,3′-dichlorobenzidine dihydrochloride: RA. Used primarily in the manufacture of pigments for printing ink, paint, paper, plastics, rubber, and textiles, and as a curing agent for isocyanate-containing polymers and solid urethane plastics. Human exposure is through inhalation of airborne dust, ingestion of contaminated well water near hazardous waste sites, and skin contact. Tumors at multiple tissue sites and leukemia occurred in laboratory animals administered the compound. No adequate data are available to evaluate the carcinogenicity in humans.

dichlorodiphenyltrichloroethane (DDT): RA. Used extensively as an insecticide until 1972, when it was banned for the majority of uses in the United States. Later used only under official supervision for public health emergencies or for health quarantine. Although residue levels have been declining, DDT is still being detected in air, soil, rain, water, animal and plant tissues, food, and the work environment, and can be ingested in small amounts from some foods. Tumors at multiple tissue sites occurred in laboratory animals administered DDT. There is inadequate evidence for the carcinogenicity in humans.

1,2-dichloroethane (ethylene dichloride): RA. Used primarily to produce vinyl chloride, although it has been used as a solvent, degreaser, insect fumigant, and general anesthetic, among other uses. Human exposure is through inhalation, ingestion, and skin contact. Tumors at multiple tissue sites occurred in laboratory animals administered 1,2-dichloroethane. No adequate data are available to evaluate carcinogenicity in humans.

dichloromethane (methylene chloride): RA. Used primarily as a solvent in paint removers. Used also as an aerosol propellant; as a processing solvent in the manufacture of steroids, antibiotics, vitamins, and tablet coatings; as a degreasing agent; in electronics manufacturing, and as a polyurethane foam blowing agent. Also used in spray shoe polish, water repellents, spot removers, cleaners, glues, adhesive removers, and lubricants, among other products. Human exposure is through inhalation, ingestion, and, to a limited degree, skin absorption. Increased incidences of alveolar/bronchiolar neoplasms, hepatocellular neoplasms, and fibroadenoma of the mammary gland occurred in laboratory animals when administered by inhalation. No adequate data are available to evaluate the carcinogenicity in humans.

1,3-dichloropropene (technical grade): RA. Used in the manufacture of 3,3-dichloro-1-propene and other pesticides, such as Telone II, a widely used agricultural soil fumigant for parasitic nematodes. Human exposure is through inhalation of vapors, ingestion of contaminated foods and water, and skin contact. A variety of tumors occurred in laboratory animals when Telone II was administered by stomach tube, and injection-site fibrosarcomas occurred when administered by injection. No adequate data are available to evaluate the carcinogenicity in humans.

diepoxybutane: RA. Not produced commercially in the United States since 1978; however, may be used in small quantities for research, as a curing agent for polymers, in textile fabrics, and to synthesize erythritol and other pharmaceuticals. Human exposure is through inhalation and skin contact. Skin cancer occurred in laboratory animals when applied topically; local fibrosarcomas and lung tumors occurred when administered by injection. No adequate data are available to evaluate the carcinogenicity in humans.

diesel exhaust particulates: RA. Come from vehicles, oil and gas production facilities, stationary engines, repair yards, chemical manufacturing, and electric utilities. The type and condition of the engine, fuel composition and additives, operating conditions, and emission control devices determine the composition and quantity of the emissions from an engine. Limited evidence of increased risk for lung cancer has been found in human studies.

diethyl sulfate: RA. Used primarily in dyes, pigments, textiles, and carbonless papers. Also used in cosmetics, household products, pharmaceuticals, agricultural chemicals, and some laboratory chemical processes. Human exposure is through inhalation and skin contact. Administration by injection induced local sarcomas in laboratory animals and tumors of the nervous system in their offspring; tumors of the forestomach occurred when administered by stomach tube. Limited evidence is available for the carcinogenicity in humans; a study found excess mortality from laryngeal cancer in workers exposed to high concentrations of diethyl sulfate.

diethylstilbestrol: K. Originally used as synthetic estrogen, and then widely prescribed for other uses in human medicine. Its use has since been reduced because of its cardiovascular toxicity and its link to a rare vaginal cancer in female offspring and possibly to testicular cancer among male offspring when given to pregnant mothers. Used in clinical trials for treatment of prostate and breast cancer and in biochemical research.

diglycidyl resorcinol ether: RA. Used as a liquid spray epoxy resin and in other epoxy resins used in electrical, tooling, adhesive, and laminating applications. Also used in polysulfide rubber and in certain pavements, and as a coating for metal. Human exposure is through inhalation and skin contact. Tumors of the forestomach of laboratory animals occurred when administered by stomach tube. No adequate data is available to evaluate the carcinogenicity in humans.

3,3´-dimethoxybenzidine and dyes metabolized to 3,3´-dimethoxybenzidine: RA. Used in production of dyes and pigments, as well as in the production of *o*-dianisidine diisocyanate for use in adhesives and as a component of polyurethanes. Human exposure is through inhalation and skin contact. Tumors at multiple tissue sites occurred in laboratory animals when administered 3,3′dimethoxybenzidine. No adequate data are available to evaluate the carcinogenicity in humans.

4-dimethylaminoazobenzene: RA. No longer produced or used commercially in the United States; previously used to color polishes and other wax products, polystyrene, and soap. Human exposure is through inhalation and skin contact. Tumors at multiple tissue sites occurred in laboratory animals when administered 4-dimethylaminoazobenzene. No adequate data are available to evaluate the carcinogenicity in humans.

3,3´-dimethylbenzidine and dyes metabolized to 3,3´-dimethylbenzidine: RA. Used in production of dyes and pigments, as well as in the production of polyurethane based high-strength elastomers, coatings, and rigid plastics. Also used in clinical laboratories in test tapes for the detection of blood and by water companies and swimming pool owners to test for chlorine in water or air. Human exposure is through inhalation, ingestion, and skin contact. Tumors at multiple tissue sites occurred in laboratory animals when administered 3,3′dimethylbenzidine. No adequate data are available to evaluate the carcinogenicity in humans.

dimethylcarbamoyl chloride: RA. Used primarily in the production of dyes, pharmaceuticals, and pesticides. Human exposure is through inhalation and skin contact. Skin cancer was induced in laboratory animals when applied topically, local sarcomas when injected, and tumors of the nasal tract when inhaled. No adequate data are available to evaluate the carcinogenicity in humans.

1,1-dimethylhydrazine: RA. Used primarily as a component of jet and rocket fuels. Also used in organic peroxide fuel additives, in photography, as an absorbent for acid gases, and as a plant growth control agent. Human exposure is through inhalation, ingestion, and skin contact. Increased incidences of lung tumors occurred in laboratory animals when administered by stomach tube, and angiosarcomas in various organs and tumors of the kidneys, lungs, and liver when administered in drinking water. No adequate data are available to evaluate the carcinogenicity in humans.

dimethyl sulfate: RA. Used in the manufacture of dyes, drugs, perfumes, pesticides, phenol derivatives, and other organic chemicals. Also used in polyurethane-based adhesives, in the analysis of auto fluids, and as a solvent for the separation of mineral oils. Human exposure is through inhalation and skin contact. Squamous cell carcinomas of the nasal cavity occurred in laboratory animals when administered by inhalation, local sarcomas when administered by injection, and tumors of the nervous system in offspring when administered by intravenous injection to pregnant animals. There is inadequate evidence for the carcinogenicity in humans; however, cases of bronchial carcinoma, pulmonary carcinoma, and choroidal melanoma have been reported in some humans exposed to dimethyl sulfate.

dimethylvinyl chloride: RA. Not used commercially; only for research. Human exposure is through inhalation. Cancers of the nasal cavity, oral cavity, esophagus, and forestomach have occurred in laboratory animals when administered by stomach tube. No data are available to evaluate the carcinogenicity in humans.

1,6-dinitropyrene: RA. Not used commercially; available for research purposes. Found in particulate emissions from combustion sources, especially diesel exhaust. Studies have determined malignant tumor formation at multiple sites in laboratory animals when exposed to 1,6-dinitropyrene by multiple routes. Human studies show limited evidence of increased risk for lung cancer when exposed to diesel exhaust particulates; however, it has not been determined whether 1,6-dinitropyrene is responsible.

1,8-dinitropyrene: RA. Not used commercially; available for research purposes. Found in particulate emissions from combustion sources, especially diesel exhaust. Human studies show limited evidence of increased risk for lung cancer when exposed to diesel exhaust particulates; however, it has not been determined whether 1,8-dinitropyrene is responsible. Studies have determined malignant tumor formation at multiple sites in laboratory animals when exposed to 1,8-dinitropyrene by multiple routes.

1,4-dioxane: RA. Used primarily as a stabilizer in chlorinated solvents; also used as a solvent, in textile processing, and in laboratory research and testing. Human exposure is through inhalation, ingestion, and skin contact. Increased incidence of cancers of the nasal turbinates, liver, gallbladder, lung, and skin occurred in laboratory animals exposed to 1,4-dioxane. Inadequate evidence for the carcinogenicity in humans.

Disperse Blue 1: RA. An anthraquinone dye used in hair color formulations and in coloring fabrics and plastics. Human exposure is through inhalation and skin contact. Tumor development in the urinary bladder and liver occurred in laboratory animals exposed to Disperse Blue 1. There is inadequate evidence for the carcinogenicity in humans.

epichlorohydrin: RA. Used in the production of epoxy resins, synthetic glycerin, elastomers, and other synthetic materials. Has also been used to cure propylene base rubbers, as a solvent for cellulose esters and ethers, and in resins for the paper industry; also widely used as a stabilizer. Human exposure is through ingestion, inhalation, and skin contact. Tumors of the forestomach occurred in laboratory animals when administered by stomach tube, tumors of the nasal cavity when administered by inhalation, and local sarcomas when administered by injection. There is inadequate evidence for the carcinogenicity in humans.

erionite: K. Belonging to a group of minerals called zeolites, erionite is no longer mined or marketed for commercial purposes. Domestic uses for natural zeolite are pet litter, animal feed, horticultural applications, oil absorbent, odor control, desiccant, pesticide carrier, water purification, aquaculture, wastewater cleanup, gas absorbent, and other miscellaneous applications. The use of other zeolites may result in potential human exposure to erionite. Deposits of fibrous erionite are found in Arizona, Nevada, Oregon, and Utah, and erionite fibers have been detected in road dust in Nevada, potentially exposing humans to erionite in ambient air. Mesothelioma and lung cancer have been linked to erionite exposure.

estrogens, steroidal: K. Most commonly used for estrogen replacement therapy or in combination with a progestogen for hormone replacement therapy. Also used in oral contraceptives; to treat breast cancer, prostate cancer, and other medical conditions; and for biomedical research. Unopposed estrogens have been shown to cause uterine endometrial cancer; however, addition of a progestogen greatly diminishes that risk. Some evidence also suggests an increased risk of breast cancer.

ethylene oxide: K. Used primarily in the production of several industrial chemicals, such as ethylene glycol (antifreeze), nonionic surfactants (detergents and dishwashing formulations), glycol ethers (solvents), ethanolamines (used in soaps, detergents, and textile chemicals), diethylene glycol (used in resins, plasticizers, and acrylate), triethylene glycol (used in dehydration of natural gas), polyethylene glycol (osmotic laxative), urethane polyols, fumigants, sterilizing agents, disinfectants, and insecticides. Human exposure is through inhalation and ingestion; very low risk of exposure from skin contact. An association between exposure to ethylene oxide and an increased risk of leukemia, stomach cancer, breast cancer, and lymphatic and hematopoietic cancers has been reported.

ethylene thiourea: RA. Used primarily in neoprene and polyacrylate rubbers. Also used in pesticides, dyes, pharmaceuticals, and synthetic resins, and in electroplating baths and antioxidant production. Human exposure is through inhalation, ingestion, and skin contact. Cancer of the thyroid, liver, and pituitary gland occurred in laboratory animals exposed to ethylene thiourea.

di(2-ethylhexyl) phthalate: RA. Used as a plasticizer in polyvinyl chloride (PVC) resins for fabricating flexible vinyl products; also used to manufacture non-PVC plasticizer. A variety of miscellaneous uses for di(2ethylhexyl) phthalate exist. Human exposure is through inhalation, ingestion, and skin contact, and through medical procedures. Tumors of the liver occurred in laboratory animals when administered in the diet. No adequate data are available to evaluate the carcinogenicity in humans.

ethyl methanesulfonate: RA. Used in laboratory research; not produced commercially in the United States. Tumors of the lung and kidney occurred in laboratory animals exposed to ethyl methanesulfonate. No adequate data are available to evaluate the carcinogenicity in humans.

formaldehyde (gas): RA. Used primarily for the production of urea-formaldehyde and phenolic resins (adhesives in pressed-wood products and building materials); also used to make other chemicals, household products, preservatives, permanent press fabrics, and paper product coatings. Human exposure is through inhalation and skin contact. Some studies have shown excess incidences of nasopharyngeal cancers in humans exposed to formaldehyde (gas).

furan: RA. Used primarily in the production of tetrahydrofuran (solvent), pyrrole, and thiophene. Also used in the formation of lacquers, as a solvent for resins, and in the production of agricultural chemicals (insecticides), pharmaceuticals, and stabilizers. Human exposure is through inhalation. Liver cancers and leukemia occurred in laboratory animals when administered by stomach tube. No adequate data are available to evaluate the carcinogenicity in humans.

glass wool (respirable size): RA. Used primarily in acoustical, electrical, and thermal insulation; filtration media; and weatherproofing. Human exposure is through inhalation and skin or eye contact. Various tumors and mesotheliomas occurred in laboratory animals when exposed to glass wool. There is inadequate evidence for the carcinogenicity in humans.

glycidol: RA. Used in many pharmaceutical and fine chemical applications, in the manufacture of vinyl polymers and natural oils, and in the synthesis of glycerol, glycidyl ethers, and amines. Also used as an alkylating agent, as a demulsifer, as a dye-leveling agent, and for sterilizing milk of magnesia. Human exposure is through inhalation, skin and eye contact, and ingestion. Tumors at multiple sites occurred in laboratory animals when administered by stomach tube. No adequate data are available to evaluate the carcinogenicity in humans.

hepatitis B virus (HBV): K. A virus that infects liver cells, causing acute or chronic hepatitis B. May be transmitted via injection or transfusion, via sexual contact, from mother to infant at time of birth, and through health care practices. Studies have demonstrated that chronic HBV infection causes liver cancer.

hepatitis C virus (HCV): K. A virus that causes most non-B viral hepatitis, acute or chronic. May be transmitted via injection (intravenous drug use), transfusion, or sexual contact; from mother to infant at time of birth; and through health care practices. Studies have demonstrated that chronic HCV infection causes malignant tumors of the liver.

heterocyclic amines (2-amino-3,4-dimethylimidazo[4,5-*f*] quinoline (MeIQ), 2-amino-3,8-dimethylimidazo[4,5-*f*] quinoxaline (MeIQx), 2-amino-3-methy-limidazo [4,5-*f*]quinoline (IQ), 2-amino-1-methyl-6-phenylimidazo[4,5-*b*]pyridine (PhIP)): RA. Formed naturally when muscle-derived foods (meat and fish) are browned during cooking. Sufficient evidence of carcinogenicity in experimental animals exists, with tumors resulting at multiple tissue sites; however, no adequate epidemiology studies have been reported that indicate a human cancer risk.

hexachlorobenzene: RA. Has not been produced commercially in the United States since the late 1970's; however, it is produced as a by-product or impurity during the synthesis of several chlorinated solvents and pesticides. Human exposure is through ingestion, inhalation, and skin contact. Tumors of the liver and thyroid occurred in laboratory animals when administered in the diet. There is inadequate evidence for the carcinogenicity in humans.

hexachloroethane: RA. Used to improve the quality of various metals and alloys, as an ignition suppressant, by the military for smoke munitions, and in various other applications. Human exposure is through inhalation, ingestion of contaminated drinking water or fish, and skin absorption. Increased incidences of tumors of the kidney, adrenal gland, and liver occurred in laboratory animals when administered by stomach tube. Few data are available to evaluate the carcinogenicity in humans.

hexamethylphosphoramide: RA. Used as a solvent, a polymerization catalyst, a stabilizer against thermal degradation in polystyrene, an additive to resins to protect against degradation by ultraviolet light, a de-icing additive for jet fuels, and a rodenticide. Human exposure is through inhalation, ingestion, and skin contact. Nasal tumors occurred in laboratory animals when administered by inhalation. There is inadequate evidence for the carcinogenicity in humans.

human papillomaviruses (HPV), some genital-mucosal types: K. Viruses that infect the genital skin and genital and nongenital mucosa; transmitted primarily through sexual contact. Low-risk HPV viruses can cause genital warts or cervical abnormalities; high-risk HPV viruses can cause cervical cancer. Evidence also suggests associations between HPV infection and cancer of the vulva, as well as some cancers of the head and neck, especially, the oropharynx (the soft palate, tonsils, and back of the tongue and throat).

hydrazine and hydrazine sulfate: RA. Used primarily to produce agricultural chemicals, spandex fibers, and antioxidants. Also used as rocket fuel, a water treatment chemical, a polymerization catalyst, a reducing agent, and a blowing agent. Additionally used for plating metals on glass and plastics and in fuel cells, solder fluxes, photographic chemicals, pharmaceuticals, textile dyes, and various other products. Human exposure is through ingestion, inhalation, and skin contact. Potential for general population exposure is low. A variety of tumors occurred when administered to laboratory animals. There is inadequate evidence for the carcinogenicity in humans.

hydrazobenzene: RA. Used primarily in the dye manufacturing industry; also used in the manufacture of pharmaceuticals and hydrogen peroxide, in the reclamation of rubber, as an additive in motor oil, as a desuckering agent for tobacco plants, in resin compositions, and in polymerization reactions. Human exposure is through inhalation, ingestion, and skin contact. A variety of tumors occurred in laboratory animals exposed to hydrazobenzene.

iron dextran complex: RA. Used to treat iron-deficiency anemia when oral treatment has failed; also used in veterinary medicine to treat baby pigs. Human exposure is through inhalation, skin contact, and treatment by injection. Local tumors occurred in laboratory animals when administered by injection. There is inadequate evidence for the carcinogenicity in humans; however, tumors at probable sites of injection in humans have been reported.

isoprene: RA. Used primarily to produce cis-1,4polyisoprene (rubber); also used to produce butyl rubber (isobutene-isoprene copolymer) and thermoplastic, elastomeric co-block (SIS) polymers. Isoprene is emitted through human breath, from tobacco smoke, and from plants and trees, resulting in low concentrations in the environment. A variety of tumors occurred in laboratory animals when exposed to isoprene through inhalation. There is inadequate evidence for the carcinogenicity in humans.

Kepone (chlordecone): RA. No longer used in the United States; used until 1978 as an insecticide for leaf-eating insects, ants, and cockroaches, and as a larvicide for flies. Human exposure is through inhalation, ingestion, and skin contact. Tumors of the liver occurred in laboratory animals when administered in the diet. There is inadequate evidence for the carcinogenicity in humans.

lead and lead compounds: RA. Lead is used largely in lead-acid storage batteries for motor vehicles and general industry; also used for ammunition, cable covering, piping, brass and bronze, bearing metals for machinery, and sheet lead. There are many lead compounds (soluble, insoluble, and organic) with many and varied uses, such as in water repellant, cotton dyes, varnishes, chrome pigments, asbestos clutch or brake linings, flame retardants, matches, explosives, paints, rubber, and plastics. Human exposure is through inhalation, ingestion, and skin contact. Tumors of the kidney, brain, hematopoietic system, and lung were reported in laboratory animals exposed to lead; lead exposure has been associated with an increased risk of lung, stomach, and bladder cancer in humans.

lindane and other hexachlorocyclohexane isomers: RA. Used primarily as an insecticidal treatment for hardwood logs and lumber, seed grains, and livestock. Also used as an insecticide for fruit and vegetable crops, and as a scabicide and pediculicide for humans in the form of a lotion, cream, or shampoo. Human exposure is through ingestion, inhalation, and skin contact. Tumors of the liver and thyroid occurred in laboratory animals when administered in the diet. There is inadequate evidence for the carcinogenicity in humans.

melphalan: K. Used to treat cancer and other medical conditions; also used as an insect chemosterilant. Studies have found that patients treated with melphalan for bone marrow cancer, breast cancer, and ovarian cancer have an increased risk of leukemia.

methoxsalen with ultraviolet A therapy (PUVA): K. Used to treat alopecia areata, atopic dermatitis, cutaneous T-cell lymphoma, lichen planus, mycosis fungoides, severe psoriasis, urticaria pigmentosa, vitiligo, and some forms of photosensitivity. Human exposure is through skin contact and ingestion. Studies have found that patients treated with PUVA have an increased risk of skin cancer.

2-methylaziridine (propylenimine): RA. Used in the adhesive, oil-additive, paper, pharmaceutical, rubber, and textile industries. Human exposure is through inhalation, ingestion, and skin contact. Leukemia and a variety of tumors have occurred in laboratory animals when administered by stomach tube or in the diet. No adequate data are available to evaluate the carcinogenicity in humans.

4,4´-methylenebis(2-chloroaniline): RA. Used primarily in the manufacture of castable urethane rubber products; has also been used in the laboratory as a model compound for studying carcinogens. Human exposure is through inhalation, skin contact, and ingestion. Liver cancer and a variety of tumors have occurred in laboratory animals exposed to 4,4´-methylenebis-(2-chloroaniline). There is inadequate evidence for the carcinogenicity in humans.

4-4´-methylenebis(*N,N*-dimethyl)benzenamine: RA. Used in manufacture of dyes, including basic yellow 2, basic orange 14, and solvent yellow 34; also used to process hydrochloride salt and as an analytical reagent for lead. Human exposure is through inhalation and skin contact. Tumors of the liver and thyroid occurred in laboratory animals when administered in the diet. No adequate data are available to evaluate the carcinogenicity in humans.

4,4´-methylenedianiline and its dihydrochloride salt: RA. 4,4´-Methylenedianiline is used in the production of 4,4´-methylenedianiline diisocyanate and polyisocyanates, which are used to produce a variety of polymers and resins. Dihydrochloride is used as a research chemical. Human exposure is through inhalation and skin contact. Increased incidences of tumors of the thyroid, liver, and adrenal gland occurred in laboratory animals when administered methylenedianiline dihydrochloride in the drinking water. No adequate data are available to evaluate the carcinogenicity in humans.

methyleugenol: RA. Used as a flavoring agent in jellies, baked goods, candy, chewing gum, nonalcoholic beverages, pudding, relish, and ice cream. Has also been used as an anesthetic in rodents and as an insect attractant in combination with insecticides. Human exposure is through ingestion and inhalation. A variety of tumors occurred in laboratory animals when administered orally. No adequate data are available to evaluate the carcinogenicity in humans.

methyl methanesulfonate: RA. Used experimentally as a research chemical and in the manufacturing of synthetic chemicals. Has been tested as a cancer treatment; potentially could be used to control insect populations and as a human male contraceptive. Human exposure is limited to laboratory research personnel. Studies have determined malignant tumor formation at multiple sites in laboratory animals exposed to methyl methanesulfonate by multiple routes. No adequate data are available to evaluate the carcinogenicity in humans.

***N*-methyl-*N*-nitro-*N*-nitrosoguanidine (MNNG): RA.** Has no known commercial use; it is used as a research chemical. Human exposure is most likely limited to research scientists. Studies have determined malignant tumor formation at multiple sites in laboratory animals exposed to MNNG by multiple routes. There is inadequate evidence available to evaluate the carcinogenicity in humans.

metronidazole: RA. Used primarily for the treatment of infections due to protozoan parasites; has also been used to treat Vincent's infection, acne rosacea, invasive intestinal amoebiasis, and amoebic hepatic abscess. Human exposure is through ingestion or topical application when used in medical treatment. Lymphomas as well as lung, mammary, pituitary, testicular, and liver tumors occurred in laboratory animals when administered orally. There is inadequate evidence available to evaluate the carcinogenicity in humans.

Michler's ketone [4,4´-(dimethylamino)benzophenone]: RA. Used in the production of at least thirteen dyes and pigments used to dye paper, leather, and textiles; one is also used as an antiseptic fungicide. Human exposure is through inhalation and skin contact. Increased incidences of liver tumors and hemangiosarcomas occurred in laboratory animals when administered orally in the diet. No adequate data are available to evaluate the carcinogenicity in humans.

mineral oils (untreated and mildly treated): K. Used primarily as lubricant base oils to produce further refined oil products used in the manufacturing, automotive, mining, construction, and other miscellaneous industries. Human exposure is through inhalation, ingestion, and skin contact. Exposure to mineral oils is strongly associated with a variety of cancers.

mirex: RA. All uses of mirex were suspended in 1977. Its primary use was as a fire-retardant additive under the name Dechlorane; it was also used as an insecticide to control fire ants in southeastern states. Mirex is very persistent in the environment and highly resistant to degradation; therefore, potential exposure to low concentrations still exists. Human exposure is through ingestion of fish caught from contaminated water, and for populations that live near a former manufacturing or waste disposal site, or live in areas where mirex was extensively used to control fire ants. Increased incidences of liver cancer, tumors of the adrenal gland, and leukemia occurred in laboratory animals when administered by stomach tube and then in the diet. No adequate data are available to evaluate the carcinogenicity in humans.

mustard gas: K. A blister-inducing agent that has been used in chemical warfare; used in research. Human exposure is through inhalation and skin contact, with military personnel being at the greatest risk. Mustard gas is associated with an increased risk of lung, laryngeal, pharyngeal, and upper respiratory tract cancers.

naphthalene: RA. Used in the production of insect repellents, phthalate plasticizers, pharmaceuticals, and other materials. Has also been used in the production of 1-naphthyl-*N*-methylcarbamate insecticides, beta-naphthol, moth repellents, surfactants, synthetic leather tanning chemicals, and toilet bowl deodorants. Human exposure is through inhalation and skin contact. Nasal tumors, neuroblastomas in the brain, and lung tumors occurred in laboratory animals when administered by inhalation. No adequate data are available to evaluate the carcinogenicity in humans.

2-naphthylamine: K. Used only in laboratory research; formerly used in the manufacture of dyes, rubber, and 2-chloronaphthylamine. Potential for human exposure is low; however, may occur through inhalation of emissions from sources where nitrogen-containing organic matter is burned, such as coal furnaces and cigarettes. Studies have shown that 2-naphthylamine causes bladder cancer.

neutrons: K. Used medically in external beam therapy, in boron neutron capture therapy, and to make radioisotopes. Also used in oil-well logging, nuclear reactors, neutron activation analysis and radiography, sterilization of materials, radiometric dating of rocks, and scientific and engineering research. Human exposure occurs naturally from cosmic radiation originating from outer space; however, additional exposure occurs in cancer patients receiving radiation therapy, nuclear industry workers, airline crews and passengers, and survivors of atomic bomb blasts. Studies show that neutron radiation induces chromosomal aberrations, mutations, deoxyribonucleic acid (DNA) damage, and many various tumors.

nickel compounds: K. Includes stainless steel, copper–nickel alloys, and other corrosion-resistant alloys. Human exposure occurs through inhalation, ingestion, and skin contact. Studies have shown an increased risk of death from lung cancer and nasal cancer.

nickel (metallic): RA. Used in alkaline batteries, coins, electrical contacts and electrodes, electroplating, machinery parts, magnets, spark plugs, surgical and dental prostheses, and welding products. Human exposure occurs through inhalation, ingestion, and skin contact. An increased incidence of malignant tumors at multiple tissue sites occurred in laboratory animals exposed to metallic nickel powder. No adequate data are available to evaluate the carcinogenicity in humans.

nitrilotriacetic acid: RA. Used primarily as a chelating agent and as a laundry detergent builder. Also used in water and textile treatment, metal plating and cleaning, pulp and paper processing, leather tanning, the manufacture of pharmaceuticals, photographic development, synthetic rubber production, and herbicide formulations and micronutrient solutions in agriculture. Human exposure is through inhalation, ingestion, and skin contact. Tumors of the kidney, ureter, urinary bladder, adrenal gland, and liver occurred in laboratory animals when administered in the diet. No adequate data are available to evaluate the carcinogenicity in humans.

***o*-nitroanisole: RA.** Used primarily in the synthesis of azo dyes; has also been used in the pharmaceutical industry. Human exposure is through skin contact, ingestion, and inhalation. Leukemia and tumors of the urinary bladder, kidney, large intestine, and liver occurred in laboratory animals when administered in the diet. No adequate data are available to evaluate the carcinogenicity in humans.

nitrobenzene: RA. Used primarily in the manufacture of aniline; also used in the manufacture of azobenzene, benzidine, dyes, isocyanates, lubricating oils, pesticides, pharmaceuticals, pyroxylin compounds, quinoline, rubber chemicals, soaps, and shoe and metal polishes. Human exposure is through inhalation, ingestion, and skin contact. Increased incidences of tumors at multiple tissue sites occurred in laboratory animals when administered by inhalation. No adequate data are available to evaluate the carcinogenicity in humans.

6-nitrochrysene: RA. Not used commercially; available for research purposes. Found in particulate emissions from combustion sources, especially diesel exhaust. Limited evidence of increased risk for lung cancer when exposed to diesel exhaust particulates has been found in human studies. Studies have determined malignant tumor formation at multiple sites in laboratory animals exposed to 6-nitrochrysene.

nitrofen (2,4-dichlorophenyl-*p*-nitrophenyl ether): RA. No longer used commercially; was used as an herbicide to control annual grasses and broadleaf weeds on various food and ornamental crops. Human exposure is through inhalation, skin contact, and ingestion. Tumors of the liver, spleen, and pancreas occurred in laboratory animals when administered in the diet. No adequate data are available to evaluate the carcinogenicity in humans.

nitrogen mustard hydrochloride: RA. Used to treat neoplastic diseases; also used to control pleural, peritoneal, and pericardial effusions caused by metastatic tumors, and has been used in clinical trials for rheumatoid arthritis, in tissue transplantation studies, and for other nonmalignant diseases. Human exposure is through injection, inhalation, and skin contact. Tumors in various organs occurred in laboratory animals exposed to nitrogen mustard hydrochloride. There is limited evidence of carcinogenicity in humans, including skin cancer, leukemia, and various other malignant tumors.

nitromethane: RA. Used primarily in the making of nitromethane derivatives, which are used as agri-cul-tural soil fumigants, industrial antimicrobials, and pharmaceuticals. Also used as a fuel or fuel additive. Human exposure is through inhalation, especially of motor vehicle exhaust and cigarette smoke; ingestion of contaminated water; and skin contact. Tumors of the harderian gland, lung, liver, and mammary gland occurred in laboratory animals when administered by inhalation. No adequate data are available to evaluate the carcinogenicity in humans.

2-nitropropane: RA. Used primarily as a solvent in adhesives, inks, paints, polymers, varnishes, and synthetic materials, and used in the manufacture of 2-nitro-2methyl-1-propanol and 2-amino-2-methyl-1-propanol. Also used in explosives and propellants, and in fuels for internal combustion engines. Human exposure is through inhalation, ingestion, and skin contact. Liver cancer occurred in laboratory animals when administered by inhalation. No adequate data are available to evaluate the carcinogenicity in humans.

1-nitropyrene: RA. Limited use in the production of 1-azidopyrene, which is used in photosensitive printing; available for research purposes in the United States. Found in particulate emissions from combustion sources, especially diesel exhaust. Limited evidence of increased risk for lung cancer when exposed to diesel exhaust particulates has been found in human studies; however, it has not been determined whether 1-nitropyrene is responsible. Studies have determined malignant tumor formation at multiple sites in laboratory animals exposed to 1-nitropyrene by multiple routes.

4-nitropyrene: RA. Used only as a laboratory chemical. Found in particulate emissions from combustion sources, especially diesel exhaust. Limited evidence of increased risk for lung cancer when exposed to diesel exhaust particulates has been found in human studies; however, it has not been determined whether 4-nitropyrene is responsible. Studies have determined malignant tumor formation at multiple sites in laboratory animals exposed to 1-nitropyrene.

***N*-nitrosodi-*n*-butylamine: RA.** Used primarily as a research chemical; once used in the synthesis of di-*n*butylhydrazine. Human exposure is through ingestion, inhalation, and skin contact. Leukemia and a variety of tumors occurred in laboratory animals exposed to *N*-nitrosodi-*n*-butylamine. No adequate data are available to evaluate the carcinogenicity in humans.

***N*-nitrosodiethanolamine: RA.** No longer used commercially; however, it is widespread in the environment; used as a research chemical. Human exposure is through skin contact, ingestion, and inhalation. Nitrosodiethanolamine is a known contaminant of anti-freeze, cosmetics, lotions, cutting fluids, shampoos, some pesticides, and tobacco. Tumors of the liver and kidney occurred in laboratory animals when administered in the drinking water, and tumors of the nasal cavity, trachea, liver, and injection site occurred when administered by injection. No adequate data are available to evaluate the carcinogenicity in humans.

***N*-nitrosodiethylamine: RA.** Used primarily as a research chemical. Also used as an antioxidant, copolymer softener, gasoline and lubricant additive, fiber industry solvent, and stabilizer in plastics, and in the synthesis of 1,1-diethylhydrazine. Human exposure is through ingestion, inhalation, and skin contact. A variety of tumors occurred in laboratory animals exposed to *N*-nitrosodiethylamine. No adequate data are available to evaluate the carcinogenicity in humans.

***N*-nitrosodimethylamine: RA.** Used primarily as a research chemical; also used to control nematodes (worms) and inhibit nitrification in soil. Used in rubber and acrylonitrile polymers, fluoride polymers, copolymers, high-energy batteries, and lubricants; as a solvent in the fiber and plastics industry; and as an antioxidant. Human exposure is through ingestion, inhalation, and skin contact. A variety of tumors occurred in animals exposed to *N*-nitrosodimethylamine.

No adequate data are available to evaluate the carcinogenicity in humans.

***N*-nitrosodi-*n*-propylamine: RA.** Not used commercially; used in laboratory research. Human exposure is through ingestion, inhalation, and skin contact. A variety of tumors occurred in laboratory animals exposed to *N*nitrosodi-*n*-propylamine. No adequate data are available to evaluate the carcinogenicity in humans.

***N*-nitroso-*N*-ethylurea: RA.** Used to synthesize diazoethane in the laboratory. Human exposure is limited; however, occupational exposure may occur through inhalation or skin contact. Leukemia and tumors at multiple sites occurred in laboratory animals when exposed to *N*-nitroso-*N*-ethylurea. No adequate data are available to evaluate the carcinogenicity in humans.

4-(*N*-nitrosomethylamino)-1-(3-pyridyl)-1-butanone (NNK): RA. Used as a laboratory chemical. Human exposure is through the inhalation of tobacco smoke or during tobacco chewing or oral snuff use. Tumors of the nasal cavity, lung, liver, and trachea occurred in laboratory animals when exposed to NNK. No adequate data are available to evaluate the carcinogenicity in humans.

***N*-nitroso-*N*-methylurea: RA.** Used in research; has been used to synthesize diazomethane in the laboratory and has been studied as a chemotherapeutic agent in cancer treatment. Human exposure is limited; however, occupational exposure may occur through inhalation or skin contact. Leukemia and tumors at multiple sites occurred in laboratory animals when exposed to *N*-nitroso-*N*-methylurea. No adequate data are available to evaluate the carcinogenicity in humans.

***N*-nitrosomethylvinylamine: RA.** Used as a research chemical. Human exposure is primarily limited to researchers; however, *N*-nitroso compounds have been identified in a variety of food products and can therefore be ingested. Tumors of the esophagus, tongue, pharynx, nasal cavity, and skin have occurred in laboratory animals when exposed to *N*-nitrosomethylvinylamine. No adequate data are available to evaluate the carcinogenicity in humans.

***N*-nitrosomorpholine: RA.** Not used commercially; however, patents have been issued for its use in the production of *N*-aminomorpholine and as a solvent for polyacrylonitrile. A variety of tumors occurred in laboratory animals exposed to *N*-nitrosomorpholine. No adequate data are available to evaluate the carcinogenicity in humans.

***N*-nitrosonornicotine: RA.** Used as a research chemical. Human exposure is through the use of tobacco products or the inhalation of sidestream smoke. Tumors of the esophagus, nasal cavity, trachea, and lung occurred in laboratory animals exposed to *N*-nitrosonornicotine. No adequate data are available to evaluate the carcinogenicity in humans.

***N*-nitrosopiperidine: RA.** Used as a research chemical. Human exposure is limited; however, exposure may occur from cigarette smoke and certain meats and fish. A variety of tumors occurred in animals exposed to *N*-nitrosopiperidine. No adequate data are available to evaluate the carcinogenicity in humans.

***N*-nitrosopyrrolidine: RA.** Used primarily as a research chemical; not used commercially. *N*-nitrosopyrrolidine is produced when foods preserved or contaminated with nitrites, especially fatty foods, are heat prepared; human exposure occurs through ingestion of these foods or inhalation of vapors released during cooking. Leukemia and a variety of tumors occurred in laboratory animals when administered in the drinking water. No adequate data are available to evaluate the carcinogenicity in humans.

***N*-nitrososarcosine: RA.** Not used commercially; has limited use in research. Human exposure is through inhalation, ingestion, and skin contact. Skin cancer of the nasal region and tumors of the esophagus and liver occurred in laboratory animals when exposed to *N*-nitrososarcosine. No adequate data are available to evaluate the carcinogenicity in humans.

norethisterone: RA. Used primarily as the progestin in progestin-estrogen combination oral contraceptives. Also used in medicines used to treat amenorrhea, dysmenorrhea, dysfunctional uterine bleeding, endometriosis, premenstrual tension, and inoperable malignant tumors of the breast. Human exposure is through ingestion, skin contact, and inhalation. Tumors of the pituitary, mammary gland, and ovaries occurred in laboratory animals when exposed to norethisterone. No adequate data are available to evaluate the carcinogenicity in humans.

ochratoxin A: RA. Not used commercially; it is an experimental teratogen and carcinogen. Human exposure is probably widespread through ingestion of food and handling of animal feed since ochratoxin A is a naturally occurring mycotoxin. Tumors of the liver, kidney, and mammary gland occurred in laboratory animals exposed to ochratoxin A. No adequate data are available to evaluate the carcinogenicity in humans.

4,4´-oxydianiline: RA. Used in the production of polyimide and poly(ester)imide resins, which are used in the manufacture of temperature-resistant products (such as wire enamels, coatings, and adhesives). Human exposure is through inhalation and through eye and skin contact. Tumors of the harderian gland, liver, and thyroid occurred in laboratory animals exposed to 4,4′oxydianiline. No adequate data are available to evaluate the carcinogenicity in humans.

oxymetholone: RA. A steroid hormone used to treat many conditions, including hypogonadism, delayed puberty, hereditary angioneurotic edema, and carcinoma of the breast. Also used to stimulate the formation of red blood cells (especially to treat anemias), to promote a positive nitrogen balance following surgery or injury, and to counteract weakness and promote weight gain during debilitating diseases. Human exposure is through ingestion and skin contact. Increased incidences of liver tumors occurred in laboratory animals when exposed to oxymetholone. Cases of liver tumors have been reported in patients treated for long periods with oxymetholone; however, a causal relationship cannot be established.

phenacetin: RA. Was used as an analgesic and fever reducing drug until it was implicated in kidney disease and withdrawn from the U.S. market in 1983; it was also once used in hair-bleaching preparations. Human exposure was through ingestion, with occupational exposure through inhalation and skin contact. Tumors of the urinary tract and nasal cavity occurred in laboratory animals when phenacetin was administered in the diet. There is limited evidence for the carcinogenicity in humans because phenacetin was usually taken mixed with other drugs.

phenacetin-containing analgesic mixtures: K. Was used as an analgesic and fever-reducing drug until it was implicated in kidney disease and withdrawn from the U.S. market in 1983; cancers of the urinary tract, renal pelvis, and bladder have also been reported in patients using large amounts of phenacetin-containing analgesic mixtures.

phenazopyridine hydrochloride: RA. Has been used as an analgesic drug to reduce pain associated with urinary tract infections or irritation; often combined with sulfonamides and antibiotics. Human exposure is through ingestion, with occupational exposure through inhalation and skin contact. Tumors of the liver, colon, and rectum occurred in laboratory animals when administered in the diet. There is inadequate evidence for the carcinogenicity in humans.

phenolphthalein: RA. Used in various ingested products, including laxatives, as well as in some scientific applications. Human exposure is through ingestion, skin contact, and inhalation. Increased incidences of tumors in multiple tissue sites occurred in laboratory animals when exposed to phenolphthalein. There is inadequate evidence for the carcinogenicity in humans.

phenoxybenzamine hydrochloride: RA. Used primarily to treat hypertension caused by pheochromocytoma; also used to treat benign prostatic hypertrophy under certain conditions. Has been used to treat peripheral vascular disorders, hypertension, and shock. Human exposure is through ingestion during its medical use and skin contact during its production. Peritoneal tumors and lung tumors occurred in laboratory animals when administered by injection. No adequate data are available to evaluate the carcinogenicity in humans.

phenytoin: RA. An anticonvulsant drug used to treat grand mal epileptic patients with focal and psychomotor seizures; has been used to treat various other conditions. Also used to control seizures occurring during neurosurgery, to prevent postcountershock arrhythmias in digitalized patients, and to reverse digitalis-induced arrhythmias. Human exposure is through injection, ingestion, inhalation, and skin contact. Thymic, generalized, and mesenteric lymphomas; liver tumors; and leukemias occurred in laboratory animals exposed to phenytoin. There is inadequate evidence for the carcinogenicity in humans; however, there is limited evidence suggesting that phenytoin may be a transplacental carcinogen in humans.

polybrominated biphenyls (PBBs): RA. Used as flameretardant additives in synthetic fibers and molded plastics. Human exposure is through ingestion, inhalation, and skin contact. Liver tumors occurred in laboratory animals when exposed to a PBB. No adequate data are available to evaluate the carcinogenicity in humans.

polychlorinated biphenyls (PCBs): RA. Uses are confined to closed systems, such as electrical capacitors, gas-transmission turbines, and vacuum pumps; exemptions are granted to individual petitioners for use as a mounting medium in microscopy, an immersion oil in low fluorescence microscopy, or an optical liquid, and for research and development. Human exposure is through ingestion, inhalation, and skin contact. Liver tumors occurred in laboratory animals when exposed to Aroclor 1260, Aroclor 1254, and Kanechlor 500 (all PCBs). There is inadequate evidence for the carcinogenicity in humans; however, an increase in the incidence of cancer, particularly skin cancer and cancers of the digestive system and of the lymphatic and hematopoietic tissues, has been reported in men exposed to PCBs.

polycyclic aromatic hydrocarbons (PAHs), (benz[*a*]anthracene, benzo[*b*]fluoranthene, benzo[*j*]fluoranthene, benzo[*k*]fluoranthene, benzo[*a*]pyrene, dibenz[*a,h*] acridine, dibenz[*a,j*]acridine, dibenz[*a,h*]anthracene, 7*H*-dibenzo[*c,g*]carbazole, dibenzo[*a,e*]pyrene, dibenzo[*a,h*]pyrene, dibenzo[*a,i*]pyrene, dibenzo[*a,l*]pyrene, indeno[1,2,3-*cd*]pyrene, 5-methylchrysene): RA. Other than dibenzo[*a,h*]pyrene, dibenzo[*a,i*]pyrene, and 5-methylchrysene, which have no known uses, the other PAHs are used only in biomedical, biochemical, laboratory, and cancer research. At least eight of those are found in coal tar and coal tar products, which include coal tar pitch and creosote. Human exposure is through inhalation of contaminated air, tobacco smoke, and wood smoke, and ingestion of contaminated water and foods, especially smoked, barbecued, and charcoal-broiled foods. Studies have determined malignant tumor formation at multiple sites in laboratory animals exposed to PAHs by multiple routes. There is inadequate evidence for the carcinogenicity in humans; however, many studies show increased incidences of cancer, including lung, skin, and genitourinary cancers, in humans exposed to mixtures of PAHs.

procarbazine hydrochloride: RA. Used in combination with other anticancer medications to treat Hodgkin disease, non-Hodgkin lymphoma, malignant melanoma, and small-cell carcinomas of the lung. Human exposure is through ingestion, inhalation, and skin contact. Leukemia, lymphomas, hemangiosarcomas, and tumors at multiple sites occurred in laboratory animals when exposed to procarbazine hydrochloride. There is inadequate evidence for the carcinogenicity in humans; however, the use of procarbazine hydrochloride in combination with other chemotherapeutic medications for the treatment of Hodgkin disease has repeatedly been shown to lead to the appearance of acute nonlymphocytic leukemia.

progesterone: RA. A naturally occurring steroidal hormone secreted by female ovaries, the placenta in pregnant females, and the adrenal cortex; used as a contraception and to treat secondary amenorrhea and dysfunctional uterine bleeding. Has also been used to treat dysmenorrhea and premenstrual tension, habitual and threatened abortion, preeclampsia and toxemia of pregnancy, female hypogonadism, mastodynia, uterine fibroma, and tumors of the breast and endometrium. Human exposure is through ingestion, injection, implantation, skin contact, and inhalation. Cancers of the breast, ovaries, endometrium, cervix, vagina, and genital tract occurred in female laboratory animals, including neonatal and newborn animals, when exposed to progesterone through injections and implants. No adequate data are available to evaluate the carcinogenicity in humans.

1,3-propane sultone: RA. Used in the production of fungicides, insecticides, some resins, dyes, detergents, lathering agents, bacteriostats, a variety of other chemicals, and untempered steel. Human exposure is through ingestion and inhalation. Brain tumors, breast tumors, and increased incidences of leukemia, tumors of the small intestine, and skin cancer of the ear occurred in laboratory animals when administered by stomach tube, and injection site tumors occurred when administered by injection. No adequate data are available to evaluate the carcinogenicity in humans.

β-propiolactone: RA. Has been used to sterilize blood plasma, vaccines, tissue grafts, surgical instruments, and enzymes; to kill spores of vegetative bacteria, pathogenic fungi, and viruses; and to manufacture acrylic acid and esters. Has also been used as a vapor-phase disinfectant in enclosed spaces, and in organic synthesis. Human exposure is limited because it is no longer used as a sterilant in medical procedures or in food; however, occupational exposure may occur through inhalation and skin contact when used as a chemical intermediate in industrial facilities. Tumors of the forestomach and skin cancer occurred in laboratory animals exposed to β-propiolactone. No adequate data are available to evaluate the carcinogenicity in humans.

propylene oxide: RA. Used primarily in the production of polyurethane polyols (used to make polyurethane foams), propylene glycols (used to make polyester resins for the textile and construction industries, as well as in drugs, cosmetics, solvents and emollients in food, plasticizers, heat transfer and hydraulic fluids, and antifreezes), glycol ethers, and specialty chemicals, including pesticides. May also be used in fumigation chambers for the sterilization of packaged foods. Human exposure is through ingestion; inhalation, and skin contact. Tumors of the nasal cavity, adrenal gland,

and peritoneum occurred in laboratory animals when administered by inhalation; local tumors and tumors of the forestomach when administered by stomach tube; and local tumors when administered by injection. No adequate data are available to evaluate the carcinogenicity in humans.

propylthiouracil: RA. Used as an antithyroid agent for the treatment of hyperthyroidism. Human exposure is primarily through ingestion as a drug. Tumors of the pituitary gland and thyroid occurred in laboratory animals when ingested. No adequate data are available to evaluate the carcinogenicity in humans.

radon: K. Used primarily for research; however, it is produced in nature by radioactive decay of radium and is released from soil into the air and groundwater. Human exposure is through inhalation and ingestion. An increased risk of lung cancer, as well as tracheal and bronchial cancer, is associated with exposure to radon.

reserpine: RA. A naturally occurring alkaloid used to lower blood pressure and reduce the heart rate and as a tranquilizer and sedative. Human exposure is through ingestion and skin contact. Tumors of the adrenal gland, breast, and seminal vesicles occurred in laboratory animals when resperine was administered in the diet and by injection. No adequate data are available to evaluate the carcinogenicity in humans.

safrole: RA. Has been used in drugs, beverages, foods, soap, and perfumes, and in the manufacture of heliotropin and piperonyl butoxide. Human exposure is through ingestion and skin contact. Liver tumors and lung tumors occurred in laboratory animals when administered safrole. No adequate data are available to evaluate the carcinogenicity in humans.

selenium sulfide: RA. Used in antidandruff shampoos and fungicides. Human exposure is through skin contact and inhalation. Liver tumors and alveolar/bronchiolar tumors occurred in laboratory animals when administered by stomach tube. No adequate data are available to evaluate the carcinogenicity in humans.

silica, crystalline (respirable size): K. Used in the production of quartzite, tripoli, gannister, chert, and novaculite; occurs naturally as agate, amethyst, chalcedony, cristobalite, flint, quartz, tridymite, and sand. Sand is used in the manufacture of glass, ceramics, foundry castings, abrasives, sandblasting materials, silicon, and ferrosilicon metals; as a filter in municipal water and sewage treatment plants; and in hydraulic fracturing in oil and gas recovery. Human exposure is through inhalation and ingestion. An increased risk of lung cancer is associated with exposure to respirable crystalline silica.

solar radiation: K. Emitted by the sun; has been determined to cause skin cancer and may also cause melanoma of the eye and non-Hodgkin lymphoma.

soots: K. Unwanted by-products of the incomplete combustion or burning of organic materials; have been used as fertilizer to provide small amounts of nitrogen and essential trace metals to plants, as a slug deterrent, as a soil conditioner, and in the recovery of trace metals in the metallurgical industry. Human exposure is through inhalation, ingestion, and skin contact. Increased risks, of scrotal cancer, lung cancer, and leukemia, as well as total lymphatic and hematopoietic cancer and cancer of the esophagus, liver, prostate, and bladder, are associated with exposure to soots.

streptozotocin: RA. Used in the treatment of metastasizing pancreatic islet cell tumors and malignant carcinoid tumors. Tumors of the kidney, lung, uterus, pancreas, liver, peritoneum, and bile ducts occurred in laboratory animals when exposed to streptozotocin. No adequate data are available to evaluate the carcinogenicity in humans.

strong inorganic acid mists containing sulfuric acid: K. Produced during the manufacture or use of sulfuric acid, sulfur trioxide, or oleum. The following industries use sulfuric acid: fertilizer, mining and metallurgy, ore processing, petroleum refining, inorganic and organic chemicals, cellulose fibers and films, inorganic pigments and paints, synthetic rubber and plastics, pulp and paper, soap and detergents, and water treatment. Lead-acid batteries are the primary consumer products containing sulfuric acid, which is also used as a general purpose food additive. Human exposure is through inhalation, ingestion, and skin contact. Exposure to strong inorganic acid mists containing sulfuric acid is associated with laryngeal and lung cancer in humans.

styrene-7,8-oxide: RA. Used in the production of styrene glycol and its derivatives, cosmetics, surface coatings, agricultural and biological chemicals, epoxy resins, and cross-linked polyesters and polyurethanes. Has also been used in the production of 2-phenylethanol used in perfumes, in the treatment of fibers and textiles, and in hydraulic fluids, chlorinated cleaning compositions, petroleum distillates, dielectric fluids, and acidsensitive polymers and copolymers. Human exposure is through contact with contaminated air or water. Tumors of the forestomach and liver occurred in laboratory animals when administered by stomach tube. No adequate data are available to evaluate the carcinogenicity in humans.

sulfallate: RA. Was used as an herbicide to control particular annual grasses and broadleaf weeds around vegetable and fruit crops; however, manufacture of sulfallate products was discontinued in the early 1990's. Potential for further human exposure is low. Tumors of the breast, forestomach, and lung occurred in laboratory animals when administered in the diet. No adequate data are available to evaluate the carcinogenicity in humans.

sunlamps or sun beds, exposure to: K. Emit primarily ultraviolet A (UVA) and ultraviolet B (UVB) radiation; have been determined to increase risk of skin cancer.

tamoxifen: K. Used primarily in the treatment of breast cancer; has also been tested as a possible treatment for other cancers. Human exposure is through ingestion and inhalation. An increased risk of endometrial cancer (cancer of the uterus) has been associated with exposure to tamoxifen.

2,3,7,8-tetrachlorodibenzo-*p*-dioxin (TCDD); "Dioxin": K. Used as a research chemical. Has no known commercial applications; however, is inadvertently produced by incineration of municipal, toxic, and hospital wastes; by paper and pulp bleaching; in PCB-filled electrical transformer fires; in smelters; and during production of chlorophenoxy herbicides. Human exposure is through inhalation, ingestion (especially of meat, fish, and dairy products), and skin contact. Studies have determined that a significant increased risk for all cancers combined, lung cancer, and non-Hodgkin lymphoma is associated with exposure to TCDD.

tetrachloroethylene (perchloroethylene): RA. Used primarily as a cleaning solvent (especially in the dry cleaning industry) and as a chemical precursor for fluorocarbons. Also used as an insulating fluid and cooling gas in electrical transformers; in adhesive formulations, leather treatments, paint removers, printing inks, and paper coatings; in aerosol formulations such as water repellants, automotive cleaners, spot removers, and silicone lubricants; as an extractant for pharmaceuticals; and as an agent that kills parasitic worms. As tetrachloroethylene is widely distributed in the environment, human exposure is through inhalation and ingestion of contaminated water or food; skin contact may also occur. Leukemia and tumors of the liver and kidney occurred in laboratory animals exposed to tetrachloroethylene. There is limited evidence for the carcinogenicity in humans. Studies have reported increased incidences of lymphosarcomas, leukemias, and cancers of the skin, colon, lung, urogenital tract, larynx, and urinary bladder in laundry and dry cleaning workers, however, these workers are also exposed to petroleum solvents and other dry cleaning agents. There is evidence as well for consistent positive associations between tetrachloroethylene exposure and nonHodgkin lymphoma and esophageal and cervical cancer.

tetrafluoroethylene (TFE): RA. Used primarily in the synthesis of polytetrafluoroethylene; also used to produce copolymers with monomers such as ethylene and hexafluoropropylene. Human exposure is primarily through inhalation. Leukemia and tumors of the liver and kidney occurred in laboratory animals when administered by inhalation. No adequate data are available to evaluate the carcinogenicity in humans.

tetranitromethane: RA. Used in rocket propellants, explosives, and diesel fuel, and as an organic reagent. Human exposure is through inhalation. A dose-related increase in alveolar/bronchiolar tumors occurred in laboratory animals when administered by inhalation. No adequate data are available to evaluate the carcinogenicity in humans.

thioacetamide: RA. Used as a replacement for hydrogen sulfide in qualitative analyses; has also been used as an organic solvent. Human exposure is through inhalation and skin contact. Tumors of the liver and bile duct have occurred in laboratory animals. No adequate data are available to evaluate the carcinogenicity in humans.

4,4′-thiodianaline: RA. Was used in the production of C.I. Mordant Yellow 16 dye, Milling Red G dye, and Milling Red FR dye; however, has not been used since the early 1990's. Human exposure may have been through skin contact, accidental ingestion, and inhalation. Tumors of the liver, thyroid, Zymbal gland, uterus, and colon occurred in laboratory animals when exposed to 4,4′-thiodianaline. No adequate data are available to evaluate the carcinogenicity in humans.

thiotepa: K. Used to treat a variety of cancers, including bladder, brain, breast, ovarian, and lung, and lymphomas. Studies have determined that patients treated with thiotepa are at increased risk to develop secondary leukemia.

thiourea: RA. Has been used in the synthesis of pharmaceuticals and insecticides, in boiler water treatment, as a photographic toning agent, as a dry cleaning agent, in hair preparations, and as a reagent for bismuth and selenite. Human exposure is through inhalation and skin contact. No adequate data are available to evaluate the carcinogenicity in humans.

thorium dioxide: K. Used in high-temperature ceramics, gas mantles, crucibles, nuclear fuel, flame spraying, medicines, nonsilica optical glass, and thoriated tungsten filaments. Concerns over its naturally occurring radioactivity have led to its substantially decreased use. Human exposure is through inhalation, intravenous injection, ingestion, and skin contact. Studies have determined a significantly increased risk of liver tumors, leukemia, and bone cancer for those exposed to thorium dioxide.

tobacco, smokeless: K. Main forms are chewing tobacco and snuff. Has been determined to cause tumors of the oral cavity, especially at the site of placement.

tobacco, smoking: K. Used in cigarettes, pipes, cigars, and bidis. Has been determined to cause cancer of the lung, urinary bladder, renal pelvis, oral cavity, pharynx, larynx, esophagus, lip, and pancreas. Sufficient evidence exists for the carcinogenicity of cigarette smoking and cancers of the nasal cavities and nasal sinus, stomach, liver, kidney, and uterine cervix, as well as myeloid leukemia.

tobacco smoke, environmental: K. Passive exposure (sidestream smoke) produced from tobacco products (cigarettes, pipes, cigars, and bidis) has been determined to cause lung cancer and cancers of the nasal cavity.

toluene diisocyanate: RA. Used primarily in the synthesis of polyurethane foams, which are used in furniture, bedding, and insulation. Also used in floor finishes, wood finishes, paints, concrete sealants, adhesive and sealant compounds, automobile parts, shoe soles, roller skate wheels, pond liners, and blood bags, and in oil fields and mines. Human exposure is through inhalation and skin contact. Tumors at multiple sites occurred in laboratory animals exposed to toluene diisocyanate. No adequate data are available to evaluate the carcinogenicity in humans.

***o*-toluidine and *o*-toluidine hydrochloride: RA.** Used primarily in the manufacture of dyes and pigments; also used in the manufacture of synthetic rubber, rubber vulcanizing chemicals, pharmaceuticals, and pesticides, as well as in organic synthesis and glucose analysis. Human exposure is through inhalation and skin contact. Tumors at multiple sites occurred in laboratory animals when administered in the diet. There is limited evidence for the carcinogenicity in humans. An excess of bladder cancers has been reported in workers exposed to *o*-toluidine; however, they were also exposed to other potential bladder carcinogens at the same time.

toxaphene: RA. Was used primarily as a pesticide, especially on cotton crops, until it was banned in the United States in 1990; was also used to control insect pests on livestock and poultry. Human exposure is through ingestion of contaminated food and water, skin contact, and inhalation. Tumors of the liver and thyroid occurred in laboratory animals when administered in the diet. No adequate data are available to evaluate the carcinogenicity in humans.

trichloroethylene (TCE): RA. Used primarily as a degreaser for metal parts, mainly by industries that manufacture furniture and fixtures, fabricated metal products, electrical and electronic equipment, transport equipment, and other miscellaneous products; it is also used in adhesives, lubricants, paint strippers, paints, varnishes, pesticides, and cold metal cleaners. Human exposure is through ingestion of food and water and through inhalation. Malignant tumor formation at multiple sites occurred in laboratory animals when exposed to TCE. There is limited evidence for the carcinogenicity in humans; studies have consistently showed an increased risk for kidney cancer, liver cancer, Hodgkin disease, non-Hodgkin lymphoma, and cervical cancer with occupational exposure to TCE.

2,4,6-trichlorophenol: RA. Has been used primarily in pesticides and wood preservatives; has also been used in fungicides, glue preservatives, insecticides, bactericides, and antimildew agents for textiles; however, most uses have been discontinued in the United States except in fungicides. Human exposure is through ingestion of contaminated food and water, inhalation of contaminated air, and skin contact. Increased incidences of leukemias, lymphomas, and liver cancer occurred in laboratory animals when administered in the diet. There is limited evidence for the carcinogenicity in humans, including soft-tissue sarcomas and non-Hodgkin lymphomas, when exposed to chlorophenols, which contain 2,4,6-trichlorophenol as well as tetrachlorodibenzo-*p*-dioxin (TCDD), which is a known carcinogen.

1,2,3-trichloropropane: RA. Used in the production of polysulfone liquid polymers and dichloropropene, and in the synthesis of hexafluoropropylene and polysulfides; it also was used as a solvent and extractive agent, and in the manufacture of a soil fumigant. Human exposure is through inhalation of vapors, skin contact, and ingestion of contaminated water. Malignant tumor formation at multiple sites occurred in laboratory animals when administered by stomach tube. No adequate data are available to evaluate the carcinogenicity in humans.

ultraviolet A radiation (UVA), ultraviolet B radiation (UVB), and ultraviolet C radiation (UVC): RA. All are components of broad-spectrum ultraviolet radiation (UVR); exposure is through solar radiation (except for UVC, which is absorbed by the ozone layer) and artificial devices emitting broad-spectrum UVR, such as sunlamps and sun beds. Exposure to each of these components induced skin tumors in laboratory animals; limited evidence shows that each of these components causes DNA damage in human tissue, which may lead to skin cancer.

ultraviolet radiation (UVR), broad spectrum: K. Exposure is through solar radiation and artificial devices emitting broad-spectrum UVR, such as sunlamps and sun beds. Has been determined to cause skin cancer.

urethane: RA. Used in the preparation of amino resins, which are used in permanent press textiles; also used in the manufacture of pesticides, fumigants, cosmetics, and pharmaceuticals, and in biochemical research. Human exposure is through inhalation, ingestion, and skin contact. Leukemias and tumors at multiple sites occurred in laboratory animals when exposed to urethane. No adequate data are available to evaluate the carcinogenicity in humans.

vinyl bromide: RA. Used primarily in the production of polymers and copolymers, which are used as flame retardants, and in the production of carpet-backing material, fabrics, home furnishings, granular products, films, laminated fibers, and rubber substitutes; also used in leather and fabricated metal products and in the production of pharmaceuticals and fumigants. Human exposure is through inhalation and skin contact. Tumors of the liver and Zymbal gland occurred in laboratory animals when vinyl bromide was administered by inhalation. No adequate data are available to evaluate the carcinogenicity in humans.

vinyl chloride: K. Used mainly by the plastics industry to produce polyvinyl chloride (PVC) and copolymers. Common items containing PVC include automotive parts and accessories, battery cell separators, containers, credit cards, electrical insulation, flooring, furniture, medical supplies, windows, wrapping film, and videodiscs. Vinyl chloride-vinyl acetate copolymers are used to produce films and resins. Human exposure is through inhalation of contaminated air, ingestion of contaminated foods and water, and skin contact. Studies indicate that vinyl chloride causes a rare tumor of the liver (angiosarcoma), as well as other tumors.

4-vinyl-1-cyclohexene diepoxide: RA. Used to dilute other diepoxides and for epoxy resins. Exposure is through inhalation and especially through skin contact. Skin cancer at the site of application and tumors of the ovary occurred in laboratory animals when exposed to 4-vinyl-1-cyclohexene diepoxide. No adequate data are available to evaluate the carcinogenicity in humans.

vinyl fluoride: RA. Used primarily in the production of polyvinyl fluoride and other fluoropolymers, which are commonly used as building materials. Human exposure is primarily by inhalation, but skin and eye contact may also occur. A variety of tumors have occurred in laboratory animals when administered by inhalation. No adequate data are available to evaluate the carcinogenicity in humans.

wood dust: K. Usually produced as a by-product of manufacturing wood products; commercially used in wood composts. Human exposure is through inhalation. Studies have determined that cancer of the nasal cavities and paranasal sinuses is associated with wood dust exposure, with limited evidence for cancer of the nasopharynx and larynx and Hodgkin disease.

X radiation and gamma radiation: K. Used in medicine (radiotherapy, computed tomography, positron emission tomography), the nuclear power industry, the military (nuclear weapons), scientific research, industry (well logging, sterilizing products, irradiating foods), and various consumer products (smoke detectors, televisions, radioluminescent clocks and watches, selfluminous signs). Exposure to X radiation and gamma radiation is strongly associated with leukemia and cancer of the thyroid, breast, and lung; cancer of the bladder, central nervous system, colon, salivary glands, skin, stomach, and ovary have also been reported.

▶ Glossary

ABCD rating: A system used to describe the stages of prostate cancer, with "A" and "B" describing cancer that is confined to the prostate, "C" for cancer that has grown out of the prostate but has not metastasized or spread to lymph nodes, and "D" for cancer that has metastasized or spread to lymph nodes.

ablation: The removal, destruction, or severing of diseased or damaged tissue, body part, or its functionality through surgery, drugs, heat, hormones, radiofrequency, or other means.

abscess: A pus-filled cavity that is usually swollen and inflamed and is a result of bacterial infection.

acquired immunodeficiency syndrome (AIDS): A disease of the immune system, caused by the human immunodeficiency virus (HIV), that causes a substantially increased risk for developing certain cancers and infections.

acromegaly: A rare disorder of adults in which an overproduction of growth hormones causes an enlargement of the bones of the hands, feet, nose, jaw, and head, as well as various other signs and symptoms.

actinic keratosis: Precancerous patches of skin that are thick and scaly. (Also called solar keratosis and senile keratosis.)

acute: That which begins and worsens quickly.

adeno-: Referring to a gland.

adenoma: A tumor of glandular origin or of a glandular structure that is not cancerous.

adenopathy: Swollen or large lymph glands.

adenosine triphosphate (ATP): The chemical compound in all living cells that provides the energy needed for metabolic processes.

adenosquamous carcinoma: A malignant tumor that contains both glandular cells and squamous cells.

adjunct therapy: Another treatment used in addition to a primary treatment to aid the primary treatment and increase the chance for a cure, such as chemotherapy used in addition to surgery.

adnexal mass: A growth of tissue in the uterine adnexa, usually in the ovary or Fallopian tube; it includes ovarian cysts, benign or malignant tumors, and ectopic (tubal) pregnancies.

adrenal glands: Small endocrine glands located on top of both kidneys that make and secrete adrenaline and noradrenaline, the steroid hormones that help control heart rate, blood pressure, and other body functions. (Also called suprarenal glands.)

adrenalectomy: Surgical removal of one or both adrenal glands.

adrenocortical: Pertaining to the outer layer of the adrenal gland.

adult T-cell leukemia/lymphoma (ATLL): A fast-growing T-cell non-Hodgkin lymphoma, which is a cancer of the immune system's T cells; it is believed to be caused by the human T-cell leukemia/lymphotropic virus type 1 (HTLV-1).

aggravating factor: Something that makes a medical condition worse, more serious, or more severe.

aggressive: That which grows, develops, or spreads quickly. agnogenic myeloid metaplasia (AMM): A slow-developing, long-term disease that occurs when bone marrow is replaced by fibrous tissue, making the bone marrow unable to manufacture blood cells properly and creating a condition in which blood is then made in organs such as the liver and the spleen; this may lead to the enlargement of these organs and progressive anemia.

AIDS: *See* aquired immunodeficiency syndrome.

AJCC staging system: Developed by the American Joint Committee on Cancer, this system describes the extent of cancer in a patient's body using T to describe the size of the tumor and if it has invaded nearby tissue, N to describe any nearby lymph nodes that are involved, and M to describe distant metastasis (spread of the cancer to another part of the body).

alanine aminopeptidase (AAP): An enzyme that is used as a biomarker to detect kidney damage and that can be used to help diagnose certain kidney disorders; high levels occur in the urine when there are problems with the kidney.

alanine transferase: An enzyme found in the liver and various bodily tissues and which, when present in abnormally high levels in the blood, may be a sign of liver damage, cancer, or other diseases.

allogeneic bone marrow transplantation: A procedure in which stem cells derived from the bone marrow are transferred to the cancer patient from a genetically similar but not identical donor, such as a brother or sister.

allogeneic stem cell transplantation: A procedure in which blood-forming stem cells are transferred to the cancer patient from a genetically similar but not identical donor, such as a brother or sister.

allopathic medicine: *See* conventional medicine.

amelanotic melanoma: A cancerous skin lesion that has little or no color, although it may appear red, pink, or white, and has an asymmetrical shape with an irregular faintly pigmented border that may be light brown, tan, or gray.

ampullary cancer: Cancer of the ampulla of Vater, which is the area where the pancreatic duct and the common bile duct (from the liver) join together and enter the small intestine.

analgesic: A drug, such as aspirin, acetaminophen, and ibuprofen, that reduces pain.

anaphylactic shock: The most severe and sometimes lifethreatening whole-body allergic reaction during which a person may experience itchy skin, edema, collapsed blood vessels, fainting, difficulty in breathing, and then death if medical treatment is not received promptly.

anaplastic: Rapidly dividing cancer cells with an abnormal appearance.

anaplastic large cell lymphoma (ALCL): A fast-growing non-Hodgkin lymphoma, that is usually a cancer of the immune system's T cells and that may occur in the lymph nodes of the neck, armpit, or groin, as well as in the bones, liver, lungs, soft tissues, or skin.

anaplastic thyroid cancer: A rare and aggressive thyroid cancer consisting of abnormal-looking cancer cells. anastomosis: A surgical procedure in which healthy sections of tubular structures in the body are connected together after a diseased portion has been surgically removed.

androblastoma: A rare ovarian tumor that secretes a male sex hormone, usually causing physical characteristics of men to appear in women.

anesthetic: A medical substance that puts the patient to sleep, causing a loss of feeling and awareness when administered systemically (general anesthetics) or causing a loss of feeling in only part of the body when applied locally.

angioimmunoblastic T-cell lymphoma: A fast-growing T-cell non-Hodgkin lymphoma that causes enlarged lymph nodes and increased antibodies in the blood, and may also cause a skin rash, fever, weight loss, and night sweats.

angiomyolipoma: A benign tumor of fat and muscle tissue usually found in the kidney and that may bleed or grow painfully large enough to cause kidney failure but otherwise rarely causes any symptoms.

anorexia: An abnormal loss of appetite.

anterior mediastinotomy: A procedure in which a tube is inserted through an incision next the breastbone to view the tissues and organs in the area between the breastbone and heart and between the lungs.

anterior pelvic exenteration: The surgical removal of the uterus, cervix, vagina, urethra, lower part of the ureters, and bladder.

anterior urethral cancer: Cancer of the part of the urethra (the tube that carries urine from the bladder to the outside of the body) that is closest to the outside of the body.

antiangiogenic: That which reduces the growth of new blood vessels.

antibody: A specific type of protein created by plasma cells (white blood cells) as an immune response to a specific antigen (foreign substance, such as a virus or bacterium) that may be a threat to the body, to neutralize or destroy that antigen. (Also called an immunoglobulin.)

antibody therapy: A medical treatment that uses an antibody to kill specific tumor cells, either directly or by stimulating the immune system to kill the tumor cells. anticoagulant: A drug used to aid in the prevention of blood clots. (Also called a blood thinner.)

antiemetic: A drug used to prevent or reduce nausea and vomiting.

antigen: A substance that stimulates a specific immune response, namely the production of antibodies.

antiglobulin test: A laboratory test used to determine blood type and to diagnose blood disorders in which antibodies are produced that destroy a patient's own red blood cells or platelets.

antimitotic agent: A drug used to treat cancer by stopping cell division (mitosis) and thereby blocking cell growth.

apheresis: A procedure in which blood is withdrawn from a patient or donor, the blood is passed through an apparatus that separates out one or more components from the blood, and then the remaining blood is transfused back into the patient or donor.

aromatase inhibitor: A drug that interferes with the role of the aromatase enzyme in the production of estradiol, a female hormone; it is used as hormone therapy for postmenopausal women who have hormone-dependent breast cancer.

arterial access device: A semipermanent implantable device, such as a port, chemo-port, port-a-cath, or PICC line, that allows a medical professional direct access to an artery without having to put a needle into the artery every time treatment is given, making administration of chemotherapy easier and reducing the risk of certain chemotherapy-related complications.

arteriogram: An X ray of arteries taken after the injection into the arteries of a special dye.

aspiration: The removal of a sample of tissue or fluid for examination by suctioning through a needle attached to a syringe, or the accidental inhalation of a foreign substance into the lungs.

assay: A laboratory test that finds and measures the quantity of one or more components within a specific substance.

ataxia: Loss of the ability to coordinate voluntary muscle movements.

atypical teratoid/rhabdoid tumor: An aggressive and rare pediatric cancer involving the central nervous system, kidney, or liver.

autoimmune hemolytic anemia: A condition in which the body's immune system interferes with the formation of red blood cells; it may occur in patients with chronic lymphocytic leukemia (CLL).

autologous bone marrow transplantation: A procedure in which a patient's own bone marrow is removed, stored, and then returned back to that person's body after intensive treatment, such as high-dose chemotherapy. autologous stem cell transplantation: A procedure in which a patient's own blood-forming stem cells are removed, stored, and then returned back to that person's body.

autonomic nervous system (ANS): The part of the nervous system that controls muscles of internal organs (such as the blood vessels, heart, lungs, intestines, and stomach) and glands (such as sweat glands and salivary glands) and affects involuntary, reflexive functions, such as heart rate, respiration rate, digestion, perspiration, and salivation. It consists of three parts: the parasympathetic nervous system, which induces fight-orflight responses in emergencies or stressful situations; the sympathetic nervous system, which allows the body to rest and digest; and the enteric nervous system, which controls the gastrointestinal system.

B cell: A white blood cell that makes antibodies and helps fight infections.

B-cell acute lymphocytic leukemia: With this leukemia, the most common type of acute lymphoblastic leukemia (ALL), abnormal immature white blood cells (B-cell lymphoblasts) crowd out the normal white blood cells, red blood cells, and platelets the body needs. (Also called B-cell acute lymphoblastic leukemia and precursor B-lymphoblastic leukemia.)

B-cell lymphoma: A type of non-Hodgkin lymphoma that affects B cells (immature white blood cells) and may be either slow-growing or fast-growing; there are many types of B-cell lymphomas.

barbiturate: A drug that depresses the central nervous system, causing a sedative effect that can be used to relieve anxiety before surgery and to treat insomnia, seizures, and convulsions.

barium swallow: *See* esophagram.

Bellini duct carcinoma (BDC): A rare, fast-growing, and fast-spreading kidney cancer that begins in the duct of Bellini in the kidney.

Bench Jones protein: A protein produced by plasma cells that is found in the urine of patients with certain diseases, especially multiple myeloma.

benign: Not cancerous.

Biafine cream: A cream applied topically by patients receiving radiation treatment to reduce the risk of and to treat skin reactions to the radiation.

bilateral cancer: Cancer that occurs in both the left and right organs, such as both breasts or both ovaries.

biliary: Pertaining to the liver, bile ducts, and gallbladder. biological response modifier (BRM) therapy: A treatment that uses monoclonal antibodies, growth factors, and vaccines to enhance or restore the immune system's ability to fight infections, cancer, and other diseases, as well as to reduce certain side effects that may be caused by some cancer treatments.

biomedicine: *See* conventional medicine.

biopsy: The removal of cells, tissues, or entire lumps or suspicious areas for microscopic examination by a pathologist.

blood-brain barrier (BBB): A network of blood vessels with closely spaced cells that prevents many potentially toxic substances, including anticancer drugs, from leaving the bloodstream and crossing the protective blood vessel walls into the brain tissues.

blood-brain barrier disruption (BBBD): The use of drugs to create gaps between the cells of the barrier so that anticancer drugs may be delivered to a brain tumor via an artery that goes into the brain.

blood cell count: *See* complete blood count (CBC).

blood thinner: *See* anticoagulant.

blood urea nitrogen (BUN): A substance in the blood that occurs naturally as a result of the breakdown of protein in liver and that is usually filtered out of the blood and into the urine by the kidneys; a high level of urea nitrogen in the blood may indicate a kidney problem.

bolus infusion: A single dose of drug given quickly by intravenous injection.

bone metastasis: Cancer that has spread to the bone from the original tumor.

bone-seeking radioisotope: A substance that gives off low-level radiation, which kills cancer cells; it is administered through a vein, then collects in bone cells and tumor cells that have spread to the bone.

brain stem gliomas: Tumors of the brain stem (the part of the brain that connects to the spinal cord).

breast-conserving surgery: The surgical removal of the breast cancer without removing all of the breast. The surgery may involve the removal of the lump (lumpectomy); the removal of one quarter, or quadrant, of the breast (quadrantectomy); or the removal of the tumor and some of the breast tissue around the tumor, as well as the lining over the chest muscles below the tumor (segmental mastectomy). (Also called breast-sparing surgery.)

breast duct endoscopy: A procedure in which a thin, flexible tube attached to a camera is inserted through the nipple and into the breast ducts deep into the breast to look for abnormal tissue in the lining of the breast ducts; samples of tissue and fluid may be removed during the procedure.

bronchogenic carcinoma: Lung cancer that begins in the lining of the airways of the lungs (bronchi) and includes small-cell and non-small cell lung cancer.

bronchoscopy: A procedure in which a thin, flexible tube with a light and lens is inserted through the nose or mouth and into the trachea, bronchi (airways of the lungs), and lungs to look for signs of cancer, remove tissue for microscopic examination by a pathologist, or perform treatment procedures.

Burkitt lymphoma: A rare, aggressive leukemia (cancer of the blood) in which an excess of white blood cells (B lymphocytes) forms in the blood and bone marrow; it has been linked to infection with the Epstein-Barr virus.

cancer: A group of diseases in which abnormal cells divide without control and then can invade nearby tissues and may even spread to other locations in the body via the blood and lymph systems.

cancer of the adrenal cortex: A rare cancer of the outer part of the adrenal gland that may or may not make more than a normal amount of certain hormones (aldosterone, cortisol, estrogen, or testosterone).

carbogen: A mixture of oxygen and carbon dioxide that is inhaled and induces an increased sensitivity of tumor cells to the effects of radiation therapy.

carcinogen: A substance that causes cancer.

carcinogenesis: The process in which normal cells are transformed into cancer cells.

carcinoma: A malignant tumor that begins in the skin or in the tissues that line or cover the internal organs (epithelial tissue).

carcinoma of unknown primary origin (CUP): A cancer in which cancer cells have spread and been found in the body; however, the initial location where the cells first started growing cannot be established.

carcinosarcoma: A malignant tumor containing both epithelial tissue (such as skin or tissue that lines or covers internal organs) and connective tissue (such as bone, cartilage, or fat).

cardiac sarcoma: A rare cancer in heart tissue. (Also called heart cancer.)

catheter: A flexible tube used to inject or withdraw fluids from the body.

cauterize: To destroy tissue by using extreme heat or cold, an electric current, or caustic chemicals.

CBC: *See* complete blood count (CBC).

cellular adoptive immunotherapy: A treatment in which the T cells (white blood cells) of a cancer patient are collected, grown, and multiplied in number in the laboratory, then given back to the patient to help the patient's immune system fight the cancer.

central nervous system primitive neuroectodermal tumor: A cancer that originates from a particular type of cell in the brain or spinal cord.

central nervous system prophylaxis: A preventive medical treatment in which chemotherapy or radiation is administered to the central nervous system to kill cancer cells that may be undetectable in the brain and spinal cord. cerebellar hemangioblastoma: A benign, slow-growing tumor in the posterior part of the brain (cerebellum).

cervical intraepithelial neoplasia (CIN): The formation of abnormal cells on the surface of the cervix.

chemoimmunotherapy: The use of chemotherapy to kill or slow cancer cell growth, combined with immunotherapy to restore the immune system's ability to fight cancer.

chemoprotective agent: A drug used to protect healthy tissues in the body from the toxic effects of anticancer drugs.

chemoradiation: A medical treatment that combines chemotherapy and radiation therapy.

chemotherapy: A drug treatment used to kill cancer cells. chloroma: *See* granulocytic sarcoma. cholangiocarcinoma: A rare cancer that occurs in the lining of the bile ducts in the liver.

cholangiosarcoma: A tumor of the connective tissues of the bile ducts in the liver.

chondrosarcoma: A cancer that forms in cartilage.

chorioadenoma destruens: A cancer that typically forms after fertilization of an egg and that grows into the muscular wall of the uterus.

choroid plexus tumor: A rare cancer that develops in the ventricles of the brain and usually occurs in children younger than two years old.

chronic: A disease or condition that continues, slowly progresses, or returns, often over a long period of time.

clear cell adenocarcinoma: A rare tumor, especially of the female genital tract, that contains cells that look clear inside when viewed under a microscope.

clinical resistance: An unsuccessful reduction in the amount of a cancer after treatment.

colorectal: Pertaining to the colon and the rectum.

complete blood count (CBC): A laboratory test that determines the number of red blood cells, white blood cells, and platelets in a sample of blood. (Also called blood cell count.)

complete hysterectomy: The surgical removal of the uterus and the cervix.

complete metastasectomy: The surgical removal of all tumors formed from cancerous cells that have spread from the original tumor.

complete remission: A period during which any clinical signs of a disease disappear in response to a treatment; however, this does not necessarily mean that the disease has been cured.

computed tomography (CT) scan: A series of detailed pictures of structures within the body, created by a computer that takes the data from multiple X-ray images taken from different angles and turns them into pictures on a screen. (Also called computerized axial tomography scan, tomography scan, computerized tomography, and CAT scan.)

concurrent therapy: A medical treatment given at the same time as another.

congenital mesoblastic nephroma: A kidney tumor, containing connective tissue cells, that may spread to nearby tissue or the other kidney and that is found in a fetus before birth or in an infant within the first three months of life.

consolidation therapy: A high-dose chemotherapy given after induction therapy as the second phase of a cancer treatment regimen, to help further reduce the presence of cancer cells in the body. (Also called intensification therapy.)

contraindication: Something, such as a medical condition or a symptom, that makes a particular treatment inadvisable because of the increased likelihood of a bad reaction.

contrast material: A dye or other substance that is given to a patient by intravenous injection, enema, or mouth and used with X rays, computed tomography (CT) scans, magnetic resonance imaging (MRI), or other imaging tests to show abnormal areas inside the body.

conventional medicine: A system of medicine in which symptoms and diseases are treated using drugs, radiation, or surgery by medical doctors with the assistance of other health care professionals, such as nurses, pharmacists, and therapists. (Also called allopathic medicine and biomedicine.)

CT scan: *See* computed tomography (CT) scan.

cystoprostatectomy: The surgical removal of the bladder and the prostate; the seminal vesicles are also removed in a radical cystoprostatectomy.

cystosarcoma phyllodes (CSP): Tumors that occur in breast tissue and are usually benign but may be malignant.

cystourethrectomy: The surgical removal of the bladder and the urethra.

cytopenia: A deficiency of blood cells.

debulking: Surgically removing as much of a tumor as possible.

desmoplastic melanoma: A rare form of skin cancer, specifically a variant of malignant melanoma, that is characterized by nonpigmented lesions on sun-exposed areas of the body, especially on the head and neck.

diffuse hyperplastic perilobar nephroblastomatosis (DHPLN): Abnormal tissue growth on the outer part of one or both kidneys that occurs during childhood and that may develop into Wilms' tumor (childhood kidney cancer) if not treated.

diffuse large B-cell lymphoma: A fast-growing cancer of the immune system (a non-Hodgkin lymphoma) that is characterized by tumors in the lymph nodes, bone marrow, liver, spleen, and other organs, as well as fever, night sweats, and weight loss.

distant metastasis: The spread of cancer from the original site to distant organs or distant lymph nodes.

donor lymphocyte infusion: A therapy in which lymphocytes (a type of white blood cell) are taken from the blood of the stem cell transplant donor and given to the recipient patient to kill remaining cancer cells.

ductal carcinoma: Cancer that begins in the cells that line the milk ducts in the breast, which is the most common type of breast cancer.

durable power of attorney: A legal document that gives one person the authority to make medical, legal, or financial decisions for another person until that person dies or cancels it; it may go into effect immediately or when that person is incapable of making those decisions.

early-stage cancer: Cancer that is in the beginning stage of its growth and has not spread to other parts of the body. ectomesenchymoma: A rare, fast-growing tumor of the nervous system or soft tissue that may form in the abdomen, head, neck, limbs, perineum, or scrotum in children and young adults.

-ectomy: Surgical removal.

endocrine: Pertaining to tissues, such as the pituitary, thyroid, and adrenal glands, which make hormones and release them throughout the body via the bloodstream; these hormones control the actions of other cells or organs.

endoscopic ultrasound (EUS): A procedure in which a thin, tubelike instrument (an endoscope) is inserted into the body and a probe at the end of the endoscope uses high-energy sound waves (ultrasound) to make a picture (sonogram) of internal organs. (Also called endosonography.)

epithelial carcinoma: Cancer that originates in the cells that line an organ.

epithelial ovarian cancer: Cancer that occurs in the cells on the outside of the ovary.

erythrocyte sedimentation rate (ESR): The distance red blood cells travel in one hour in a sample of blood as they settle to the bottom of a test tube; this rate increases when inflammation, infection, cancer, diseases of the blood and bone marrow, and rheumatic diseases are present. erythroleukemia: Cancer of the blood-forming tissues in which an excess of immature, abnormal red blood cells is found in the blood and bone marrow.

erythroleukoplakia: Potentially cancerous patches of red and white tissue that form on mucous membranes in the mouth; alcohol and tobacco (smoking or chewing) increase the risk of erythroleukoplakia.

esophageal stent: A metal mesh, plastic, or silicone tube that is placed in the esophagus to keep a blocked area open so that the patient can swallow soft food and liquids; it may be used in the treatment of esophageal cancer.

esophagram: A series of X rays of the esophagus taken after the patient drinks a barium solution. (Also called barium swallow and upper GI series.)

Ewing family of tumors (EFTs): A group of tumors that all come from the same type of stem cell and include Ewing tumor of bone (ETB or Ewing sarcoma of bone), extraosseous Ewing (EOE) tumors, Askin tumors (PNET of the chest wall), and primitive neuroectodermal tumors (PNET or peripheral neuroepithelioma).

excision: Removal by surgery.

excisional biopsy: The surgical removal of a lump or suspicious area for microscopic examination by a pathologist.

excisional skin surgery: The surgical removal of cysts, moles, other skin growths, and skin cancer (including some of the healthy tissue around it) using local anesthesia.

extracranial germ-cell tumor: A rare cancer that originates in reproductive cells (germ cells) in the ovary or testicle, or in germ cells that have traveled to areas of the body other than the brain, such as the abdomen, chest, or tailbone.

extrahepatic bile duct cancer: A rare cancer that occurs in the part of the bile duct that is outside the liver. extrapleural pneumonectomy: The surgical removal of a diseased lung, part of the membrane covering the heart (pericardium), part of the muscle between the lungs and the abdomen (diaphragm), and part of the membrane lining the chest (parietal pleura); this surgery is often used to treat malignant mesothelioma.

familial adenomatous polyposis (FAP): An inherited condition in which many growths (polyps) form on the inside walls of the colon and rectum; this condition increases the risk for colorectal cancer.

familial dysplastic nevi: A hereditary condition in which at least two members of a family have atypical moles (dysplastic nevi) and are at very high risk for developing melanoma.

familial isolated hyperparathyroidism (FIHP): A rare inherited condition characterized by a loss of calcium in the bones, an elevated calcium level in the blood (hypercalcemia), and an excessive amount of parathyroid hormone (PTH) being produced because of one or more tumors in the parathyroid glands.

familial medullary thyroid cancer: An inherited form of cancer that develops in the cells of the thyroid that make the hormone calcitonin.

fast-neutron beam radiation: A type of radiation therapy in which a machine (a cyclotron) focuses a beam of high-energy neutrons to kill cancer cells.

fibroid: A benign smooth-muscle tumor most often found in the uterus or gastrointestinal tract. (Also called leiomyoma.)

fibromatosis: A condition in which many benign tumors grow in connective tissues.

fine needle aspiration (FNA) biopsy: The removal of a sample of tissue or fluid for examination under a microscope by suctioning through a thin needle attached to a syringe.

fluoroscopy: An imaging technique that allows a physician to see internal organs in motion by the use of a fluoroscope (a machine that transmits an X-ray beam through a patient so that it strikes a fluorescent plate that is attached to a television camera, causing the images to be visible live on a television monitor); this technique is often used to observe the digestive tract.

FOLFOX: A chemotherapy drug combination of folinic acid (leucovorin), fluorouracil, and oxaliplatin that is used to treat colorectal cancer.

follicular large-cell lymphoma: A rare, slow-growing cancer of the lymphatic system (a non-Hodgkin lymphoma) with large cancer cells.

follicular lymphoma: A cancer of the immune system (a B-cell non-Hodgkin lymphoma) in which tumor cells grow as groups to form nodules.

follicular mixed-cell lymphoma: A slow-growing cancer of the lymphatic system (a B-cell non-Hodgkin lymphoma) with both large and small cancer cells.

follicular thyroid cancer: A slow-growing, highly treatable cancer of the follicular cells in the thyroid.

functional magnetic resonance imaging (fMRI): A noninvasive diagnostic tool that uses a powerful magnetic field, radio waves, and a computer to produce detailed pictures of the brain, spinal cord, or other organs and allows physicians to measure the metabolic changes that are taking place by detecting changes in blood flow and blood oxygenation.

fungating lesion: A type of skin lesion that develops when an underlying malignant tumor increases in size and extends through the epithelium, leaving a visible ulceration with tissue necrosis (death of living tissue), infection, and odor, and that may occur in many types of cancer, especially in advanced disease.

gamma irradiation: A type of radiation therapy that uses a high-energy radiation different from X rays called gamma radiation.

gastrectomy: Surgical removal of all or part of the stomach.

gastroscopy: Examination of the inside of the stomach by passing a thin, tubelike instrument with a light and lens for viewing through the mouth and esophagus into the stomach. (Also called upper endoscopy.)

germinoma: A germ-cell tumor that is most often found in the brain.

glial tumors: Tumors of the central nervous system, which include astrocytomas, ependymal tumors, glioblastoma multiforme, and primitive neuroectodermal tumors.

glucagonoma: A fast-growing tumor of the central nervous system originating in the glial tissue of the brain and spinal cord.

graft-versus-host (GVD) disease: An antitumor effect in which immune system cells in transplanted tissue from a donor (for example, bone marrow or peripheral blood) attack and help eliminate the recipient patient's tumor cells.

granulocytic sarcoma: A malignant, green-colored tumor composed of immature white blood cells (myeloblasts) and often associated with myelogenous leukemia. (Also called chloroma.)

health care proxy (HCP): A legal document that gives one person the authority to make health care decisions for another person when that person loses the ability to make those decisions.

heart cancer: *See* cardiac sarcoma.

hematoma: A mass of clotted or partially clotted blood that forms in a tissue, an organ, or a body space as a result of a broken blood vessel.

hematopoiesis: The production of new blood cells.

hemilaryngectomy: The surgical removal of one side of the larynx (voice box).

hemorrhage: Extensive blood loss from damaged blood vessels, usually within a short amount of time.

hepatectomy: Surgical removal of all or part of the liver.

hepatic: Pertaining to the liver.

hepatic arterial occlusion: A blockage in the blood flow to the liver; can be caused intentionally using drugs or other agents to help kill cancer cells growing in the liver or inadvertently while providing chemotherapy through a catheter in the hepatic artery.

hepatic veno-occlusive disease: A blockage in some of the veins in the liver, which is a common complication of high-dose chemotherapy given before a bone marrow transplant and which causes increases in weight, liver size, and blood levels of bilirubin.

hepatobiliary: Pertaining to the liver, bile ducts, and gallbladder.

hepatoblastoma: A malignant liver tumor of infants and young children.

hepatocellular carcinoma: The most common type of liver tumor; it originates in the hepatocytes, the major type of cell in the liver, and is usually caused by cirrhosis (scarring of the liver).

hepatoma: A tumor of the liver.

hereditary nonpolyposis colorectal cancer (HNPCC): An inherited cancer syndrome in which a person has a very high risk of developing colorectal cancer and an above-normal risk of other cancers, including uterus, ovary, stomach, small intestine, biliary system, urinary tract, brain, and skin. (Also called Lynch syndrome.)

high-dose chemotherapy: An intensive anticancer drug treatment that also destroys bone marrow and may cause other severe side effects; bone marrow or stem cell transplantation to rebuild the bone marrow usually follows this type of chemotherapy.

high-dose radiation (HDR) therapy: A greater amount of radiation than in typical radiation therapy is directed precisely at the tumor, so as to kill more cancer cells in fewer treatments without damaging healthy tissue.

high dose rate remote radiation therapy: A radiation treatment that involves placing a radiation source inside the body as close as possible to the cancer cells and then removing it between treatments.

high-energy photon therapy: A radiation therapy in which high-energy photons (units of light energy) penetrate deeply into tissues to attack tumors while imparting less radiation to superficial tissues, such as the skin.

high-grade lymphoma: A cancerous tumor of lymphoid tissue that grows and spreads quickly and has severe symptoms.

high-grade squamous intraepithelial lesion (HSIL): A precancerous condition in which there are abnormal cells of the uterine cervix.

high-risk cancer: A cancer that is likely to spread or come back.

homeopathic medicine: An alternative system of medicine based on the belief that a substance that causes particular symptoms in a healthy person can be used in minute doses to cure those symptoms in an ill person. Hurthle cell neoplasm: A type of thyroid tumor that is un-common and may be either benign or malignant.

hyper-: Excessive; above normal.

hyperalimentation: The intravenous feeding of nutrients to patients who cannot ingest or digest food through the alimentary tract.

hyperfractionation: The practice of giving smaller doses (fractions) of radiation more often than the standard radiation dose of once a day, resulting in fewer side effects.

hypernephroma: Kidney cancer that originates in the lining of the renal tubules in the kidney; it is the most common type of kidney cancer. (Also called renal cell cancer.)

hypersensitivity: An abnormal or excessive response by the immune system to a drug or other substance.

hyperuricemia: Presence of an excessive amount of uric acid in the blood, which is sometimes a side effect of anticancer drugs.

hypo-: Less than normal.

hypofractionation: The practice of giving larger doses (fractions) of radiation less often and over a shorter period of time than the standard radiation dose of once a day.

hypopharyngeal cancer: Cancer that originates in the bottom part of the throat (hypopharynx).

idiopathic pneumonia syndrome: A condition characterized by pneumonia-like symptoms, such as fever, chills, coughing, and breathing difficulties, with no obvious infection in the lung; it can occur after a stem cell transplant.

immature teratoma: A rare germ-cell tumor often containing different tissues, such as bone, hair, and muscle.

immunoglobulin: *See* antibody.

implantable pump: A small device that is implanted under the skin and that administers a steady dose of drugs. incidence: The number of new cases of a disease diagnosed in a specific population during a specified period (usually a year).

incision: A cut or wound in body tissue, especially that made with a surgical instrument.

incisional biopsy: Surgical removal of a part of a lump or suspicious area for examination under a microscope.

incontinence: Inability to control the discharge of urine (urinary incontinence) or feces (fecal incontinence).

indolent: Slow to develop or progress.

indolent lymphoma: *See* low-grade lymphoma.

induction therapy: The initial treatment used in an effort to make subsequent treatments, such as surgery or radiotherapy, more effective and to evaluate the response to drugs or other agents.

infiltrating cancer: Cancer that has spread into nearby, healthy tissue. (Also called invasive cancer.)

intensification therapy: *See* consolidation therapy.

inter-: Between or among.

interstitial radiation therapy: Radiation treatment in which radioactive material sealed in needles, wires, seeds, or catheters is inserted into tissue at or near the tumor site.

intra-: Within, during, or between layers of. intracranial tumor: A tumor situated in the brain. intrahepatic infusion: The administration of drugs directly into the blood vessels of the liver.

intraluminal intubation and dilation: A procedure in which a tube (plastic or metal) is inserted through the mouth into the esophagus to keep it open; it is used especially during radiation therapy for esophageal cancer.

intramuscular (IM): Within or into muscle.

intraoperative radiation therapy (IORT): A procedure in which a concentrated beam of radiation is aimed directly at a tumor while it is exposed during surgery.

intraperitoneal (IP): Within the peritoneal (abdominal) cavity.

intraperitoneal chemotherapy: Treatment in which anticancer drugs are delivered directly into the peritoneal (abdominal) cavity through a thin tube.

intraperitoneal infusion: The administration of drugs and fluids directly into the peritoneal (abdominal) cavity through a thin tube.

intraperitoneal radiation therapy: Treatment in which a radioactive liquid is delivered directly into the peritoneal (abdominal) cavity through a thin tube.

intrathecal chemotherapy: Treatment in which anticancer drugs are delivered by injection directly into the fluidfilled space between the thin layers of tissue that cover the brain and spinal cord.

intravenous pyelogram (IVP): A series of X rays taken of the kidneys, ureters, and bladder after intravenous administration of a dye that collects in and is excreted by the kidneys.

intraventricular infusion: The administration of a drug into the fluid-filled cavity within the heart or brain.

invasive cancer: *See* infiltrating cancer.

inverted papilloma: A tumor of the mucosal membrane of the nasal cavity, paranasal sinus, or urinary tract in which the epithelial cells grow downward into the underlying supportive tissue.

irradiation: The use of high-energy radiation to kill cancer cells and shrink tumors. (Also called radiation therapy.)

isolated hepatic perfusion: A procedure in which the liver's blood supply is temporarily separated from blood circulating throughout the rest of the body by the placement of a catheter into the artery that provides blood to the liver and the placement of a second catheter into the vein that takes blood away from the liver, so that high doses of anticancer drugs can be directed to the liver only.

isolated limb perfusion: A procedure in which a tourniquet is used to stop the flow of blood to and from a limb (arm or leg) temporarily so that high-dose anticancer drugs can be delivered directly to the limb where the cancer is situated.

isolated lung perfusion: A surgical procedure during which high-dose anticancer drugs are delivered directly to tumors in the lungs after separating the circulation of blood to the lungs from the circulation of blood through the rest of the body.

-itis: A suffix denoting inflammation or inflammatory disease.

J-pouch coloanal anastomosis: The surgical attachment of the colon to the anus after the removal of the rectum, performed by forming a J-shaped pouch from a 2to 4-inch section of the colon as a replacement for the rectum.

jaundice: A condition in which the liver is not working properly or a bile duct is blocked, causing the skin and the whites of the eyes to yellow, the urine to darken, and the color of the stool to become lighter than normal.

juvenile myelomonocytic leukemia (JMML): A rare childhood cancer of the blood or bone marrow in which cancer cells spread into tissues such as the skin, lungs, and intestines.

Kahler disease: A cancer of plasma cells (immune system cells in bone marrow that produce antibodies).

keratoacanthoma: A quick-growing, rounded skin tumor that occurs on sun-exposed areas of the body, especially on the head and neck, and that tends to heal on its own.

Klatskin tumor: A cancer of the lining of the bile ducts in the liver at the junction where the left and right ducts meet; it is a type of cholangiocarcinoma.

large-cell carcinoma: The uncontrolled growth of large, cancerous cells of the lung.

late-stage cancer: A cancer that has been growing for a while and has spread to the lymph nodes or other parts of the body.

leiomyoma: *See* fibroid.

leukemia: A cancer of the blood or bone marrow that is characterized by an abnormal increase in the number of white blood cells in the tissues of the body and may also include an increase of those in the circulating blood; leukemias are classified according to the type of white blood cell most noticeably involved.

ligation: The surgical process of tying up a blood vessel to stop blood from reaching a tumor or part of the body. light-emitting diode (LED) therapy: A therapy in which a special type of light is used to activate specific drugs that react when exposed to the light, enabling them to kill the cancer cells.

limited-stage small-cell lung cancer: Lung cancer in which cancer cells are found in one lung, only nearby lymph nodes, and the tissues between the lungs.

lipoma: A benign tumor consisting of fat cells.

localized cancer: Cancer that is confined to the original site without evidence of having spread.

locally advanced cancer: Cancer that has spread to nearby tissue or lymph nodes.

low-grade lymphoma: Cancer of immune system cells that grows and spreads slowly, inducing few symptoms. (Also called indolent lymphoma.)

low-grade squamous intraepithelial lesion (LSIL): Slight changes in the size and shape of the cells on the surface of the uterine cervix that are considered mild abnormalities caused by human papillomavirus (HPV) infection.

lower gastrointestinal (GI) series: A group of X rays taken of the colon and rectum following a barium enema; it is used to diagnose abnormalities in the large intestine.

lymph nodes: Glands that are located along the lymphatic system in many areas throughout the body and that filter impurities, such as cancer cells or bacteria, from the lymphatic fluid that flows through the nodes.

lymphoepithelioma: A cancer that originates in the tissues covering the nasopharynx (the upper part of the throat behind the nose).

lymphography: An X-ray study of lymphatic vessels and lymph nodes after injection of a special dye.

lymphoma: A malignant tumor of the lymph nodes or other lymphatic tissues.

lymphoscintigraphy: An imaging technique used in conjunction with a radioactive substance injected at the site of the tumor to identify the first draining lymph node near a tumor so that a physician can determine which lymph node to remove for examination.

Lynch syndrome: *See* hereditary nonpolyposis colon cancer (HNPCC).

lytic lesion: An area of bone that has been destroyed from a disease process, such as cancer.

magnetic resonance imaging (MRI): An imaging method using magnetism, radio waves, and a computer to produce images of organs and soft tissues; it provides spatial information about the size and shape of a tumor.

magnetic resonance perfusion imaging: A diagnostic technique that is used in conjunction with an injected dye to produce computerized images of blood flow through tissues; it is a special type of magnetic resonance imaging (MRI).

magnetic resonance spectroscopic imaging (MRSI): An imaging method that detects and measures activity at the cellular level, providing metabolic information; it is used in conjunction with magnetic resonance imaging (MRI).

magnetic-targeted carrier: A tiny bead containing iron and carbon particles that is attached to an anticancer drug and used to direct the drug to the tumor site with the use of a magnet outside the body, allowing a larger dose of the drug at the tumor site for a longer period of time, and protecting healthy tissue from the side effects of chemotherapy.

maintenance therapy: Treatment that is given to help a primary treatment continue working and to help keep cancer in remission.

malignant: Cancerous.

malignant ascites: An accumulation in the abdomen of fluid containing cancer cells.

malignant meningioma: A rare, fast-growing tumor that arises from the meninges (membranes that cover and protect the brain and spinal cord) and that may spread to other areas of the body.

malignant mesothelioma: A cancerous tumor of the lining of the lung and chest cavity (pleura) or lining of the abdomen (peritoneum); it is often caused by sustained exposure to airborne particles of asbestos.

malignant mixed Müllerian tumor (MMMT): A rare tumor containing carcinoma and sarcoma cells and often occurring in the uterus.

malignant peripheral nerve sheath tumor (MPNST): A soft-tissue tumor arising from a protective sheath (covering) around peripheral nerves (nerves outside the central nervous system).

malignant pleural effusion: A condition in which cancer, most often lung cancer, breast cancer, lymphoma, and leukemia, causes an abnormal accumulation of fluid in the lining of the lung and the wall of the chest cavity.

MALT: *See* mucosa-associated lymphoid tissue lymphoma.

Mammotome: A minimally invasive device used to perform a breast biopsy.

margin: The edge of the tissue removed in cancer surgery, which is examined for cancer cells to determine whether all the cancer has been removed.

marginal zone lymphoma (MZL): A slow-growing B-cell non-Hodgkin lymphoma that originates in the outer edges of lymph tissue.

mature T-cell lymphoma: A fast-growing non-Hodgkin lymphoma (malignant tumor of the lymphoid tissue) that originates in mature T lymphocytes.

mature teratoma: A benign germ-cell tumor often containing different tissues, such as bone, hair, and muscle. maximum inspiratory pressure test (MIP test): A test in which a person inhales and exhales through a manometer, a device that measures the strength of the muscles used in breathing.

maximum tolerated dose: The highest dose of a drug or treatment that a person can tolerate before unacceptable side effects begin to occur.

mean survival time: The average time that patients in a clinical study stayed alive, beginning with the time of diagnosis or with the start of treatment.

median survival time: The length of time from diagnosis or start of treatment by which half of the patients with a specific disease have died.

medical nutrition therapy: Therapy in which appropriate foods or nutrients are used in the treatment of conditions such as diabetes, heart disease, and cancer, and which may include changes in a person's diet or intravenous or tube feeding.

medullary thyroid cancer: Cancer of the C cells of the thyroid, which make calcitonin (a hormone that helps maintain a healthy blood calcium level).

Merkel cell cancer: *See* trabecular cancer.

melanoma: A cancer that originates in pigmented tissues, such as the skin (in the form of a mole), in the eye, or in the intestines.

metaplastic carcinoma: A cancer that originates in cells that have changed into an abnormal form for that tissue; it is usually found in the alimentary or upper respiratory tract or in the breast.

metastasectomy: Surgical removal of one or more tumors that have formed from cells that have spread from the original (primary) tumor.

metastasize: To spread, especially cancer cells, from the original site in the body to another area of the body. metronomic therapy: Low doses of anticancer drugs given continuously or frequently, usually in conjunction with other therapy methods.

mixed glioma: A brain tumor consisting of more than one type of cell.

modified radical mastectomy: Surgical removal of the breast, lymph nodes under the arm, the lining over the chest muscles, and sometimes part of the chest wall muscles.

molar pregnancy: A slow-growing tumor that originates in the cells (trophoblastic) that aid in embryo attachment to the uterus and in placenta formation after fertilization of an egg by a sperm; it is usually benign but can become invasive, as well as malignant (then called a choriocarcinoma).

molecular marker: A distinctive biological molecule found in the body that indicates a specific process, condition, or disease, and that may be used to determine the body's response to a treatment for that disease or condition.

MRI: *See* magnetic resonance imaging.

mucosa-associated lymphoid tissue (MALT) lymphoma: A cancer (non-Hodgkin lymphoma) that originates in B cells in mucosal tissue that are involved in antibody production.

Müllerian tumor: A rare cancer of the uterus, ovary, or Fallopian tubes.

multidisciplinary: Involving a number of different specialties (disciplines), especially in the approach to planning treatment and the team of experts who oversee that treatment.

neck dissection: Surgical removal of lymph nodes and other tissues in the neck.

necrosis: Death of living tissues.

negative axillary lymph node: A cancer-free lymph node in the armpit.

neoadjuvant therapy: Treatment given before the primary treatment to help the primary treatment, such as drugs given to shrink an inoperable tumor so that surgery is possible.

neoplasm: *See* tumor.

nephrectomy: Surgical removal of a kidney.

nephrotomogram: A series of X rays of the kidneys taken from different angles.

nephrotoxic: Poisonous to the kidney.

nephroureterectomy: Surgical removal of a kidney and its ureter.

nerve block: The injection of a local anesthetic around a nerve or into the spine to block pain.

nerve-sparing radical prostatectomy: Surgical removal of the prostate with an attempt at saving the nerves that help cause penile erections.

neuroendocrine carcinoma of the skin: *See* trabecular cancer.

neuroma: A tumor that originates in nerve cells.

neuropathy: An abnormal or degenerative condition of the nervous system that causes pain, tingling, numbness, swelling, or muscle weakness, usually beginning in the hands or feet and spreading to different parts of the body over time; physical injury, infection, toxic substances, disease (including cancer), or drugs (including anticancer drugs) may be the cause.

neurotoxic: Poisonous or damaging to the nervous system. non-small-cell lung cancer: A group of lung cancers in which the cells, when viewed under a microscope, are not the small-cell type, and which include adenocarcinoma, large-cell carcinoma, and squamous cell carcinoma.

nonfunctioning tumor: A tumor occurring in the endocrine tissue that does not make hormones.

nonseminoma: A group of testicular cancers that begin in the cells that give rise to sperm (germ cells) and include choriocarcinoma, embryonal carcinoma, teratoma, and yolk sac carcinoma.

occult primary tumor: Cancer in which the original tumor site is unknown, and the metastases of which are mostly found in the head and neck.

ocular melanoma: A rare cancer of the eye occurring in the cells that produce the pigment melanin (melanocytes).

oligoastrocytoma: A brain tumor that is a type of mixed glioma (consists of more than one type of cell).

omentectomy: Surgical removal of all or part of the omentum (a fold of the lining of the abdomen).

open biopsy: A procedure in which tissues or lumps are removed through an incision in the skin to be examined by a pathologist.

open colectomy: Surgical removal of all or part of the colon through an incision in the wall of the abdomen. operable: Referring to a condition that can be treated by surgery.

opportunistic infection: An infection caused by an organism that usually does not cause disease but can do so in people with weakened immune systems.

oral: Pertaining to the mouth.

osteosarcoma: Bone cancer, usually of the large bones of the arm or leg.

ostomy: An operation in which an artificial passage is created from an area inside the body to the outside for bodily elimination, such as in a colostomy, ileostomy, or urostomy.

ovarian ablation: Surgery, a drug treatment, or radiation therapy to prevent the functioning of the ovaries.

oxygen therapy: The administration of oxygen through a nose tube, mask, or tent.

Pancoast tumor: A type of lung cancer that forms at the very top (apex) of a lung and invades nearby tissues, such as the chest wall, ribs, and vertebrae.

papillary serous carcinoma: A fast-growing cancer that spreads rapidly and usually affects the uterus/endometrium, ovary, or peritoneum.

papillary thyroid cancer: A common type of slowgrowing thyroid cancer that originates in the follicular cells in the thyroid.

papillary tumor: A mushroom-shaped tumor, the stem of which is attached to the inner lining (epithelial layer) of an organ.

papilledema: Swelling around the optic disk as a result of increased brain pressure, sometimes caused by a brain tumor.

paraganglioma: A rare tumor that arises from cells of the paraganglia and is usually found in the abdomen, thorax, or head or neck region.

parathyroidectomy: Surgical removal of one or more of the parathyroid glands.

parotidectomy: Surgical removal of all or part of the parotid gland (a salivary gland).

partial cystectomy: Surgical removal of part of the bladder.

partial hysterectomy: Surgical removal of the uterus only.

partial laryngectomy: Surgical removal of part of the larynx (voice box).

partial mastectomy: Surgical removal of a tumor of the breast, as well as some of the tissue around the tumor, the lining over the chest muscles below the tumor, and usually some of the lymph nodes under the arm. (Also called segmental mastectomy.)

partial nephrectomy: Surgical removal of part of a kidney or a kidney tumor.

partial oophorectomy: Surgical removal of part of one ovary or part of both ovaries.

partial remission: A decrease in the amount of cancer in the body or the size of a tumor as a result of treatment received.

partial vulvectomy: Surgical removal of part of the vulva.

pathologic fracture: A break in the bone due to a disease, especially the spread of cancer to the bone.

pathology report: A written report prepared by a pathologist describing the cells and tissues of a biopsy specimen after viewing under a microscope; it is used to help the primary physician make a diagnosis of a patient's condition.

patient advocate: A person who speaks on behalf of a patient to doctors, insurance companies, employers, case managers, or lawyers to protect the patient's rights and to help that patient resolve issues about health care, medical bills, and job discrimination as a result of the patient's medical condition.

patient-controlled analgesia (PCA): A method of pain relief in which a preset dose of pain medicine is automatically administered to the patient when that patient presses a button on a computerized pump, allowing pain relief as needed. The pump also monitors the amount of medicine the patient is receiving within a certain time period and limits that amount when needed to prohibit an overdose.

pelvic exenteration: Surgical removal of the lower colon, rectum, and bladder, as well as the cervix, vagina, ovaries, and nearby lymph nodes in women; then an opening is created through which urine and stool can pass out of the body.

pelvic lymphadenectomy: Surgical removal of lymph nodes in the pelvis for microscopic examination by a pathologist.

penectomy: Surgical removal of part or all of the penis.

percutaneous ethanol injection: An injection of ethanol (pure alcohol) through the skin directly into the tumor, using a very thin needle with the help of ultrasound or computed tomography visual guidance, to destroy cancer cells.

percutaneous transhepatic cholangiodrainage (PTCD): A procedure in which a stent is placed in the liver to drain bile and to relieve pressure in the bile ducts caused by a blockage; the bile may then drain through the stent into the small intestine or into a collection bag outside the body.

periampullary cancer: A cancer that occurs near the ampulla of Vater (the area where the pancreatic duct and the common bile duct from the liver join together and enter the small intestine).

perineal colostomy: An operation in which an artificial passage is created surgically to allow the colon to exit the body through the perineum (the area between the anus and the vulva in females and between the anus and the scrotum in males) after part of the colon has been removed.

perineal prostatectomy: Surgical removal of the prostate through an incision in the perineum (the area between the scrotum and the anus).

peripheral blood lymphocyte therapy: A treatment in which lymphocytes from a sibling donor are infused into a patient who is suffering from Epstein-Barr virus infection or overgrowth of white blood cells after an organ or bone marrow transplant.

peripheral venous catheter: A small, flexible tube inserted into a vein, usually in the back of the hand or forearm, taped in place and used to administer fluids into the body.

peritoneal cancer: A rare cancer that originates in the tissues that line the inside of the abdomen and cover the organs in the abdomen.

peritonitis: Inflammation of the peritoneum (the tissues that line the inside of the abdomen and cover the organs in the abdomen) as a result of infection, injury, or a disease.

photo-beam radiation: A radiation treatment that uses high-energy X rays to reach deep tumors.

photocoagulation: Sealing off blood vessels or destroying tissue with a high-energy beam of light.

photopheresis: A procedure in which blood is removed from the body so that it can be treated with ultraviolet light and drugs that become active when exposed to light, and then is returned to the body.

pineocytoma: A slow-growing brain tumor occurring in or near the pineal gland, which is near the center of the brain.

plaque radiotherapy: A type of radiation therapy used to treat eye tumors that involves sewing to the outside wall of the eye a thin piece of metal with radioactive seeds attached, leaving it there for several days, and then removing it at the end of treatment.

plasma cell myeloma: A cancer that originates in plasma cells (white blood cells that produce antibodies).

plasma cell tumor: A tumor that originates in plasma cells (white blood cells that produce antibodies); includes multiple myeloma, monoclonal gammopathy of undetermined significance (MGUS), and plasmacytoma.

plasmacytoma: A tumor that originates in plasma cells (white blood cells that produce antibodies) and may turn into multiple myeloma.

pleurectomy: Surgical removal of part of the pleura (the thin layer of tissues that covers, protects, and cushions the lungs).

pneumatic larynx: A device that uses air to produce sound to help a person whose larynx (voice box) has been removed to talk.

port: An implantable device that allows a medical professional direct access to an artery without having to put a needle into the artery every time treatment is given or blood is withdrawn.

positive axillary lymph node: A lymph node in the armpit area in which cancer cells are detected.

posterior pelvic exenteration: Surgical removal of the lower part of the bowel, rectum, cervix, uterus, ovaries, Fallopian tubes, and vagina; some pelvic lymph nodes may also be removed.

posterior urethral cancer: Cancer in the part of the urethra that connects to the bladder.

postremission therapy: Anticancer drugs given after remission induction therapy to kill any remaining cancer cells.

post-transplant lymphoproliferative disorder (PTLD): A condition in which a group of B-cell lymphomas occurs in a patient with a weakened immune system after an organ transplant; it is usually associated with patients who have also been infected with Epstein-Barr virus and may progress to non-Hodgkin lymphoma.

power of attorney: A legal document that gives one person the authority to make medical, legal, or financial decisions for another person; it may go into effect immediately or when that person is incapable of making those decisions.

precancerous: Pertaining to a condition that may become cancer.

precancerous dermatitis: A skin disease characterized by thickened or scaly patches on the skin, usually on sun-exposed areas, and often caused by prolonged exposure to arsenic.

precursor B-lymphoblastic leukemia: *See* B-cell acute lymphocytic leukemia.

preventive mastectomy: Surgical removal of one or both breasts to reduce the risk of developing breast cancer.

primary tumor: The original tumor.

primitive neuroectodermal tumor (PNET): A tumor that may develop in the brain or central nervous system (CNS-PNET), or in sites outside the brain such as the limbs, pelvis, and chest wall (peripheral PNET).

proctoscopy: Visual examination of the rectum by inserting a thin, tubelike instrument with a light and lens (a proctoscope) into the rectum.

proctosigmoidoscopy: Visual examination of the lower colon by inserting a thin, tubelike instrument with a light and lens (a sigmoidoscope) into the rectum.

prognosis: The most likely outcome of a disease, including the probability of recovery or recurrence.

progression-free survival: The length of time for which a patient's disease remains stable and does not progress both during and after treatment, often used in a clinical study or trial as a measure of how well a new treatment works.

prophylactic cranial irradiation: Radiation therapy to the head to prevent the spread of cancer to the brain. prophylactic surgery: Surgical removal of a cancer-free organ or gland as a preventive step for a person with a high risk of developing cancer in that organ or gland.

prostate-specific antigen (PSA) bounce: A brief increase and then decrease in the blood level of PSA; an increased level of PSA occurs in men with disease or infection of the prostate, and that level may briefly rise and fall again one to three years after receiving radiation treatment for prostate cancer as a result of PSA being released from destroyed cancer cells or from normal prostate tissue exposed to the radiation treatment, not because the cancer has come back.

prostate-specific antigen (PSA) failure: An increase in the blood level of PSA after treatment with surgery or radiation for prostate cancer; it may indicate a recurrence of the cancer.

prosthesis: An artificial replacement for part of the body, such as a leg or an arm.

pruritus: Itching.

psoralen and ultraviolet A therapy (PUVA therapy): A type of photodynamic therapy in which psoralen (a drug that becomes active when exposed to light) is administered either by mouth or topically to the skin and then followed by ultraviolet A radiation to treat skin conditions such as psoriasis, vitiligo, and skin nodules of cutaneous T-cell lymphoma.

punch biopsy: Removal of a small cylinder of tissue, using a sharp, hollow instrument, for microscopic examination by a pathologist.

quadrantectomy: Surgical removal of approximately onequarter of the breast—the quarter that contains the cancer. quality of life: Degree of well-being and ability to perform daily activities.

radiation dermatitis: A painful skin condition in which the skin becomes red, itchy, and blistered as a side effect of radiation therapy.

radiation enteritis: A complication of radiation therapy to the abdomen, pelvis, or rectum in which the small intestine becomes inflamed, causing nausea, vomiting, abdominal pain and cramping, watery or bloody diarrhea, fatty stools, and weight loss.

radiation fibrosis: Scar tissue caused by radiation therapy. radiation necrosis: Death of healthy tissue as a result of radiation therapy; this dead tissue may form at the site of an irradiated tumor months or even years after the radiation therapy has ended and may require surgery to be removed.

radiation surgery: A type of radiation therapy in which special equipment is used to position the patient so that a single large dose of radiation can accurately target a tumor; it is often used to treat brain tumors.

radiation therapy: *See* irradiation.

radical cystectomy: Surgical removal of the bladder and nearby tissues and organs.

radical hysterectomy: Surgical removal of the uterus, cervix, and part of the vagina; may also include removal of the ovaries, Fallopian tubes, and nearby lymph nodes.

radical local excision: Surgical removal of a tumor and a large area of surrounding normal tissue; nearby lymph nodes may also be removed.

radical lymph node dissection: Surgical removal of most or all of the lymph nodes that drain lymph from the area around a tumor for microscopic examination by a pathologist.

radical nephrectomy: Surgical removal of a kidney, the nearby adrenal gland and lymph nodes, and surrounding tissue.

radical perineal prostatectomy: Surgical removal of the prostate through an incision in the perineum (the area between the scrotum and the anus); nearby lymph nodes may also be removed through another incision in the wall of the abdomen.

radical retropubic prostatectomy: Surgical removal of the prostate and nearby lymph nodes through an incision in the wall of the abdomen.

radical vulvectomy: Surgical removal of the vulva and nearby lymph nodes.

radioimmunoguided surgery: Surgical removal of tumors that have been located using radioactive substances.

radiologic exam: An imaging procedure that uses radiation (such as X rays) to help diagnose certain cancers and other abnormalities.

radiology: The branch of medicine in which X rays, ultrasound, magnetic resonance imaging, and other imaging technologies are used to diagnose and sometimes treat certain diseases, such as cancer.

rectal reconstruction: Surgery in which the rectum is rebuilt using a section of the colon following the surgical removal of the rectum due to cancer or other diseases.

refractory cancer: Cancer that is resistant to treatment.

regional lymph node dissection: Surgical removal of some of the lymph nodes that drain lymph from the area around a tumor for microscopic examination by a pathologist.

regression: A decrease in the amount of cancer in the body or the size of a tumor.

remission: A reduction or cessation of any signs and symptoms of cancer, even though the cancer may still exist.

remission induction therapy: The initial treatment with anticancer drugs to bring about a reduction or cessation of signs and symptoms of cancer.

renal cell cancer: *See* hypernephroma.

resection: Surgical removal of tissue or part or all of an organ.

retropubic prostatectomy: Surgical removal of the prostate through an incision in the wall of the abdomen. rhabdoid tumor: A malignant tumor found in either the kidney or the central nervous system.

risk factor: Something that increases the likelihood of developing a certain disease, such as family history, exposure to tobacco products or other cancer-causing agents, obesity, and age.

sarcoma: A malignant tumor of bone, cartilage, fat, muscle, blood vessels, or other connective or supportive tissue.

sarcomatoid carcinoma: Cancer that contains long spindle-shaped cells and that originates in the skin or in the lining or covering of internal organs. (Also called spindle cell cancer.)

scintimammography: A supplemental imaging technique that uses a radioactive substance (technetium 99) and a gamma camera to detect cancer cells in a breast with dense breast tissue or that has produced an abnormal mammogram.

segmental mastectomy: *See* partial mastectomy.

segmental resection: Surgical removal of part of an organ or gland.

seminal vesicle biopsy: Needle aspiration of fluid or tissue from the seminal vesicles (glands in the male reproductive tract that produce part of the semen) for microscopic examination by a pathologist.

seminoma: Cancer of the testicles that has the potential to spread to the bone, brain, liver, or lung.

senile keratosis: *See* actinic keratosis.

sestamibi scan: An imaging technique in which a radioactive substance (technetium bound to sestamibi) injected into a patient can be detected by a gamma camera when it collects in overactive parathyroid glands, cancer cells in the breast, or diseased heart muscle.

shave biopsy: Removal of a skin abnormality with a thin layer of surrounding skin for microscopic examination by a pathologist by using a small blade in such a way that stitches are not needed.

shunt: A passage that diverts a bodily fluid from one area of the body to another.

side-to-end coloanal anastomosis: The surgical attachment of the side of the colon to the anus after the removal of the rectum, by forming a small J-shaped pouch from a 2-inch section of the colon as a replacement for the rectum.

signet ring cell carcinoma: A highly malignant cancer containing cells that resemble signet rings and are usually found in the glandular cells that line the digestive organs.

skinning vulvectomy: Surgical removal of the top layer of skin of the vulva.

sleeve lobectomy: A lung-saving procedure in which a tumor in a central lobe of the lung is surgically removed along with a part of the main bronchus; then the ends of the bronchus are rejoined and remaining lobes are reattached to the bronchus.

small-cell lung cancer: A fast-growing cancer of the lung that can spread to other parts of the body.

smoldering myeloma: A slow-growing myeloma in which abnormal plasma cells produce too much of a specific protein (monoclonal antibody); this is an asymptomatic condition that could progress to fully developed multiple myeloma.

soft-tissue sarcoma: A malignant tumor that originates in the muscle, fat, fibrous tissue, blood vessels, or other supporting tissue of the body.

solar keratosis: *See* actinic keratosis.

solid tumor: A benign or malignant mass of tissue, usually free of any cysts or liquid areas; includes carcinomas, sarcomas, and lymphomas.

somatostatin receptor scintigraphy (SRS): An imaging technique in which a radioactive drug (octreotide) injected into a patient attaches to tumor cells, which can then be detected by a radiation-measuring device;

a picture is then created that shows where the tumor cells are in the body.

spindle cell cancer: *See* sarcomatoid carcinoma.

spiral computed tomography (CT) scan: A series of detailed pictures of structures within the body, created by a computer linked to an X-ray machine that scans the body in a spiral path.

stromal tumor: A tumor that occurs in the supporting connective tissue of an organ.

subcutaneous port: A semipermanent device implanted just under the skin that allows a medical professional direct access to an artery without having to put a needle into the artery every time intravenous fluids or drugs need to be administered or blood samples need to be taken.

supraglottic laryngectomy: Surgical removal of the supraglottis (the part of the larynx that is above the vocal cords).

suprarenal glands: *See* adrenal glands.

syngeneic: Pertaining to individuals or tissues from those individuals containing identical genes, such as identical twins.

systemic therapy: Treatment that affects cells all over the body by traveling through the bloodstream.

T-cell depletion: Treatment that destroys T cells, especially from a donor's bone marrow graft, to reduce the risk of an immune reaction against the recipient's tissues.

T-cell lymphoma: Cancer of T-lymphocytes (cells of the lymph system).

terminal disease: An incurable disease that will lead to death.

thermal ablation: The removal, destruction, or severing of a diseased or damaged tissue, body part, or its function through the use of heat.

thermotherapy: The use of heat in the treatment of a disease.

third-line therapy: Treatment that is given after both an initial and a subsequent treatment fail or become ineffective.

three-dimensional conformal radiation therapy: A procedure in which a tumor is subjected to the highest possible dose of radiation while surrounding tissue is spared; accomplished by using a computer-generated three-dimensional picture of the tumor.

thrombectomy: Surgical removal of a thrombus (blood clot) from a blood vessel.

thrombolysis: Dissolving or breaking up a thrombus (blood clot), especially through the use of drugs.

thyroidectomy: Surgical removal of part or all of the thyroid.

time to progression: The length of time following diagnosis or treatment until the disease begins to get worse.

tissue flap reconstruction: Breast reconstruction using a flap of tissue surgically removed from another area of the body and formed into a new breast mound.

tomography: The process of creating a series of detailed pictures of structures within the body, by a computer linked to an X-ray machine.

tongue cancer: Cancer that originates in the tongue.

topical: Pertaining to the surface of the body.

topical chemotherapy: The application of anticancer drugs directly on the skin in the form of a lotion, an ointment, or a cream.

total-body irradiation: Radiation therapy to the whole body to kill cancer cells throughout the body and to destroy the bone marrow and immune system in preparation for bone marrow or stem cell transplantation.

total mastectomy: Surgical removal of the breast.

total nodal irradiation: Radiation therapy to the neck, chest, spleen, and lymph nodes under the arms, in the upper abdomen, and in the pelvic area.

total pancreatectomy: Surgical removal of the pancreas, as well as nearby lymph nodes, the common bile duct, the gallbladder, the spleen, and part of the stomach and small intestine.

total parenteral nutrition (TPN): The intravenous feeding of nutrients to patients who cannot ingest or digest food through the alimentary tract.

total skin electron beam radiation therapy (TSEB radiation therapy): Radiation therapy that directs electrons at the entire surface of the body, allowing the radiation into the outer layers of the skin but not penetrating deeper into the tissues or organs below the skin.

trabecular cancer: A rare cancer of the skin that may form on or just below the skin, especially in parts of the body exposed to the sun and in older people and those with weakened immune systems. (Also called Merkel cell cancer and neuroendocrine carcinoma of the skin.)

transperineal biopsy: Removal of a sample of tissue from the prostate, using a thin needle inserted through the skin between the scrotum and the rectum, for microscopic examination by a pathologist.

transrectal biopsy: Removal of a sample of tissue from the prostate, using a thin needle inserted through the rectum, for microscopic examination by a pathologist.

transsphenoidal surgery: Surgery in which part of the brain is accessed through the nose and the sphenoid bone (a bone at the base of the skull); this type of surgery is common when removing tumors of the pituitary gland.

transurethral biopsy: Removal of a sample of tissue from the prostate by inserting a thin tube with a cutting loop attachment through the urethra and into the prostate; the sample is then examined under a microscope by a pathologist.

transurethral resection of the prostate (TURP): Surgical removal of tissue from the prostate using an instrument inserted through the urethra.

treatment field: The area of the body at which the radiation beam is aimed during radiation therapy.

tubulovillous adenoma: An abnormal growth of tissue (polyp), in the colon, the gastrointestinal tract, or other parts of the body, that may become cancerous.

tumor: A new mass of tissue resulting from uncontrolled cell division and that serves no physiological function; it may be benign or malignant. (Also called neoplasm.)

tumor load: Pertaining to the size of a tumor, the number of cancer cells, or the amount of cancer in the body. tumor volume: The amount of space taken up by a tumor.

ultrasound-guided biopsy: Surgical removal of a sample of tissue, using an ultrasound imaging device to locate and guide the removal of that tissue, for microscopic examination by a pathologist.

unilateral: Pertaining to one side of the body.

unilateral salpingo-oophorectomy: Surgical removal of the ovary and Fallopian tube on one side of the body.

unresectable gallbladder cancer: Gallbladder cancer that has spread to nearby areas, such as the lymph nodes, liver, stomach, pancreas, and intestine, so that it cannot be surgically removed.

unsealed internal radiation therapy: Radiation therapy in which a radioactive substance that has not been sealed in a container is injected into the body or swallowed.

upper endoscopy: *See* gastroscopy.

upper GI series: *See* esophagram.

urinary diversion: A surgical procedure to create an alternative passage for urine to exit the body; it may include redirecting urine into the colon, draining the bladder through the use of catheters, or making an incision in the abdomen and collecting urine in a bag outside the body.

vaginectomy: Surgical removal of part or all of the vagina.

ventilator: A machine that helps a patient breathe.

video-assisted resection: Surgery in which a video camera projects and enlarges the surgical field onto a television screen, allowing the surgeon an enhanced view of the surgical field.

villous adenoma: An abnormal growth of tissue (polyp) in the colon, the gastrointestinal tract, or other parts of the body that may become cancerous.

visual pathway glioma: A tumor that occurs along the optic nerve (the nerve that sends messages from the eye to the brain).

wedge resection: Surgical removal of a triangle-shaped piece of tissue or a tumor with some of the normal tissue around it.

Whipple procedure: Surgical removal of the head of the pancreas, the duodenum, part of the stomach, and other nearby tissues to treat pancreatic cancer.

whole genome association study (WGA study): A study in which the deoxyribonucleic acid (DNA) of people with a disease or medical condition is compared to the DNA of people without it in an effort to discover the genes that are involved in the disease and to aid medical professionals in the prevention, diagnosis, and treatment of the disease.

wide local excision: Surgical removal of the cancer along with healthy tissue around it.

X-ray therapy: Radiation therapy that uses X rays to shrink tumors and kill cancer cells.

▶ Bibliography

2008 Physical Activity Guidelines for Americans. Centers for Disease Control and Prevention. Retrieved from http://www.cdc.gov/physicalactivity/downloads/pa_fact_sheet_adults.pdf

Abbas, Abul & Lichtman, Andrew. (2015). *Cellular and molecular immunology* (8th ed.). Philadelphia, PA: Elsevier/Saunders.

Abegaz, E. M. "Aspartame Not Linked to Cancer." *Environmental Health Perspectives* 115, no. 1 (January, 2007): A16-17.

Abeloff, M. D., et al. *Clinical Oncology.* 3rd ed. Edinburgh, Scotland: Churchill Livingstone, 2004.

_______, et al. *Clinical Oncology.* 3rd ed. Orlando, Fla.: Churchill Livingstone, 2004.

Abeloff, Martin D., et al. *Clinical Oncology.* 3rd ed. Philadelphia: Churchill Livingstone/Elsevier, 2004.

Ablin, R. J., & Piana, R. (2014). *The great prostate hoax: How big medicine hijacked the PSA test and caused a public health disaster.* Basingstoke, England: Palgrave Macmillan.

Abner, A. "Approach to the Patient Who Presents with Superior Vena Cava Obstruction." *Chest* 103 (1993): 394S-397S.

About the Chemopreventive Agent Development Research Group. National Cancer Institute: Division of Cancer Prevention. Retrieved from http://prevention.cancer.gov/research-groups/chemopreventive-agent-development/about-chemopreventive

Aboutalebi, S., and F. M. Strickland. "Immune Protection, Natural Products, and Skin Cancer: Is There Anything New Under the Sun?" *Journal of Drugs in Dermatology* 5 (2006): 512-517.

Abraham, J., Gulley. J. L., & Allegra, C. J. (2014). *The Bethesda handbook of clinical oncology* (4th ed.). Philadelphia, PA: Lippincott Williams & Wilkins.

Abrahm, J. L. "Assessment and Treatment of Patients with Malignant Spinal Cord Compression." *Journal of Supportive Oncology* 2, no. 5 (2004): 377-388, 391.

Abrams, D. I., & Weil, A. (Eds.). (2014). *Integrative Oncology* (2nd ed.). New York: Oxford University Press. https://global.oup.com/academic/product/integrative-oncology-9780199329724? cc=us&lang=en&#

Accardi, F., Toscani, D., Bolzoni, M., Dalla Palma, B., Aversa, F. & Giuliani, N. (2015). Mechanism of action of bortezomib and the new proteasome inhibitors on myeloma cells and the bone microenvironment: Impact on myeloma-induced alterations of bone remodeling. *Biomed Research International*, v. 2015, Article ID 172458, 13 pages.

Acton, Ashton, (Ed.). (2013). Herpes simplex virus: New insights for the healthcare professional. *Atlanta, GA: ScholarlyEditions.*

Adair, Thomas H., & Montani, Jean-Pierre. (2010). *Angiogenesis.* San Rafael (CA): Morgan & Claypool Life Sciences. Available at: http://www.ncbi.nlm.nih.gov/books/NBK53238.

Adamo, V., et al. "Overview and New Strategies in Metastatic Breast Cancer (MBC) for Treatment of Tamoxifen-Resistant Patients." *Annals of Oncology* 18, suppl. 6 (June, 2007): 53-57.

Adams, J. (2003). The proteasome: structure, function, and role in the cell. *Cancer Treatment Reviews*, 29(suppl 1): 3–9.

Adams, Val R., and Thomas G. Burke, eds. *Camptothecins in Cancer Therapy.* Totowa, N.J.: Humana Press, 2005.

"Adjuvant Therapy for Breast Cancer." *NIH Consensus Statement* 17, no. 4 (November 1-3, 2000): 1-35.

Adler, Elizabeth M. *Living with Lymphoma: A Patient's Guide.* Baltimore: Johns Hopkins University Press, 2005.

Adler, E. M. (2015). *Living with lymphoma: A patient's guide.* Baltimore: Johns Hopkins University Press.

Adler, L., and P. Sykes. "How Little Is Known About Cervical Cancer in Pregnancy?" *Annals of Oncology (European Society for Medical Oncology)* 16, no. 3 (2005): 341-343.

Adrouny, R. *Understanding Colon Cancer.* Jackson: University of Mississippi Press, 2002.

Agnew, Karen L., Barbara A. Gilchrist, and Christopher B. Bunker. *Skin Cancer.* Oxford, England: Health Press, 2005.

Aguirre-Molina, Marilyn, Molina, Carlos, & Zambrana, Ruth Enid. (Eds.). (2001). *Health issues in the Latino community.* San Francisco: Jossey-Bass.

Ahmed, M., & Rahman, N. (2006). ATM and breast cancer susceptibility. *Oncogene,* 25: 5906-5911.

Ahmed, S., et al. "Breast Reconstruction." *British Medical Journal* 330 (2005): 943-948.

Ahnen, Dennis J., & Axell, Lisen. (2015). Lynch syndrome (hereditary nonpolyposis colorectal cancer): Clinical manifestations and diagnosis. In J. Thomas Lamont and Shilpa Grover (Eds.), *UpToDate.* Retrieved at: www.uptodate.com.

Ajani, Jaffer A., et al., eds. *Gastrointestinal Cancer*. New York: Springer, 2005.

Ajithkumar, T. V., A. L. Minimole, M. M. John, and O. S. Ashokkumar. "Primary Fallopian Tube Carcinoma." *Obstetrics and Gynecological Survey* 60 (2005): 247-252.

Akechi, T., & Furukawa, T.A. (2016). Depressed with cancer can respond to antidepressants, but further research is needed to confirm and expand on these findings. *Evidence Based Mental Health.* Retrieved from http://ebmh.bmj.com on February 11, 2016.

Akopov, A. L., et al. "Thoracoscopic Collagen Pleurodesis in the Treatment of Malignant Pleural Effusions." *European Journal of Cardiothoracic Surgery* 28, no. 5 (2005): 750-753.

Alam, M., and D. Ratner. "Cutaneous Squamous-Cell Carcinoma." *New England Journal of Medicine* 344 (2001): 975-983.

Albert, Daniel M., and Arthur Polans, eds. *Ocular Oncology*. New York: Marcel Dekker, 2003.

Alberts, B., Johnson, A., Lewis, J., Morgan, D., Raff, M., Roberts, K., & Walter, P. (2014). *Molecular biology of the cell* (6th ed.). New York: Garland Science.

Albini A, & Tímár J. (2010). Genomics of metastatic progression. Clinical and Experimental Metastasis, 27(6):453. http://www.ncbi.nlm.nih.gov/pubmed/20711639

Albritton, K. H. "Sarcomas in Adolescents and Young Adults." *Hematology/Oncology Clinics of North America* 19 (2005): 527-546.

Aldrich, Matthew. *Stop Smoking*. Chicago: Contemporary Books, 2006.

Alfassa, Shelomo. (Ed.). (2006). *Ethnic Sephardic Jews in the Medical Literature*. New York, NY: International Sephardic Leadership Council.

Ali, Abrar Ashraf, et al. "Carcinoma Breast: A Dilemma for Our Society." *Ann King Edward Medical College* 9, no. 2 (June, 2003): 87-89.

Ali-Osman, Francis, ed. *Brain Tumors*. Totowa, N.J.: Humana Press, 2003.

Alirol, E., and J. C. Martinou. "Mitochondria and Cancer: Is There a Morphological Connection?" *Oncogene* 25(2006): 4706-4716.

Allard, W.J., Matera, J., Miller, C.J., Repollet, M., Connelly, M.C., Rao, C. Terstappen, L. W. M. M. (2004). Tumor cells circulate in the peripheral blood of all major carcinomas but not in healthy subjects or patients with nonmalignant diseases. *Clinical Cancer Research*, 10(20): 6897-6904.

Allen, J. I., et al. "Best Practices: Community-Based Gastroenterology Practices." *Clinical Gastroenterology and Hepatology* 4 (2006): 292-295.

Allen, P. J., et al. "Merkel Cell Carcinoma: Prognosis and Treatment of Patients from a Single Institution." *Journal of Clinical Oncology* 23, no. 10 (April 1, 2005): 2300-2309.

Allis, C. D., Caparros, M-L., Jenuwein, T., Reinberg, D., & Lachlin M. (Eds.). (2015). *Epigenetics*. Cold Spring Harbor Laboratory, NY: Cold Spring Harbor Laboratory Press.

Al-Nafussi, Awatif. *Tumor Diagnosis: Practical Approach* and Pattern Analysis. New York: Oxford University Press, 2005.

Althuis, M. D. "Uterine Cancer After Use of Clomiphene Citrate to Induce Ovulation." *American Journal of Epidemiology* 161 (2005): 607-615.

Altman, Arnold J., ed. *Supportive Care of Children with Cancer: Current Therapy and Guidelines from the Children's Oncology Group*. Boston: Johns Hopkins University Press, 2004.

Amaravadi, R.K., Lippincott, S. J., Yin, X. M., Weiss, W. A., Takebe, N., Timmer, W., DiPaola, R.S., White, E. (2011). Principles and current strategies for targeting autophagy for cancer treatment. *Clinical Cancer Research*, 17(4): 654-666.

Amendola, B. E., et al. "Pineal Tumors: Analysis of Treatment Results in Twenty Patients." *Journal of Neurosurgery* 102 (January, 2005): 175-179.

American Cancer Society. *Cancer Facts and Figures*. Atlanta: American Cancer Society, 2005.

American Cancer Society. "Cancers Linked to Infectious Disease." In *Cancer Facts and Figures*. Atlanta: Author, 2005.

American Cancer Society. *Cancer Facts and Figures*. Atlanta: American Cancer Society, 2005.

American Cancer Society. *The American Cancer Society's Healthy Eating Cookbook: A Celebration of Food, Friends, and Healthy Living*. 3rd ed. Atlanta: American Cancer Society, 2005.

American Cancer Society and National Comprehensive Cancer Network. *Colon and Rectal Cancer: Treatment Guidelines for Patients*. Version IV. Atlanta: American Cancer Society, 2005. Available online at http://www.nccn.org.

American Cancer Society. (2007). *Cancer facts and Figures for African Americans*. Atlanta: American Cancer Society.

American Cancer Society. *Imaging*. Atlanta: Author, 2007.

American Cancer Society. *Quick Facts Colon Cancer: What You Need to Know—Now*. Atlanta: Author, 2007.

American Cancer Society. *Cancer Facts and Figures 2008*. Atlanta: Author, 2008.

American Cancer Society. *Cancer Facts and Figures for African Americans*. Atlanta: American Cancer Society, 2007.

American Cancer Society (2012). Cancer Facts & Figures 2012: American Cancer Society. http://www.cancer.org/research/cancerfactsfigures/cancerfactsfigures/cancer-facts-figures-2012

American Cancer Society. (2014). Genes and cancer. Retrieved from http://www.cancer.org/acs/groups/cid/documents/webcontent/002550-pdf.pdf

American Cancer Society. (2014 November 21). Rhabdomyosarcoma. Retrieved on February 10, 2016 from http://cancer.org/cancer/rhabdosarcoma /detailed-guide/rhabdomyosarcoma-what-is-rhabdomyosarcoma. This article provides a less detailed description of rhabdomyosarcoma.

American Cancer Society. (2015). Facts and Figures for Hispanics/Latinos, 2015-2017. Atlanta. Retrieved from http://m.cancer.org/acs/groups/content/@research/documents/document/acspc-046405.pdf

American Cancer Society. (2016). Surgery for Breast Cancer. Retrieved from http://www.cancer.org/cancer/breastcancer/detailedguide/breast-cancer-treating-surgery.

American College of Radiology. (2015). *Manual on Contrast Media* (Vol. 10.1). Retrieved from http://www.acr.org/quality-safety/resources/contrast-manual

American Cancer Society. "How Are Lung Carcinoid Tumors Staged?" Available online at http://www .cancer.org.

American Cancer Society. *Detailed Guide: Colon and Rectum Cancer Surgery*. Available online at http://www.cancer.org.

American College of Sports Medicine. *ACSM's Guide to Exercise and Cancer Survivorship*. Champaign, IL: Human Kinetics, 2012.

American College of Sports Medicine. *ACSM's Guidelines for Exercise Testing and Prescription*. Baltimore: Wolters Kluwer/Lippincott Williams and Wilkins, 2014. (pp 264-273)

American Conference of Governmental Industrial Hygienists. *1999 TLVs and BEIs: Threshold Limit Values for Chemical Substances and Physical Agents—Biological Exposure Indices*. Cincinnati, Ohio: Author, 1999.

American Dental Association. *ADA Guide to Dental Therapeutics*. 4th ed. Chicago: Author, 2006.

American Heart Association. "2005 American Heart Association Guidelines for Cardiopulmonary Resuscitation and Emergency Cardiovascular Care." *Journal of the American Heart Association* 112, no. 24 (December 13, 2005).

American Industrial Hygiene Association. *The AIHA 1998 Emergency Response Planning Guidelines and Workplace Environmental Exposure Level Guides Handbook*. Fairfax, Va.: Author, 1998.

American Institute for Cancer Research. *Diet and Health Recommendations for Cancer Prevention: Healthy Living and Lower Cancer Risk*. Washington, D.C.: Author, 2006.

_______. *The New American Plate Cookbook: Recipes for a Healthy Weight and a Healthy Life*. Berkeley: University of California Press, 2005.

American Joint Committee on Cancer. *AJCC Cancer Staging Manual*. 5th ed. Philadelphia: Lippincott-Raven, 1997.

American Journal of Medical Genetics. (2014). Connection found between lack of PRC2 gene and B-cell acute lymphoblastic leukemia. *American Journal of Medical Genetics Part A*, 164(8): x-xi.

American Medical Association. *American Medical Association Guide to Home Caregiving*. New York: John Wiley & Sons, 2001.

American Medical Association. *Health Professions Career and Educational Directory 2007-2008*. 35th ed. Chicago: AMA Press, 2007.

American Psychiatric Association. (2013). *Diagnostic and Statistical Manual of Mental Disorders: DSM-5* (5th ed.). Washington, D.C.: Author.

American Society of Clinical Oncology. *Optimizing Cancer Care: The Importance of Symptom Management*. Dubuque, Iowa: Kendall/Hunt, 2001.

American Society of Clinical Oncology. (2015). Managing the cost of cancer care: Practical guidance for patients and families. http://www.cancer.net/sites/cancer.net/files/cost_of_care_booklet.pdf

American Society of Clinical Oncology. (n.d.) Retrieved from http://www.cancer.net/cancer-types/lynch-syndrome

Amin, A., & Buratovich, M. A. (2009). New platinum and ruthenium complexes – the latest class of potential chemotherapeutic drugs – a review of new developments in the field. *Mini Reviews in Medicinal Chemistry*, 9(13): 1489-1503.

Anderson, E. M., et al. "Multidetector Computed Tomography Urography (MDCTU) for Diagnosing Urothelial Malignancy." *Clinical Radiology* 62, no. 4 (April, 2007): 324-332.

Anderson, Greg. *Cancer: Fifty Essential Things to Do*. New York: Penguin Books, 1999.

Anderson, Kenneth C., and Irene Ghobrial, eds. *Multiple Myeloma*. New York: Informa Healthcare, 2007.

Andersson, B. U., E. Tani, U. Andersson, and J. I. Henter. "Tumor Necrosis Factor, Interleukin 11, and Leukemia Inhibitory Factor Produced by Langerhans Cells in Langerhans Cell Histiocytosis." *Journal of Pediatric Hematology Oncology* 26, no. 11 (2004): 706-711.

Andoh, Toshiwo, ed. *DNA Topoisomerases in Cancer Therapy: Present and Future*. New York: Kluwer Academic/Plenum, 2003.

Anestakis D., Petanidis S., Kalyvas S., Nday C.M., Tsave O., Kioseoglou E., & Salifoglou A. (2015). Mechanisms and applications of interleukins in cancer immunotherapy. *International Journal of Molecular Science*, 16(1):1691-710. http://www.ncbi.nlm.nih.gov/pubmed/25590298

Answers.com. "Tumor Grading." In *Oncology Encyclopedia*. Available online at http://www.answers.com/topic/tumor-grading.

"Antiperspirants Don't Cause Breast Cancer." *Harvard Women's Health Watch* 10, no. 5 (2003): 7.

Applegate, K. "Pregnancy Screening of Adolescents and Women Before Radiologic Testing: Does Radiology Need a National Guideline?" *Journal of American College of Radiology* 4, no. 8 (August, 2007): 533-536.

Aqui, N., & O'Doherty, U. (2015). Leukocytapheresis for the treatment of hyperleukocytosis secondary to acute leukemia. *Hematology,* 2014(1): 457-460.

Arambula, J. F., Preihs, C., Borthwick, D., Madga, D., & Sessler, J. L. (2011). Texaphyrins: Tumor localizing redox active expanded porphyrins. *Anticancer Agents in Medicinal Chemistry*, 11: 222-232.

Arjona, D., et al. "Early Genetic Changes Involved in Low-Grade Astrocytic Tumor Development." *Current Molecular Medicine* 6 (September, 2006): 645-650.

Armanios M., & Greider, C.W. (2005). Telomerase and cancer stem cells. *Cold Spring Harbor Symposia on Quantitative Biology*, 70: 205-208.

Armstrong, G. L., et al. "The Prevalence of Hepatitis C Virus Infection in the United States, 1999 Through 2002." *Annals of Internal Medicine* 144 (2006): 705-714.

Armstrong, Sue. (2014). P53: The gene that cracked the cancer code. New York: Bloomsbury Sigma.

Arnal, J. F., et al. "Understanding the Controversy About Hormonal Replacement Therapy: Insights from Estrogen Effects on Experimental and Clinical Atherosclerosis." *Archives des maladies du coeur et des vaisseaux* 100, nos. 6/7 (June/July, 2007): 554-562.

Aronovitch, Sharon. "Changing a Bowel Diversion Ostomy Appliance: Pouching a Stoma." In *Delmar's Fundamental and Advanced Nursing Skills*. 2d ed. New York: Delmar Learning, 2004.

Arora, M., Cutler, C.S., Jagasia, M.H., Pidala, J., Chai, X., Martin, P.J., ... Lee, S.J. (2016). Late acute and chronic graft-versus-host disease after allogeneic hematopoietic cell transplantation. *Biology of Blood and Marrow Transplantation*, 22, 449-455.

Arrowsmith, C. H., Bountra, C., Fish, P. V., Lee, K., & Schapira, M. (2012). Epigenetic protein families: a new frontier for drug discovery. *Nature Reviews Drug Discovery,* 11(5): 384–400.

Ashby, L. S., and T. C. Ryken. "Management of Malignant Glioma: Steady Progress with Multimodal Approaches." *Neurosurgical Focus* 20, no. 4 (2006): E6.

Attfield, M. D., Schleiff, P. L., Lubin, J. H., Blair, A., Stewart, P. A., Vermeulen, R., Silverman, D. T. (2012). The diesel exhaust in miners study: A cohort mortality study with emphasis on lung cancer. *JNCI Journal of the National Cancer Institute, 104*(11), 869–883. http://doi.org/10.1093/jnci/djs035

Avalare Health. (2012, March). Total cost of cancer care by site of service: Physician office vs outpatient hospital. http://www.communityoncology.org/pdfs/avalere-cost-of-cancer-care-study.pdf

Avgustinova, A., & Benitah, S. A., (2016). The epigenetics or tumour initiation: Cancer stem cells and their chromatin. *Current Opinion of Genetics and Development*, 36, 8-15.

Awad, Atif B., and Peter G. Bradford, eds. *Nutrition and Cancer Prevention*. Boca Raton, Fla.: CRC, Taylor & Francis, 2006.

Ayhan, A. "Association Between Fertility Drugs and Gynecologic Cancers, Breast Cancer, and Childhood Cancers." *Acta Obstetricia et Gynecologica Scandinovica* 83 (2004): 1104-1111.

Aziz, Khalid, and George Y. Wu. *Cancer Screening: A Practical Guide for Physicians*. Totowa, N.J.: Humana Press, 2002.

Aziz, Z., et al. "Socioeconomic Status and Breast Cancer Survival in Pakistani Women." *Journal of the Pakistan Medical Association* 54, no. 9 (September, 2004): 448-453.

Baaj, Y., Magdelaine, C., Ubertelli, V., Valat, C., Talini, L., Soussaline, F., ... Sturtz, F. G. (2008). A highly specific microarray method for point mutation detection. *BioTechniques*, 44(1), 119–126. A paper that describes a new technique for using microarrays to detect mutations in patients with neurological diseases.

Babovic-Vuksanovic, Dusica, et al. "Familiar Occurrence of Carcinoid Tumors and Association with

Other Malignant Neoplasms." *Cancer Epidemiology Biomarkers and Prevention* 8 (August, 1999): 715-719.

Backes, Michael. (2014). *Cannabis Pharmacy.* New York, New York: Black Dog and Leventhal Publishers. Presents a scientific discussion of medicinal marijuana and how it has been used by individuals with more than 25 health conditions.

Badger, T. M., M. J. Ronis, R. C. Simmen, and F. A. Simmen. "Soy Protein Isolate and Protection Against Cancer." *Journal of the American College of Nutrition* 24, no. 2 (April, 2005): 146S-149S.

Baerlocher G. M., Leibundgut, E. O., Ottmann, O. G., Spitzer, G., Odenike, O., McDevitt, M. A., Snyder, D. S. (2015). Telomerase Inhibitor Imetelstat in Patients with Essential Thrombocythemia. *New England Journal of Medicine*, 373(10): 920-928.

Baert, A. L., C. Bartolozzi, and R. Lencioni. *Liver Malignancies: Diagnostic and Interventional Radiology.* New York: Springer, 2003.

Baez-Escudero, José L., John N. Greene, Ramon L. Sandin, and Albert L. Vincent. "Pneumocystis Carinii Pneumonia in Cancer Patients." *Abstracts in Hematology and Oncology* 7, no. 1 (2005).

Bahn, Duke, et al. "Focal Prostate Cryoablation: Initial Results Show Cancer Control and Potency Preservation." *Journal of Endourology* 20, no. 9 (2006): 688-692.

Bai, R. K., et al. "Mitochondrial Genetic Background Modifies Breast Cancer Risk." *Cancer Research* 67, no. 10 (2007): 4687-4694.

Baider, L., & Surbone, A. (2014). Universality of ageing: family caregivers for elderly cancer patients. *Frontiers in Psychology*, 5, 744. doi:10.3389/fpsyg.2014.00744.

Bailey, Eric J. *Medical Anthropology and African American Health.* Westport, Conn.: Bergin & Garvey, 2000.

Baker, Laurence H., ed. *Soft Tissue Sarcomas.* Boston: Martinus Nijhoff, 1983.

Baker, T. (2012). *Non-Hodgkin lymphoma. Seattle*, WA: Amazon Digital Services LLC.

Baker, Vicki V. "Gestational Trophoblastic Disease." In *Clinical Oncology*, edited by Martin D. Abeloff et al. 2d ed. Philadelphia: Churchhill Livingstone, 2000.

Balinsky, Warren L. *Home Care: Current Problems and Future Solutions.* San Francisco: Jossey-Bass, 1994.

Ball, Edward D., and Gregory A. Lelek. *One Hundred Questions and Answers About Leukemia.* Sudbury, Mass.: Jones and Bartlett, 2003.

Ballantyne, Jane C., ed. *The Massachusetts General Hospital Handbook of Pain Management.* 3rd ed. Philadelphia: Lippincott Williams & Wilkins, 2006.

Ballantyne, J. C. "Opioid Analgesia: Perspectives on Right Use and Utility." *Pain Physician* 10, no. 3 (May, 2007): 479-491.

Barbui T, Thiele, J., Vannucchi, A. M., & Tefferi, A. (2015). Rationale for revision and proposed changes of the WHO diagnostic criteria for polycythemia vera, essential thrombocythemia and primarily myelofibrosis. *Blood Cancer Journal,* 5(8):e337. This article reviews proposed 215 changes to WHO classification of myeloproliferative neoplasms to accommodate newer information on disease-specific mutations and distinguishing morphologic features.

Barbui, T., & Tefferi, A. (Eds.). (2012). *Myeloproliferative neoplasms: Critical concepts and management (Hematologic Malignances).* New York: Springer. This book discusses myeloproliferative neoplasms including polycythemia vera, essential thrombycythemia, and primary myelofibrosis. This book includes recent advances and practical issues for physicians, including contemporary diagnostic approaches.

Bard, R. L. (2014). *The prostate cancer revolution: Beating prostate cancer without surgery.* New York: Morgan James Publishing

Bardos, A. P., ed. *Trends in Ovarian Cancer Research.* Hauppauge, N.Y.: Nova Science, 2004.

Barnard, C. F. J. (1989). Platinum anticancer agents: Twenty years of continuing development. *Platinum Metals Review*, 33(4): 162-167.

Barnea, Eytan R., Eric Jauniaux, and Peter E. Schwartz, eds. *Cancer and Pregnancy.* London: Springer, 2001.

Barnes, D. M., and L. A. Newman. "Pregnancy-Associated Breast Cancer: A Literature Review." *Surgical Clinics of North America* 87 (2007): 417-430.

Barnett, Gene H., ed. *High-Grade Gliomas: Diagnosis and Treatment.* Totowa, N.J.: Humana, 2007.

Barnett, Laura, ed. *When Death Enters the Therapeutic Space: Existential Perspectives in Psychotherapy and Counseling.* New York: Routledge, 2008.

Barnhill, Raymond, Michael Piepkorn, and Klaus Busam. *Pathology of Melanocytic Nevi and Malignant Melanoma.* 2d ed. New York: Springer, 2006.

Baron-Faust, Rita, and Jill P Buyon. *The Autoimmune Connection: Essential Information for Women on Diagnosis, Treatment, and Getting on with Life.* Chicago: Contemporary Books, 2003.

Barraclough, Jennifer. *Cancer and Emotion: A Practical Guide to Psycho-Oncology.* New York: Wiley, 1999.

Barraclough, Jennifer, ed. *Enhancing Cancer Care: Complementary Therapy and Support.* New York: Oxford University Press, 2007.

Barras, M. A., Hughes, D., & Ullner, M. (2016). Direct oral anticoagulants: New drugs with practical problems. How can nurses help prevent patient harm? *Nursing and Health Sciences,* doi: 10.1111/nhs.12263.

Barry, Joanne. "Reaching Out to Educate." *Canadian Nurse* 103, no. 8 (October, 2007): 34-35.

Barry, Michael S. *The Art of Caregiving: How to Lend Support and Encouragement to Those with Cancer.* Colorado Springs, Colo.: Life Journey, 2007.

Bartlett, John M. S. *Ovarian Cancer: Methods and Protocols.* Totowa, N.J.: Humana Press, 2000.

Barton-Burkey, Margaret, and Gail M. Wilkes. *Cancer Therapies.* Sudbury, Mass.: Jones and Bartlett, 2006.

Bartrip, Peter. *Beyond the Factory Gates: Asbestos and Health in Twentieth Century America.* New York: Continuum, 2006.

Bashey, A., Abonour, R., & Huston, J. A. (2012). *100 questions & answers about myeloma.* Burlington, MA: Jones & Bartlett Learning.

Battacharyua, Prosun, et al., eds. *Biogeochemical Interactions, Health Effects, and Remediation.* Vol. 9 in *Arsenic in Soil and Groundwater Environment.* Cambridge, Mass.: Elsevier, 2007.

Battaglia, A., et al. "Comparisons of Growth Patterns of Acoustic Neuromas with and Without Radiosurgery." *Otology and Neurotology* 27 (2006): 705-712.

Baum, A. (Eds.). *Psychosocial interventions for cancer.* American Psychological Association (2001).

Baumann, Nicole, and Danielle Pham-Dinh. "Biology of Oligodendrocyte and Myelin in the Mammalian Central Nervous System." *Physiological Reviews* 18, no. 2 (2001): 871-927.

Baylin, Stephen B. (2005). Review of: DNA Methylation and Gene Silencing in Cancer. *Nature Clinical Practice Oncology*, 2, S4-S11.

Bazell, Robert. (1998). *Her-2: The Making of Herceptin, a Revolutionary Treatment for Breast Cancer.* New York: Random House.

Beaber, E.F., Buist, D.S.M., Barlow, W.E., Malone, K. E., Reed, S. D., & Li, C. I. (2014). Recent oral contraceptive use by formulation and breast cancer risk among women 20 to 49 years of age. *Cancer Research,* 74: 4078-4089.

Bearison, David J., and Raymond K. Mulhern, eds. *Pediatric Psychooncology: Psychological Perspectives on Children with Cancer.* New York: Oxford University Press, 1999.

Beeran, A.A., Maliyakkal, N., Rao, C.M., & Udupa, N. (2015). The enriched fraction of *Elephantopus scaber* triggers apoptosis and inhibits multidrug resistance transporters n human epithelial cancer cells. *Pharmacognosy Magazine,* 11(42). doi: 10.4103/0973-1296.153077.

Beers, Mark H., and Robert Berkow. *Merck Manual of Geriatrics.* Rahway, N.J.: Merck Sharp & Dohme Research Laboratories, 2000.

______, et al., eds. *The Merck Manual of Medical Information, Second Home Edition.* Whitehouse Station, N.J.: Merck Research Laboratories, 2003.

Beers, M. H., and R. Berkow, eds. "Cystosarcoma Phyllodes." In *The Merck Manual of Diagnosis and Therapy.* Whitehouse Station, N.J.: Merck Research Laboratories, 2004.

Beers, Mark H., ed. *The Merck Manual of Diagnosis and Therapy.* 18th ed. Whitehouse Station, N.J.: Merck, 2006.

Beeson, W. L., Abbey, D. E., & Knutsen S. F. (1998). Long-term concentrations of ambient air pollutants and incident lung cancer in California adults. *Environmental Health Perspectives*, 106: 813-822.

Begley, Sharon. "Science Journal: Nature's Quirks Limit DNA-Based Drug Possibilities." *Pittsburg Post Gazette*, November 11, 2005.

Behl, D., and A. Jatoi. "Pharmacological Options for Advanced Cancer Patients with Loss of Appetite and Weight." *Expert Opinion on Pharmacotherapy* 8, no. 8 (June, 2007): 1085-1090.

Behrens, Barbara J. & Beinert, Holly. (2014). *Physical Agents: Theory and Practice.* Philadelphia: F.A. Davis Company. O'Sullivan, Susan B., Schmitz, Thomas J., & Fulk, George. (2014). *Physical Rehabilitation.* Philadelphia: F.A. Davis Company.

Being a Young Adult With Cancer (2015). Cance.Net. Retrieved from http://www.cancer.net/navigating-cancer-care/young-adults/being-young-adult-cancer

Bell, Ruth, et al. *Changing Bodies, Changing Lives: A Book for Teens on Sex and Relationships.* 3rd ed. New York: Times Books, 1998.

Bellenir, Karen, ed. *Cancer Sourcebook.* 4th ed. Detroit: Omnigraphics, 2003.

_______, ed. *Cancer Survivor Sourcebook.* Detroit: Omnigraphics, 2007.

_______, ed. *Tobacco Information for Teens: Health Tips About the Hazards of Using Cigarettes, Smokeless Tobacco, and Other Nicotine Products.* Detroit: Omnigraphics, 2007.

Ben Simon, G. J., R. M. Schwarcz, R. Douglas, et al. "Orbital Exenteration: One Size Does Not Fit All." *American Journal* of *Ophthalmology* no. 139, no. 6 (2005): 7-11.

Benedet, J. L., et al. "FIGO Staging Classifications and Clinical Practice Guidelines in the Management of Gynecologic Cancers." *International Journal of Gynecology and Obstetrics* 70 (2000): 209-262.

Benedet, Rosalind. *Understanding Lumpectomy: A Treatment Guide for Breast Cancer*. Omaha, Nebr.: Addicus Books, 2003.

Benn, Diana E., et al. "Clinical Presentation and Penetrance of Pheochromocytoma/Paraganglioma Syndromes." *Journal of Clinical Endocrinology and Metabolism* 91, no. 3 (2005): 827-836.

Bennet, J. W., and M. Klich. "Mycotoxins." *Clinical Microbiology Reviews* 16, no. 3 (2003): 497-516.

Bennett, John E., Dolin, Raphael, & Blazer, Martin J. (Eds.). Principles and practice of infectious diseases (8th ed.). Philadelphia, PA.: Saunders.

Benson, Ellis S., Barbara F. Atkinson, and Martin Alax. *Career Guide in Pathology*. Chicago: American Society for Clinical Pathology, 1998.

Berek, J. S., and N. F. Hacker. *Practical Gynecologic Oncology*. Philadelphia: Lippincott Williams & Wilkins, 2005.

Beres, Samantha. *Pesticides: Critcal Thinking About Environmental Issues*. Farmington Hills, Mich.: Greenhaven Press, 2002.

Berg, J. W., P. S. Appelbaum, C. W. Lidz, and L. S. Parker. *Informed Consent: Legal Theory and Clinical Practice*. New York: Oxford University Press, 2001.

Berger, Mitchel S., and Charles B. Wilson, eds. *The Gliomas*. Philadelphia: W. B. Saunders, 1999.

Bergquist, Thomas H. *MRI of the Musculoskeletal System*. 4th ed. Philadelphia: Lippincott Williams & Wilkins, 2001.

Berkowitz, Ross S., and Donald P. Goldstein. "Gestational Trophoblast Neoplasia." In *Practical Gynecologic Oncology*, edited by Jonathan S. Berek and Neville F. Hacker. 4th ed. Philadelphia: Lippincott Williams & Wilkins, 2004.

Berman, Joel. *Understanding Surgery: A Comprehensive Guide for Every Family*. Wellesley, Mass.: Branden Books. 2001.

Bernardes de Jesus, B., Schneeberger, K., Vera, E., Tejera, A., Harley, C. B., & Blasco, M. A. (2011). The telomerase activator TA-65 elongates short telomeres and increases health span of adult/old mice without increasing cancer incidence. *Aging Cell* 10(4): 604–621.

Berndtsson, Ina, et al. "Long-Term Outcome After Ileal Pouch Anal Anastomosis: Function and Health-Related Quality of Life." *Diseases of the Colon & Rectum* 50 (2007): 1545-1552.

Bernick, P. E., and W. D. Wong. "Staging: What Makes Sense? Can the Pathologist Help?" *Surgical Oncology Clinics of North America* 9 (2000): 703-720.

Bernstein, Charles N. *Inflammatory Bowel Disease Yearbook 2004*. London: Remedica, 2004.

Bernstein, J., ed. *Musculoskeletal Medicine*. Rosemont, Ill.: American Academy of Orthopedic Surgeons, 2003.

Bernstein M., & Berger, M.S. (Ed.). (2014). *Neuro-Oncology: The essentials (3rd ed.)*. New York, NY: Thieme Publishing Group.

Berry, Daniel J., and Scott P. Steinmann. *Adult Reconstruction*. Philadelphia: Lippincott Williams & Wilkins, 2007.

Bertagna, Xavier, ed. *Adrenal Cancer*. Montrouge, France: John Libbey Eurotext, 2006.

Best Companies: Eli Lilly and Company (2012, August 20). *Working Mother*. Retrieved from http://www.workingmother.com/best-companies/eli-lilly-and-company

Betancourt, Marian, and Joseph F. Dooley. *The Coming Cancer Breakthroughs: What You Need to Know About the Latest Cancer Treatment Options*. New York: Kensington Books, 2003.

Bettocchi, S., et al. "What Does 'Diagnostic Hysteroscopy' Mean Today? The Role of the New Techniques." *Current Opinions in Obstetrics and Gynecology* 15, no. 4 (August, 2003): 303-308.

Bevilacqua, José Luiz B., et al. "Doctor, What Are My Chances of Having a Positive Sentinel Node? A Validated Nomogram for Risk Estimation." *Journal of Clinical Oncology* 25, no. 24 (August 20, 2007): 3670-3679.

Bigbee W., and R. B. Herberman. "Tumor Markers and Immunodiagnosis." In *Cancer Medicine*, edited by James F. Holland and Emil Frei. 6th ed. Hamilton, Ont.: BC Decker, 2003.

Bignold, Leon. *Principles of Tumors*. San Diego, CA: Academic Press, 2015.

Bilezikian, J. "Management of Acute Hypercalcemia." *New England Journal of Medicine* 326 (1992): 1196-1203.

Birchard, Stephen J., and Robert G. Sherding. *Saunders' Manual of Small Animal Practice*. 3rd ed. Philadelphia: Elsevier, 2006.

Bishop, D. T. "*BRCA1* and *BRCA2* and Breast Cancer In cidence: A Review." *Annals of Oncology* 10, suppl. 6 (1999): S113-S119.

Bishop, J. Michael. How to Win the Nobel Prize. Cambridge, Mass.: Harvard University Press, 2003.

Bjorkholm, Magnus. "Lymphoplasmacytic Lymphoma/Waldenström's Macroglobulinemia." In *The*

Lymphomas, edited by George P. Canellos, T. Andrew Lister, and Bryan D. Young. Philadelphia: Elsevier/Saunders, 2006.

Black, P. and C. Hyde. *Diverticular Disease*. Hoboken, N.J.: John Wiley & Sons, 2005.

Black, Peter McL. *Living with a Brain Tumor: Dr. Peter Black's Guide to Taking Control of Your Treatment*. New York: Henry Holt, 2006.

Blanc, Paul D. *How Everyday Products Make People Sick: Toxins at Home and in the Workplace*. Berkeley: University of California Press, 2007.

Blay, J. Y., et al. "Consensus Meeting for the Management of Gastrointestinal Stromal Tumors: Report of the GIST Consensus Conference of 20-21 March 2004, Under the Auspices of ESMO." *Annals of Oncology* 16, no. 4 (2005): 566-578.

Bleiker, T. O., N. Nicolaou, J. Traulsen, and P. E. Hutchinson. "'Atrophic Telogen Effluvium' from Cytotoxic Drugs and a Randomized Controlled Trial to Investigate the Possible Protective Effect of Pretreatment with a Topical Vitamin D_3 Analogue in Humans." *British Journal of Dermatology* 153, no. 1 (2005): 103-112.

Blevins, Lewis, S., ed. *Cushing's Syndrome*. New York: Springer, 2002.

Bloch, A. *Nutrition Management of the Cancer Patient*. Sudbury, Mass.: Jones and Bartlett, 1990.

Bloch, Abby, et al., eds. *Eating Well, Staying Well During and After Cancer*. Atlanta: American Cancer Society, 2004.

Block, Keith. (2009). *Life over cancer: The block center program for integrative cancer treatment*. New York: Bantam.

BLS for Health Care Providers. Dallas: American Heart Association, 2006.

Bodey, Gerald P., ed. *Candidiasis*. 2d ed. New York: Raven Press, 1993.

Boffetta, P., Couto, E., Wichmann, J., Ferrari, P., Trichopoulos, D., Bueno de Mesquita, H. B., Trichopoulou, A. (2010). Fruit and vegetable intake and overall cancer risk in the European Prospective Investigation into Cancer and Nutrition (EPIC). *Journal of the National Cancer Institute,* 102, 529-537.

Bogot, N. R., and L. E. Quint. "Imaging of Thymic Disorders." *Cancer Imaging* 5 (December 15, 2005): 139-149.

Bohle, A. "Long-Term Followup of a Randomized Study of Locally Advanced Prostate Cancer Treated with Combined Orchiectomy and External Radiotherapy Versus Radiotherapy Alone." *International Brazillian Journal of Urology* 32, no. 6 (November/December, 2006): 739.

Bone, M., P. Critchley, and D. Buggy. "Gabapentin in Postamputation Phantom Limb Pain: A Randomized, Double-Blind Placebo-Controlled, Cross-Over Study." *Regional Anesthesia and Pain Medicine* 27, no. 5 (2002): 481.

Bonnet, F., et al. "Malignancy-Related Causes of Death in Human Immunodeficiency Virus-Infected Patients in the Era of Highly Active Antiretroviral Therapy." *Cancer* 101 (July 15, 2004): 317-324.

Bonner, J. A., et al. "Radiotherapy plus Cetuximab for Squamous-Cell Carcinoma of the Head and Neck." *New England Journal of Medicine* 354 (2006): 567-578.

Boog, Kathryn M., and Claire Tester. *A Practical Guide to Palliative Care: Finding Meaning and Purpose in Life and Death*. New York: Elsevier, 2008.

Booker, N.W., Pharm, D., & Zuckerman, D. (2015). Antioxidants and cancer risk: The good, the bad, and the unknown. Retrieved from http://www.stopcancerfund.org/pz-diet-habits-behaviors/antioxidants-and-cancer-risk-the-good-the-bad-and-the-unknown/

Bosanquet, Nick, and Karol Sikora. *The Economics of Cancer Care*. Cambridge: Cambridge University Press, 2006.

Boshoff, Chris, and Robin Weiss. *Kaposi Sarcoma Herpesvirus: New Perspectives*. New York: Springer-Verlag, 2006.

Boshoff, C., and R. A. Weiss, eds. "Kaposi Sarcoma Herpesvirus: New Perspectives." *Current Topics in Microbiology and Immunology* 312 (2007).

Bospene, Edwin B., ed. *Eye Cancer Research Progress*. New York: Nova Science, 2007.

Boston Women's Health Book Collective. *Our Bodies, Ourselves: Menopause*. New York: Simon & Schuster, 2006.

Bostwick, D. G., et al. "Human Prostate Cancer Risk Factors." *Cancer* 101, suppl. 10 (2004): 2371-2490.

Botha, M. H., & Kruger, T. F. (2012). A review of the incidence and survival of childhood and adolescent cancer and the effects of treatment on future fertility and endocrine development.(Report). *South African Journal of Obstetrics and Gynaecology*. South African Medical Association. Retrieved March 02, 2016 from HighBeam Research: https://www.highbeam.com/doc/1G1-288874072.html

Bourgeois, P., O. Leduc, and A. Leduc. "Imaging Techniques in the Management and Prevention of Posttherapeutic Upper Limb Edemas." *Cancer* 83 (December 15, 1998): 2805-2813.

Bourke, B., Broderick, A., & Bohane, T. (2006). Peutz-Jeghers syndrome and management recommendations. *Clinical Gastroenterology and Hepatology,* 4(12): 1550.

Boursi, B., Sella, T., Liberman, E., Shapira, S., David, M., Kazanov, D., Kraus, S. (2013). The APC p.I1307K polymorphism is a significant risk factor for CRC in average risk Ashkenazi Jews. *European Journal of Cancer,* 49(17): 3680-3685.

Bowcock, Anne M, ed. *Breast Cancer: Molecular Genetics, Pathogenesis, and Therapeutics*. Totowa, N.J.: Humana Press, 1999.

Bowker, Michael. *Fatal Deception: The Untold Story of Asbestos—Why It Is Still Legal and Still Killing Us*. Emmaus, Pa.: Rodale, 2003.

Boyiadzis, Michael, et al. *Hematology-Oncology Therapy*. New York: McGraw-Hill, 2006.

Bozzone, Donna M. *Causes of Cancer*. New York: Chelsea House, 2007.

Braasch, W. F. *Early Days in the Mayo Clinic*. Springfield, Ill.: Thomas, 1969.

Brady L. Stein, Brandon J McMahon. *Contemptorary management of myeloproliferative neoplasms.* 1st Edition. This book is a comprehensive guide to diagnosis and management of MPN. Jaypee Brothers Meidcal Pub, 2015.

Brady, Mary S. "Current Management of Patients with Merkel Cell Carcinoma." *Dermatologic Surgery* 30, no. 2 (February, 2004): 321-325.

Brandenberg, R. O., et al. "Report of the WHO/ISFC Task Force on Definition and Classification of Cardiomyopathies." *Circulation* 64 (1981): 437A.

Brandon, M., P. Baldi, and D. C. Wallace. "Mitochondrial Mutations in Cancer." *Oncogene* 25, no. 34 (2005): 4647-4662.

Brandt, A. M. *The Cigarette Century: The Rise, Fall, and Deadly Persistence of the Product That Defined America*. New York: Basic Books, 2007.

Brandt-Rauf, Sherry I., et al. "Ashkenazi Jews and Breast Cancer: The Consequences of Linking Ethnic Identity to Genetic Disease." *American Journal of Public Health* 96, no. 11 (2006): 1979-1988.

Brant, William E., and Clyde A. Helms. *Fundamentals of Diagnostic Radiology*. Baltimore: Williams and Wilkins, 1994.

Braverman, Lewis E. *Diseases of the Thyroid*. 2d ed. Totowa, N.J.: Humana Press, 2003.

________, and Robert D. Utiger, eds. *Werner and Ingbar's The Thyoid: A Fundamental and Clinical Text*. 7th ed. New York: Lippincott-Raven, 1991.

Breitbart, W. "Spirituality and Meaning in Supportive Care: Spirituality- and Meaning-Centered Group Psychotherapy Interventions in Advanced Cancer." *Journal of Supportive Care in Cancer* 10, no. 4 (2002): 272-280.

Brennan, F., D. B. Carr, and M. Cousins. "Pain Management: A Fundamental Human Right." *Anesthesia & Analgesia* 105, no. 1 (July, 2007): 205-221.

Brennan, James. *Cancer in Context: A Practical Guide to Supportive Care*. New York: Oxford University Press, 2004.

Brenner, Malcolm & Hung, Mien-Chie. (Eds.). (2014). *Cancer gene therapy by viral and non-viral vectors.* Hoboken, NY: John Wiley & Sons.

Brian, G., M., et al. "International Uniform Response Criteria for Multiple Myeloma." *Leukemia* 20, no. 9 (2006): 1467.

Bridget, S. Wilkins, and Dennis H. Wright. *Illustrated Pathology of the Spleen*. New York: Cambridge University Press, 2000.

Brinton, L. "Long-Term Effects of Ovulation-Stimulating Drugs on Cancer Risk." *Reproductive BioMedicine Online* 15 (2007): 38-44.

Brinton, L. A., et al. "Ovarian Cancer Risk After the Use of Ovulation-Stimulating Drugs." *Obstetrics and Gynecology* 103 (2004): 1194-1203.

Brinton Wolbarst, Anthony. *Looking Within: How X-Ray, CT, MRI, Ultrasound, and Other Medical Images Are Created and How They Help Physicians Save Lives*. Berkeley: University of California Press, 1999.

Brito-Zerón P., & Ramos-Casals M. (2014). Advances in the understanding and treatment of systemic complications in Sjögren's syndrome. *Current Opinions in Rheumatology,* 26(5), 520-527.

Broadbent, V., H. Gadner, D. M. Komp, and S. Ladisch. "Histiocytosis Syndromes in Children: II. Approach to the Clinical and Laboratory Evaluation of Children with Langerhans Cell Histiocytosis." *Medical and Pediatric Oncology* 17, no. (1989): 492-495.

Brockstein, Bruce, and Gregory Masters, eds. *Head and Neck Cancer*. Boston: Kluwer Academic, 2003.

Brody, T. (2011). *Clinical trials: Study design, endpoints and biomarkers, drug safety, and FDA and ICH Guidelines.* Waltham, MA: Elsevier.

Broom, M. A., et al. "Successful Umbilical Cord Blood Stem Cell Transplantation in a Patient with Rothmund-Thomson Syndrome and Combined Immunodeficiency." *Clinical Genetics* 69, no. 4 (April, 2006): 337-343.

Brower, V. (2015, April 1). The CAR T-cell race. *The Scientist*, 29(4). Retrieved from http://www.the-scientist.com/?articles.view/articleNo/42462/title/The-CAR-T-Cell-Race/.

Brown, Gina. (2007). *Colorectal cancer.* New York: Cambridge University Press.

Brown, L., M. M. Rhead, K. C. C. Bancroft, and N. Allen. "Model Studies of the Degradation of Acrylamide Monomer." *Water Research* 14, no. 7 (1980): 775-778.

Brown, M. L., G. F. Riley, N. Schussler, and R. D. Etzioni. "Estimating Health Care Costs Related to Cancer Treatment from SEER-Medicare Data." *Medical Care* 40, suppl. 8 (August, 2002): IV-104-117.

Brown, M. L., J. Lipscomb, and C. Snyder. "The Burden of Illness of Cancer: Economic Cost and Quality of Life." *Annual Review of Public Health* 22 (2001): 91-113.

Bruce, J. N., and A. T. Ogden. "Surgical Strategies for Treating Patients with Pineal Region Tumors." *Journal of Neurooncology* 69, nos. 1-3 (August/September, 2004): 221-236.

Brunekreef, B., Beelen, R., Hoek, G., Schouten, L., Bausch-Goldbohm, S., Fischer, P., van den Brandt, P. (2009). Effects of long-term exposure to traffic-related air pollution on respiratory and cardiovascular mortality in the Netherlands: the NLCS-AIR study. *Research Report (Health Effects Institute)*, 139: 5–71.

Bruno, M. K., and J. Raizer. "Leptomeningeal Metastases from Solid Tumors (Meningeal Carcinomatosis)." *Cancer Treatment and Research* 125 (2005): 31-52.

Brunt, L. M. "Endoscopic Parathyroid and Thyroid Surgery." In *Current Review of Minimally Invasive Surgery*, edited by D. C. Brooks. Philadelphia: Current Medicine, 1998.

Brunzel, Nancy A. *Fundamentals of Urine and Body Fluid Analysis*. 2d ed. Philadelphia: W. B. Saunders, 2004.

Brusic, V., O. Marina, C. J. Wu, and E. L. Reinherz. "Proteome Informatics for Cancer Research: From Molecules to Clinic." *Proteomics* 7 (2007): 976-991.

Buckley, John F., and Nicole D. Prysby. *2005 State by State Guide to Managed Care Law*. New York: Aspen, 2005.

Buffart, L. M., van Uffelen, J. G., Riphagen, I. I., Brug, J., van Mechelen, W., Brown, W. J., & Chinapaw, M. J. (2012). Physical and psychosocial benefits of yoga in cancer patients and survivors, a systematic review and meta-analysis of randomized controlled trials. *BMC Cancer*, 12: 559.

Bulatao, Randy A., & Anderson, Norman B. (2004). *Understanding racial and ethnic differences in health in late life: A research agenda*. Washington, D.C.: National Academies Press, 2004.

Bullwinkle, E. (2015). Abstract 3203: Multiple myeloma microenvironment and obesity. *Cancer Research*, 75(15 Supplement), 3203-3203. doi:10.1158/1538-7445.AM2015-3203

Burger-Szabo, A., Gabos-Greu, M., Theodor, M., Hajnal, F., Ferencz, M, Gabos-Grecu, C., & Gabos-Grecu, I. (2015). Pain and distress in cancer patients. *Acta Medica Marisensis,* 61(3): 213-216. doi: 10.1515/amma-2015-0057.

Burns, C. A., and M. D. Brown. "Imiquimod for the Treatment of Skin Cancer." *Dermatology Clinics* 23, no. 1 (2005): 151-164.

Burotto, M., Ali, S. A., & O'Sullivan Coyne, G. (2014). Class act: safety comparison of approved tyrosine kinase inhibitors for non-small-cell lung carcinoma. *Expert Opinion on Drug Safety*, 14(1): 97-110.

Burton, A. W., et al. "Chronic Pain in the Cancer Survivor: A New Frontier." *Pain Medicine* 8, no. 2 (March, 2007): 189-198.

Busby, J. E., and C. A. Pettaway. "What's New in the Management of Penile Cancer?" *Current Opinion in Urology* 15, no. 5 (September, 2005): 350-357.

Bushong, Stewart C. *Diagnostic Ultrasound*. New York: McGraw-Hill, 1999.

Buthiau, Didier, and David Khayat. *CT and MRI in Oncology*. New York: Springer-Verlag, 1998.

Butler, J., Healy, C., Toner, M., & Flint, S. (2005). Gardner syndrome: Review and report of a case. *Oral Oncology Extra,* 5(41), 89-92.

Butterfield, L. H. "Recent Advances in Immunotherapy for Hepatocellular Cancer." *Swiss Medical Weekly* 137 (2007): 83-90.

Byers, Tim, Susan J. Curry, Maria Elizabeth Hewitt, and National Cancer Policy Board. *Fulfilling the Potential of Cancer Prevention and Early Detection*. Washington, D.C.: National Academies Press, 2003.

Byrd, W. Michael, and Linda A. Clayton. *A Medical History of African Americans and the Problem of Race, Beginnings to 1900*. Foreword by Robert J. Blendon. New York: Routledge, 2000-2002.

Cabrero, M., Jabbour, E., Ravandi, F., Bohannan, Z., Pierce, S., Kantarjian, H. M., & Garcia-Manero, G. (2015). Discontinuation of hypomethylating agent therapy in patients with myelodysplastic syndromes or acute myelogenous leukemia in complete remission or partial response: Retrospective analysis of survival after long-term follow-up. *Leukemia Research*, 39(5):520-524.

Cahill, Bridget A. "Management of Patients Who Have Undergone Hepatic Artery Chemoembolization." *Clinical Journal of Oncology Nursing* 9, no. 1 (2005): 69-75.

Calder, Kimberly J., and Karen Pollitz. *What Cancer Survivors Need to Know About Health Insurance*. Silver

Springs, Md.: National Coalition for Cancer Survivorship, 2006.

Caligaris-Cappio, F., and R. Dalla-Favera, eds. *Chronic Lymphocytic Leukemia*. New York: Springer, 2005.

Calva, D. & Howe, J. (2008). Harmartomatous polyposis syndromes. *The Surgical Clinics of North America,* 88(4): 779–817.

Campanacci, M. *Bone and Soft Tissue Tumors*. New York: Springer, 1990.

Campanacci, M., et al. "Giant Cell Tumor of the Bone." *Journal of Bone Joint Surgery* 69A (1987): 106-114.

Campbell, J. J., Clark, R. A., Watanabe. R., & Kupper, T. S. (2010. Sézary syndrome and mycosis fungoides arise from distinct T-cell subsets: A biological rationale for their distinct clinical behaviors. *Blood,* 116(5), 767-771.

Campbell, Steven C., et al. *One Hundred Questions and Answers About Kidney Cancer*. Sudbury, Mass.: Jones and Bartlett, 2009.

Canale, S. Terry, ed. *Campbell's Operative Orthopaedics*. 9th ed. St. Louis, Mo.: Mosby, 1998.

Canavan, T. P., and N. R. Doshi. "Endometrial Cancer." *American Family Physician* 59, no. 11 (June, 1999): 3069-3077.

Cancer Network Editors. (2015). Coffee and Cancer Risk. *Cancer Network: Home of the Journal Oncology*. http://www.cancernetwork.com/articles/coffee-and-cancer-risk

Cancer Prevention: Putting It Together. American Institute for Cancer Research Retrieved from http://www.aicr.org/reduce-your-cancer-risk/cancer-prevention/?referrer=https://www.google.com/

Cancer Research Now: Adolescent and Young Adult Cancer. National Cancer Institute. Retrieved from https://www.youtube.com/watch?v=XRNwluM10FI

Cancer.net. (2014 February). Rhabdomyosarcoma-Childhood. Retrieved on February 10, 2016 from Http://www.cancer.net/cancer-types/rhabdomyosarcoma-childnood/view-all. This article discusses all aspects of care, including grouping and staging.

Cannon, Geneva. *Caring for Your Loved One Who Is Ill at Home: A Comprehensive Guide and Planner for Family Caregivers and Personal Home Care Assistants*. Salisbury, Md.: Avenegg, 2006.

Capossela, Cappy, and Sheila Warnock. *Share the Care: How to Organize a Group to Care for Someone Who Is Seriously Ill*. Rev. ed. New York: Simon and Schuster, 2004.

Cappello, Mary (2009). *Called Back: My reply to cancer, my return to life*. New York City, NY: Alyson Books.

Carcinogens. Davenport, Iowa: Mangan Communications, 2007.

Cardiovascular Care Made Incredibly Visual. Philadelphia: Lippincott Williams & Wilkins, 2007.

Carey, Nessa. (2013). *The epigenetics revolution: How modern biology is rewriting our understanding of genetics, disease, and inheritance*. NY: Columbia University Press.

Caris, Lauren. (2015, July 6) Three Things Cancer Taught Me at Age 28. *Huffpost Living Healthy*. Retrieved from http://www.huffingtonpost.com/lauren-caris-/on-friendship-and-coping_b_7714818.html

Carlson, Karen J., Stephanie A. Eisenstat, and Terra Ziporyn. *The New Harvard Guide to Women's Health*. Cambridge, Mass.: Harvard University Press, 2004.

Carmignani, C. P., and P. H. Sugarbaker. "Synchronous Extraperitoneal and Intraperitoneal Dissemination of Appendix Cancer." *European Journal of Surgical Oncology* 30, no. 8 (October, 2004): 864-868.

Carney, Jan K. *Public Health in Action: Practicing in the Real World*. Sudbury, Mass.: Jones and Bartlett, 2006.

Carpenter, G., ed. *The EGF Receptor Family: Biologic Mechanisms and Role in Cancer*. Amsterdam: Elsevier Academic Press, 2004

Carpenter, Malcolm B. *Core Text of Neuroanatomy*. 2d ed. Baltimore: Williams & Wilkins, 1981.

Carper, E., and M. Hass. "Advanced Practice Nursing in Radiation Oncology." *Seminars in Oncology Nursing* 22, no. 4 (November, 2006): 203-211.

Carper, Elise. *One Hundred Questions and Answers About Head and Neck Cancer*. Sudbury, Mass.: Jones and Bartlett, 2007.

Carper, Elise, Kenneth Hu, and Elena Kuzin. *One Hundred Questions and Answers About Head and Neck Cancer*. Sudbury, Mass.: Jones and Barlett, 2008.

Carrier, Ewa, and Gracy Ledinham. *One Hundred Questions and Answers About Bone Marrow and Stem Cell Transplantation*. Sudbury, Mass.: Jones and Bartlett, 2003.

Carson, Rachel. *Silent Spring*. 1962. Reprint. Boston: Mariner Books, 2007.

Casper, Janina K., and Raymond H. Colton. *Clinical Manual for Laryngectomy and Head/Neck Cancer Rehabilitation*. 2d ed. San Diego, Calif.: Singular, 1998.

Cassidy, Jim, Johnston, Patrick, & van Cutsem, Eric. (Eds.). (2007). *Colorectal cancer*. New York: Informa Healthcare.

Castillo, J. J., Sa, S. D', Lunn, M. P., Minnema, M. C., Tedeschi, A., Lansigan, F., … Treon, S. P. (2015). Central nervous system involvement by Waldenström macroglobulinaemia (Bing-Neel syndrome): A multi-institutional retrospective study, *British Journal of Haematology*, doi: 10.1111/bjh.13883.

Catovsky, D., Fooks, J., & Richards, S. (1989). Prognostic factors in chronic lymphocytic leukaemia: The importance of age, sex, and response to treatment in survival. *British Journal of Haematology,* 72, 141-149.

Caulkins, Jonathan P., Kilmer, Beau, & Kleinman, Mark A. R. (2016). *Marijuana Legalization: What Everyone Needs to Know.* New York, New York: Oxford University Press. The authors describe marijuana legalization, medicinal marijuana laws, and the broader sociopolitical context of policy around marijuana use.

Cavalli, F., Kaye, S. B., Hansen, H. H., Armitage, J. O., Piccart-Gebhart, M. (Eds.). (2009). *Textbook of medical oncology* (4th ed.). United Kingdom: Taylor & Francis Ltd., 2009.

Cavalli, F., et al., eds. *Textbook of Medical Oncology*. 3rd ed. New York: Informa Healthcare, 2004.

Centeno, Arthur S., and Gary Onik. *Prostate Cancer: A Patient's Guide to Treatment.* Omaha, Nebr.: Addicus, 2004.

Center for Young Women's Health. (2014). Medical uses of the birth control pill. Retrieved from http://youngwomenshealth.org/2011/10/18/medical-uses-of-the-birth-control-pill/.

Centers for Disease Control and Prevention. *Targeting Tobacco Use: The Nation's Leading Cause of Death, 2005.* Bethesda, Md.: Author, 2005.

Centers for Disease Control. *U.S. Cancer Statistics: 2004 Incidence and Mortality*. Washington, D.C.: Author, 2004.

Central Brain Tumor Registry of the United States. *Primary Brain Tumors in the United States: Statistical Report, 1992-1997.* Chicago: Author, 2000.

Cerhan, James R. (2006). Oral contraceptive use and breast cancer risk: Current status. *Mayo Clinic Proceedings,* 81(10): 1287-1289.

Chabner, B. A., & Longo, D. L. (Eds.). (2010). Cancer chemotherapy and biotherapy: Principles and practice (5th ed.). Philadelphia: Lippincott Williams & Wilkin.

Chabner, Bruce A., and Dan L. Longo, eds. *Cancer Chemotherapy and Biotherapy: Principles and Practice.* Philadelphia: Lippincott Williams & Wilkins, 2006.

Chakrabarti, I., A. P. Amar, W. Couldwell, and M. H. Weiss. "Long-Term Neurological, Visual, and Endocrine Outcomes Following Transnasal Resection of Craniopharyngioma." *Journal of Neurosurgery* 102 (2005): 650-657.

Chan, Helen S. L. *Understanding Cancer Therapies.* Jackson: University of Mississippi Press, 2007.

Chandwani, K., Ryan, J. L., Peppone, L. J., Janelsins, M. M. Sprod, L. K., Devine, K., ...Mustian, K. M. (2012). Cancer-related stress and complementary and alternative medicine: A review. *Evidence-Based Complementary and Alternative Medicine,* Volume 2012 (2012), Article ID 979213, 15 pages. http://dx.doi.org/10.1155/2012/979213

Chang, J., et al. "Prediction of Clinical Outcome from Primary Tamoxifen by Expression of Biologic Markers in Breast Cancer Patients." *Clinical Cancer Research* 6 (2000): 616-621.

Chang, Jae C., and H. Bradford Hawley. "Neutropenic Fever of Undetermined Origin (N-FUO): Why Not Use the Naproxen Test?" *Cancer Investigation* 13 (1995): 448-450.

Chang, S., et al. "Estimating the Cost of Cancer: Results on the Basis of Claims Data Analyses for Cancer Patients Diagnosed with Seven Types of Cancer During 1999 to 2000." *Journal of Clinical Oncology* 22, no. 17 (September 1, 2004): 3524-3530.

Chatterjee, A., E. Mambo, and D. Sidransky. "Mitochondrial DNA Mutations in Human Cancer." *Oncogene* 25, no. 34 (2006): 4663-4674.

Chauhan, D., Hideshima, T., & Anderson, K. C. (2005). Proteasome inhibition in multiple myeloma: Therapeutic implication. *Annual Reviews of Pharmacology and Toxicology*, 45, 465-476.

Cheah, P. Y. "Hypothesis for the Etiology of Colorectal Cancer: An Overview." *Nutrition and Cancer* 14 (1990): 5-13.

Chen, C. I. "Treatment for Waldenström's Macroglobulinemia." *Annals of Oncology* 15 (2004): 550-558.

Chen, D., Frezza, M, Schmitt, S, Kanwar, J. & Dou, Q.P. (2011). Bortezomib as the first proteasome inhibitor anticancer drug: Current status and future perspectives. *Current Cancer Drug Targets*, 11(3): 239-253.

Chen, J., & Chen, T. (2004). *Chinese medical herbology and pharmacology*. City of Industry, CA: Art of Medicine Press. http://www.aompress.com/book_herbology/pdfs/RenShen.pdf

Chen, W. Y., and G. A. Colditz. "Risk Factors and Hormone-Receptor Status: Epidemiology, Risk-Prediction Models and Treatment Implications for Breast Cancer." *Nature Clinical Practice Oncology* 4 (2007): 415-423.

Chen, Y. C., Y. J. Chang, Y. C. Tsou, M.C. Chen, and Y. C. Pai. Effectiveness of Nurse Case Management Compared with Usual Care in Cancer Patients at a Single Medical Center in Taiwan: A Quasi-Experimental Study. BMC Health Services Research. 31 May 2013. doi: 10.1186/1472-6963-13-202. Available at http://www.biomedcentral.com/1472-6963/13/202.

Chen, Y. T., et al. "Sunlamp Use and the Risk of Cutaneous Malignant Melanoma: A Population-Based Case-Control Study in Connecticut, USA." *International Journal of Epidemiology* 27 (1998): 759-765.

Cheung, W. Y., et al. "Appropriateness of Testicular Cancer Management: A Population-Based Cohort Study." *Canadian Journal of Urology* 14, no. 3 (June, 2007): 3542-3550.

Childers, Linda. Oncology Case Managers Help Patients, Families. Nurse.Com. 21 November 2014. Available at https://news.nurse.com/2014/11/21/oncology-case-managers-help-patients-families/.

Chin, K., et al. "In Situ Analyses of Genome Instability in Breast Cancer." *Nature Genetics* 36 (2004): 984-988.

Chinyama, Catherine N. *Benign Breast Diseases: Radiology, Pathology, Risk Assessment*. New York: Springer, 2004.

Chiou, S. M., et al. "Stereotactic Radiosurgery of Residual or Recurrent Craniopharyngioma, After Surgery, with or Without Radiation Therapy." *Neuro-oncology* 3 (2001): 159-166.

Cho, Chi Hin, and Vishnudutt Purohit, eds. *Alcohol, Tobacco, and Cancer*. New York: Karger, 2006.

Cho, W. C. S. "Contribution of Oncoproteomics to Cancer Biomarker Discovery." *Molecular Cancer* 6 (2007): 25-37.

Christian, Paul E., and Kristen M. Waterstram-Rich, eds. *Nuclear Medicine and PET: Technology and Techniques*. 6th ed. St. Louis: Mosby/Elsevier, 2007.

Christiansen, Charles H., and Kathleen M. Matuska, eds. *Ways of Living: Adaptive Strategies for Special Needs*. Bethesda, Md.: American Occupational Therapy Association, 2004.

Chu, Edward, and Vincent T. DeVita. *Physicians' Cancer Chemotherapy Drug Manual 2007*. Sudbury, Mass.: Jones and Bartlett, 2007.

Chu, E., & DeVita, V. T. (2014). Physicians' cancer chemotherapy drug manual (15th ed.). Burlington, MA: Jones & Bartlett Learning.

Chung, Leland. *Prostate Cancer: Biology, Genetics, and New Therapeutics*. Totowa, N.J.: Humana Press, 2001.

Church, James. *Hereditary Colorectal Cancer Syndromes*. Malden, Mass.: Blackwell, 2006.

Cibus, Edmund S., and Barbara S. Ducatman. *Cytology: Diagnostic Principles and Clinical Correlates*. 2d ed. Philadelphia: Saunders, 2003.

Clancy, S. (2008). DNA damage and repair: Mechanisms for maintaining DNA integrity. *Nature Education* 1(1):103.

Clark, Orlo H. *Endocrine Tumors*. Hamilton, Ont.: BC Decker, 2003.

Clarke, C. A., and S. L. Glaser. "Changing Incidence of Non-Hodgkin Lymphomas in the United States." *Cancer* 94 (2002): 2015-2023.

Claus, E. B., et al. "Epidemiology of Intracranial Meningioma." *Neurosurgery* 57 (2005): 1088-1095.

Clayman, G. L., et al. "Mortality Risk from Squamous Cell Skin Cancer." *Journal of Clinical Oncology* 23 (2005): 759-765.

Clayton, G., A. Omasta-Martin, and M. Bower. "The Effects of HAART on AIDS-Related Kaposi's Sarcoma and Non-Hodgkin's Lymphoma." *Journal of HIV Therapy* 11, no. 3 (September, 2006): 51-53.

ClinicalTrials.gov. (2015). Study of orally administered AG-120 in subjects with advanced solid tumors, including glioma, with an IDH1 mutation. https://clinicaltrials.gov/ct2/show/NCT02073994

Cockerell, Clay, and Alvin Friedman-Kien. *Color Atlas of AIDS*. Philadelphia: W. B. Saunders, 1996.

Coghlin C, & Murray GI. (2014). The role of gene regulatory networks in promoting cancer progression and metastasis. Future Oncology, 10(5): 735-48. http://www.ncbi.nlm.nih.gov/pubmed/24799055

Cohen, J., et al. "Quality Indicators for Esophagogastroduodenoscopy." *American Journal of Gastroenterology* 101 (2006): 886-891.

Cohen, M. Michael. "Malformations of the Craniofacial Region: Evolutionary, Embryonic, Genetic, and Clinical Perspectives. *American Journal of Medical Genetics* 115 (2002):245-268.

Cohen, M. Michael. "Beckwith-Wiedemann Syndrome: Historical, Clinicopathological, and Etiopathogenetic Perspectives." *Pediatric and Developmental Pathology* 8 (2005): 287-304.

Cohen, S. R., D. K. Payne, and R. S. Tunkel. "Lymphedema: Strategies for Management." *Cancer* 92 (August 15, 2001): 980-987.

Colborn, T., D. Dumanoski, and J. P. Myers. *Our Stolen Future*. New York: Dutton Press, 1995.

Colditz, Graham A., and Cynthia J. Stein. *Handbook of Cancer Risk Assessment and Prevention*. Boston: Jones and Bartlett, 2004.

Coleman, R. E. "Clinical Features of Metastatic Bone Disease and Risk of Skeletal Morbidity." *Clinical Cancer Research* 12, no. 20, pt. 2 (2006): 6243s-6249s.

Colen, B. D. *The Essential Guide to a Living Will: How to Protect Your Right to Refuse Medical Treatment*. New York: Prentice Hall, 2001.

Colice, G. L., et al. "Medical and Surgical Treatment of Parapneumonic Effusions: An Evidence-Based Guideline." *Chest* 118 (2000): 1158-1171.

Collins, Catherine Fisher. *African American Women's Health and Social Issues*. Foreword by Vivian W. Pinn. Westport, Conn.: Praeger, 2006.

Colver, Graham. *Skin Cancer: A Practical Guide to Management*. London: Martin Dunitz, 2002.

Comeau, C. "I get by with a little help from my friends: The role of the support group in breast cancer survivorship." *Journal of Oncology Navigation & Survivorship* 5, no. 3 (June, 2014): 30-31.

Committee on EPA's Exposure and Human Health Reassessment of TCDD and Related Compounds. Board on Environmental Studies and Toxicology. Division on Earth and Life Studies. National Research Council of the National Academies. *Health Risks from Dioxin and Related Compounds: Evaluation of the EPA Reassessment*. Washington, D.C.: National Academies Press, 2006.

Committee on Infectious Diseases, American Academy of Pediatrics. (2006). Herpes simplex. In L. K. Pickering, C. J. Baker, S. S. Long, & J. A. McMillan (Eds.), *Red Book: 2006 Report of the Committee on Infectious Diseases* (27th ed.)(pp. 361-370). Elk Grove Village, Ill.: American Academy of Pediatrics.

Compostella, A., et al. "Prognostic Factors for Anaplastic Astrocytomas." *Journal of Neuro-Oncology* 81 (February, 2007): 295-303.

Connelly, J. M., and M. G. Malkin. "Environmental Risk Factors for Brain Tumors." *Current Neurology and Neuroscience Reports* 7 (2007): 208-214.

Conner, Kristine, and Lauren Langford. *Ovarian Cancer: Your Guide to Taking Control*. Sebastopol, Calif.: O'Reilly, 2003.

Cook, Allan R., ed. *The New Cancer Sourcebook*. Vol. 12. Detroit: Omnigraphics, 1996.

Cook, K.M., & Figg, W.D. (2010). Angiogenesis inhibitors: current strategies and future prospects. *CA: A Cancer Journal for Clinicians*, 60(4): 222-243. http://dx.doi.org/10.3322%2Fcaac.20075

Cooke, Robert. (2001). *Dr. Folkman's War*. New York: Random House, Inc.

Cooper, Geoffrey M. *The Cancer Book: A Guide to Understanding the Causes, Prevention, and Treatment of Cancer*. Boston: Jones and Bartlett, 1993.

Cooper, G.M., & Hausman, R.E. (2016). *The Cell: A Molecular Approach* (7th ed.). Sunderland (MA): Sinauer Associates.

Cooper, Jill, ed. *Occupational Therapy in Oncology and Palliative Care*. Hoboken, N.J.: Whurr, 2006.

Cooper, Laura D. *Insurance Solutions: Plan Well, Live Better—A Workbook for People with Chronic Illnesses or Disabilities*. New York: Demos Medical, 2002.

Cooper, Sue, ed. *Tracheostomy Care*. Hoboken, N.J.: John Wiley & Sons, 2006.

Copstead, Lee-Ellen C., and Jacquelyn Banasik. *Pathophysiology: Biological and Behavioral Perspectives*. 3rd ed. Philadelphia: Saunders, 2005.

Corbridge, Roger, and Nicholas Steventon. *Oxford Handbook of ENT and Head and Neck Surgery*. New York: Oxford University Press, 2006.

Cordts, G. (2013). Palliative care. In S. Durso & G. Sullivan (Eds), Geriatrics Review Syllabus, 8th edition (pp119-127). New York: American Geriatrics Society.

Corner, Jessica, and Christopher Bailey, eds. *Cancer Nursing: Care in Context*. Malden, Mass.: Blackwell, 2008.

Cornetta K., Lauglin M., Carter S., Wall D., Weinthal, J., Delaney, C., Chao, N. (2005). Umbilical cord blood transplantation in adults: Results of the prospective cord blood transplantation (COBLT). *Biology of Blood and Marrow Transplantation,* 11(2), 149-160.

Corrigan, Patricia, Humberto Fagundes, and Alan P. Lyss. *Chemotherapy and Radiation for Dummies*. Hoboken, N.J.: John Wiley & Sons, 2005.

Cortes, Jorge, and Michael Deininger, eds. *Chronic Myeloid Leukemia*. New York: Informa Healthcare, 2007.

Corthay, A. (2010). How do Regulatory T Cells Work?" *Scandinavian Journal of Immunology*, 70(4): 759-767.

Cotterchio, M., et al. "Colorectal Screening Is Associated with Reduced Colorectal Cancer Risk: A Case-Control Study Within the Population-Based Ontario Familial Colorectal Cancer Registry." *Cancer Causes & Control* 16, no. 7 (2005): 865-875.

Coughlin, S. S., et al. "Nonadherence to Breast and Cervical Cancer Screening: What Are the Linkages to Chronic Disease Risk?" *Preventing Chronic Disease* 1, no. 1 (January, 2004): A04.

Coumoul, Xavier, and Chu-Xia Deng. "Roles of FGF Receptors in Mammalian Development and Congenital Diseases." *Birth Defects Research* 69 (2003): 286-304.

Couriel, Daniel, et al. "Ancillary Therapy and Supportive Care of Chronic Graft-Versus-Host Disease: National Institutes of Health Consensus Development Project on Criteria for Clinical Trials in Chronic Graft-Versus-Host Disease—V. Ancillary Therapy and Supportive Care Working Group Report." *Biology of Blood and Marrow Transplantation* 12, no. 4 (2006): 375-396.

Cousins, Norman. *Anatomy of an Illness as Perceived by the Patient*. New York: W. W. Norton, 1979.

Couturaud, F., Leroyer, C., Julian, J. A., Kahn, S. R., Ginsberg, J. S., Wells, P. S., Kearon, C. (2009). Factors that Predict Risk of Thrombosis in Relatives of

Patients with Unprovoked Venous Thromboembolism. *Chest,* 136(6): 1537-1545.

Covolo, L., Rubinelli, S., Ceretti, E., & Gelatti, U. (2015). Internet-based direct-to-consumer genetic testing: A systematic review. *Journal of Medical Internet Research, 17(12), e279.*

Craig, Jordan V., and Barrington J. A. Furr, eds. *Hormone Therapy in Breast and Prostate Cancer*. Totowa, N.J.: Humana Press, 1999.

Cranston, R. D., et al. "The Prevalence, and Predictive Value, of Abnormal Anal Cytology to Diagnose Anal Dysplasia in a Population of HIV-Positive Men Who Have Sex with Men." *International Journal of STD and AIDS* 18, no. 2 (February, 2007): 77-80.

Crawford, C., et al. "Relationship Between Changes in Hemoglobin Level and Quality of Life During Chemotherapy in Anemic Cancer Patients Receiving Erythropoietin Therapy." *Cancer* 95 (2002): 888-895.

Crawford, Dorothy, Johnannessen, Ingolfur, & Rickinson, Alan B. (2014). *Cancer virus: The discovery of the Epstein-Barr virus.* New York: Oxford University Press.

Crawford, L., Walker, B., & Levine, A. (2011). Proteasome inhibitors in cancer therapy. *Journal of Cell Communication and Signaling*, 5(2): 101–110.

Creasman, W. T., F. Odicino, and P. Maigonnueve. "FIGO Annual Report on the Results of Treatment in Gynecological Cancer: Carcinoma of the Corpus Uteri." *Journal of Epidemiology and Biostatistics* 23 (1998): 35-61.

Creasman, W. T., J. L. Phillips, and H. R. Menck. "The National Cancer Data Base Report on Cancer of the Vagina." *Cancer* 83 (1998): 1033-1040.

Cross, Jeff, & Ellwanger, Julia. (2015). Takeda announces consolidation of U.S. vaccine sites in Boston/Cambridge area. *Takeda News*. Retrieved from https://www.takeda.com/news/2015/20150603_7012.html

Cruciferous Vegetables and Cancer Prevention. National Cancer Institute. Retrieved from http://www.cancer.gov/about-cancer/causes-prevention/risk/diet/cruciferous-vegetables-fact-sheet

Crul, B., L. Blok, and J. van Egmond. "The Present Role of Percutaneous Cervical Cordotomy for Treatment of Cancer Pain." *Journal of Headache Pain* 6, no. 1 (February, 2005): 24-29.

Crumley, R. L. "Unilateral Recurrent Laryngeal Nerve Paralysis." *Journal of Voice* 8, no. 1 (March, 1994): 79-83.

Cukier, Daniel. *Coping with Chemotherapy and Radiation Therapy*. 4th ed. New York: McGraw-Hill, 2004.

_______ et al. *Coping with Chemotherapy and Radiation Therapy*. 4th ed. New York: McGraw-Hill, 2004.

Cunha, Burke A., ed. "Fever." *Infectious Disease Clinics of North America* 10 (1996): 1-222.

Cunha, Burke A., ed. *Pneumonia Essentials*. Royal Oak, Mich.: Physicians' Press, 2007.

Cunningham, A. J., et al. "A Randomized Controlled Trial of the Effects of Group Psychological Therapy on Survival in Women with Metastatic Breast Cancer." *Psycho-oncology* 7 (1998): 508-517.

Curcio, K. R., Lambe, C., Schneider, S., & Khan, K. (2012). Evaluation of a cancer survivorship protocol: Transitioning patients to survivors. *Clinical Journal of Oncology Nursing*, 16(4): 400-406.

Curry, Thomas S., III, James E. Dowdey, and Robert C. Murry, Jr. *Christensen's Physics of Diagnostic Radiology*. 4th ed. Philadelphia: Lea & Febiger, 1990.

Curtin, Nicola. "DNA repair dysregulation from cancer driver to therapeutic target." *Nature Reviews/Cancer* 12 (December 2012): 801-818.

Cutler, S. J., & Cutler, H. G. (2000). *Biologically Active Natural Products: Pharmaceuticals.* Boca Raton, Fla.: CRC Press. This book explores the use of plants and plant products in pharmaceutical development, including evaluation of plant extracts for anticancer treatment.

D'Amico, Anthony V., Jay S. Loeffler, and Jay R. Harris, eds. *Image-Guided Diagnosis and Treatment of Cancer*. Totowa, N.J.: Humana Press, 2003.

D'Souza, G., et al. "Case-Control Study of Human Papillomavirus and Oropharyngeal Cancer." *New Enland Journal of Medicine* 357 (2007): 1944-1956.

Da Rocha, A. B., Lopes, R. M. & Schwartsmann, G. (2001). Natural products in anticancer therapy. *Current Opinion in Pharmacology*, 1(4): 364-369.

Dabbs, David J., ed. *Diagnostic Immunohistochemistry*. 2d ed. Philadelphia: Elsevier Churchill Livingstone, 2006.

Damania, B., & Pipas, J. (Eds.). (2009). *DNA tumor viruses*. New York: Springer.

Damjanov, Ivan, and Fang Fan, eds. *Cancer Grading Manual*. New York: Springer, 2007.

Damron, Timothy A., ed. *Oncology and Basic Science*. Philadelphia: Lippincott Williams & Wilkins, 2008.

Dana-Farber Cancer Institute. (2014, April). Link between Down syndrome, leukemia uncovered. *ScienceDaily.* www.sciencedaily.com/releases/2014/04/140420131810.htm

Darwish, H., Trejo. I. E., Shapira, I., Oweineh, S., Sughayer, M., Baron, L., Arber, N. (2002). Fighting colorectal cancer: molecular epidemiology differences among Ashkenazi and Sephardic Jews and Palestinians. *Annals of Oncology,* 13(9): 1497-1501.

Das, P., C. H. Crane, and J. A. Ajani. "Current Treatment for Localized Anal Carcinoma." *Current Opinions in Oncology* 19, no. 4 (July, 2007): 396-400.

Dassonneville, L., Bonjean, K., De Pauw-Gillet, M-C., Colson, P., Houssier, C., Quetin-Leclercq, J., Bailly, C. (1999). Stimulation of topoisomerase II-mediated DNA cleavage by three DNA-intercalating plant alkaloids: Cryptolepine, Matadine, and Serpentine. *Biochemistry*, 38(24): 7719-7726. http://pubs.acs.org/doi/abs/10.1021/bi990094t

Davies, A. A., Davey Smith, G., Harbord, R., Bekkering, G. E., Sterne, J. A., Beynon, R., & Thomas, S. Nutritional interventions and outcome in patients with cancer or preinvasive lesions: Systematic review. *Journal of the National Cancer Institute*, 98, 961-963. http://www.ncbi.nlm.nih.gov/pubmed/16849679

Davies, H., et al. "Mutations of the *BRAF* Gene in Human Cancer." *Nature* 417 (2002): 949-954. Shaw, Gina. "BRAF Mutations Predict Tumor Response." *Drug Discovery and Development* 8 (2005): 8.

Davis, Carol M., ed. *Complementary Therapies in Rehabilitation*. 2d ed. Thorofare, N.J.: Slack, 2004.

Davis, D. W., R. S. Herbst, and J. L. Abbruzzese. (Eds.). (2007). *Antiangiogenic cancer therapy*. New York: CRC Press.

Davison, K. P., et al. "Who talks? The social psychology of illness support groups." *American Psychologist* 55, no. 2 (February, 2000): 205-217.

de Magalhães, J. P. (2013). How ageing processes influence cancer. *National Reviews Cancer*, 13(5), 357-365. doi: 10.1038/nrc3497.

De Pergola, G., & Silvestris, F. (2013). Obesity as a Major Risk Factor for Cancer. *Journal of Obesity*, 2013, 291546. doi:10.1155/2013/291546

De Vito, Vincent T., Samuel Hellman, and Steven A. Rosenberg, eds. *Cancer: Principles and Practice of Oncology*. Philadelphia: Lippincott Williams and Wilkins, 2005.

De Vos, M., et al. "Novel *PMS2* Pseudogenes Can Conceal Recessive Mutations Causing a Distinctive Childhood Cancer Syndrome." *American Journal of Human Genetics* 74 (2004): 954-964.

DeCava, Judith A. *The Real Truth About Vitamins and Antioxidants*. 2d ed. Fort Collins, Colo.: Selene River Press, 2006.

Deeg, H. J., et al. *Hematologic Malignancies: Myelodysplastic Syndromes*. New York: Springer, 2006.

Definition of Tumor, MedicineNet.com http://www.medicinenet.com/script/main/art.asp?articlekey=14066 http://www.nytimes.com/health/guides/disease/tumor/overview.html

DeGregorio, Michael W., and Valerie J. Wiebe. *Tamoxifen and Breast Cancer*. New Haven, Conn.: Yale University Press. 1996.

Delaini, Gian D., ed. *Rectal Cancer: New Frontiers in Diagnosis, Treatment, and Rehabilitation*. New York: Springer, 2005.

Delamarre, L, Mellman, I. & Yadav, M. (2015). Neo approaches to cancer vaccines. *Science*, 348(6236): 760-761.

DeLaney, Thomas F., and Hanne M. Kooy, eds. *Proton and Charged Particle Radiotherapy*. Philadelphia: Lippincott Williams & Wilkins, 2008.

Delfino, Michelangelo, and Mary E. Day. *We Live and Die by Radiation*. Mountain View, Calif.: MoBeta, 2006.

Della Rocca, Robert, Edward H. Bedrossian, Jr., and Bryan Arthurs, eds. *Ophthalmic Plastic Surgery: Decision Making and Techniques*. New York: McGraw-Hill, 2002.

DeMatteo, R., et al. *One Hundred Questions and Answers About Gastrointestinal Stromal Tumor (GIST)*. Boston: Jones & Bartlett, 2006.

Dembic, Zlatko. (2015). *The cytokines of the immune system.* Waltham, MA: Elsevier.

Deming, S. (2015, August). New gene therapy for bladder cancer shows promise. *OncoLog*, 60(8). https://www.mdanderson.org/publications/oncolog/august-2015/new-gene-therapy-for-bladder-cancer-shows-promise.html

DeMonte, Franco, et al., eds. *Tumors of the Brain and Spine*. New York: Springer, 2007.

Dempsey, Sharon. *My Brain Tumour Adventures: The Story of a Little Boy Coping with a Brain Tumour*. London: Jessica Kingsley, 2003.

DeNelsky, Garland Y. *Stop Smoking Now! The Rewarding Journey to a Smoke-Free Life*. Cleveland, Ohio: Cleveland Clinic Press, 2007.

Dennerstein, Lorraine, Carl Wood, and Ann Westmore. *Hysterectomy: New Options and Advances*. New York: Oxford University Press, 1995.

Dennis, Leslie K., and Deborah Dawson. "Meta-analysis of Measures of Sexual Activity and Prostate Cancer." *Epidemiology* 13, no. 1 (January, 2002): 72-79.

Denniston, Alastair K. O., and Phillip I. Murray. *Oxford Handbook of Ophthalmology*. New York: Oxford University Press, 2006.

Desai R, Collett D, Watson CJ, Johnson P, Evans T, Neuberger J. "Estimated risk of cancer transmission from organ donor to graft recipient in a national transplantation registry." *Br J Surg* 101, no. 7 (June 2014):768-774.

Desai, Sujal R., ed. *Lung Cancer*. New York: Cambridge University Press, 2007.

Detterbeck, F. C. "Clinical Value of the WHO Classification System of Thymoma." *Annals of Thoracic Surgery* 81, no. 6 (June, 2006): 2328-2334.

Deusberg, P., R. Li, A. Fabarius, and R. Hehlmann. "The Chromosomal Basis of Cancer." *Cellular Onocology* 27 (2005): 293-318.

DeVita Jr., V.T., & Chu, E. (2008). A History of Cancer Chemotherapy. *Cancer Research,* 68: 8643-8653. This is a review article discussing the history of chemotherapy to treat different kinds of cancers.

Devita, Vincent T., Jr., Samuel Hellman, and Steven A. Rosenberg, eds. *Cancer: Principles and Practice of Oncology*. 7th ed. Philadelphia: Lippincott Williams & Wilkins, 2005.

DeVita, Vincent T., Jr., Samuel Hellman, and Steven A. Rosenberg, eds. *Cancer: Principles and Practice of Oncology—Pancreatic Cancer*. Philadelphia: Lippincott Williams & Wilkins, 2006.

DeVita, Vincent T., Lawrence, Theodore S., & Rosenberg, Steven A. (Eds.). (2015). *DeVita, Hellman, and Rosenberg's cancer: Principles & practice of oncology* (10th ed.). Philadelphia: Wolters Kluwer.

DeVita, Vincent. T & DeVita-Raeburn, Elizabeth. (2015). *The death of cancer: After fifty years on the front lines of medicine, a pioneering oncologist reveals why the war on cancer is winnable--and how we can get there*. New York: Sarah Crichton Books.

Devoy, A., Soane, T., Welchman, R., & Mayer, R.J. (2005). The ubiquitin-proteasome system and cancer. *Essays in Biochemistry*, 41: 187–203.

Dewar, J. A., R. Arriagada, S. Benhamous, et al. "Local Relapse and Contralateral Tumor Rates in Patients with Breast Cancer Treated with Conservative Surgery and Radiotherapy." *Cancer* 76 (1995): 2260-2265.

Di Lorenzo, G., et al. "Management of AIDS-Related Kaposi's Sarcoma." *Lancet Oncology* 8, no. 2 (February, 2007): 167-176.

Diaconescu R., Flowers C., Storer B., Sorror, M. L., Maris, M. B., Maloney, D. G. Storb, R. (2004). Morbidity and mortality with nonmyeloablative compared with myeloablative conditioning before hematopoietic cell transplantation from HLA-matched related donors. *Blood,* 104(5), 1550-1558.

Diamandis, E. P., et al., eds. *Tumor Markers: Physiology, Pathobiology, Technology, and Clinical Applications*. Washington, D.C.: AACC Press, 2002.

Dias Pereira, A., A. Suspiro, and P. Chaves. "Cancer Risk in Barrett's Oesophagus." *European Journal of Gastroenterology and Hepatology* 19 (2007): 915-918.

Diaz, José I., Linda B. Mora, and Ardeshir Hakam. "The Mainz Classification of Renal Cell Tumors." *Cancer Control: Journal of the Moffitt Cancer Center* 6 (November/December, 1999): 571-579.

Diaz-Montero, C. M., Finke, J., & Montero, A. J. (2014). Myeloid-derived suppressor cells in cancer: Therapeutic, predictive, and prognostic implications. *Seminars in Oncology*, 41(2), 174-184.

Dickman, P. W., and H. O. Adami. "Interpreting Trends in Cancer Patient Survival." *Journal of Internal Medicine* 260, no. 2 (August, 2006): 103-117.

Diefenbach, Russell J., & Fraefel, Cornel. (Eds.). (2014). *Herpes simplex virus: Methods and protocols (Methods in molecular biology) 2014 Edition*. New York: Humana Press.

Dietel, M., ed. *Targeted Therapies in Cancer*. New York: Springer, 2007.

Dimitrov, L., Hong, C. S., Yang, C., Zhuang, Z., & Heiss, J. D. (2015). New developments in the pathogenesis and therapeutic targeting of the IDH1 mutation in glioma. *International Journal of Medical Sciences*, 12(3): 201-213.

Dinerello, Charles A., and Jeffrey A. Gelfand. "Fever and Hyperthermia." In *Harrison's Principles of Internal Medicine*, edited by Dennis L. Kasper et al. 16th ed. New York: McGraw-Hill, 2005.

"Disorders of the Oral Region: Neoplasms." In *The Merck Manual of Diagnosis and Therapy*, edited by Mark H. Beers and Robert Berkow. 17th ed. Whitehouse Station, N.Y.: Merck Research Laboratories, 1999.

Dixon, Danielle. (2014). *Cervical cancer causes, symptoms, stages & treatment guide: Cure cervical cancer with a positive outlook.* Seattle, WA: Amazon Digital Services.

Dizon, Don S. *One Hundred Questions and Answers About* Ovarian Cancer. 2d ed. Sudbury, Mass.: Jones and Bartlett, 2006.

Dodd, Marilyn J. *Managing the Side Effects of Chemotherapy and Radiation*. 2d ed. San Francisco: Regents University of California School of Nursing, 2001.

Doheny, K. (2015).Coffee May Lower Endometrial Cancer Risk. *WebMD News from Health Day.* http://www.webmd.com/cancer/news/20150206/coffee-linked-to-possible-lower-endometrial-cancer-risk

Doherty, Gerard M., and Lawrence W. Way, eds. *Current Surgical Diagnosis and Treatment*. 12th ed. New York: Lange Medical Books/McGraw-Hill, 2006.

Dokmanovic, M., Clarke, C., & Marks, P. A. (2007). Histone deacetylase inhibitors: Overview and perspectives. *Molecular Cancer Research*, 5: 981-989. http://mcr.aacrjournals.org/content/5/10/981.full

Dollinger, Malin, Ernest H. Rosenbaum, and Greg Cable. *Cancer Therapy*. Kansas City: Andrews and McMeel, 1994.

Dollinger, M., et al. *Everyone's Guide to Cancer Therapy: How Cancer Is Diagnosed, Treated, and Managed Day to Day*. 4th ed. Kansas City, Mo.: Andre McMell, 2002.

Dollinger, Malin, et al. *Everyone's Guide to Cancer Therapy*. 4th rev. ed. Kansas City, Mo.: Andrews & McMeel, 2002.

Domalpally A., Ip, M. S., & Ehrlich, J. S. (2015). Effects of intravitreal ranibizumab on retinal hard exudate in diabetic macular edema: Findings from the RIDE and RISE phase III clinical trials. *Ophthalmology,* 122(4): 779-86.

Dombret, H., & Gardin, C. (2016). An update of current treatments for adult acute myeloid leukemia. *Blood,* 127(1):53-61. Treatment guidelines for AML in adults patients.

Dominik, D., et al. "Multiple Myeloma: A Review of the Epidemiologic Literature." *International Journal of Cancer* 120, suppl. 12 (2007): 40-61.

Dong, S.T., Butow, P.N., Tong, A., Agar, M., Boyle, F., Forster … Lovell, M.R. (2016). *Support Care Cancer,* 24: 1374-1386. doi: 10.1107/s00520-015-2913-4.

Donnerer, Josef, ed. *Antiemetic Therapy*. New York: Karger, 2003.

Donnez, Jacques, ed. *Atlas of Operative Laparoscopy and Hysteroscopy*. 3rd ed. New York: Informa Healthcare, 2007.

Dores, G. M., T. R. Coté, and L. B. Travis. "New Malignancies Following Hodgkin Lymphoma, Non-Hodgkin Lymphoma, and Myeloma." In *New Malignancies Among Cancer Survivors: SEER Cancer Registries, 1973-2000*, edited by R. E. Curtis et al. NIH Publication 05-5302. Bethesda, Md.: National Cancer Institute, 2006.

Dorgan, J. F., et al. "Serum Hormones and the Alcohol-Breast Cancer Association in Postmenopausal Women." *Journal of the National Cancer Institute* 93 (2001): 710-715.

Dotinga, R. (2014, April 16). Cancer "vaccine" for advanced disease passes early hurdle. *Health Day Reporter.* Retrieved from http://consumer.healthday.com/cancer-information-5/mis-cancer-news-102/cancer-vaccine-for-advanced-disease-passes-early-hurdle-686863.html

Downing, Robin. *Pets Living with Cancer: A Pet Owner's Resource*. Lakewood, Colo.: AAHA, 2000.

Dreifus, C. (2014, March 3). Arming the immune system against cancer. *The New York Times*, pp. D2. Retrieved from http://www.nytimes.com/2015/03/03/science/arming-the-immune-system-against-cancer.html

Drop, A., et al. "The Modern Methods of Gastric Imaging." *Annales Universitatis Mariae Curie-Skuodowska* 59, no. 1 (2004): 373-381.

Drug Facts and Comparisons 2008. 62d ed. St. Louis: Wolters Kluwer Health, 2008.

Du Vivier, Anthony, and Phillip H. McKee. *Atlas of Clinical Dermatology*. 3rd ed. Edinburgh: Churchill Livingston, 2002.

Duffy, Jim. "Cancer Clusters." *Ecologist* 37, no. 5 (June, 2007): 9-18.

Dummer, R. "Future Perspectives in the Treatment of Cutaneous T-cell Lymphoma (CTCL)." *Seminars in Oncology* 33, no. 1 (2006): S33-S36.

Dunetz, Gary N. *Bladder Cancer: A Resource Guide for Patients and Their Families*. Bloomington, Ind.: AuthorHouse, 2006.

Dunn, Jancie. "Toxic Overload: Teflon, Pesticides on Golf Courses, Plastic Bottles—An Explosion of Research Is Investigating Environmental Links and Breast Cancer." *Vogue*, October, 2006, 326ff.

Dupuis, M. J. M., and C. Verellen-Dumoulin. "Gastrointestinal Polyposis and Nonpolyposis Syndromes." *New England Journal of Medicine* 332 (1995): 1518.

Duran, Eduardo. *Healing the Soul Wound: Counseling with American Indians and Other Native Peoples*. New York: Teachers College Press, 2006.

Duwe, Beau V., Daniel H. Sterman, and Ali I. Musani. "Tumors of the Mediastinum." *Chest* 128 (2005): 2893-2909.

Dwyer, J. W., L. L. Clarke, and M. K. Miller. "The Effect of Religious Concentration and Affiliation on County Cancer Mortality Rates." *Journal of Health and Social Behavior* 31 (1990): 185-202.

Dynlacht, B. (1997). Regulation of transcription by proteins that control the cell cycle. *Nature,* 389(6647):149-152.

Eapen M., Klein J., Ruggeri A., Spellman S., Lee, S. J., Anasetti, C., … Center for International Blood and Marrow Transplant Research, Netcord, Eurocord, and the European Group for Blood and Marrow Transplantation. (2014). Impact of allele-level HLA matching on outcomes after myeloablative single unit umbilical cord Blood transplantation for hematologic malignancy. *Blood,* 123(1), 133-140.

Eaton, D. L., and J. D. Groopman. *The Toxicology of Aflatoxins*. New York: Academic Press, 1994.

Eble, John N., Guido Sauter, Jonathan Epstein, and Isabell Sesterhenn, eds. *Pathology and Genetics of Tumours of the Urinary System and Male Genital Organs*. Vol. 7 in *World Health Organization Classification of Tumours*. Lyon, England: International Agency for Research on Cancer Press, 2003.

Eckardt, John R., and Julia E. Kimmis. *Understanding Lung Cancer: A Guide for Patients and Their Families*. Manhasset, N.Y.: CMP Healthcare Media, 2005.

Eckman, Margaret & Labus, Diana. (Eds.). (2008). Clinical pharmacology made incredibly easy (3rd ed.). Philadelphia: Lippincott Williams & Wilkins. This book provides clear descriptions of mechanisms of action of drugs and their interactions in treatment and disease.

Edlick, R. F., et al. "Advances in Breast Reconstruction After Mastectomy." *Journal of Long-Term Effects of Medical Implants* 15 (2005): 197-207.

Edmonds, C. V., G. A. Lockwood, and A. J. Cunningham. "Psychological Response to Long-Term Group Therapy: A Randomized Trial with Metastatic Breast Cancer Patients." *Psycho-oncology* 8 (1999): 74-91.

Egan, Conleth A., et al. "Anti-Epiligrin Cicatricial Pemphigoid and Relative Risk for Cancer." *The Lancet* 357, no. 9271 (June 9, 2001): 1850.

Egan, Tracie. *Skin Cancer: Current and Emerging Trends in Detection and Treatment*. New York: Rosen Publishing Group, 2006.

Egger, Gerda & Arimondo, Paola. (Eds.). (2016). *Drug discovery in cancer epigenetics*. Waltham, MA: Academic Press.

Ehrlich, Melanie. (12 August 2002). Review of: DNA Methylation in Cancer: Too Much, But Also Too Little. *Oncogene*, 21(35), 5400-5413.

Eiser, Christine. *Children with Cancer: The Quality of Life*. Mahwah, N.J.: Lawrence Erlbaum Associates, 2004.

Eldredge, Debra M., and Margaret H. Bonham. *Cancer and Your Pet: The Complete Guide to the Latest Research, Treatments, and Options*. Sterling, Va.: Capital Books, 2005.

Eli Lilly and Company. *The New York Times*. Retrieved from http://topics.nytimes.com/top/news/business/companies/lilly_eli_and_company/index.html

Elliott, Frederick C. *The Birth of the Texas Medical Center: A Personal Account*. College Station: Texas A&M University Press, 2004.

Elliott, Laura, Laura L. Molseed, and Paula Davis McCallum, eds. *The Clinical Guide to Oncology Nutrition*. 2d ed. Chicago: American Dietetic Association, 2006.

Ellis, Lee M., et al. *Radiofrequency Ablation for Cancer: Current Indication, Techniques, and Outcomes*. New York: Springer, 2003.

Ellis, Neal C., ed. *Inherited Cancer Syndromes: Current Clinical Management*. New York: Springer, 2003.

Ellis, T. L., V. W. Stieber, and R. C. Austin. "Oligodendroglioma." *Current Treatment Options in Oncology* 4, no. 6 (2003): 479-490.

Ellsworth, Pamela. *One Hundred Questions and Answers About Bladder Cancer*. Sudbury, Mass.: Jones & Bartlett, 2005.

Ellsworth, Pamela, and Anthony Caldamone. *The Little Black Book of Urology*. Sudbury, Mass.: Jones and Bartlett, 2007.

Ellsworth, Pamela, and Brett Carswell. *One Hundred Questions and Answers About Bladder Cancer*. Sudbury, Mass.: Jones and Bartlett, 2006.

Ellsworth, Pamela, John Heaney, and Cliff Gill. *One Hundred Questions and Answers About Prostate Cancer*. Sudbury, Mass.: Jones & Bartlett, 2003.

Elmore, S. (2007). Apoptosis: A review of programmed cell death. *Toxicologic Pathology*, 35(4): 495-516.

Emili, Andrew & Wodak, Shoshana. (Eds.). (2014). *Systems analysis of chromatin related protein complexes in cancer.* New York: Springer Science-Business Media.

Enders, G. (2010). *Cell cycle deregulation in cancer.* New York: Springer.

Engelsen, I. B., et al. "Pathologic Expression of *p53* or *p16* in Preoperative Curettage Specimens Identifies High-Risk Endometrial Carcinomas." *American Journal of Obstetrics and Gynecology* 195, no. 4 (October, 2006): 979-986.

Ennis, Don G. (2001). Mutagenesis. Encyclopedia of life sciences. Retrieved on February 15, 2016 from http://www.els.net/WileyCDA/ELSarticle/refid-a0000559.html. This author describes the different types of mutations.

EPA; Progress Cleaning the Air and Improving People's Health (2015). http://www.epa.gov/clean-air-act-overview/progress-cleaning-air-and-improving-peoples-health#pollution

Epstein, Samuel S. *Cancer-Gate: How to Win the Losing Cancer War*. Amityville, N.Y.: Baywood, 2005.

Ercan, S., et al. "Does Esophagogastric Anastomic Technique Influence the Outcome of Patients with Esophageal Cancer?" *Journal of Thoracic and Cardiovascular Surgery* 129 (2005): 623-631.

Erickson, V. S., et al. "Arm Edema in Breast Cancer Patients." *Journal of the National Cancer Institute* 93, no. 2 (January 17, 2001): 96-111.

Ersoy, O., B. Sivri, and Y. Bayraktar. "How Helpful Is Capsule Endoscopy to Surgeons?" *World Journal of Gastroenterology* 13, no. 27 (July 21, 2007): 3671-3676.

Esposito, N. N., et al. "Phyllodes Tumor: A Clinicopathologic and Immunohistochemical Study of Thirty Cases." *Archives of Pathology and Laboratory Medicine* 130, no. 10 (2006): 1516-1521.

Estala, E. M. "Proposed Screening Recommendations for Male Breast Cancer." *The Nurse Practitioner* 31, no. 2 (2006): 62-63.

Etkin, Nina L. (2008). *Edible Medicines: An Ethnopharmacology of Food.* Tucson, Arizona: University of Arizona Press. This book discusses the use of food as medicines, including the historical uses of medicinal plants.

Ettinger, Stephen J., and Edward C. Feldman. "Section X: Cancer." In *Textbook of Veterinary Internal Medicine.* 6th ed. Philadelphia: Elsevier, 2005.

Etzioni, D. A., et al. "Measuring the Quality of Colorectal Cancer Screening: The Importance of Follow-Up." *Diseases of the Colon and Rectum* 49, no. 7 (July, 2006): 1002-1010.

Evans, A., & Blum, Kristie A. (Eds.). (2015). *Non-Hodgkin Lymphoma: Pathology, Imaging, and Current Therapy* (Cancer Treatment and Research). New York: Springer.

Even-Sapir, E. "Imaging of Malignant Bone Involvement by Morphologic, Scintigraphic, and Hybrid Modalities." *Journal of Nuclear Medicine* 46, no. 8 (2005): 1356-1367.

Eyre, Harmon, and Dianne Partie Lange, eds. *Informed Decisions: The Complete Book of Cancer Diagnosis, Treatment, and Recovery.* 2d ed. Atlanta: American Cancer Society, 2002.

_______, et al., eds. *Informed Decisions: The Complete Book of Cancer Diagnosis, Treatment, and Recovery.* 2d ed. Atlanta, Ga.: American Cancer Society, 2002.

Ezzo, J. M., M. A. Richardson, and A. Vickers. "Acupuncture Point Stimulation for Chemotherapy-Induced Nausea or Vomiting." *The Cochrane Database of Systematic Reviews* 2 (2007).

Ezzone, Susan, & Schmit-Pokorny, Kim. (Eds.). (2007). *Blood and marrow stem cell transplantation: Principles, practices, and nursing insights.* Sudbury, MA: Jones and Bartlett. An encyclopedic treatment of stem cell transplants for blood-based cancers and diseases.

Fabbro, Doriano, and Frank McCormick, eds. *Protein Tyrosine Kinases: From Inhibitors to Useful Drugs.* Totowa, N.J.: Humana Press, 2006.

"Facts About Cancer." In *American Medical Association Family Medical Guide.* 4th ed. Hoboken, N.J.: John Wiley, 2004.

Faden, R. R., and T. L. Beauchamp. *A History and Theory of Informed Consent.* New York: Oxford University Press, 1986.

Fader, A. N., and R. G. Rose. "Role of Surgery in Ovarian Carcinoma." *Journal of Clinical Oncology* 25, no. 20 (July 10, 2007): 2873-2883.

Faguet, G. B. *Chronic Lymphocytic Leukemia: Molecular Genetics, Biology, Diagnosis, and Management.* Totowa, N.J.: Humana Press, 2003.

Faigel, Douglas O., and David R. Cave, eds. *Capsule Endoscopy.* Philadelphia: Saunders Elsevier, 2008.

Faigel, D. O., et al. "Quality Indicators for Gastrointestinal Endoscopic Procedures: An Introduction." *American Journal of Gastroenterology* 101 (2006): 866-872.

Falker, E. S. *The Ultimate Insider's Guide to Adoption: Everything You Need to Know About Domestic and International Adoption.* New York: Hachette USA, 2006.

Farhadi, J., et al. "Reconstruction of the Nipple-Areola Complex: An Update." *Journal of Plastic, Reconstructive & Aesthetic Surgery* 59 (2006): 40-53.

Fast Stats Deaths: Final Data for 2013 Table 10. Centers for Disease Control and Prevention. Retrieved from http://www.cdc.gov/nchs/data/nvsr/nvsr64/nvsr64_02.pdf

Fauce, S. R., Jamieson, B. D., Chin, A. C., Mitsuyasu, R. T., Parish, S. T., Ng, S. T., … Effros, R. B. (2008). Telomerase-based pharmacologic enhancement of antiviral function of human CD8+ T lymphocytes." *Journal of Immunology* 181(10): 7400-7406.

Fauci, A., et al., eds. *Harrison's Principles of Internal Medicine.* New York: McGraw-Hill Health, 1998.

Fawzy, F. I., N. W. Fawzy, L. A. Arndt, and R. O. Pasnau. "Critical Review of Psychosocial Interventions in Cancer Care." *Archives of General Psychiatry* 52 (1995): 100-113.

Fazekas de St. Groth, B. "DCs and Peripheral T Cell Tolerance." *Seminars in Immunology* 13, no. 5 (2001): 311-322.

FDA Sheds Light Sunscreens. U.S. Food and Drug Administration. Retrieved from http://www.fda.gov/ForConsumers/ConsumerUpdates/ucm258416.htm

FDA. (2010). Trastuzumab (Herceptin) prescribing information. Retrieved from http://www.accessdata.fda.gov/drugsatfda_docs/label/2010/103792s5250lbl.pdf

Fearon, Kenneth C., Anne C. Voss, and Deborah S. Hustead. "Definition of Cancer Cachexia: Effect of Weight Loss, Reduced Food Intake, and Systemic Inflammation on Functional Status and Prognosis." *American*

Journal of Clinical Nutrition 83, no. 6 (June, 2006): 1345-1350.

Feigal, Ellen, et al., eds. *AIDS-Related Cancers and Their Treatment*. New York: Marcel Dekker, 2000.

Fein, Alan, et al. *Diagnosis and Management of Pneumonia and Other Respiratory Infections*. Caddo, Okla.: Professional Communications, 1999.

Fekrat, Sharon, and Jennifer S. Weizer, eds. *All About Your Eyes*. Durham, N.C.: Duke University Press, 2006.

Feld, Stanley. *AACE Clinical Practice Guidelines for the Diagnosis and Management of Thyroid Nodules*. New York: American Association of Clinical Endocrinologists, 1996.

Fentiman, I. S., and H. Hamed. "Breast Reconstruction." *International Journal of Clinical Practice* 60 (2006): 471-474.

Fenton, J. J., et al. "Specificity of Clinical Breast Examination in Community Practice." *Society of General Internal Medicine* 22 (January 9, 2007): 332-337.

Fenton, J. J., et al. "Delivery of Cancer Screening: How Important Is the Preventive Health Examination?" *Archives of Internal Medicine* 167, no. 6 (March 26, 2007): 580-585.

Ferner, R. E. "Neurofibromatosis 1." *European Journal of Human Genetics*. 15 (2007): 131-138.

Ferrandon, S., Malleval, C., El Hamdani, B., Battiston-Montagne, P., Bolbos, R., Langlois. J-P., … Poncet, D. (2015). Telomerase inhibition improves tumor response to radiotherapy in a murine orthotopic model of human glioblastoma. *Molecular Cancer*, 14: 134.

Ferrer, Jaume. "Predictors of Pleural Malignancy in Patients with Pleural Effusion Undergoing Thoracoscopy." *Chest* 127 (2005): 1017-1022.

Ferreri, A. J., et al. "Therapeutic Management of Ocular Adnexal MALT Lymphoma." *Expert Opinion on Pharmacotherapy* 8, no. 8 (June, 2007): 1073-1083.

Feuerstein, Michael, and Patricia Findley. *The Cancer Survivor's Guide: The Essential Handbook to Life After Cancer*. New York: Marlowe, 2006.

Field, Michael, ed. *Diarrheal Diseases*. New York: Elsevier, 1991.

Field, S. S. Shanley, and J. Kirk. "Inherited Cancer Susceptibility Syndromes in Paediatric Practice." *Journal of Paediatrics and Child Health* 43, no. 4 (April, 2007): 219-229.

Figg, William, & Folkman, Judah. (Eds.). (2008). *Angiogenesis: An Integrative Approach from Science to Medicine*. New York: Springer.

Figlin, Robert A., ed. *Kidney Cancer*. Boston: Kluwer Academic, 2003.

Filippakopoulos, Panagis. (2012). "Histone recognition and large-scale structural analysis of the human bromodomain family." *Cell* 149(1): 214-231.

Fincannon, Joy L., and Katherine V. Bruss. *Couples Confronting Cancer: Keeping Your Relationship Strong*. Atlanta: American Cancer Society, 2003.

Finkel, Madelon L. *Understanding the Mammography Controversy: Science, Politics, and Breast Cancer Screening*. Westport, Conn.: Praeger, 2005.

Finlay, I. & Capel, M. (2010). Palliative medicine for the elderly patient. In H. Fillet, K. Rockwood, & K. Woodhouse (Eds.), *Brocklehurst's Textbook of Medicine and Gerontology,* 7th edition (pp. 973-982). Philadelphia: Saunders Elsevier.

Finn, Olivera J. "Cancer Vaccines: Between the Idea and the Reality." *Nature Reviews Immunology* 3, no. 8 (August, 2003): 630-641.

Finn, O. J. (2012). Immuno-oncology: Understanding the function and dysfunction of the immune system in cancer. *Annals of Oncology* 23(suppl 8): iiv6-iiv9. http://annonc.oxfordjournals.org/content/23/suppl_8/viii6.full

Finn, William G., and LoAnn C. Peterson, eds. *Hematopathology in Oncology*. Boston: Kluwer Academic, 2004.

Fiore, Neil. *The Road Back to Health: Coping with the Emotional Aspects of Cancer*. Berkeley, Calif.: Celestial Arts, 1990.

Firat, Y., A. Kizilay, G. Sogutlu, and B. Mizrak. "Primary Mucosa-Associated Lymphoid Tissue Lymphoma of Hypopharynx." *Journal of Craniofacial Surgery* 18, no. 5 (September, 2007): 1189-1193.

Firmin, M. W., Pathammavong, M. B., Johnson, C. B., & Trudel, J. F. (2013). Anxiety experienced by individuals with cancer in remission. *Psychology, Health & Medicine*, 19(2): 153-158.

Fisch, Michael J., and Allen W. Burton, eds. *Cancer Pain Management*. New York: McGraw-Hill, 2007.

Fischbach, Frances Talaska, and Marshall Barnett Dunning III. *A Manual of Laboratory and Diagnostic Tests*. 7th ed. Philadelphia: Lippincott Williams & Wilkins, 2004.

Fischer, David S., et al. *The Cancer Chemotherapy Handbook*. 6th ed. St. Louis: Mosby, 2003.

Fisher, Stephen. *Colon Cancer and the Polyps Connection*. Tuscon, Ariz.: Fisher Books, 1995.

Fizazi, Karim, ed. *Carcinoma of an Unknown Primary Site*. New York: Taylor & Francis, 2006.

Flaxseeds and breast cancer. *Oncology Nutrition*. Retrieved from https://www.oncologynutrition.org/erfc/hot-topics/flaxseeds-and-breast-cancer/

Fleming, M., Ravula, S., Tatishchev, S. F., & Wang, H. L. (2012). Colorectal carcinoma: Pathologic aspects. *Journal of Gastrointestinal Oncology,* 3(3), 153–173. http://doi.org/10.3978/j.issn.2078-6891.2012.030

Fleury, I., Chevret, S., Pfreunschuh, M., Salles, G., Coiffer, B., van Oers, M., … Thieblemont, C. (2015). Rituximab and risk of second primary malignancies in patients with non-Hodgkin lymphoma: A systematic review and meta-analysis. *Annals of Oncology*, doi: 10.1093/annonc/mdv616.

Florescu, Maria, et al. (2013) Chemotherapy-induced cardiotoxicity. Maedica (Buchar). 2013; 8(1): 59-67. http://www.ncbi.nlm.nih.gov/pmc/articles/PMC3749765

Foley, John R., Julie M. Vose, and James O. Armitage. *Current Therapy in Cancer*. Philadelphia: W. B. Saunders, 1994.

Foley, K. M., et al. *When the Focus Is on Care: Palliative Care and Cancer*. Atlanta: American Cancer Society, 2005.

Folkman, J. (1971). Tumor angiogenesis: Therapeutic implications. *New England Journal of Medicine*, 285: 1182-1186.

Forough, Reza. (Ed.). (2006). *New Frontiers in Angiogenesis*. Dordrecht, The Netherlands: Springer.

FORTUNE magazine. (2005). *Genentech, FORTUNE magazine, 100 Best Companies to Work For 2015*. http://fortune.com/best-companies/genentech-9

Fossel, Michael B. *Cells, Aging, and Human Disease*. New York: Oxford University Press, 2004.

Fossel, Michael B. *Cells, Aging, and Human Disease*. Oxford, England: Oxford University Press, 2004.

Foulkes, William D., and Shirley V. Hodgson, eds. *Inherited Susceptibility to Cancer: Clinical, Predictive, and Ethical Perspectives*. New York: Cambridge University Press, 1998.

Fox, R. I., & Fox, C. M. (Eds.) (2011). *Sjögren's syndrome: Practical guidelines to diagnosis and therapy.* Springer Publishing Company: New York.

Fox, Stuart I. *Human Physiology*. 10th ed. New York: McGraw-Hill, 2007.

Frank, Eugene D., Bruce W. Long, and Barbara J. Smith. *Merrill's Atlas of Radiographic Positions and Radiologic Procedures*. 11th ed. St. Louis: Mosby/Elsevier, 2007.

Frank, Thomas S., and Mark H. Skolnick. "Testing for Hereditary Cancer Risk: Pandora or Prometheus?" *Journal of Clinical Endocrinology and Metabolism* 84, no. 6 (1999): 1882-1885.

Frankel, David H., ed. *Field Guide to Clinical Dermatology*. Philadelphia: Lippincott Williams & Wilkins, 2006.

Freedman, Jeri. *Lymphoma: Current and Emerging Trends in Detection and Treatment*. New York: Rosen, 2006.

Frei, Balz, ed. *Natural Antioxidants in Human Health and Disease*. San Diego, Calif.: Academic Press, 2006.

Frequently Asked Questions About Genetic Counseling. National Institutes of Health (NIH): National Human Genome Research Institute. Retrieved from http://www.genome.gov/19016905

Friberg, S,, & Mattson, S. (1997), On the growth rates of human malignant tumors: Implications for medical decision making. *Journal of Surgical Oncology,* 65(4), 284-97.

Friedberg, Errol, et al. *DNA Repair and Mutagenesis*. Washington, DC: ASM Press, 2006.

Friedenson Bernard. "The BRCA1/2 pathway prevents hematologic cancers in addition to breast and ovarian cancers." *BMC Cancer*. 2007;7:152. doi:10.1186/1471-2407-7-152.

Friedman, L. M., Furberg, C. D., DeMets, D. L., Roboussin, D. M., & Granger, C. B. (2015). *Fundamentals of clinical trials* (5th ed.). New York, NY: Springer.

Friedman, P. J., A. A. Liebow, and J. Sokoloff. "Eosinophilic Granuloma of Lung: Clinical Aspects of Primary Pulmonary Histiocytosis in the Adult." *Medicine* 60 (1981): 385.

Frohnmayer, Lynn. *Fanconi Anemia: A Handbook for Families and Their Physicians*. Eugene, Oreg.: Fanconi Anemia Research Fund, 2000.

Fromer, Margot Joan. (1998). *Surviving childhood cancer: A guide for families*. Oakland, CA: New Harbinger.

Frost, Floyd J. *Cancer Risks Associated with Elevated Levels of Drinking Water Arsenic Exposure*. Washington, D.C.: AWWA Research Foundation and U.S. Environmental Protection Agency, 2004.

Fu, M. R. "Breast Cancer Survivors' Intentions of Managing Lymphedema." *Cancer Nursing* 28, no. 6 (2005): 446-457.

Fuller, Arlan F., Jr., Robert H. Young, and Michael V. Seiden. *Uterine Cancer*. Hamilton, Ont.: BC Decker, 2004.

Fung-Kee-Fung, M., et al. "Follow-Up After Primary Therapy for Endometrial Cancer: A Systematic Review." *Gynecologic Oncology* 101, no. 3 (June, 2006): 520-529.

Gabrilovich, D. I., & Nagaraj, S. (2009). Myeloid-derived suppressor cells as regulators of the immune system. *Nature Reviews Immunology*, 9(3), 162-174.

Gaillard, Rolf C., ed. *The ACTH Axis: Pathogenesis, Diagnosis, and Treatment*. New York: Springer, 2003.

Galateau-Sallé, Françoise, ed. *Pathology of Malignant Mesothelioma*. London: Springer, 2006.

Gallagher, R. P., J. J. Spinelli, and T. K. Lee. "Tanning Beds, Sunlamps, and Risk of Cutaneous Malignant Melanoma." *Cancer Epidemiology Biomarkers and Pre*vention 14, no. 3 (2005): 562-566.

Gallegos-Hernández, José-Francisco, et al. "The Number of Sentinel Nodes Identified as Prognostic Factor in Oral Epidermoid Cancer." *Oral Oncology* 41, no. 9 (October, 2005): 947-952.

Galloway, D. "Treating Patients with Cancer Requires Looking Beyond the Tumor." *OncoLog* 49, nos. 7/8 (July/August, 2004).

Gallus, S., et al. "Artificial Sweeteners and Cancer Risk in a Network of Case-Control Studies." *Annals of Oncology* 18, no. 1 (January, 2007): 40-44.

Galvin, Jan C., and Scherer Marcia J., eds. *Evaluating, Selecting, and Using Appropriate Assistive Technology*. Austin, Tex.: Pro-Ed, 2004.

Gandini, S., H. Merzenich, C. Robertson, and P. Boyle. "Meta-analysis of Studies on Breast Cancer Risk and Diet: The Role of Fruit and Vegetable Consumption and the Intake of Associated Micronutrients." *European Journal of Cancer* 36 (March, 1990).

Ganschow, Pamela, et al., eds. *Breast Health and Common Breast Problems: A Practical Approach*. Philadelphia: American College of Physicans, 2004.

Garber, K. "Energy Boost: The Warburg Effect Returns in a New Theory of Cancer." *Journal of the National Cancer Institute* 96, no. 24 (2004): 1805-1806.

_______. "Energy Deregulation: Licensing Tumors to Grow." *Science* 312 (2006): 1158-1159.

Garcia-Manero, G. (2015). Myelodysplastic syndromes: 2015 update on diagnosis, risk-stratification and management. *American Journal of Hematology*, 90(9): 831-841.

Gardner, E. J. "A Genetic and Clinical Study of Intestinal Polyposis, a Predisposing Factor for Carcinoma of the Colon and Rectum." *American Journal of Human Genetics* 3, no. 2 (June, 1951): 167-176.

Garner, John C. *Health Insurance Answer Book*. 7th ed. New York: Aspen, 2006.

Garrè, M. L., and A. Cama. "Craniopharyngioma: Modern Concepts in Pathogenesis and Treatment." *Current Opinions in Pediatrics* 19 (2007): 471-479.

Garrett, Andrea, and Michael A. Quinn. "Hormonal Therapies and Gynaecological Cancers." *Best Practice & Research Clinical Obstetrics & Gynaecology* 22, no. 2 (April, 2008): 407-421.

Garrison, Kevin S. *It's Just a Matter of Balance*. Baltimore: Gateway Press, 2005.

Gatchel, Robert, and Mark Ooordt. *Clinical Health Psychology and Primary Care*. Washington, D.C.: American Psychological Association, 2003.

Gatrell, A. C. *Geographies of Health: An Introduction*. Malden, Mass.: Blackwell, 2002.

Gaynor, Mitchell L. *The Healing Power of Sound: Recovery from Illness by Using Sound, Voice, and Music*. Boulder, Colo.: Shambhala, 2002.

Geiger, Brian F., et al. "Using Technology to Teach Health: A Collaborative Pilot Project in Alabama." *Journal of School Health* 72, no. 10 (December, 2002): 401-407.

Geisinger, K. R., et al. "Soft-Tissue Sarcoma." *New England Journal of Medicine* 353 (2005): 2303-2304.

Genden, Eric M., and Mark A. Varvares, eds. *Head and Neck Cancer: An Evidence-Based Team Approach*. New York: Thieme, 2008.

Genentech. (2015). The 2015 Genentech oncology trend report: Perspectives from managed care, specialty pharmacies, oncologists, practice managers, and employers. 7th ed. South San Francisco, CA: Genentech. https://www.genentech-forum.com/content/dam/gene/managedcare/forum/pdfs/Oncology-Trends/2015-genentech-oncology-trend-report.pdf

Genetic Consultation. National Library of Medicine. Retrieved from http://ghr.nlm.nih.gov/handbook/consult

Genetic Counseling. (2009). *Understanding Genetics: A New York, Mid-Atlantic Guide for Patients and Health Professionals*. Genetic Alliance; The New York-Mid-Atlantic Consortium for Genetic and Newborn Screening Services. Washington (DC): Genetic Alliance. Retrieved from http://www.ncbi.nlm.nih.gov/books/NBK115552/

George, Andrew J. T., and Catherine E. Urch, eds. *Diagnostic and Therapeutic Antibodies*. Totowa, N.J.: Humana Press, 2000.

Gerald, K., Iwasa, J., & Marshall, W. (2015). *Karp's cell and molecular biology* (8th ed.). New York City, NY: John Wiley.

Getz, K., & Borfitz, D. (2002). *Informed consent: The consumer's guide to the risks and benefits of volunteering for clinical trials*. Boston, MA: CenterWatch.

Ghert, M. A., et al. "The Surgical and Functional Outcome of Limb-Salvage Surgery with Vascular Reconstruction for Soft-Tissue Sarcoma of the Extremity." *Annals of Surgical Oncology* 12 (2005): 1102-1110.

Gierisch, J.M., Coeytaux, R.R., Urrutia, R.P., Havrilesky, L. J., Moorman, P. G., Lowery, W. J., … Myers, E. R. (2013). Oral contraceptive use and risk of breast, cervical, colorectal, and endometrial cancers: A systematic review. *Cancer Epidemiology, Biomarkers & Prevention*, 22: 1931-1943.

Gil, F., Costa, G., Hilker, I., & Benito, L. (2012). First anxiety, afterwards depression: Psychological distress in cancer patients at diagnosis and after medical treatment. *Stress and Health*, 28: 362-367.

Gilbar, Ora, and Hasida Ben-Zur. *Cancer and the Family Caregiver: Distress and Coping*. Springfield, Ill.: Charles C Thomas, 2002.

Gilbert, S. G. *A Small Dose of Toxicology: The Health Effects of Common Chemicals*. Boca Raton, Fla.: CRC Press, 2004.

Giller, C. A. "The Neurosurgical Treatment of Pain." *Archives of Neurology* 60 (2003): 1537-1540.

Gilligan, David, and Robert Rintoul. *Your Guide to Lung Cancer*. London: Hodder Arnold, 2007.

Ginès, Pere, et al., eds. *Ascites and Renal Dysfunction in Liver Disease: Pathogenesis, Diagnosis, and Treatment*. 2d ed. Malden, Mass.: Blackwell Publishing, 2005.

Gingerich, Barbara Stover, and Deborah Anne Ondeck, eds. *Clinical Pathways for the Multidisciplinary Home Care Team*. Gaithersburg, Md.: Aspen, 1997.

Ginsberg, Gregory, et al. *Clinical Gastrointestinal Endoscopy*. Philadelphia: Elsevier Saunders, 2005.

Girardi, M., P. W. Heald, and L. D. Wilson. "The Pathogenesis of Mycosis Fungoides." *The New England Journal of Medicine* 350, no. 19 (2004): 1978-1988.

Gislason, Stephen J. *Food and Digestive Disorders: Irritable Bowel Syndrome, Crohn's Disease, Celiac Disease, Ulcerative Colitis, Ulcers, Reflux and Motility Disorders*. Sechelt, B.C.: Environmed Research, 2003.

Giulano, A., D. M. Kirgan, J. M. Guenther, et al. "Lymphatic Mapping and Sentinel Lymphadenectomy for Breast Cancer." *Annals of Surgery* 220 (1994): 439-442.

Giusti, F., Marini, F., & Luisa Brandi, M. (2015). Multiple endocrine neoplasia I. In R. A. Pagon, M. P. Adam, H. H. Ardinger, S. E. Wallace, A. Amemiya, L. J. H. Bean, T. D. Bird, C-T. Fong, H. C. Mefford, R. J. H. Smith, & K. Stephens (Eds.), *Gene reviews*. Seattle, WA: University of Washington. Available from: http://www.ncbi.nlm.nih.gov/books/NBK1538/

Givan, Alice Longobardi. *Flow Cytometry: First Principles*. 2d ed. New York: Wiley-Liss, 2001.

Goldberg, A.L., Elledge, S.J. & Harper, J.W. (2001). The cellular chamber of doom. *Scientific American*, 284(1): 56–61.

Goldblatt, L., ed. *Aflatoxin: Scientific Background, Control, and Implications*. New York: Academic Press, 1969.

Goldblum, John R., Folpe, Andrew L., & Weiss, Sharon W. (2014). *Enzinger and Weiss's soft-tissue tumors* (6th ed.). Philadelphia: Elsevier Saunders.

Goldman, Larry, Thomas Wise, and David Brody. *Psychiatry for Primary Care Physicians*. Chicago: American Medical Association, 1998.

Goldman, Larry, Wise, Thomas, & Brody, David. (2004). *Psychiatry for primary care physicians* (2nd ed.). Chicago: American Medical Association.

Goldman, Lee, & Schafer, Andrew L. (Eds.). (2015). Goldman-Cecil Medicine, 25th ed. Philadelphia, PA, Saunders.

Goldmann, David R., and David A. Horowitz, eds. *American College of Physicians Complete Home Medical Guide*. New York: DK, 2003.

Golen, Kenneth van. *The Rho GTPases in Cancer.* New York: Springer, 2010.

Golshan, M., and B. Smith. "Prevention and Management of Arm Lymphedema in the Patient with Breast Cancer." *Journal of Supportive Oncology* 4, no. 8 (2006): 381-386.

Gómez, H. L., Neciosup, S., Tosello, C., Mano, M., Bines, J., Ismael, G., (2016). A phase II randomized study of lapatinib combined with capecitabine, vinorelbine, or gemcitabine in patients with HER2-positive metastatic breast cancer with progression after a taxane. *Clinical Breast Cancer,* 16(1): 38–44.

Goodman, Richard, and Arno G. Motulsky, eds. *Genetic Diseases Among Ashkenazi Jews*. New York: Raven Press, 1979.

Goodwin, Pamela J. "Support Groups in Advanced Breast Cancer." *Cancer* 104, suppl. 11 (December 1, 2005): 2596-2601.

_______. "Support Groups in Breast Cancer: When a Negative Result Is Positive." *Journal of Clinical Oncology* 22, no. 21 (November 1, 2004): 4244-4246.

Goodwin, Scott C., Michael S. Broder, and David Drum. *What Your Doctor May Not Tell You About Fibroids: New Techniques and Therapies—Including Breakthrough Alternatives to Hysterectomy*. New York: Warner Books, 2003.

Gordis, L. *Epidemiology*. Philadelphia: Elsevier/Saunders, 2004.

Gordon, Serena. "Oral Sex Implicated in Some Throat and Neck Cancer." *Washington Post*, August 27, 2007.

Gore, Martin E., and Douglas Russell. *Primary Care and Cancer*. Edited by Paul F. Engstrom. New York: Informa Healthcare, 2003.

Gore, R. M., et al. "Upper Gastrointestinal Tumours: Diagnosis and Staging." *Cancer Imaging* 29, no. 6 (December, 2006): 213-217.

Gornik, H., M. Gerhard-Herman, and J. Beckman. "Abnormal Cytology Predicts Poor Prognosis in Cancer Patients with Pericardial Effusion." *Journal of Clinical Oncology* 23, no. 22 (August 1, 2005): 5211-5216.

Gott, Peter H. *Live Longer, Live Better: Taking Care of Your Health After Fifty*. Sanger, Calif.: Quill Driver Books, 2004.

Gottlieb, B., et al. "Cancer support groups: A critical review of empirical studies." *Psycho-Oncology* 16, no. 5 (May, 2007): 379-400.

Gourzones-Dmitriev, C., Kassambara, A., Sahota, S., Rème, T., Moreaux, J., Bourquard, P., … Klein, B. (2013). DNA repair pathways in human multiple myeloma: Role in oncogenesis and potential targets for treatment. *Cell Cycle* 12(17): 2760–2773.

Gozani, O., & Shi, Y. (2014). Histone methylation in chromatin signaling. In J. L. Workman & A. M. Abmayr (Eds.), *Fundamentals of chromatin* (pp. 213–256). New York, NY: Springer.

Gragert, L., Eapen, M., Williams, E., Freeman, J., Spellman, S., Baitty, R., … Maiers, M. (2014). HLA match likelihoods for hematopoietic stem-cell grafts in U.S. registry. *The New England Journal of Medicine,* 371(4), 339-348.

Grand, J. A., (Ed.). (2001). *Viruses, cell transformation, and cancer.* New York: Elsevier.

Granet, Roger. *Surviving Cancer Emotionally: Learning How to Heal*. New York: John Wiley & Sons, 2001.

Grant, A., and J. Neuberger, for the British Society of Gastroenterology. "Guidelines for the Use of Liver Biopsy in Clinical Practice." *Gut* 45, suppl. 4 (1999): IV1-IV11.

Gray, S. G. (2001). "Targeting Huntington's disease through histone deacetylases." *Clinical Epigenetics* 2: 257-277.

Gray, Steven. (Ed.). (2015). *Epigenetic Cancer Therapy*. Waltham, MA: Academic Press.

Green, A., and R. Marks. "Squamous Cell Carcinoma of the Skin (Non-Metastatic)." *Clinical Evidence* 14 (2005): 2086-2090.

Green, Lawrence W., and Marshall W. Kreuter. *Health Promotion Planning: An Educational and Ecological Approach*. 3rd ed. Mountain View, Calif.: Mayfield, 1999.

Green M, Covington S, Taranto S, Wolfe C, Bell W, Biggins SW, Conti D, DeStefano GD, Dominguez E, Ennis D, Gross T, Klassen-Fischer M, Kotton C, LaPointe-Rudow D, Law Y, Ludrosky K, Menegus M, Morris MI, Nalesnik MA, Pavlakis M, Pruett T, Sifri C, Kaul D. "Donor-derived transmission events in 2013: a report of the Organ Procurement Transplant Network Ad Hoc Disease Transmission Advisory Committee." *Transplantation* 99, no. 2 (February 2015): 282-287.

Green, S., Benedetti, J., Smith, A., & Crowley, J. (2012). *Clinical trials in oncology* (3rd ed.). Boca Raton, FL: CRC Press.

Green, W. B., ed. *Netter's Orthopedics*. Philadelphia: Saunders/Elsevier, 2006.

Greenberg, Mark S. *Handbook of Neurosurgery*. 6th ed. New York: Theime Medical, 2006.

Greenberg, Michael R. *Environmental Policy Analysis and Practice*. New Brunswick, N.J.: Rutgers University Press, 2007.

Greene, F. L. "Updates to Staging System Reflect Advances in Imaging, Understanding." *Journal of the National Cancer Institute* 22 (2002): 1664-1666.

_______, et al., eds. *American Joint Committee on Cancer Staging Manual*. 6th ed. New York: Springer, 2002.

_______. "Updating the Strategies in Cancer Staging." *American College of Surgeons Bulletin* 87 (2002): 13-15.

Greer, John P., et al., eds. *Wintrobe's Clinical Hematology*. 11th ed. Philadelphia: Lippincott Williams & Wilkins, 2004.

Greider, Carol W., & Blackburn, Elizabeth H. (2009). Telomeres, telomerase and cancer. *Scientific American*. Retrieved from http://www.scientificamerican.com/article/telomeres-telomerase-and/

Greten, Tim F., and Elizabeth M. Jaffe. "Cancer Vaccines." *Journal of Clinical Oncology* 17, no. 3 (March, 1999): 1047-1060.

Grimes, D. A. "Economy KE: Primary Prevention of Gynecologic Cancers." *American Journal of Obstetrics and Gynecology* 172 (1995): 227.

Griner, Erin and Dan Theodorescu. "The faces and friends of RhoGDI2." *Cancer and Metastasis Review* (December 2012) 31(3): 519-528.

Grobstein, Ruth H. *The Breast Cancer Book: What You Need to Know to Make Informed Decisions*. New Haven, Conn.: Yale University Press, 2005.

Groenwald, Susan L., et al. *Cancer Symptom Mangement*. Boston: Jones and Bartlett, 1996.

Grossman, Robert I., and David M. Yousem. *Neuroradiology: The Requisites*. St. Louis: Mosby-Year Book, 1994.

Grosvenor, M. B., & Smolin, L. A. (2012). *Visualizing: Nutrition Everyday Choices* (2nd ed.). Hoboken, NJ: John Wiley & Sons Inc.

Grotenhermen, Franjo, & Russo, Ethan (Eds.). (2002). *Cannabis and Cannabinoids: Pharmacology, Toxicology, and Therapeutic Potential*. Binghamton, N.Y.: Haworth Press. A pharmacologic examination of marijuana and its derivatives; how they work, side-effects, and potential therapeutic uses.

Grubbs, S. S., Polite, B. N., Carney, J., Bowser, W., Rogers, J., Katurakes, N., … Paskett, E. D. (2013). Eliminating racial disparities in colorectal cancer in the real world: It took a village. *Journal of Cancer Oncology*, 31: 1928-1930.

Grunberg, S. M. "Antiemetic Activity of Corticosteroids in Patients Receiving Cancer Chemotherapy: Dosing, Efficacy, and Tolerability Analysis." *Annals of Oncology* 18, no. 2 (February, 2007): 233-240.

Guermazi, A., ed. *Imaging of Kidney Cancer*. New York: Springer, 2006.

"Guidelines for the Prevention and Treatment of Infection in Patients with an Absent or Dysfunctional Spleen." *BMJ* 312 (1996): 430-434. Also available at http://www.bmj.com.

Gullatte, M. M. (2005). *Clinical guide to antineoplastic therapy: A chemotherapy handbook*. Philadelphia, PA: Oncology Nursing Society.

Gunabushanam, G., Subramanian, S., & Seith, A. (2006). Peutz-Jeghers syndrome. *Pediatric Radiology,* 36(8): 888-889.

Gupta, Renu. *Skin-Care*. Delhi, India: Diamond Pocket Books, 2000.

Gupta, S. P. (Ed.). (2014). *Cancer-causing viruses and their inhibitors*. Boca Raton, FL: CRC Press.

Gururangan, S., et al. "High-Dose Chemotherapy with Autologous Stem-Cell Rescue in Children and Adults with Newly Diagnosed Pineoblastomas." *Journal of Clinical Oncology* 21, no. 11 (June 1, 2003): 2187-2191.

Haas, Adelaide, and Susan L. Puretz. *The Woman's Guide to Hysterectomy: Expectations and Options*. Berkeley, Calif.: Celestial Arts, 2002.

Haas, Marilyn L., et al. *Radiation Therapy: A Guide to Patient Care*. St. Louis: Mosby/Elsevier, 2007.

Hackney, D. B. "Neoplasms and Related Disorders." *Topics* in Magnetic Resonance Imaging 4 (1992): 37-61.

Hagga, John R., and Charles F. Lanzieri. *Computed Tomography and Magnetic Resonance Imaging of the Whole Body*. 4th ed. St. Louis: Mosby, 2003.

Haggar, F. A., & Boushey, R. P. (2009). Colorectal cancer epidemiology: Incidence, mortality, survival, and risk factors. *Clinics in Colon and Rectal Surgery,* 22(4), 191–197. http://doi.org/10.1055/s-0029-1242458

Haighton, L. A., et al. "An Evaluation of the Possible Carcinogenicity of Bisphenol A to Humans." *Regulatory Toxicology and Pharmacology* 35 (2002): 238-254.

Hainaut, Pierre, & Wiman, Klas G. (1999). Twenty-five years of p53 research. New York: Springer.

Hales, D. (2014). *An Invitation to Health*. 16th ed. Boston, MA: Cengage Learning.

Half, E., Bercovich, D., & Rozen, P. (2009). Familial adenomatous polyposis. *Orphanet Journal of Rare Diseases,* 4, 22.

Halliwell, B. "Oxidative Stress and Cancer: Have We Moved Forward?" *Biochemistry Journal* 401 (2007): 1-11.

Hamad, G. G., M. T. Brown, and J. A. Clavijo-Alvarez. "Postoperative Video Debriefing Reduces Technical Errors in Laparoscopic Surgery." *American Journal of Surgery* 194 (2007): 110-114.

Hamaoka, T., et al. "Bone Imaging in Metastatic Breast Cancer." *Journal of Clinical Oncology* 22, no. 14 (2004): 2942-2953.

Hamas, Edward A. *How to Write Your Own Living Will*. Naperville, Ill.: Sphinx, 2002.

Hamilton, S. R., et al. "The Molecular Basis of Turcot's Syndrome." *New England Journal of Medicine* 332 (1995): 839-847.

Hamilton, William, and Tim J. Peters. *Cancer Diagnosis in Primary Care*. New York: Churchill Livingstone/Elsevier, 2007.

Hammerly, Milton, and Cheryl Kimball. *When the Doctor Says It's PCOS (Polycystic Ovarian Syndrome)*. Beverly, Mass.: Fair Winds Press, 2003.

Hanahan D., and R. A. Weinberg. "The Hallmarks of Cancer." *Cell* 100 (2000): 57-70.

________. (2011). Hallmarks of cancer: The next generation. *Cell,* 144(5), 646–674.

Hanna, N., Shepherd, F. A., Fossella, F. V., Pereira, J.R., De Marinis. F., von Pawel, J., … Bunn, P. A. Jr. (2004). Randomized phase III trial of pemetrexed versus docetaxel in patients with non–small-cell lung cancer previously treated with chemotherapy. *Journal of Clinical Oncology* 22(9): 1589-1597.

Hannah, S., Lynch, V., Guldi, D. M., Gerasimchuk, N., MacDonald, C. L. B., Magda, D., & Sessler, J. L. (2002). Late first-row transition-metal complexes of texaphyrin. *Journal of the American Chemical Society,* 124: 8416-8427.

Hannon, M. J. (2007). Metal-based anticancer drugs: From a past anchored in platinum chemistry to a post-genomic future of diverse chemistry and biology. *Pure Applied Chemistry*, 79(12): 2243-2261Johnstone, T. C., Park, G. Y., & Lippard, S. J. (2014). Understanding and improving platinum anticancer drugs – phenanthriplatin. *Anticancer Research*, 34(1): 471-476.

Hansen, Ruth, et al. "Fibroblast Growth Factor Receptor 2, Gain-of-Function Mutations, and Tumourigenesis:

Investigating a Potential Link." *Journal of Pathology* 207 (2005): 27-31.

Hansmann, A., Adolph, C., Vogel, T., Unger, A., & Moeslein, G. (2004). High-dose tamoxifen and sulindac as first-line treatment for desmoid tumors. *Cancer,* 100(3), 612-620.

Hara, A. K., et al. "Imaging of Small Bowel Disease: Comparison of Capsule Endoscopy, Standard Endoscopy, Barium Examination, and CT." *Radiographics* 25, no. 3 (May/June, 2005): 697-711.

Hardell, L., M. Hansson, and M. Carlberg. "Case-Control Study on the Use of Cellular and Cordless Phones and the Risk for Malignant Brain Tumours." *International Journal in Radiation Biology* 78 (2002): 931-936.

Harding, Fred. *Breast Cancer: Cause—Prevention—Cure*. Rev. ed. London: Tekline Publishing, 2007.

Hargrave, D. R., and S. Zacharoulis. "Pediatric CNS Tumors: Current Treatment and Future Directions." *Expert Review of Neurotherapeutics* 7, no. 8 (August, 2007): 1029-1042.

Harmey, Judith H., ed. *VEGF and Cancer*. New York: Kluwer Academic/Plenum, 2004.

Harper, Peter S. *First Years of Human Chromosomes: The Beginnings of Human Cytogenetics*. Bloxham, England: Scion, 2006.

Harpham, Wendy Schlessel. *When a Parent Has Cancer: A Guide to Caring for Your Children*. New York: Perennial Currents, 2004.

Harpman, Wendy Schlessel. (1994). *After cancer: A guide to your new life*. New York: W. W. Norton.

Harris, L. V., and I. A. Kahwa. "Asbestos: Old Foe in Twenty-First Century Developing Countries." *Science of the Total Environment* 307, nos. 1-3 (2003): 1-9.

Harti, D. M., and D. F. Brasnu. "Recurrent Laryngeal Nerve Paralysis: Current Concepts and Treatment." *Ear, Nose and Throat Journal* 79, no. 12 (December, 2000): 918.

Hartmann, D., et al. "Capsule Endoscopy: Technical Impact, Benefits, and Limitations." *Langenbecks Archives of Surgery* 389, no. 3 (June, 2004): 225-233.

Hartmann, Lynn C., and Charles L. Loprinzi. *Mayo Clinic Guide to Women's Cancers*. New York: Kensington, 2005.

_______, eds. *Mayo Clinic Guide to Women's Cancers*. Rochester, Minn.: Mayo Clinic, 2005.

Hartwell, L., et al. "Cancer Biomarkers: A Systems Approach." *Nature Biotechnology* 24 (2006): 905-908.

Harvey, P. W., and D. J. Everett. "Significance of the Detection of Esters of P-hydroxybenzoic Acid (Parabens) in Human Breast Tumours." *Journal of Applied Toxicology* 24 (2004): 1-4.

Harvie, M., Howell, A., Vierkant, R. A., Kumar, N., Cerhan, J. C., Kelemen, L. E., … Sellers, T. A. (2005). Association of gain and loss of weight before and after menopause with risk of postmenopausal breast cancer in the Iowa women's health study. *Cancer Epidemiology Biomarkers & Prevention*, 14, 656-66. doi:10.1158/1055-9965.

Hashibe, Mia, et al. "Alcohol Drinking in Never Users of Tobacco, Cigarette Smoking in Never Drinkers, and the Risk of Head and Neck Cancers: Pooled Analysis in the International Head and Neck Cancer Epidemiology Consortium." *Journal of the National Cancer Institute* 99 (2007): 777-789.

Hass, Jennifer S., et al. "Do Physicians Tailor Their Recommendations for Breast Cancer Risk Reduction Based on Patient's Risk?" *Journal of General Internal Medicine* 19, no. 4 (2004): 302-309.

Hassan, M. N., et al. "Risk Factors for Pancreatic Cancer: Case-Control Study." *American Journal of Gastroenterology* 102, no. 12 (August, 2007): 2696-2707.

Hasumi, H., Baba, M., Hasumi, Y., Furuya, M. & Yao, M. (2015), Birt–Hogg–Dubé syndrome: Clinical and molecular aspects of recently identified kidney cancer syndrome. *International Journal of Urology,* 23(3), 204-210. doi: 10.1111/iju.13015

Hawkins, Rebecca. "Clinical Focus: Ascites." *Clinical Journal of Oncology Nursing* 5, no. 1 (January/February, 2001).

Hayat, M. A., ed. *Cancer Imaging, Volume 1: Lung and Breast Carcinomas*. Oxford, England: Elsevier Academic Press, 2007.

_______. *Cancer Imaging, Volume 2: Instrumentation and Applications*. Oxford, England: Elsevier Academic Press, 2007.

Haynes, M. Alfred, and Brian D. Smedley, eds. *The Unequal Burden of Cancer: An Assessment of NIH and Research Programs for Ethnic Minorities and the Medically Underserved*. Washington, D.C.: National Academy Press, 1999.

Head, Barbara Anderson, ed. *Study Guide for the Hospice and Palliative Nursing Assistant*. Dubuque, Iowa: Kendall/Hunt, 2004.

Hearing, Vincent J., and Stanley P. L. Leong, eds. *From Melanocytes to Melanoma: The Progression to Malignancy*. Totowa, N.J.: Humana Press, 2006.

Hearle. N., Schumacher, V., Menko, F. H., Olschwang, S., Boardman, L. A., Gille, J. J., … Houlston, R. S. (2006). Frequency and spectrum of cancers in the Peutz-Jeghers Syndrome. *Clinical Cancer Research,* 12(10): 3209-3215.

Heath, Angela. *Long Distance Caregiving: A Survival Guide for Far Away Caregivers*. Atascadero, Calif.: American Source Books, 1993.

Heathcote, E.J., Shiffman, M.L., Cooksley, W.G., Dusheiko, G.M., Lee, S.S., Balart, L., Reindollar, R., Reddy, R.K., Wright, T.L., Lin, A., Hoffman, J., De Pamphilis, J. (2000). Peginterferon alfa-2a in patients with chronic hepatitis C and cirrhosis. *New England Journal of Medicine,* 343(23): 1673-1680.

Heft, E., & Blanco, J. G. (2016). Anthracycline-related cardiotoxicity in patients with acute myeloid leukemia and Down syndrome: A literature review. *Cardiovascular Toxicology,* 16(1): 5-13.

Heim, Sverre, and Felix Mitelman. *Cancer Cytogenetics*. 2d ed. New York: Wiley-Liss, 1995.

Hellstr-Lindberg, E., and L. Malcovati. "Supportive Care, Growth Factors, and New Therapies in Myelodysplastic Syndromes." *Blood Reviews* 22, no. 2 (March, 2008): 75-91.

Hemingway, Jean. "An Overview of Pesticide Resistance." *Science* 5, no. 298 (October 4, 2003): 96-97.

HemOnc Today. (2009, July 10). Phasing out anthracyclines in breast cancer: Is it time? *Healio*, http://www.healio.com/hematology-oncology/breast-cancer/news/print/hemonc-today/%7Bb-ccf5629-277b-4591-b4d1-65320a4063e9%7D/phasing-out-anthracyclines-in-breast-cancer-is-it-time

Henderson, I. Craig, ed. *Adjuvant Therapy of Breast Cancer*. Boston: Kluwer Academic, 1992.

Hendrix, C.C., Bailey,Jr., D.E., Steinhauser, K.E., Olsen, M.K., Stechuchak, K.M., Lowman, S.G. ... Tulsky, J.A. (2016). Effects of enhanced caregiver training program on cancer caregiver's self-efficacy, preparedness, and psychological well-being. *Support Care Cancer,* 24: 327-336. doi: 10.1007/s00520-015-2797-3.

Hennessey, Maya. *If Only I'd Had This Caregiving Book*. Bloomington, Ind.: AuthorHouse, 2006.

Hennessy, B. T., et al. "New Approaches in the Treatment of Myelofibrosis." *Cancer* 103, no. 1 (January 1, 2005): 32-43.

Heppell, Jacques. "Surgical Management of Inflammatory Bowel Disease." *UptoDate*, January, 2008.

Herdman, Roger, and Leonard Lichtenfeld, eds. *Fulfilling the Potential of Cancer Prevention and Early Detection: An American Cancer Society and Institute of Medicine Symposium*. Washington, D.C.: National Academies Press, 2004.

Herrera, Lemuel, ed. *Familial Adenomatous Polyposis*. New York: A. R. Liss, 1990.

Hiatt, Jonathan R., Edward H. Phillips, and Leon Morgenstern, eds. *Surgical Diseases of the Spleen*. New York: Springer, 1997.

Hickey, Joanne V. *The Clinical Practice of Neurological and Neurosurgical Nursing*. 5th ed. Philadelphia: Lippincott Williams & Wilkins, 2003.

Higdon, J. (Spring/Summer 2006). Cruciferous Vegetables and Cancer Risk. *The Linus Pauling Institute Research Newsletter*. pp. 7-9. Retrieved from http://lpi.oregonstate.edu/files/pdf/newsletters/ss06.pdf

Hill, David, J. Mark Elwood, and Dallas R. English, eds. *Prevention of Skin Cancer*. Boston: Kluwer Academic, 2004.

Hind, D., et al. "Hormonal Therapies for Early Breast Cancer: Systematic Review and Economic Evaluation." *Health Technology Assessment* 11, no. 26 (July, 2007).

Hinz, A., Mehnert, A., Kocalevent, R.-D., Brahler, E., Forkman, T., Singer, S., & Schulte. (2016). Assessment of depression severity with the PHQ-9 in cancer patients and in the general population. *Psychiatry,* 16(22): doi: 10.1186/s12888-016-0728-6.

Hisham, Abdullah, and Cheng-Har Yip. "Overview of Breast Cancer in Malaysian Women: A Problem with Late Diagnosis." *Asian Journal of Surgery* 27, no. 2 (April, 2004): 130-133.

Hoadley, J., Summer, L., Hargrave, E., Cubanski, J., & Neuman T. (2014, August 18). Medicare Part D in Its Ninth Year: The 2014 Marketplace and Key Trends, 2006-2014. The Henry J. Kaiser Family Foundation. Retrieved from http://kff.org/medicare/report/medicare-part-d-in-its-ninth-year-the-2014-marketplace-and-key-trends-2006-2014/

Hobart, Julie A., and Douglas R. Smucker. "The Female Athlete Triad." *American Family Physician* 61, no. 11 (June 1, 2000).

Hodgson, N. C. "Merkel Cell Carcinoma: Changing Incidence Trends." *Journal of Surgical Oncology* 89, no. 1 (January, 2005): 1-4.

Hoffman, Barbara, ed. *A Cancer Survivor's Almanac: Charting Your Journey*. Minneapolis: National Coalition for Cancer Survivorship, 1996.

Hoffman, R., Benz, E. J., Silberstain, L. E., Heslop, H., Weitz, J., & Anastasi, J. (2013). Hematology: Basic principles and practice (6th ed.). New York: Churchill Livingstone.

Hoffman, Ronald. (2005). *Hematology: Basic principles and practice* (4th ed.). St. Louis: Elsevier Churchill Livingstone.

_______, et al. *Hematology: Basic Principles and Practice*. 4th ed. Philadelphia: Churchill Livingstone, 2005.

_______, et al. *Hematology: Basic Principles and Practice*. 4th ed. Orlando, Fla.: Churchill Livingstone, 2005.

Hofman, Maarten, et al. "Cancer-Related Fatigue: The Scale of the Problem." *The Oncologist* 12 (May, 2007): 4-10.

Holdsworth, M. T. "State of Oncology Pharmacotherapy." *The Annals of Pharmacotherapy* 40, no. 12 (December, 2006): 2238-2239.

Holen, Kyle, & Chung, Ki Young. (2008). *Dx/Rx: Colorectal cancer.* Sudbury, MA: Jones and Bartlett.

Holland, Jimmie C., and Sheldon Lewis. *The Human Side of Cancer*. New York: HarperCollins, 2000.

Holland, Jimmie C., et al., eds. *Psycho-Oncology*. New York: Oxford University Press, 1998.

Holman, Peter, Jodi Garrett, and William Jansen. *One Hundred Questions and Answers About Lymphoma*. Sudbury, Mass.: Jones and Bartlett, 2004.

Holtz, Carol, ed. *Global Health Care: Issues and Policies*. Sudbury, Mass.: Jones and Bartlett, 2008.

Hong, I., Lee, H., & Kang, K. (2014). Mescenchymal stem cells and cancer: Friends or enemies? *Mutation Research/Fundamental and Molecular Mechanisms of Mutagenesis,* 768, 98 – 106.

Hope, Mari, et al. "Sporadic Colorectal Cancer: Role of the Commensal Microbiota." *FEMS Microbiology Letters* 244 (2005): 1-7.

Horner, Peter. "O.R. in the O.R.: Saving Lives as Well as Money, Memorial Sloan-Kettering Center Earns the Edelman with Breakthrough Modeling and Computational Techniques for Treating Prostate Cancer." *OR/MS Today* 34, no. 3 (June, 2007): 18-22.

Hosaka, K. "Radiological Investigation of the Mucosae Around Early Gastric Cancers." *Journal of Gastroenterology* 41, no. 10 (October, 2006): 943-953.

Hoskin, P. J., and P. Bownes. "Innovative Technologies in Radiation Therapy: Brachytherapy." *Seminars in Radiation Oncology* 16, no. 4 (October, 2006): 209-217.

Hoskin, P. J., K. Motohashi, P. Bownes, L. Bryant, and P. Ostler. "High Dose Rate Brachytherapy in Combination with External Beam Radiotherapy in the Radical Treatment of Prostate Cancer: Initial Results of a Randomized Phase Three Trial." *Radiotherapy & Oncology* 84, no. 2 (August, 2007): 114-120.

Hottinger, A. F., and Y. Khakoo. "Update on the Management of Familial Central Nervous System Tumor Syndromes." *Current Neurology and Neuroscience Reports* 7, no. 3 (May, 2007): 200-207.

Houlihan, Nancy G. *Lung Cancer*. Pittsburgh: Oncology Nursing Society, 2004.

Houts, Peter S., and Julia A. Bucher, eds. *Caregiving: A Step by Step Resource for Caring for the Person with Cancer at Home*. Rev. ed. Atlanta: American Cancer Society, 2003.

Houts, Peter, ed. *Home Care Guide for Cancer*. Philadelphia: American College of Physicians, 1996.

Howard, D. H., Back P. B., Berndt, E. R., & Conti, R. M. (2015). Pricing in the market for anticancer drugs. *Journal of Economic Perspectives* 29(1):139-162. http://pubs.aeaweb.org/doi/pdfplus/10.1257/jep.29.1.139

Howe, G. Melvyn, ed. *Global Geocancerology: A World Geography of Human Cancers*. New York: Churchill Livingstone, 1986.

Howlader, N., Noone, A. M., Krapcho, M., Garshell, J., Miller, D., Altekruse, S. F., ... Cronin, K. A. (Eds.). (2015). SEER Cancer Statistics Review, 1975-2012, National Cancer Institute. Bethesda, MD, http://seer.cancer.gov/csr/1975_2012/, based on November 2014 SEER data submission, posted to the SEER web site, April 2015.

Huang, Suming, Litt, Michael D., & Blakey, C. A. (Eds.). (2015). *Epigenetic gene expression and regulation*. Waltham, MA: Academic Press.

Huang, Tsai-Wang, et al. "Middle Mediastinal Thymoma." *Re*spirology 12, no. 6 (2007): 934-936.

Huber, W. W., B. Grasl-Kraupp, and R. Schulte-Hermann. "Hepatocarcinogenic Potential of Di(2-ethylhexyl) Phthalate in Rodents and Its Implications on Human Risk." *Critical Reviews in Toxicology* 26 (1996): 365-481.

Huettel, Scott, et al. *Functional Magnetic Resonance Imaging*. Sunderland, Mass.: Sinauer Associates, 2004.

Hughes, D. C., Darby, N., Gonzalez, K., Boggess, T., Morris, R. M., & Ramirez, A. G. (2015). Effect of a six-month yoga exercise intervention on fitness outcomes for breast cancer survivors. *Physiotherapy Theory and Practice*, 31(7): 451-60.

Hughes, Sally Smith. (2013). *Genentech: The beginnings of biotech*. Chicago, IL: University of Chicago Press.

Hughes, Timothy P., David M. Ross & Melo, Junia V. (2014). *Handbook of chronic myeloid leukemia*. New York: Springer.

Huh, Jung Wook, et al. "A Diverting Stoma Is Not Necessary When Performing a Handsewn Coloanal Anastomosis for Lower Rectal Cancer." *Diseases of the Colon & Rectum* 50 (2007): 1040-1046.

Hulbert-Williams, N., Neal, R., Morrison, V., Hood, K., & Wilkinson, C. (2012). Anxiety, depression, and quality of life after cancer diagnosis: What psychosocial variables best predict how patients adjust? *Psycho-Oncology,* 21: 857-867. doi: 10.1002/pon.1980.

Hunt, Ian, Martin Muers, and Tom Treasure, eds. *ABC of Lung Cancer*. Malden, Mass.: Blackwell, 2008.

Hunt, Kelly K., Geoffrey L. Robb, Eric A. Strom, and Naoto T. Ueno. *Breast Cancer*. M. D. Anderson Cancer Care Series. New York: Springer, 2001.

Hunter, Brenda. *Staying Alive: Life-Changing Strategies for Surviving Cancer*. Colorado Springs, Colo.: WaterBrook Press, 2004.

Hunter, Carrie P., Karen A. Johnson, and Hyman B. Muss. *Cancer in the Elderly*. New York: Marcel Dekker, 2000.

Hunter, John, John Savin, and Mark Dahl. *Clinical Dermatology*. 3rd ed. Malden, Mass.: Blackwell, 2002.

Hupp, James R., Edward Ellis, and Myron R. Tucker. *Contemporary Oral and Maxillofacial Surgery*. 5th ed. Philadelphia: Elsevier Health Sciences, 2008.

Huscher, C. G., et al. "Laparoscopic Versus Open Subtotal Gastrectomy for Distal Gastric Cancer: Five-Year Results of a Randomized Prospective Trial." *Annals of Surgery* 241, no. 2 (2005): 232-237.

Hussain, R., D. Christie, V. Gebski, et al. "The Role of the Gallium Scan in Primary Extranodal Lymphoma." *Journal of Nuclear Medicine* 39, no. 1 (1998): 95-98.

Hussain, S. P., L. J. Hofseth, and C. C. Harris. "Radical Causes of Cancer." *Nature Reviews. Cancer* 3 (2003): 276-285.

Hutter, A., et al. "Brain Neoplasms: Epidemiology, Diagnosis, and Prospects for Cost-Effective Imaging." *Neuroimaging Clinics of North America* 13 (2003): 237-250.

Hyangsook, L., K. Schmidt, and E. Ernst. "Acupuncture for the Relief of Cancer-Related Pain: A Systematic Review." *European Journal of Pain* 9, no. 4 (August, 2005): 437-444.

Ichimura K. (2012). Molecular pathogenesis of IDH mutations in gliomas. *Brain Tumor Pathology*, 29(3): 131-139.

Icon Health. *Angiogram: A Medical Dictionary, Bibliography, and Annotated Research Guide to Internet References*. San Diego, Calif.: Author, 2004.

Icon Health. *Esophagitis: A Medical Dictionary, Bibliography, and Annotated Research Guide to Internet References*. San Diego, Calif.: Author, 2004.

Icon Health. *Ewing's Sarcoma: A Medical Dictionary, Bibliography, and Annotated Research Guide to Internet References*. San Diego, Calif.: Author, 2004.

Icon Health. *Gallbladder Cancer: A Medical Dictionary, Bibliography, and Annotated Research Guide to Internet References*. San Diego, Calif.: Author, 2004.

Icon Health. *Hairy Cell Leukemia: A Medical Dictionary, Bibliography, and Annotated Research Guide to Internet References*. San Diego, Calif.: Author, 2004.

Icon Health. *Horner's Syndrome: A Medical Dictionary, Bibliography, and Annotated Research Guide to Internet References*. San Diego, Calif.: Author, 2004.

Icon Health. *Metastasis: A Medical Dictionary, Bibliography, and Annotated Research Guide to Internet References*. San Diego, Calif.: Author, 2004.

Icon Health. *Ovarian Cancer: A Medical Dictionary, Bibliography, and Annotated Research Guide to Internet References*. San Diego, Calif.: Author, 2004.

Icon Health. *Ovarian Cysts: A Medical Dictionary, Bibliography, and Annotated Research Guide to Internet References*. San Diego, Calif.: Author, 2004.

Icon Health. *Smokeless Tobacco: A Medical Dictionary, Bibliography, and Annotated Research Guide to Internet References*. San Diego, Calif.: Author, 2004.

Icon Health. *The Official Patient's Sourcebook on Carcinoma of Unknown Primary: A Revised and Updated Directory for the Internet Age*. San Diego, Calif.: Author, 2002.

Icon Health. *The Official Patient's Sourcebook on Progressive Multifocal Leukoencephalopathy: A Revised and Updated Directory for the Internet Age*. San Diego, Calif.: Author, 2003.

Icon Health. *The Official Patient's Sourcebook on Salivary Gland Cancer: A Revised and Updated Directory for the Internet Age*. San Diego, Calif.: Author, 2004.

Icon Health. *The Official Patient's Sourcebook on Small Intestine Cancer: Directory for the Internet Age*. San Diego, Calif.: Author, 2004.

Iizasa, H., Nanbo, A., Nishikawa, J. Jinushi, M., & Yoshiyama, H. (2012). Epstein-Barr virus (EBV)-associated gastric carcinoma. *Viruses,* 4, 3420-3439.

Im, A. P. (2014). DNMT3A and IDH mutations in acute myeloid leukemia and other myeloid malignancies: associations with prognosis and potential treatment strategies. *Leukemia* 28: 1774-1783.

Imperiale, T. F., et al. "Fecal DNA Versus Fetal Occult Blood for Colorectal Cancer Screening in an Average-Risk Population." *New England Journal of Medicine* 351, no. 26 (2004): 2704-2714.

IMS Institute for Healthcare Informatics. (2015, May). Developments in cancer treatments, market dynamics, patient access and value: Global oncology trend report. http://www.imshealth.com/en/thought-leadership/ims-institute/reports/global-oncology-trend-2015

Institute of Medicine of the National Academies. (2007). *Cancer-related genetic testing and counseling: Workshop proceedings*. Washington, D.C.: National Academies Press.

Institute of Medicine of the National Academies. Board on Population Health and Public Health Practices. Committee on Asbestos: Selected Health Effects. *Asbestosis: Selected Cancers*. Washington, D.C.: National Academies Press, 2006.

"Interventional Radiology for the Cancer Patient." In *Cancer Medicine*, edited by Donald W. Kufe et al. 6th ed. Hamilton, Ont.: BC Decker, 2003. Also available online at http://www.ncbi.nlm.nih.gov/books.

Intner, Riki, and Roberta Cole. *Caregiving from the Heart:* Tales of Inspiration. San Francisco: Elders Academy Press, 2006.

Ishikawa, S., et al. "Mass Screening of Multiple Abdominal Solid Organs Using Mobile Helical Computed Tomography Scanner: A Preliminary Report." *Asian Journal of Surgery* 30, no. 2 (April, 2007): 118-121.

Itano, J. K., and K. N. Toaka. *Core Curriculum for Oncology Nursing*. 4th ed. Philadelphia: Elsevier/Saunders, 2005.

Izakson, Orna. "Farming Infertility: Country Living May Be Hazardous to Your Potency." *E/The Environmental Magazine* 15, no. 1 (January/February, 2004): 40-41.

Jackisch, C., Kim, S. B., Semiglazov, V., Melichar. B., Pivot, X. Hillenbach, C. … Ismael, G. (2015). Subcutaneous versus intravenous formulation of trastuzumab for HER2-positive early breast cancer: updated results from the phase III HannaH study. *Annals of Oncology*, 26: 320-325.

Jackman, Ann L., ed. *Antifolate Drugs in Cancer Therapy*. Totowa, N.J.: Humana Press, 1999.

Jacobs, Hollye & Messina, Elizabeth (2014). *The Silver Lining: A supportive & insightful guide to breast cancer* (Kindle edition). Retrieved from http://www.amazon.com/The-Silver-Lining-Supportive-Insightful/dp/1476743711

Jacobs, Léa K., ed. *Coping with Cancer*. New York: Nova Science, 2008.

Jacobs, T. W., et al. "Fibroepithelial Lesions with Cellular Stroma on Breast Core Needle Biopsy: Are There Predictors of Outcome on Surgical Excision?" *American Journal of Clinical Pathology* 124, no. 3 (2005): 342-354.

Jaeckel, E., Cornberg, M., Wedemeyer, H., Santantonio, T., Mayer, J., Zankel, M., Pastore, G., Dietrich, M., Trautwein, C., Manns, M.P.; German Acute Hepatitis CTherapy Group. (2001). Treatment of acute hepatitis C with interferon alfa-2b. *New England Journal of Medicine*, 345(20): 1452-1457.

Jaeckle, K. A. "Improving the Outcome of Patients with Leptomeningeal Cancer: New Clinical Trials and Experimental Therapies." *Cancer Treatment and Research* 125 (2005): 181-193.

Jain, N. (2015). New developments in Richter Syndrome. *Clinical Advances in Hematology & Oncology,* 13(4), 220-222.

James, C., Thomas, M., Lillie-Blanton, M. D., & Garfield, R. (2003). Key facts: Race, ethnicity, and medical care. Menlo Park, CA: Henry J. Kaiser Family Foundation. http://files.kff.org/attachment/report-key-facts-race-ethnicity-and-medical-care

James, John W., Russell Freidman, and Leslie Matthews. *When Children Grieve: For Adults Who Help Children Deal with Death, Divorce, Pet Loss, Moving, and Other Losses*. New York: HarperCollins, 2001.

Jandu, H., Aluzaite, K., Fogh, L., Thrdane, S.W., Noer, J.B., Proszek, J., … Stenvang, J. (2016). Molecular characterization of iriotecan (SN-38) resistant breast cancer cell lines. *BioMedCentral,* 16(34). doi: 10.1186/s12885-016-2071-1.

Janes-Hodder, Honna, and Nancy Keene. *Childhood Cancer: A Parent's Guide to Solid Tumor Cancers*. 2d ed. Sebastopol, Calif.: O'Reilly, 1999.

Janeway, C. A., ed. *Immunobiology*. 5th ed. New York: Garland, 2001.

Jang, Y.Y., Cai, L., & Ye, Z. (2016). Genome editing systems in novel therapies. *Discovery Medicine*, 21(113):57-64. http://www.ncbi.nlm.nih.gov/pubmed/26896603

Jeffries, Lee P., ed. *Leading Topics in Cancer Research*. New York: Nova Science, 2007.

Jemal, A., et al. "Cancer Statistics, 2007." *CA: A Cancer Journal for Clinicians* 57, no. 1 (January/February, 2007): 43-66.

Jenkins, V., & Fallowfield, L. (2000). Reasons for accepting or declining to participate in randomized clinical trials for cancer therapy. *British Journal of Cancer,* 82, 1783-1788.

Jenks Kettmann, J. D., & Altmaier, E. M. (2008). Social support and depression among bone marrow transplant patients. *Journal of Health Psychology*, 13, 39-46.

Jennings, Lesajean McDonald. *A Guide for Men as They Walk Through the Experience of Breast Cancer with the Women in Their Lives: Specifics to Support Emotional and Relationship Health.* Auburn Hills, Mich.: Jessies Legacy, 2004.

Jimbo, M., et al. "Effectiveness of Complete Diagnostic Examination in Clinical Practice Settings." *Cancer Detection and Prevention* 30, no. 6 (2006): 545-551.

Johanson, Paula. *Frequently Asked Questions About Testicular Cancer*. New York: Rosen, 2007.

_______. *Frequently Asked Questions About Testicular Cancer*. New York: Rosen, 2008.

Johnson, B. L., and J. Gross. *Handbook of Oncology Nursing*. 3rd ed. Sudbury, Mass.: Jones and Bartlett, 1998.

Johnson, Carolyn Y. (2014). Cancer cells may guide treatment. *Boston Globe*. https://www.bostonglobe.com/news/science/2014/07/10/rare-tumor-cells-blood-can-help-target-cancer-treatment-study-shows/OlX-6CVXbNIt51T6nu3J5QM/story.html

Johnson, Lenworth N., and Michael A. Meyer. "Lumbar Puncture." In *Neuro-ophthalmology: The Practical Guide*, edited by Leonard A. Levin and Anthony C. Arnold. New York: Thieme Medical, 2005.

Johnson, Stephen A. "Waldenström's Macroglobulinemia." *Reviews in Clinical and Experimental Hematology* 6, no. 4 (2002): 421-434.

Johnson, S. B., T. Y. Eng, G. Giaccone, and C. R. Thomas, Jr. "Thymoma: Update for the New Millennium." *Oncologist* 6, no. 3 (2001): 239-246.

Jones, B., et al. "Is There Still a Role for Open Cordotomy in Cancer Pain Management?" *Journal of Pain and Symptom Management* 25, no. 2 (2003): 179-184.

Jones, Marcia L., Theresa Eichenwald, and Nancy W. Hall. *Menopause for Dummies*. 2d ed. New York: Wiley, 2006.

Jordan, K., H. J. Schmoll, and M. S. Aapro. "Comparative Activity of Antiemetic Drugs." *Critical Reviews in Oncology/Hematology* 61, no. 2 (February, 2007): 162-175.

Jorgensen, J., Pfaller, M., Carroll, K., Funke, G., Landry, M., Richter, S., & Warnock, D. (Eds.). (2015). *Manual of Clinical Microbiology,* 11th ed. Washington, DC: ASM Press.

Josefowicz, S. Z., Lu, L-F., & Rudensky, A. Y. (2012). Regulatory T cells: Mechanisms of differentiation and function. *Annual Review of Immunology*, 30: 531-564.

Jothilakshmi, P. K., A. J. Watson, and E. Jude. "Acute Alopecia Due to Metformin Treatment for Polycystic Ovarian Syndrome." *Journal of Obstetrics and Gynaecology* 26, no. 6 (2006): 584-585.

Jung, U. J., & Choi, M.-S. (2014). Obesity and Its Metabolic Complications: The Role of Adipokines and the Relationship between Obesity, Inflammation, Insulin Resistance, Dyslipidemia and Nonalcoholic Fatty Liver Disease. *International Journal of Molecular Sciences,* 15(4), 6184-6223. doi:10.3390/ijms15046184

Kaal, E. C., and C. J. Vecht. "CNS Complications of Breast Cancer: Current and Emerging Treatment Options." *CNS Drugs* 21, no. 7 (2007): 559-579.

Kaefer, C.M. & Milner, J.A. (2011). Herbs and Spices in Cancer Prevention and Treatment. Boca Raton, FL: Taylor & Francis.

Kaelin, Carolyn M., & Coltrera, Francesca. (2005). *Living through breast cancer*. New York: McGraw-Hill.

Kaithoju, Srikanth. (2014). Epigenetics and Cancer Therapy. *Journal of Cancer Biology and Research,* 2(3), 1052.

Kane, Jeff. *How to Heal: A Guide for Caregivers*. New York: Allworth Press, 2003.

Kantarjian, H. M., Wolff, R. A., & Koller, C. A. (2011). *The MD Anderson manual of medical oncology* (2nd ed.). New York: The McGraw-Hill Companies, Inc.

Kantarjian, Hagop M., et al. *The M. D. Anderson Manual of Medical Oncology*. New York: McGraw-Hill, 2006.

Kanwal, R., Gupta, K., & Gupta, S. (2014). Cancer epigenetics: An introduction. In Mukesh Verma (Ed.), *Cancer epigenetics: Risk assessment, diagnosis, treatment, and prognosis* (pp. 3-25). New York, NY: Springer.

Kappelman, Michael D., Rifas-Shiman, Sheryl L., Kleinman, Ken, Ollendorf, Dan, Bousvaros, Athos, Grand, Richard J., & Finkelstein, Jonathan A. (2007). The prevalence and geographic distribution of Crohn's disease and ulcerative colitis in the United States. *Clinical Gastroenterology and Hepatology,* 5(12), 1424-1429. An article that reported the estimation of the prevalence of Inflammatory Bowel Diseases (Crohn's Disease and Ulcerative Colitis) in the United States; the study intended to quantify the overall burden of disease and assist the planning for appropriate clinical services.

Karch, Amy M. *2008 Lippincott's Nursing Drug Guide*. Philadelphia: Wolters Kluwer/Lippincott Williams & Wilkins, 2008.

Karp, Freddie, ed. *So Far Away: Twenty Questions for Long-Distance Caregivers*. Bethesda, Md.: National Institute on Aging, National Institutes of Health, U.S. Department of Health and Human Services, 2006.

Kasper, D. L., et al. *Harrison's Principles of Internal Medicine*. 16th ed. New York: McGraw-Hill, 2005.

Katoh, H., & Watanabe, M. (2015). Myeloid-derived suppressor cells and therapeutic strategies in cancer. *Mediators of Inflammation*, doi:10.1155/2015/159269.

Katz, Anne. *Breaking the Silence on Cancer and Sexuality: A Handbook for Healthcare Providers*. Pittsburgh: Oncology Nursing Society, 2007.

Kauff, N. D., and R. R. Barakat. "Risk-Reducing Salpingo-oophorectomy in Patients with Germline Mutations in *BRCA1* or *BRCA2*." *Journal of Clinical Oncology* 25, no. 20 (July 10, 2007): 2921-2927.

Kauffman, H. M., et al. "Deceased Donors with a Past History of Malignancy: An Organ Procurement and Transplantation Network/United Network for Organ Sharing Update." *Transplantation* 84, no. 2 (July 27, 2007): 272-274.

Kaufman, Howard L. *The Melanoma Book: A Complete Guide to Prevention and Treatment*. New York: Gotham Books, 2005.

Kavanaugh, S. A., White, L. A., & Kolesar, J. M. (2010). Vorinostat: A novel therapy for the treatment of cutaneous T-cell lymphoma. *American Journal of Health System Pharmacy*, 67: 793-797.

Keane, Maureen, and Daniella Chace. *What to Eat if You Have Cancer*. 2d ed. New York: McGraw-Hill, 2007.

Keane, Maureen, and Daniella Chace. *What to Eat If You Have Cancer: Healing Foods That Boost Your Immune System*. 2d ed. New York: McGraw-Hill, 2007.

Keane, M., and D. Chace. *What to Eat If You Have Cancer: A Guide to Adding Nutritional Therapy to Your Treatment Plan*. New York: McGraw-Hill, 1996.

Kedar-Barnes, I., & Rozen, P. (2004). The Jewish people: Their ethnic history, genetic disorders, and specific cancer susceptibility. *Familial Cancer*, 3(3/4): 193-199.

Keebler, Catherine M., and Theresa M. Somrak. *The Manual of Cytotechnology*. 7th ed. Chicago: ASCP Press, 1997.

Keegan, L. *Healing with Complementary and Alternative Therapies*. Albany, N.Y.: Delmar, 2001.

Keene, Nancy. (2002). *Chemo, craziness, and comfort: My book about childhood cancer*. Washington, D.C.: Candlelighters.

Keene, Nancy. *Childhood Leukemia: A Guide for Families, Friends, and Caregivers*. 3rd ed. Sebastopol, Calif.: O'Reilly, 2002.

Keesey, John Carl. *Myasthenia Gravis: An Illustrated History*. Roseville, Calif.: Publishers Design Group, 2002.

Kehoe, J., and V. P. Khatri. "Staging and Prognosis of Colon Cancer." *Surgical Oncology Clinics of North America* 15 (2006): 129-146.

Keilberg, D. & Otterman, K. M. (2016). How *Helicobacter pylori* senses, targets, and interacts with the gastric epithelium. *Environmental Microbiology*, doi: 10.1111/1462-2920.13222. [Epub ahead of print]. This is a recent review on the mechanism of how *Helicobacter pylori* interacts with the lining of the stomach and how this bacteria affects target cells in the stomach lining. This article is available to the public and can be accessed free at http://onlinelibrary.wiley.com/doi/10.1111/1462-2920.13222/epdf

Kelleher, P. C., et al. "Beryllium Particulate Exposure and Disease Relations in a Beryllium Machining Plant." *Journal of Occupational and Environmental Medicine* 43 (2001): 238-249.

Kelley, Mark (ed.). *DNA Repair in Cancer Therapy*. Waltham, MA: Elsevier Inc., 2012.

Kelloff, Gary, Ernest T. Hawk, and Caroline C. Sigman, eds. *Cancer Chemoprevention*. 2 vols. Totowa, N.J.: Humana Press, 2004-2005.

Kelloff, Gary, Ernest T. Hawk, and Caroline C. Sigman. *Cancer Chemoprevention*. Totowa, N.J.: Humana Press, 2004.

______. *Cancer Chemoprevention*. Totowa, N.J.: Humana Press, 2005.

Kelly, Mary Olson. *Number One Best Tools and Tips from the Trenches of Breast Cancer*. Austin, Tex.: Books Beyond Borders, 2006.

Kelvin, Joanne, and Leslie Tyson. *One Hundred Questions and Answers About Cancer Symptoms and Cancer Treatment Side Effects*. Sudbury, Mass.: Jones and Bartlett, 2004.

______. *One Hundred Questions and Answers About Cancer Symptoms and Cancer Treatment Side Effects*. Sudbury, Mass.: Jones and Bartlett, 2005.

Keren, David F. *High-Resolution Electrophoresis and Immunofixation: Techniques and Interpretation*. 2d ed. Boston: Butterworth-Heinemann, 1994.

Kershaw, Michael H., Westwood, J. A., Slaney, C. Y., & Darcy, P. K. (2014). Clinical Application of Genetically Modified T Cells in Cancer Therapy. *Clinical and Translational Immunology,* 3: e16. Retrieve at http://www.nature.com/cti/journal/v3/n5/full/cti20147a.html

Keum, N., & Giovannucci, E. (2014). Vitamin D supplements and cancer incidence and mortality: A meta-analysis. *British Journal of Cancer,* 111(5), 976-80. http://www.ncbi.nlm.nih.gov/pmc/articles/PMC4150260

Kevles, Bettyann. *Naked to the Bone: Medical Imaging in the Twentieth Century*. New Brunswick, N.J.: Rutgers University Press, 1997.

Khan, M. A. Q., and R. H. Stanton. *Toxicology of Halogenated Hydrocarbons*. New York: Pergamon Press, 1980.

Khan, M. A. Q., S. F. Khan, and F. Shutari. "Ecotoxicology of Halogenated Hydrocarbons." In *Encyclopedia of Ecology*. Washington, D.C.: National Council of Science and Environment, 2007.

Khanna, Reena, Bressler, Brian, Levesque, Barrett G., Zou, Guangyong, Stitt, Larry W., Greenberg, Gordon R., ... REACT Study Investigators. (2015). Early combined immunosuppression for the management of Crohn's disease (REACT): a cluster randomised controlled trial. *The Lancet, 386*(10006), 1825-1834. The REACT Study which evaluated using an early treatment of Crohn's Disease with combined immunosuppression (immunomodulator + antibody to TNF); the results showed improved clinical outcomes (decreased need for surgery or hospital admissions and decreased Crohn's disease-related complications).

Khatri, Vijay P., ed. *Lymphadenectomy in Surgical Oncology*. Philadelphia: Saunders, 2007.

Kiernan, Stephen P. *Last Rights: Rescuing the End of Life from the Medical System*. New York: St. Martin's Press, 2006.

Kim, H-G., Cho, J-H., Yoo, S-R., Lee, J-S., Han, J-M., Lee, N-H., ... Son, C-G. (2013). Antifatigue effects of *Panax ginseng* C.A. Meyer: A randomized, double-blind, placebo-controlled trial. *PLoS One*, 8: e61271.

Kim, M., Thompson, L. A., Wenger, S. D., & O'Bryant, C. L. (2012). "Romidepsin: A histone deacetylase inhibitor for refractory cutaneous T-cell lymphoma." *Annals of Pharmacotherapy* 46(10):1340-1348.

Kimura, F. "Molecular Target Drug Discovery." *Internal Medicine* 46 (2007): 87-89.

King, Nancy. *Making Sense of Advance Directives*. Dordrecht, Netherlands: Kluwer, 1991.

King, Roger J. B., and Mike W. Robins. *Cancer Biology*. 3rd ed. New York: Pearson/Prentice Hall, 2006.

King, R. J. B. *Cancer Biology*. 2d ed. New York: Prentice Hall, 2000.

Kingsley, C. (2010, March) & Bandolin, S. (2011, April). Cultural and Socioeconomic Factors Affecting Cancer Screening, Early Detection and Care in the Latino Population. Ethnomed. Retrieved from https://ethnomed.org/clinical/cancer/cultural-and-socioeconomic-factors-affecting-cancer-screening-early-detection-and-care-in-the-latino-population

Kintzios, S. E. (2006). Terrestrial Plant-Derived Anticancer Agents and Plant Species Used in Anticancer Research. *Critical Reviews in Plant Sciences,* 25: 79-113. This is an article published in a scientific journal that reviews the literature over a 35-year period on plant-derived anticancer compounds and their potential as therapeutic agents.

Kiran, R., and V. Fazio. "Inflammatory Bowel Disease: Surgical Management." In *Fecal and Urinary Diversions: Management Principles*, edited by J. Colwell, M. Goldberg, and J. Carmel. St. Louis: Mosby, 2004.

Kirkwood, John M., ed. *Strategies in Adjuvant Therapy*. Malden, Mass.: Blackwell, 2000.

Kiuru, M., and V. Launonen. "Hereditary Leiomyomatosis and Renal Cell Cancer (HLRCC)." *Current Molecular Medicine* 4, no. 8 (December, 2004): 869-875.

Kivity, S., Arango, M. T., Ehrenfeld, M., Tehori, O., Shoenfeld, Y., Anaya, J., & Agmon-Levin, N. (2014). Infection and autoimmunity in Sjogren's syndrome: A clinical study and comprehensive review. *Journal of Autoimmunity,* 51, 17-22.

Klaassen, Curtis D., ed. *Casarett and Doull's Toxicology: The Basic Science of Poisons*. New York: McGraw-Hill, 2001.

Klaassen, C. D., M. O. Amdur, and J. Doull. *Toxicology: The Basic Science of Poisons*. New York: Macmillan, 1986.

Klag, Michael J, ed. *Johns Hopkins Family Health Book*. New York: HarperCollins, 1999.

Kleihus, P., and W. K. Cavenee. *Pathology and Genetics of Tumours of the Nervous System*. New York: Oxford University Press, 2000.

Klein, Harvey G., and David J. Anstee. *Mollison's Blood Transfusion in Clinical Medicine*. 11th ed. Malden, Mass.: Blackwell, 2005.

Klein, Karen. *Mama Said There'd Be Days like This: A Twelve-Step Guide to Surviving a Mastectomy*. Farmington, Conn.: Variegate Press, 2001.

Kleinsmith, L. J. *Principles of Cancer Biology*. New York: Pearson, Benjamin Cummings, 2006.

_______. *Principles of Cancer Biology*. San Francisco: Pearson Benjamin Cummings, 2006.

Klimaszewska-Wisniewska, A., Halas-Wisniewska, M., Tadrowski, T., Gagat, M., Grazaka, D., & Granka, A. (2016). Paclitaxel and dietary floavonoid fisetin: A synergistic combination that induces mitotic catastrophe and autophagic cell death in A549 non-small cell lung cancer cells. *Cancer Cell International,* 16(10). doi: 10.1186/s12935-016-0288-3.

Kluetz, P. G., Ning, Y. M., Maher, V. E., Zhang L., Tang, S., Ghosh D., ... Padzur, R. (2013). Abiraterone acetate in combination with prednisone for the treatment of patients with metastatic castration-resistant prostate cancer: U.S. food and drug administration drug approval summary. *Clinical Cancer Research* 19(24): 6650-6656. http://clincancerres.aacrjournals.org/content/19/24/6650

Knoepfler, Paul. (2013). *Stem cells: An insider's guide*. Hackensack, NJ: World Scientific.

Knox, Sally M. *The Breast Cancer Care Book: A Survival Guide for Patients and Loved Ones*. Grand Rapids, Mich.: Zondervan, 2004.

Knox, Sally M., and Janet K. Grant. *The Breast Cancer Care Book: A Survival Guide for Patients and Loved Ones*. Grand Rapids, Mich.: Zondervan, 2004.

Knutson, D., and E. Steiner. "Screening for Breast Cancer: Current Recommendations and Future Directions." *American Family Physician* 75, no. 11 (June 1, 2007): 1660-1666.

Ko, A., E. H. Rosenbaum, and M. Dollinger. *Everyone's Guide to Cancer Therapy: How Cancer Is Diagnosed, Treated, and Managed Day to Day*. 5th ed. Kansas City, Mo.: Andrews McMeel, 2007.

Kochman, M. L., ed. *The Clinician's Guide to Gastrointestinal Oncology*. Thorofare, N.J.: Slack, 2005.

Kogut, Valerie, and Sandra Luthringer. *Nutritional Issues in Cancer Care*. Philadelphia: Oncology Nursing Society, 2005.

Kolata, Gina. "Using Genetic Tests: Ashkenazi Jews Vanquish a Disease." *The New York Times*, February 18, 2003, Sec. F, pp. 1, 6.

Kolata, K. (2015, April 20). New blood test shows promise in cancer fight. *New York Times*, pp. A1. http://www.nytimes.com/2015/04/20/health/blood-test-shows-promise-as-alternative-to-cancer-biopsy.html?_r=0

Kongstvedt, Peter R. *Managed Care: What It Is and How It Works*. 2d ed. New York: Aspen, 2004.

Konkimalla, V. B., & Efferth, T. (2008). Evidence-based Chinese medicine for cancer therapy. *Journal of Ethnopharmacology, 116*(2): 207–210.

Konstantinopoulos, P. A., Karamouzis, M. V., & Papavassiliou, A. G. (2007) Focus on acetylation: The role of histone deactylase inhibitors in cancer therapy and beyond. *Expert Opinion on Investigational Drugs,* 16(5): 569-571. Short and somewhat technical review of the promise of HDACis as anticancer treatments.

Konstantinopoulos, P. A., R. J. Sullivan, M. V. Karamouzis, and B. J. Dezube. "Investigational Agents for Treatment of AIDS-Related Kaposi's Sarcoma." *Expert Opinion on Investigational Drugs* 16, no. 4 (April, 2007): 495-504.

Koren, G., M. Lishner, and D. Farine, eds. *Cancer in Pregnancy: Maternal and Fetal Risks*. New York: Cambridge University Press, 1996.

Korf, Bruce R., and Allan E. Rubenstein. *Neurofibromatosis: A Handbook for Patients, Families, and Health Care Professionals*. New York: Thieme Medical, 2005.

Koshy, Mary, et al. "Multiple Management Modalities in Esophageal Cancer." *The Oncologist* 9 (2004): 137-159.

Koss, Leonard G., and Myron R. Melamed. *Koss' Diagnostic Cytology and Its Histopathologic Bases*. 5th ed. Philadelphia: Lippincott/Williams and Wilkins, 2006.

Kovacs, C., S. MacDonald, C. Chik, and E. Bruera. "Hypercalcemia of Malignancy: A Treatment Strategy." *Journal of Pain and Symptom Management* 10 (1995): 224-232.

Kovner, Abba. *Sloan-Kettering: Poems*. Translated from the Hebrew by Eddie Levenston. New York: Schocken Books, 2002.

Kravdal, O. "The Impact of Marital Status on Cancer Survival." *Social Science and Medicine* 52, no. 3 (February, 2001): 357-368.

Krejci, M., Janikova, A., Folber, F., Kral, Z., & Mayer, J. (2015). Outcomes of 167 healthy sibling donors after peripheral blood stem cell mobilization with G-CSF 16μg/kg/day: Efficacy and safety. *Neoplasma,* 5(62): 787-792.

Kroemer, G. "Mitochondria in Cancer." *Oncogene* 25 (2006): 4630-4632.

Krug, K., Miksch, A., Peters-Klimm, F. Engeser, P., & Szecsenyi, J. (2016). Correlation between patient quality of life in palliative care and burden of their family caregivers: A prospective observational cohort study. *BMC Palliative Care,* 15(4). doi: 10.1186/s12904-016-0082-y.

Kruis, W., et al. *Diverticular Disease: Emerging Evidence in a Common Condition*. Norwell, Mass.: Springer and Falk Foundation, 2006.

Krychman, Michael L. *One Hundred Questions and Answers for Women Living with Cancer: A Practical Guide for Survivorship*. Sudbury, Mass.: Jones and Bartlett, 2007.

Kryger, Zol B., and Mark Sisco, eds. *Practical Plastic Surgery*. Austin: Landes Bioscience, 2007.

Krzyzanowski, M., Kunnadibbert, B., & Schneider, J. (Eds.). (2005). Health effects of transport-related air pollution. Geneva, Switzerland: World Health Organization.

Kubota, K. "From Tumor Biology to Clinical PET: A Review of Positron Emission Tomography (PET) in Oncology." *Annals of Nuclear Medicine* 15 (2001): 471-486.

Kuebler, Kim, Debra E. Heidrich, and Peg Esper. *Palliative and End of Life Care: Clinical Practice Guidelines*. 2d ed. St. Louis: Saunders/Elsevier, 2007.

Kufe, D. W., et al., eds. *Holland Frei Cancer Medicine*. 7th ed. Hamilton, Ont.: BC Decker, 2006.

Kuker, R. A., G. Mesoloras, and S. A. Gulec. "Optimization of FDG-PET/CT Imaging Protocol for Evaluation of Patients with Primary and Metastatic Liver Disease." *International Seminars in Surgical Oncology* 4 (2007): 17-21. Also available online at http://www.issoonline.com.

Kulik, L. M. "Advancements in Hepatocellular Carcinoma." *Current Opinion in Gastroenterology* 23 (2007): 268-274.

Kulkarni, P. S., and Purvish M. Parikh. "The Carcinoma of Parathyroid Gland." *Indian Journal of Cancer* 41 (April 1, 2004): 51-59.

Kumar, P., et al. "Late-Onset Rothmund-Thomson Syndrome." *International Journal of Dermatology* 46, no. 5 (May, 2007): 492-493.

Kumar, V., A. Abbas, N. Fausto, and R. Mitchels, eds. *Robbins Basic Pathology*. 8th ed. Philadelphia: Saunders/Elsevier, 2007.

Kumar, V., N. Fausto, and A. Abbas. *Robbins and Cobran Pathological Basis of Disease*. 7th ed. Philadelphia: Saunders, 2003.

Kumar, Vinay, et al., eds. *Robbins and Cotran Pathologic Basis of Disease*. Philadelphia: Elsevier Saunders, 2005.

Kunisaki, C., et al. "Outcomes of Mass Screening for Gastric Carcinoma." *Annuals Surgical Oncology* 13, no. 2 (February, 2006): 221-228.

Kurian, A. W., Lichtensztajn, D. Y., Keegan, T. H., Nelson, D. O., Clarke, C. C., & Gomez, S. L. (2014). Use of and mortality after bilateral mastectomy compared with other surgical treatments for breast cancer in California, 1998-2011. *JAMA*, 312: 902-914.

Kurth, K. H., G. H. J. Mickisch, and Fritz H. Schroder, eds. *Renal, Bladder, Prostate, and Testicular Cancer: An Update*. New York: Parthenon, 2001.

Kushi, Lawrence H., et al. "American Cancer Society Guidelines on Nutrition and Physical Activity for Cancer Prevention." *Cancer: A Cancer Journal for Clinicians* 56 (2006): 254-281.

Kuter, D. J., P. Hunt, W. Sheridan, and D. Zucker-Franklin, eds. "Thrombopoiesis and Thrombopoietins." In *Molecular, Cellular, Preclinical, and Clinical Biology*. Totowa, N.J.: Humana Press, 1997.

Kwon, H., & Pessin, J. E. (2013). Adipokines Mediate Inflammation and Insulin Resistance. *Frontiers in Endocrinology,* 4, 71. doi:10.3389/fendo.2013.00071

Labus, James B., and Alison A. Lauber. *Patient Education and Preventative Medicine*. Philadelphia: W. B. Saunders, 2001.

Lacey, J. V., et al. "Menopausal Hormone Therapy and Ovarian Cancer Risk in the NIH-AARP Diet and Health Study Cohort." *Journal of the National Cancer Institute* 98, no. 19 (2006): 1397-1405.

Lackriz, Barb. *Adult Leukemia: A Comprehensive Guide for Patients and Families*. Cambridge, Mass.: O'Reilly, 2001.

_______. *Adult Leukemia: A Comprehensive Guide for Patients and Families*. Sebastopol, Calif.: O'Reilly, 2001.

Laham, R., et al. "Pericardial Effusion in Patients with Cancer: Outcome with Contemporary Management Strategies." *Heart* 75, no. 1 (January, 1996): 67-71.

Lalloo, Fiona, ed. *Risk Assessment and Management in Cancer Genetics*. New York: Oxford University Press, 2005.

Lambert, P. F., and B. Sugden. "Viruses and Human Cancer." In *Clinical Oncology*, edited by M. D. Abeloff et al. 3rd ed. Philadelphia: Elsevier Churchill Livingstone, 2004.

Lambertini, M., Ferreira, A., Mastro, D. I., Danesi, R. & Pronzato, P. (2015). Pegfilgrastim for the prevention of chemotherapy-induced febrile neutropenia in patients with solid tumors. *Expert Opinion on Biological Therapy.*, 12(15): 1-19.

Landay, David S. *Be Prepared: The Complete Financial, Legal, and Practical Guide for Living with a Life-Challenging Condition*. New York: St. Martin's Press, 1998.

Landrigan, Phillip J. "Prevention of Occupational Cancer." *CA Cancer Journal for Clinicians* 46 (1996): 67-69.

Lang, Joan. "Making Comfort Healthy: Cancer Center's New Chef Finds Ways to Satisfy Patients' Need for Comfort." *Food Service Director* 20, no. 8 (August, 2007): 40.

Langdon, Simon P., ed. *Cancer Cell Culture: Methods and Protocols*. Totowa, N.J.: Humana Press, 2004.

Langhorne, Martha E., Janet S. Fulton, and Shirley E. Otto, eds. *Oncological Nursing*. 5th ed. St. Louis: Mosby Elsevier, 2007.

Langton, Helen. (2000). *The child with cancer: Family-centered care in practice*. New York: Baillière Tindall.

Lanyi, M. *Mammography: Diagnosis and Pathological Analysis*. New York: Springer, 2003.

Lapointe, Martin M., ed. *Adolescent Smoking and Health Research*. New York: Nova Biomedical Books, 2008.

Larson, D. M., et al. "Comparison of D&C and Office Endometrial Biopsy in Predicting Final Histopathologic Grade in Endometrial Cancer." *Obstetrics and Gynecology* 86, no. 1 (July, 1995): 38-42.

Lassere, Yvonne, and Paulo Hoff. "Management of Hand-Foot Syndrome in Patients Treated with Capecitabine (Xeloda)." *European Journal of Oncology Nursing* 8 (2004): S31-S40.

Laszlo, John, and Francis A. Neelson. *The Doctor's Doctor: A Biography of Eugene A. Stead, Jr., MD*. Durham, N.C.: Carolina Academic Press, 2006.

LaVeist, Thomas A. *Minority Populations and Health: An Introduction to Health Disparities in the United States*. San Francisco: Jossey-Bass, 2005.

Lavin, M. F., & Kozlov, S. (2007). ATM activation and DNA damage response. *Cell Cycle,* 6(8): 931-942.

Lawson, C. H., et al. "Interstitial Chemotherapy for Malignant Gliomas: The Johns Hopkins Experience." *Journal of Neuro-Oncology* 83 (2007): 61-70.

Lawson, Glenda. "Upper Airway Problems." In *Medical-Surgical Nursing*, edited by Wilma J. Phipps et al. 7th ed. St. Louis: Mosby, 2003.

Lax, Alistair, and Warren Thomas. "How Bacteria Could Cause Cancer: One Step at a Time." *Trends in Microbiology* 10 (2002): 293-299.

Lazaroff, M. *The Complete Idiot's Guide to Anatomy and Physiology*. Indianapolis, Ind.: Alpha Books, 2004.

Le, Q. T., B. W. Loo, A. Ho, et al. "Results of a Phase I Dose-Escalation Study Using Single-Fraction Stereotactic Radiotherapy for Lung Tumors." *Journal of Thoracic Oncology* 1, no. 8 (October, 2006): 802-809.

Leck, Renee. (2015, June 12). Agios announces new data from ongoing phase 1 trial of AG-120 showing durable clinical activity in patients with advanced hematologic malignancies. http://investor.agios.com/phoenix.zhtml?c=251862&p=irol-newsArticle&ID=2058807

Lee, Howard S., et al. *Cranial and Spinal MRI and CT*. 4th ed. New York: McGraw-Hill Professional, 1999.

Lee, J. H., et al. "Neuroimaging Strategies for Three Types of Horner Syndrome with Emphasis on Anatomic Location." *American Journal of Roentgenology* 188, no. 1 (January, 2007): W74-W81.

Lee, Stephanie J., Georgia Vogelsang, and Mary E. D. Flowers. "Chronic Graft-Versus-Host Disease." *Biology of Blood and Marrow Transplantion* 9, no. 4 (2003): 215-233.

Lee, S. J., et al. "American Society of Clinical Oncology Recommendations on Fertility Preservation in Cancer Patients." *Journal of Clinical Oncology* 24, no. 18 (2006): 2917-2931.

Lee, Sylvia, & Margolin, Kim. (2011). Cytokines in cancer immunotherapy. *Cancers*, 3: 3856-3893.

Lee, Y., & McKinnon, P. J. (2007). Responding to DNA double-strand breaks in the nervous system. *Neuroscience,* 145: 1365-1374.

Leibel, Steven A. *Textbook of Radiation Oncology*. 2d ed. Philadelphia: Saunders, 2004.

_______, and Theodore L. Phillips, eds. *Textbook of Radiation Oncology*. 2d ed. Philadelphia: Saunders, 2004.

Leiblum, Sandra R., ed. *Principles and Practice of Sex Therapy*. 4th ed. New York: Guilford Press, 2007.

Leifer, John, and Leifer, Lori L. (2015). *After you hear it's cancer: A guide to navigating the difficult journey ahead.* Lanham, MA: Rowman & Littlefield.

Lenhard, R. E., R. T. Osteen, and T. Gansler. *The American Cancer Society's Clinical Oncology*. Atlanta: American Cancer Society, 2001.

Leong A. S.-Y., and T. Y.-M. Leong. "Newer Developments in Immunohistology." *Journal of Clinical Pathology* 59 (2006): 1117-1126.

Leong, Anthony S.-Y., Kumarasen Cooper, and F. Joel W.-M. Leong. *Manual of Diagnostic Antibodies for Immunohistology*. 2d ed. London: Greenwich Medical Media, 2002.

Leong, Stanley P. L. *Selective Sentinel Lymphadenectomy for Human Solid Cancer*. New York: Springer, 2007.

Leslie, K. K., and C. A. Lange. "Breast Cancer and Pregnancy." *Obstetrics & Gynecology Clinics of North America* 32 (2005): 547-558.

Lethaby, Anne E., and Beverley J. Vollenhoven. "An Evidence-Based Approach to Hormonal Therapies for Premenopausal Women with Fibroids." *Best Practice & Research Clinical Obstetrics & Gynaecology* 22, no. 2 (April, 2008): 307-331.

Levin, B. *American Cancer Society's Complete Guide to Colorectal Cancer*. Atlanta: American Cancer Society, 2006.

Levine, M. S., and S. E. Rubesin. "Diseases of the Esophagus: Diagnosis with Esophagography." *Radiology* 237, no. 2 (November, 2005): 414-427.

Levine, Margie. *Surviving Cancer: One Woman's Story and Her Inspiring Program for Anyone Facing a Cancer Diagnosis*. New York: Broadway Books, 2001.

Levine, Marvin J. *The Toxic Time Bomb in Our Midst*. Westport, Conn.: Praeger, 2007.

Lewarski, Joseph. "Management of the Tracheostomy Patient in the Home." *RT for Decision Makers in Respiratory Care*, August, 2006. Available online at http://www.rtmagazine.com.

Lewis, C. S. *A Grief Observed*. New York: HarperCollins, 1961.

Lewis, Clare E., Jennifer Barraclough, and Rosalind O'Brien. *The Psychoimmunology of Cancer*. New York: Oxford University Press, 2002.

Lewis, Milton J. *Medicine and Care of the Dying: A Modern History*. New York: Oxford University Press, 2007.

Li, C. I., et al. "Changing Incidence Rate of Invasive Lobular Breast Carcinoma Among Older Women." *Cancer* 88, no. 11 (2000): 2561-2569.

Li, William. (2010). *Can we eat to starve cancer?* (TED talk). Retrieved from https://www.ted.com/talks/william_li?language=en

Li, Y & Zhu, B. (2014). Acute myeloid leukemia with DNMT3A mutations. *Leukemia and Lymphoma* 55(9): 2002-2012.

Li, Z., & Zhu, W. (2014). Targeting histone deacetylases for cancer therapy: From molecular mechanisms to clinical implications. *International Journal of Biological Sciences,* 10(7): 757-770. Technical but excellent description of how basic research can lead to clinical applications.

Liang, S.-L., and D. W. Chan. "Enzymes and Related Proteins as Cancer Biomarkers: A Proteomic Approach." *Clinica Chimica Acta* 381 (2007): 93-97.

Lichstenstein, Gary R., Hanauer, Stephen B., Sandborn, William J. & the Practice Parameters Committee of the American College of Gastroenterology. (2009). Management of Crohn's disease in adults. *American Journal of Gastroenterology,* 104(2), 465–483. This is the practice guideline developed by the American College of Gastroenterology for managing Crohn's Disease in adults. This article is available to the public and can be accessed at http://www.nature.com/ajg/journal/v104/n2/full/ajg2008168a.html.

Lichtman, M. A., et al., eds. *William's Hematology*. 7th ed. New York: McGraw-Hill, 2006.

Lichtman, M., et al. "International Society of Geriatric Oncology Chemotherapy Taskforce: Evaluation of Chemotherapy in Older Patients—An Analysis of the Medical Literature." *Journal of Clinical Oncology* 25, no. 14 (May 10, 2007): 1832-1843.

Liekweg, A., M. Westfeld, and U. Jaehde. "From Oncology Pharmacy to Pharmaceutical Care: New Contributions to Multidisciplinary Cancer Care." *Support Care Cancer* 12, no. 2 (February, 2004): 73-79.

Ligibel, J. A., Alfano, C. M., Courneya, K. S., Demark-Wahnefried, W., Burger, R. A., Chlebowski, R. T., . . . Hudis, C. A. (2014). American Society of Clinical Oncology position statement on obesity and cancer. *J Clin Oncol,* 32(31), 3568-3574. doi:10.1200/jco.2014.58.4680

Likis, Frances E., and Kerri Durnell Schuiling. *Women's Gynecologic Health*. Sudbury, Mass.: Jones and Bartlett, 2005.

Lim, U., et al. "Consumption of Aspartame-Containing Beverages and Incidence of Hematopoietic and Brain Malignancies." *Cancer Epidemiology Biomarkers and Prevention* 15 (September, 2006): 1654-1659.

Lindor, N. M., Hand, J., Burch, P. A. & Gibson, L. E. (2001). Birt-Hogg-Dubé syndrome: An autosomal dominant disorder with predisposition to cancers of the kidney, fibrofolliculomas, and focal cutaneous mucinosis. *International Journal of Dermatology,* 40(10), 653-656.

Lindorfer, M. A., Cook, E. M., Tupitza, J. C., Zent, C. S., Burack, R., de Jong, R. N., … Taylor, R. P. (2016). Real-time analysis of the detailed sequence of cellular events in mAb-mediated complement-dependent cytotoxicity of B-cell lines and of chronic lymphocytic leukemia B-cells. *Molecular Immunology*, 70: 13–23. doi: 10.1016/j.molimm.2015.12.007.

Linehan, W. M., B. Zbar, and D. R. Klausner. "Renal Carcinoma." In *The Metabolic and Molecular Bases of Inherited Disease*, edited by Charles R. Scriver, Arthur L. Beaudet, David Valle, and William S. Sly. 8th ed. New York: McGraw-Hill, 2001.

Link, John. *Breast Cancer Survival Manual: A Step-by-Step Guide for the Woman with Newly Diagnosed Breast Cancer*. 4th ed. New York: Holt, 2007.

Linus Pauling Institute. (2015, June 11). Resveratrol. *Micronutrient Information Center.* Retrieved from http://lpi.oregonstate.edu/mic/dietary-factors/phytochemicals/resveratrol

Lionel, J., N. Bathurst, D. Mohan, and D. Beckly. "Turcot's Syndrome." *Diseases of the Colon and Rectum* 31 (1998): 11.

Liotta, L. A., and I. R. Hart, eds. *Tumor Invasion and Metastasis*. Boston: Kluwer, 1982.

Lipkin, M: "Strategies for Colon Cancer Prevention." *Annals New York Academy of Sciences* 768 (September 30, 1995): 170-179.

Lippe, Scott D. "Ashkenazi Jews and Colon Cancer." *American Journal of Gastroenterology* 94, no. 10 (1999): 3085.

Lippman, Scott M., et al. "Cancer Prevention and the American Society of Clinical Oncology." *Journal of Clinical Oncology* 22, no. 19 (October 1, 2004): 3848-3851.

Lisle, D. (2012). *Imaging for students* (4th ed.). Boca Raton, FL: CRC Press. Excellent how-to book that shepherds medical students through the theory and techniques of medical imaging.

List, Thomas, Casi, Giulio, & Neri, Dario. (2014). A chemically defined trifunctional antibody-cytokine-drug conjugate with potent antitumor activity. *Molecular Cancer Therapeutics*, 13: 2641.

Litin, Scott C., Jr., ed. *Mayo Clinic Family Health Book*. 3rd ed. New York: HarperCollins, 2003.

Little, Jullian. *Epidemiology of Childhood Cancer*. IARC Scientific Publications 149. Lyon, France: International Agency for Research on Cancer, 1999.

Liu, F. S. "Molecular Carcinogenesis of Endometrial Cancer." *Taiwanese Journal of Obstetrics and Gynecology* 46, no. 1 (March, 2007): 26-32.

Liu, J., et al. "Wild-Type *p53* Inhibits Nuclear Factor-êB-Induced Matrix Metalloproteinase-9 Promoter

Activation: Implications for Soft-Tissue Sarcoma Growth and Metastasis." *Molecular Cancer Research* 4 (2006): 803-810.

Llamas, Michelle. (2015). Takeda offers $2.4 billion in Actos MDL cancer lawsuits, settles more in Nevada. *Drugwatch*, Retrieved from http://www.drugwatch.com/2015/10/23/actos-settlements-ongoing-litigation

Locker, G. Y., and H. T. Lynch. "Genetic Factors and Colorectal Cancer in Ashkenazi Jews." *Familial Cancer* 3, nos. 3/4 (2004): 215-221.

Loeb, Keith R. & Loeb, Lawrence A. (1999 September 20). Significance of multiple mutations in cancer. Retrieved on February 12, 2016 from http://www.Carcin.oxfordjournals.org/content/21/3/379.full. These authors discuss mutations in cancer in more depth.

Loeser, John D., ed. *Bonica's Management of Pain*. 3rd ed. Philadelphia: Lippincott Williams & Wilkins, 2001.

Lohmann, E., Krüger, S., Hauser, A-K., Hanagasi, H., Guven, G., Erginel-Unaltuna, N. … Gasser, T. (2015). Clinical variability in ataxia telangiectasia. *Journal of Neurology,* 262(7): 1724-1727.

Lorigan, Paul. *Lung Cancer*. Dana-Farber Cancer Institute Handbook. Philadelphia: Mosby, 2007.

_______, ed. *Lung Cancer*. Dana-Farber Cancer Institute Handbook. New York: Mosby Elsevier, 2007.

Love, Susan M., and Karen Lindsay. *Dr. Susan Love's Breast Book*. Rev. 4th ed. Cambridge, Mass.: Da Capo Press, 2005.

_______. *Dr. Susan Love's Breast Book*. 5th ed. Cambridge, Mass.: Da Capo Press, 2005.

Lowy, Andrew M., Steven D. Leach, and Philip Philip, eds. *Pancreatic Cancer*. New York: Springer, 2008.

Löwy, Ilana. (2011). *A woman's disease: The history of cervical cancer*. New York: Oxford University Press.

Lu, K. H., & Schmeler, K. M. (2015). Endometrial and ovarian cancer screening and prevention in women with Lynch syndrome (hereditary nonpolyposis colorectal cancer). In Barbara Goff and Sandy J. Falk (Eds.), *UpToDate*. Retrieved at: www.uptodate.com.

Lu, W., Dean-Clower E., Doherty-Gilman A., & Rosenthal D. S. (2008). The value of acupuncture in cancer care. *Hematology/Oncology Clinics of North America 22*(4), 631–648.

Luesly, David M., Frank Lawton, and Andrew Berchuck, eds. *Uterine Cancer*. New York: Informa Healthcare, 2005.

Lund, A. H., & van Lohuizen, M. (2004). Epigenetics and Cancer. *Genes and Development,* 18:2315-2335. http://genesdev.cshlp.org/content/18/19/2315.full

Lusis, E., and D. H. Gutmann. "Meningioma: An Update." *Current Opinion in Neurology* 17 (2004): 687-692.

Lydiatt, William M., and Perry J. Johnson. *Cancers of the Mouth and Throat: A Patient's Guide to Treatment*. Omaha, Neb.: Addicus Books, 2001.

Lyman, Gary H., and Jeffrey Crawford, eds. *Cancer Supportive Care: Advances in Therapeutic Strategies*. New York: Informa Healthcare USA, 2008.

Lynch, H. T., et al. "Cancer in Jews: Introduction and Overview." *Familial Cancer* 3, nos. 3/4 (2004): 177-192.

_______. "Familial Pancreatic Carcinoma in Jews." *Familial Cancer* 3, nos. 3/4 (2004): 233-240.

Lynn, Joanne, and Joan Harrold. *Handbook for Mortals: Guidance for People Facing Serious* Illness. New York: Oxford University Press, 1999.

Lynn, Joanne, et al. *Improving Care for the End of Life: A Sourcebook for Health Care Managers and Clinicians*. 2d ed. New York: Oxford University Press, 2008.

Lynn, Jorde, et al. *Medical Genetics,* 5th ed. Philadelphia, PA: Elsevier, 2015.

Lyons, Lyman. *Diagnosis and Treatment of Cancer*. New York: Chelsea House, 2007.

Lyss, Alan P., and Humberto M. Fagundes. *Chemotherapy and Radiation for Dummies*. Hoboken, N.J.: Wiley, 2005.

M. D. Anderson Hospital and Tumor Institute. *The First Twenty Years of the University of Texas, M. D. Anderson Hospital and Tumor Institute*. Houston: Author, 1964.

Ma, J. Y., et al. "Clinicopathologic Characteristics of Esophagectomy for Esophageal Carcinoma in Elderly Patients." *World Journal of Gastroenterology* 12, no. 8 (2006): 1296-1299.

Ma, J., McKeown, N. M., Hwang, S.-J., Hoffman, U., Jacques, P. F., & Fox, C. S. (2016). Sugar-Sweetened Beverage Consumption is Associated With Change of Visceral Adipose Tissue Over 6 Years of Follow-Up. *Circulation*. doi:10.1161/CIRCULATIONAHA.115.018704

Ma, X. J., et al. "Gene Expression Profiles of Human Breast Cancer Progression." *Proceedings of the National Academy of Sciences of the United States of America* 100 (2003): 5974-5979.

Mabayoje. O. (2009, Aug.6). Hispanics Who Move to the U.S. Face Higher Cancer Rate. The New York Times. Retrieved from http://www.nytimes.com/2009/08/07/health/07cancer.html?_r=0

Macbeth, Helen, & Shetty, Prakash. (Eds.). (2001). Health and ethnicity. London: Taylor & Francis.

MacDonald, T. H. *Third World Health: Hostage to First World Health*. Abingdon, England: Radcliffe, 2005.

Machado, Carlos R., & Menck, Carlos F.M. (1997). Human DNA repair diseases: From genome instability to cancer. *Brazilian Journal of Genetics*, 20(4) Retrieved February 10, 2016, from http://www.scielo.br/scielo.php?script=sci_arttext&pid=S0100-84551997000400032&lng=en&tlng=en.

MacKay, Judith, and Michael P. Eriksen. *The Tobacco Atlas*. Geneva: World Health Organization, 2002.

MacKenzie, D. J., et al. "Care of Patients After Esophagectomy." *Critical Care Nurse* 24, no. 1 (February, 2004): 16-31.

Mackowiak, Philip A., ed. *Fever: Basic Mechanisms and Management*. 2d ed. Philadelphia: Lippincott Williams & Wilkins, 1997.

Macky, Hazel, and Susan Nancarrow. *Enabling Independence: A Guide for Rehabilitation Workers*. Malden, Mass.: Blackwell, 2006.

Maderazo, E., N. Hickingbotham, C. Woronick, et al. "The Influence of Various Factors on the Accuracy of Gallium-67 Imaging for Occult Infection." *Journal of Nuclear Medicine* 29, no. 5 (1988): 608-615.

Magee, Sherri, and Kathy Scalzo. *Picking Up the Pieces: Moving Forward After Surviving Cancer*. Piscataway, N.J.: Rutgers University Press, 2007.

Mager, Dixie. "Bacteria and Cancer: Cause, Coincidence, or Cure? A Review." *Journal of Translational Medicine* 4 (2006): 14.

Maghfoor, I., D. C. Doll, and J. W. Yarbro. "Effusions." In *Clinical Oncology*, edited by M. D. Abeloff et al. New York: Churchill Livingstone, 2000.

Magrath, Ian T., ed. *The Non-Hodgkin's Lymphomas*. New York: Oxford University Press, 1997.

Mahowald, Mary B. "Ethnicity, Cultural Differences, and Sex Selection." In *Genes, Women, Equality*. New York: Oxford University Press, 2000.

Maitral, Anirban, et al. "The Human MitoChip: A High-Throughput Sequencing Microarray for Mitochondrial Mutation Detection." *Genome Research* 14 (2004): 812-819.

Making Sense of Your Genes: A Guide to genetic Counseling (2008). National Society of Genetic Counselors, Inc. and Genetic Alliance. Retrieved from http://www.geneticalliance.org/sites/default/files/publicationsarchive/guidetogcfinal.pdf

Malawer, Martin, and Paul H. Sugarbaker, eds. *Musculoskeletal Cancer Surgery: Treatment of Sarcomas and Allied Diseases*. Washington, D.C.: Kluwer Academic, 2001.

Malfertheiner, P., Megraud, F., O'Morain, C. A., Atherton, J., Axon, A. T., Bazzoli, F., ... The European Helicobacter Study Group. (2012). Management of *Helicobacter pylori* infection--the Maastricht IV/ Florence Consensus Report. *Gut,* 61(5), 646-664. This is a consensus report by 44 experts from 24 countries on the recommended management of *Helicobacter pylori* infection based on best current evidence at the time of their meeting. There were three subdivided workshops from the group's deliberations: (1) Indications and contraindications for diagnosis and treatment. (2) Diagnostic tests and treatment of infection. (3) Prevention of gastric cancer and other complications.

"Malignant Melanoma of the Uvea." In *AJCC Cancer Staging Manual*, edited by Frederick L. Greene et al. 6th ed. New York: Springer-Verlag, 2002.

Man, Yang-gao, Stojadinovic, A., Mason, J., Avital, I., Bilchik, A., Bruecher, B., ... Jewett, A. (2013). Tumor-infiltrating immune cells promoting tumor invasion and metastasis: existing theories. *Journal of Cancer*, 4(1): 84-95.

Manaster, B. J., and A. J. Doyle. "Giant Cell Tumors of the Bone." *Radiologic Clinics of North America* 31, no. 2 (1993): 299-323.

Mandal, A. & Viswanathan, C., (2015) Natural Killer Cells: In Health and Disease. *Hematology Oncology and Stem Cell Therapy,* 8(2): 47-55.

Mandal, A. (2013). What are antioxidants? Retrieved from http://www.news-medical.net/health/What-are-Antioxidants.aspx

Mandrell, B. N. "Secondary Breast Cancer in a Woman Treated for Hodgkin Lymphoma as a Child." *Oncology* 21 (October, 2007): 27-29.

Manni, Andrea, ed. *Endocrinology of Breast Cancer*. Totowa, N.J.: Humana Press, 1999.

Mansel, R. E., ed. *Recent Developments in the Study of Benign Breast Disease: The Proceedings of the Fifth International Benign Breast Symposium*. Park Ridge, N.J.: Parthenon, 1993.

Mappes, Thomas A., and David De Grazia. *Biomedical Ethics*. 6th ed. New York: McGraw-Hill, 2006.

Maraldo, M., Giusti, F., Vogelius, I., Lundemann, M., van der Kaaij, M. A., Ramadan, S., ... European Organisation for Research and Treatment of Cancer (EORTC) Lymphoma Group. (2015). Cardiovascular disease after treatment for Hodgkin's lymphoma: An analysis of nine collaborative EORTC-LYSA trials. *The Lancet Haematology,* 2(11): e492-e502.

Marcil, William Matthew. *Occupational Therapy: What It Is and How It Works*. Clifton Park, N.Y.: Thomson Delmar, 2007.

Marcinko, David E. *Dictionary of Health Insurance and Managed Care*. New York: Springer, 2006.

_______., and Hope R. Hetico, eds. *Dictionary of Health Insurance and Managed Care*. New York: Springer, 2006.

Marcus, R., Sweetenham, J. W., & Williams, M. E. (Eds.). (2014). *Lymphoma: Pathology, Diagnosis, and Treatment* (Cambridge Medicine). New York: Cambridge University Press.

Marincola, F. M., E. M. Jaffee, D. J. Hicklin, and S. Ferrone. "Escape of Human Solid Tumors from T-Cell Recognition: Molecular Mechanisms and Functional Significance." *Advances in Immunology* 74 (2000): 181-273.

Maris, J. M., M. D. Hogarty, R. Bagatell, and S. I. Cohn. "Neuroblastoma." *Lancet* 369, no. 9579 (June 23, 2007): 2106-2120.

Mark, Hon Fong L., ed. *Medical Cytogenetics*. Boca Raton, Fla.: CRC Press, 2000.

Markowska, A., Kasprzak, B., Jaszczyn´ska-Nowinka, K., Lubin, J., & Markowska, J. (2015). Nobel metals in oncology. *Contemporary Oncology*, 19(4): 271-275.

Marks, Sheldon. *Prostate Cancer: A Family Guide to Diagnosis, Treatment, and Survival*. Cambridge, Mass.: Fisher Books, 2000.

Marquard, J., & Eng, C., (2015). Multiple Endocrine Neoplasia Type 2. In R. A. Pagon, M. P. Adam, H. H. Ardinger, S. E. Wallace, A. Amemiya, L. J. H. Bean, T. D. Bird, C-T. Fong, H. C. Mefford, R. J. H. Smith, & K. Stephens (Eds.), *Gene reviews*. Seattle, WA: University of Washington. Available from: http://www.ncbi.nlm.nih.gov/books/NBK1257/

Marr, Kieren A., & Subramanian, Aruna K. (Eds). (2010). Infections in transplant and oncology patients. Infectious Disease Clinics of North America, 24(2): 257-529.

Martakis, Ignatius K., ed. *Cancer Research at the Leading Edge*. New York: Nova Science, 2007.

Marx, S. J. & Wells, S. A. Jr. (2012). Multiple endocrine neoplasia. In S. Melmed, K. S. Polonsky, P. R. Larsen, & M. Kronenberg (Eds.), *Williams textbook of endocrinology* (12th ed.) (pp. 1728–1767). Philadelphia, PA: Elsevier.

Maryam, M., Rusea, G. C., Yong, S. Y., & Mohd, N. (2013). Vinca Alkaloids. *International Journal of Preventive Medicine,* 4: 1231-1235. This is a scientific article that discusses the four major vinka alkaloids currently in clinical use.

Maser, R. S., and R. A. DePinho. "Connecting Chromosomes, Crisis, and Cancer." *Science* 297 (2002): 565-569. Rajagopalan, H., and C. Lengauer. "Aneuploidy and Cancer." *Nature* 432 (2004): 338-341.

Mason, W. P. "Oligodendroglioma." *Current Treatment Options in Neurology* 7, no. 4 (July, 2005): 305-314.

Master-Hunter, Tarannum, and Diana L. Heiman. "Amenorrhea: Evaluation and Treatment. " *American Family Physician* 73, no. 8 (April 15, 2006).

Mauch, P.M., Armitage, J.O., Coiffier, B., Dalla-Favera, R., Harris, N. L, (Eds.). (2004). *Non-Hodgkin's Lymphomas*. Philadelphia, PA: Lippincott Williams & Wilkins.

Mauch, Peter M., et al., eds. *Hodgkin's Disease*. Philadelphia: Lippincott Williams & Wilkins, 1999.

Maude, S. L., Frey, N., Shaw, P. A., Aplenc, R., Barrett, D. M., Bunin, N. J., … Grupp, S. A. (2014). Chimeric antigen receptor T cells for sustained remissions in leukemia. *New England Journal of Medicine*, 371, 1507-1517.

Maxwell, G. Larry. (2015). The state of advocacy in cancer. *Gynecologic Oncology*, 139, 573-579.

Mayo Clinic Staff (2014, Feb 12). *Breast cancer chemoprevention: Medicines that reduce breast cancer risk.* Mayo Clinic. Retrieved from http://www.mayoclinic.org/diseases-conditions/breast-cancer/in-depth/breast-cancer/art-20045353

Mayo Clinic. *Mayo Clinic Family Health Book*. 3rd ed. New York: HarperCollins, 2003.

Mayo Clinic. *Mayo Clinic: Guide to Women's Cancers*. New York: Kensington, 2005.

Mayur V. J., Paczulla, A. M., Klonisch, T., Dimgba, F. N., Rao, S. B., Roberg, K., Schweizer F, Lengerke C, Davoodpour P, Palicharla VR, Maddika S, Łos M. (2003). Interconnections between apoptotic, autophagic and necrotic pathways: Implications for cancer therapy development. *Journal of Cellular and Molecular Medicine*, 17(1): 12-29.

McAllister, L. D., J. H. Ward, S. F. Schulman, and L. M. DeAngelis. *Practical Neuro-Oncology: A Guide to Patient Care*. 5th ed. Boston: Butterworth-Heinemann, 2001.

McCally, Michael. *Life Support: The Environment and Human Health*. Cambridge, Mass.: MIT Press, 2003.

McCarthy, Desmond A., and Marion G. Macey, eds. *Cytometric Analysis of Cell Phenotype and Function*. New York: Cambridge University Press, 2001.

McClatchey, Kenneth D., ed. *Clinical Laboratory Medicine*. 2d ed. Philadelphia: Lippincott Williams & Wilkins, 2002.

McClay, Edward F. *One Hundred Questions and Answers About Melanoma and Other Skin Cancers*. Sudbury, Mass.: Jones and Bartlett, 2004.

_______, Mary-Eileen T. McClay, and Jodie Smith. *One Hundred Questions and Answers About Melanoma and Other Skin Cancers*. Sudbury, Mass.: Jones and Bartlett, 2004.

McCrae, Keith R., ed. *Thrombocytopenia*. New York: Taylor & Francis, 2006.

McDonald, S., D. Saslow, and M. H. Alciati. "Performance and Reporting of Clinical Breast Examination: A Review of the Literature." *CA: A Cancer Journal for Clinicians* 54 (2004): 345-361.

McDougal, W. S. "Advances in the Treatment of Carcinoma of the Penis." *Urology* 66, suppl. 5 (November, 2005): 114-117.

McGranahan, G., & Murray, F. (2003). Air pollution and health in developing Countries. London: Earthscan.

McGrath, K. G. "An Earlier Age of Breast Cancer Diagnosis Related to More Frequent Use of Antiperspirants/Deodorants and Underarm Shaving." *European Journal of Cancer Prevention* 12, no. 6 (2003): 479-485.

McIlwain, Harris H. *The Fifty-Plus Wellness Program*. Hoboken, N.J.: John Wiley and Sons, 1991.

McKay-Moffat, Stella, ed. *Disability in Pregnancy and Childbirth*. New York: Churchill Livingstone/Elsevier, 2008.

McKinnell, G. R., Parchment, R. E., Perantoni, A. O. Barry Pierce, G., & Damjanov, I. (Eds.). (2006). The biological basis of cancer (2nd ed.). New York: Cambridge University Press.. http://www.cambridge.org/us/academic/subjects/life-sciences/cell-biology-and-developmental-biology/biological-basis-cancer-2nd-edition?format=AR. ISBN-13: 000-0521606330

McLaughlin, L., Cruz, C. R., & Bollard, C. M. (2015). Adoptive T-cell therapies for refractory/relapsed leukemia and lymphoma: current strategies and recent advances. *Therapeutic Advances in Hematology*, 6(6), 295-307.

McLellan, B. (2013). How to recognize and manage hand-foot syndrome due to capecitabine or doxorubicin. *ASCO Post,* 4(10). http://www.ascopost.com/issues/june-25,-2013/how-to-recognize-and-manage-hand-foot-syndrome-due-to-capecitabine-or-doxorubicin.aspx

McNeil, D. G. (2014, April 1). Expansion in use of cancer vaccine. *The New York Times,* pp. D5. Retrieved from http://www.nytimes.com/2014/04/01/health/an-expansion-in-use-of-cancer-vaccine.html?_r=0

McPhee, Stephen J. Maxine A. Papadakis, and Lawrence M. Tierney, eds. *Current Medical Diagnosis and Treatment 2008*. New York: McGraw-Hill Medical, 2007.

McTiernan, Anne, ed. *Cancer Prevention and Management Through Exercise and Weight Control*. Boca Raton, Fla.: Taylor & Francis, 2006.

McTiernan, Anne, Julie Gralow, and Lisa Talbott. *Breast Fitness: An Optimal Exercise and Health Plan for Reducing Your Risk of Breast Cancer.* New York: St. Martin's Press, 2014.

McWhinney, S. R., Goldberg, R. M., & McLeod, H. L. (2009). Platinum neurotoxicity pharmaco-genetics. *Molecular Cancer Therapeutics*, 8(10): 10-16. http://www.ncbi.nlm.nih.gov/pmc/articles/PMC2651829/

Meade, M. S., and R. J. Earickson. *Medical Geography*. 2d ed. New York: Guilford, 2005.

Meadows, Michelle. "Robots Lend a Helping Hand to Surgeons." *FDA Consumer* 36 (2002).

Mechanisms of Carcinogenesis. International Agency for Cancer Research, 2008 https://www.iarc.fr/en/publications/pdfs-online/wcr/2008/wcr_2008_5.pdf

Medicare and Clinical Research Studies. Centers for Medicare and Medicaid Services. Retrieved from https://www.medicare.gov/Pubs/pdf/02226.pdf

Mehta, M.P., Chang, S.M., Guha, A., Newton, H.B., & Vogelbaum, M.A. (Ed.). (2011). *Principles and practice of neuro-oncology: A multidisciplinary approach*, New York, NY: Demos Medical Publishing.

Melamud, Alex, Rakhee Palekar, and Arun Singh. "Retinoblastoma." *American Family Physician* 73, no. 6 (2006): 1039-1044.

Melero, I., et al. "Immunostimulatory Monoclonal Antibodies for Cancer Therapy." *Nature Reviews Cancer* 7 (2007): 95-106.

Melero, I., Gaudemack, G., Gerritsen, W., Huber, C., Parmiani, G., Scholl, S., … Mellstedt, H. (2014). Therapeutic vaccines for cancer: An overview of clinical trials. *Nature Reviews Clinical Oncology* 11: 509–524.

Memorial Sloan-Kettering Cancer Center. "Cancer-Reducing Benefits of Preventive Surgery May Be Specific to Gene Mutation." *Science Daily*, June 5, 2006. Also available at http://www.science daily.com.

Mendelsohn, J., Howley, P. M., Israel, M. A., Gray, J. W., & Thompson, C. B. (Eds.). (2015). The molecular basis of cancer (4th ed.). Philadelphia: Elsevier/Saunders.

Mendenhall, W., et al. "Management of Acoustic Schwannoma." *American Journal of Otolaryngology* 25 (2004): 38-47.

Mendes, E. (2015). Personalized medicine: Redefining cancer and its treatment. Retrieved from: http://www.cancer.org/research/acsresearchupdates/more/personalized-medicine-redefining-cancer-and-its-treatment.

Menendez, L. R., ed. *Orthopaedic Knowledge Update: Musculoskeletal Tumors*. Rosemont, Ill.: American Academy of Orthopedic Surgeons, 2002.

Menikoff, J., & Richards, E. P. (2006). *What the doctor didn't say: The hidden truth about medical research.* New York, NY: Oxford University Press.

Merchant, T. E., et al. "Craniopharyngioma: The St. Jude Children's Research Hospital Experience, 1984-2001." *International Journal of Radiation Oncology, Biology and Physics* 53 (2002): 533-542.

Merisio, C., et al. "Endometrial Cancer in Patients with Preoperative Diagnosis of Atypical Endometrial Hyperplasia." *European Journal of Obstetrics & Gynecology and Reproductive Biology* 122, no. 1 (September 1, 2005): 107-111.

Merrick, G. S., et al. "Long Term Rectal Function After Permanent Prostate Brachytherapy." *Cancer Journal* 13, no. 2 (March/April, 2007): 95-104.

Metrosa, Elene V., ed. *Racial and Ethnic Disparities in Health and Health Care*. New York: Nova Science, 2006.

Mettler, Fred A., and Milton J. Guiberteau. *Essentials of Nuclear Medicine Imaging*. 3rd ed. Philadelphia: W. B. Saunders, 1991.

Mettler, Fred A., Jr., and Milton J. Guiberteau. *Essentials of Nuclear Medicine Imaging*. 5th ed. Philadelphia: Saunders/Elsevier, 2006.

Meuten, Donald J., ed. *Tumors in Domestic Animals*. 4th ed. Malden, Mass.: Blackwell, 2002.

Meyer, J., B. Czito, F. F. Yin, and C. Willett. "Advanced Radiation Therapy Technologies in the Treatment of Rectal and Anal Cancer: Intensity-Modulated Photon Therapy and Proton Therapy." *Clinical Colorectal Cancer* 6, no. 5 (January, 2007): 348-356.

Meyer, Jerrold S., & Quenzer, Linda F. (2013). *Psychopharmacology: Drugs, the Brain, and Behavior, 2nd Ed.* Sunderland, MA: Sinauer Associations, Inc. Provides an overview of psychopharmacology, mechanisms of action for various drugs and their effects on behavior, and a chapter focused on cannabinoids and the endocannabinoid system.

Meyer, Marie M., and Paula Derr. *The Comfort of Home: A Complete Guide for Caregivers*. Portland, Oreg.: CareTrust Publications, 2007.

Meyer, W. H., and S. L. Spunt. "Soft-Tissue Sarcomas of Childhood." *Cancer Treatment Reviews* 30 (2004): 269-280.

Micali, G., M. R. Nasca, D. Innocenzi, and R. A. Schwartz. "Penile Cancer." *Journal of the American Academy of Dermatology* 54, no. 3 (March, 2006): 369-391.

Michaels, Carol and Maria Drozda. *Exercises for Cancer Survivors.* Victoria, BC:FriesenPress, 2013.

Michiels, J. J., De Raeve, H., Berneman, Z., & Schrovens, W. (2006). The 2001 World Health Organization and updated European clinical and pathological criteria for the diagnosis, classification, and staging of the Philadelphia chromosome-negative chronic myeloproliferative disorders. *Seminars in Thrombosis and Hemostasis,* 32: 307-340.

Micsik, T., Lorincz, A., Gal, J., Schwab, R., & Petak. (2015). MDR-1 and MRP-1 activity in peripheral blood leukocytes of rheumatoid arthritis patients. *Diagnostic Pathology,* 10(216). doi: 10.1186/s13000-015-0447-1.

Mikkola, A., et al. "Ten-Year Survival and Cardiovascular Mortality in Patients with Advanced Prostate Cancer Primarily Treated by Intramuscular Polyestradiol Phosphate or Orchiectomy." *Prostate* 67, no. 4 (March 1, 2007): 447-455.

Miller, Anthony B., ed. *Advances in Cancer Screening*. Boston: Kluwer Academic, 1996.

Miller, B. A,, Kolonel, L. N., Bernstein, L., Young Jr., J. L., Swanson, G. M., West, D. … Sondik, E. J. (Eds.). (1996). Racial/ethnic patterns of cancer in the United States 1988-1992, *NIH Pub. No. 96-4104*. Bethesda, MD: National Cancer Institute.

Miller, C. R., and A. Perry. "Glioblastoma." *Archives of Pathology and Laboratory Medicine* 131 (March, 2007): 397-406.

Miller, M., and M. Brinker, eds. *Review of Orthopedics*. 4th ed. Philadelphia: W. B. Saunders, 2004.

Miller, S., Bowen, D., Croyle, R., & Rowland, J. (Eds.). (2009). *Handbook of Cancer control and behavioral science: A resource for researchers, practitioners, and policymakers.* Washington, D.C.: American Psychological Association.

Miller, William R., and James N. Ingle. *Endocrine Therapy in Breast Cancer*. New York: Informa Healthcare, 2002.

Minkin, Mary Jane, and Carol V. Wright. *A Woman's Guide to Sexual Health*. New Haven, Conn.: Yale University Press, 2004.

Mintz, Suzanne Gebben. *Love, Honor, and Value: A Family Caregiver Speaks Out About the Choices and Challenges of Caregiving*. Sterling, Va.: Capital Books, 2002.

Mirick, D. K., S. Davis, and D. B. Thomas. "Antiperspirant Use and the Risk of Breast Cancer." *Journal of the National Cancer Institute* 94, no. 20 (2002): 1578-1580.

Miskovitz, Paul A., and Marian Betancourt. *The Doctor's Guide to Gastrointestinal Health*. Hoboken, N.J.: Wiley, 2005.

Mitchell, Deborah. (2012). *The Women's Pill Book: Your Complete Guide to Prescription and Over-the-Counter Medication*. New York: St. Martin's Press.

Mitchell, I. "Patient Education at a Distance." *Radiology* 13, no. 1 (February, 2007): 30-34.

Mittelstaedt, Martin. "'Inherently Toxic' Chemical Faces Its Future." *Globe and Mail*, April 7, 2007.

Miwa, M., Ura, M., Nishida, M., Sawada, N., Ishikawa, T., Mori, K., … Ishitsuka, H. (1998). Design of a novel oral fluoropyrimidine carbamate, capecitabine, which generates 5-fluorouracil selectively in tumours by enzymes concentrated in human liver and cancer tissue. *European Journal of Cancer.* 34(8): 1274-1278.

Miyahira, A. K., Simons, J. W., & Soule, H. R. (2015). The 21st annual Prostate Cancer Foundation scientific retreat report. *The Prostate,* 75(11), 1119–1128. DOI:10.1002/pros.22993

Molgora, B., Bateman, R., Sweeney, G., Finger, D., Dimler, T., Rita B. Effros. R. B., & Hector F. Valenzuela. (2013). Functional assessment of pharmacological telomerase activators in human T cells. *Cells* 2(1): 57-66.

Moline J, & Eng C. (2011). Multiple endocrine neoplasia type 2: An overview. *Genetics in Medicine,* 13(9), 755–764. http://www.ncbi.nlm.nih.gov/pubmed/21552134

Molineux, G., M. A. Foote, and S. G. Elliott, eds. *Erythropoietins and Erythropoiesis: Molecular, Cellular, Preclinical, and Clinical Biology.* Basel, Switzerland: Birkhäuser, 2003.

Molino, D., J. Sepe, P. Anastasio, and N. G. De Santo. "The History of Von Hippel-Lindau Disease." *Journal of Nephrology* 10 (2006): S119-S123.

Montanari, F., Zdrazil, B., Digles, D., & Ecker, G.F. (2016). Selectivity profiling of BCRP versus P-gp inhibition: From automated collection of polypharmacology data to multi-label learning. *Journal of Chemiformatics,* 8(7). doi: 10.1186/s13321-016-0121-y.

Montgomery, Elizabeth, and Alan D. Aaron, eds. *Clinical Pathology of Soft-Tissue Tumors.* London: Informa Healthcare, 2001.

Montgomery, Hugh, Neil Goldsack, and Richard Marshall. *My First MRCP Book.* London: Remedica, 2003.

Moolgavkar, S., et al., eds. *Quantitative Estimation and Prediction of Human Cancer Risks.* IARC Scientific Publications 131. Lyon, France: International Agency for Research on Cancer.

Moore, K., and L. Schmais. *Living Well with Cancer: A Nurse Tells You Everything You Need to Know About Managing the Side Effects of Your Treatment.* New York: Putnam Publishing Group, 2001.

Moore, Stephen W. *Griffith's Instructions for Patients.* 7th ed. Philadelphia: Elsevier Saunders, 2005.

Moorhouse, Timothy. *Hospice Design Manual: For In-Patient Facilities.* Machiasport, Maine: Hospice Education Institute, 2006.

Moreau, P., Richardson, P.G., Cavo, M., Orlowski, R.Z., San Miguel, J.F., Palumbo, A., & Harousseau, J.L. (2012). Proteasome inhibitors in multiple myeloma: 10 years later. *Blood,* 120: 947–959.

Morgan, D. (2007). *The cell cycle: Principles of control.* Sunderland, MA: Sinauer Associates.

Morra, Marion E., and Eve Potts. *Choices.* 4th ed. New York: HarperCollins, 2003.

Morrison, Patrick J., Shirley V. Hodgson, and Neva E. Haites, eds. *Familial Breast and Ovarian Cancer: Genetics, Screening, and Management.* New York: Cambridge University Press, 2002.

Morrow, G. R. "Cancer-Related Fatigue: Causes, Consequences, and Management." *The Oncologist* 12 (May, 2007): 1-3.

Morstyn, G., Foote, M. A., & Lieschke, G. J. (Eds.). (2004). *Hematopoietic growth factors in oncology: Basic science and clinical therapeutics.* Totowa, N.J.: Humana Press.

Mortimer, P. S. "The Pathophysiology of Lymphedema." *Cancer* 83 (1998): 2798-2802.

Morton, David. *Nolo's Guide to Social Security Disability: Getting and Keeping Your Benefits.* 2d ed. Berkeley, Calif.: Nolo Press, 2003.

Mosby's Drug Consult 2007. St. Louis: Mosby Elsevier, 2007.

Moseholm, E., Rydaho-Hansen, S., Lindhardt, B.O. (2016). Under diagnostic evaluation for possible cancer affects the health-related quality of life in patients presenting with non-specific symptoms. *PLOS ONE,* 11(2). doi: 10.1371/journal.pone.0148463.

Moticka, Edward. (2016). *A historical perspective on evidence-based immunology.* Waltham, MA: Elsevier.

Mould, D. P., McGonagle, A. E., Wiseman, D. H., Williams, E. L., & Jordan, A. M. (2015). Reversible inhibitors of LSD1 as therapeutic agents in acute myeloid leukemia: Clinical significance and progress to date. *Medicinal Research Reviews,* 35: 586–618.

Mountain, C. F. "Revisions in the International System for Staging Lung Cancer." *Chest* 111 (1997): 1710-1717.

Moussa, P., Marton, J., Vidal, S. M. & Fodil-Cornu, N. (2012) Genetic dissection of NK cell responses. *Frontiers in Immunology,* 3(425): Retrieved at http://dx.doi.org/10.3389/fimmu.2012.00425.

Moynihan, T.J. (2015, March 25). HER2-positive breast cancer: What is it? Retrieved from http://www.mayoclinic.org/breast-cancer/expert-answers/faq-20058066

Mozes, A. (2015). Can Coffee Lower Risk of Colon Cancer's Return? *WebMD News from Health Day.* http://www.webmd.com/colorectal-cancer/news/20150817/can-coffee-lower-risk-of-colon-cancers-return

Mukherjee, A. K., Basu, S., Sarkar, N., & Ghosh, A. C. (2001). Advances in Cancer Therapy with Plant Based Natural Products. *Current Medicinal Chemistry,* 8(12): 1467-1486. This is a review article that discusses anticancer properties of plants, including structure, chemistry, mechanism of action, and recent advances.

Mukherjee, Siddharta. (2010). *The Emperor of All Maladies: A Biography of Cancer*. New York, NY: Scribner.

Mukhopadhyay, Tapas, Maxwell, Steven A., & Roth, Jack A. (1995). p53 suppressor gene. New York: Springer, 1995.

Mullahy, C. *The Case Manager's Handbook*. 5th ed. Sudbury, Mass.: Jones and Bartlett, 2014.

Mullan, P.B., Quinn, J. E., & Harkin, D. P. (2006). The role of BRCA1 in transcriptional regulation and cell cycle control. *Oncogene,* 25(43): 5854-5863.

Munden, Julie, et al. *Pathophysiology Made Incredibly Easy!* 4th ed. Philadelphia: Lippincott Williams & Wilkins, 2008.

Munoz, Juan Carlos, & Lambiase, Louis R. (2015). Hereditary Colorectal Cancer. In Francisco Talavera and BS Anand (Eds.), *Medscape* (April, 2015). Retrieved from http://emedicine.medscape.com/article/188613-overview

Murphy, Kathryn. (Ed.). (2015). *Children's oncology group family handbook* (Kindle edition) (2nd ed.). Monrovia, CA: The Children's Oncology Group.

Murphy, Kenneth. (2011). *Janeway's immunobiology* (8th ed.). New York: Garland Science, 2011.

Murphy, Kevin. *Adjuvant Chemotherapy Guide*. Available online at http://www.cancerguide.org.

Murray, Henry W., ed. *FUO: Fever of Undetermined Origin*. New York: Futura, 1988.

Myers, Eugene N., et al., eds. *Cancer of the Head and Neck*. 4th ed. Philadelphia: Saunders, 2003.

Mytko, J. J., and S. J. Knight. "Body, Mind, and Spirit: Towards the Integration of Religiosity and Spirituality in Cancer Quality of Life Research." *Psycho-oncology* 8 (1999): 439-450.

Nadir, Y., & Brenner, B. (2007). Hemorrhagic and thrombotic complications in bone marrow transplant recipients. *Thrombosis Research*, 120(suppl. 2), 92-98.

Nag, Subir, ed. *Principles and Practices of Brachytherapy*. Malden, Mass.: Blackwell, 1997.

Nagore, Eduardo, Amelia Insa, and Onofre Sanmartín. "Antineoplastic Therapy-Induced Palmar Plantar Erythrodysesthesia ('Hand-Foot') Syndrome: Incidence, Recognition, and Management." *American Journal of Clinical Dermatology* 1, no. 4 (2000): 225-234.

Naidu, R., et al., eds. *Managing Arsenic in the Environment: From Soil to Human Health.* Enfield, N.H.: CSIRO and Science, 2006.

Nakamichi, Takashi & Loftus, Peter. (2015). Takeda pharmaceutical to pay up to $2.4 billion to settle U.S. lawsuits. *Wall Street Journal*, Retrieved from http://www.wsj.com/articles/takeda-pharmaceutical-to-pay-up-to-2-4-billion-to-settle-u-s-lawsuits-1430270490

Nakamura, R. M., et al., eds. *Cancer Diagnostics: Current and Future Trends*. Totowa, N.J.: Humana Press, 2004.

Nastiuk, K.L., & Krolewski, J.J. (2016). Opportunities and challenges in combination gene cancer therapy. *Advances in Drug Delivery Reviews*, 98:35-40. http://www.ncbi.nlm.nih.gov/pubmed/26724249

Nathan, David G. *The Cancer Treatment Revolution: How Smart Drugs and Other New Therapies Are Renewing Our Hope and Changing the Face of Medicine*. New York: Wiley, 2007.

______. *The Cancer Treatment Revolution: How Smart Drugs and Other New Therapies Are Renewing Our Hope and Changing the Face of Medicine*. Hoboken, N.J.: John Wiley & Sons, 2007.

Nathan-Garner, L. (2013). Menopause and cancer risk: Get answers. *MD Anderson Cancer Center*. Retrieved from: http://www.mdanderson.org/patient-and-cancer-information/cancer-information/cancer-topics/prevention-and-screening/health/menopausecancer.html.

National Cancer Institute, Division of Cancer Research Resources and Centers. *The Cancer Centers Program*. Washington, D.C.: U.S. Department of Health, Education, and Welfare, Public Health Service, National Institutes of Health, 1974.

National Cancer Institute. *What You Need to Know About Cancer of the Larynx*. Bethesda, Md.: National Institutes of Health, 1995.

National Cancer Institute. *Taking Time: Support for People with Cancer and the People Who Care About Them*. Bethesda, Md.: Author, 2003.

National Cancer Institute. *Pain Control: A Guide for People with Cancer and Their Families*. NIH Publication 03-4746. Bethesda, Md.: Author, 2003.

National Cancer Institute. *Trainer's Guide for Cancer Education*. Bethesda, Md.: National Institutes of Health, National Cancer Institute, 2005.

National Cancer Institute. (2003). Biological therapy: Treatments that use your immune system to fight cancer. *NIH Publication 03-5406*. Bethesda, MD.: National Institutes of Health. Also available at http:// www .cancer.gov.

National Cancer Institute. *Chemotherapy and You*. NIH Publication No. 07-7156. Bethesda, Md.: National Institutes of Health, U.S. Department of Health and Human Services, 2007.

National Cancer Institute. (2011). 21st Century Adult Cancer Sourcebook: Chronic Myeloproliferative Disorders – Chronic Myelogenous Leukemia, Polycythemia Vera, Myelofibrosis, Thrombocythemia, Neutrophilic Leukemia. Progressive Management. This sourcebook includes information from cancer experts and includes information on signs, symptoms, treatment options, diagnostic testing, prognosis and survival.

National Cancer Institute. (2011). Chemotherapy and you: Support for people with cancer. NIH Publication No. 11-7156. Bethesda, Md.: National Institutes of Health, U.S. Department of Health and Human Services, Rev. June 2011. Available at http://www.cancer.gov/publications/patient-education/chemo-and-you.

National Cancer Institute. 21st Century Adult Cancer Sourcebook: Adult Acute Myeloid Leukemia (AML), ANLL, Myelogenous or Myeloblastic Leukemia. (2011). Patient-directed, comprehensive information from cancer experts across the nation and includes signs, symptoms, treatment options, drugs, chemotherapy, staging, biology, prognosis, and survival.

National Cancer Institute. (2012). Oral Contraceptives and Cancer Risk. Retrieved from http://www.cancer.gov/about-cancer/causes-prevention/risk/hormones/oral-contraceptives-fact-sheet.

National Cancer Institute. (2013). Surgery to Reduce the Risk of Breast Cancer. Retrieved from http://www.cancer.gov/types/breast/risk-reducing-surgery-fact-sheet.

National Cancer Institute. (2013 June 12). Biological Therapies for Cancer. Retrieved February 7, 2016 from Http://www.cancer.gov/about-cancer/treatment/types/immunotherapy/biotheraputics-fact-sheet.

National Cancer Institute. (2013, July 3). FDA approval for trastuzumab. Retrieved from http://www.cancer.gov/about-cancer/treatment/drugs/fda-trastuzumab#Anchor-Gastric

National Cancer Institute. (2015). Male Breast Cancer Treatment-for health professionals (PDQ). Retrieved from http://www.cancer.gov/types/breast/hp/male-breast-treatment-pdq.

National Cancer Institute. (2015 April 1). BRCA1 and BRCA2: Cancer risk and genetic testing. Retrieved on February 15, 2016 from http://www.cancer.net/ about-cancer/causes-prevention/genetics/brca-fact-sheet.

National Cancer Institute. (2015 December 18) Childhood Rhabdomyosarcoma Treatment. Retrieved February 10, 2016 from http://www.cancer.gov/types/soft-tissue-sarcoma/patient/rhabdosarcoma-treatments.PDQ. This article discusses the diagnosis and newer treatments of rhabdomyosarcoma.

National Cancer Institute (n.d). *Obesity and Cancer Risk*. Retrieved 15 February 2016, from http://www.cancer.gov/about-cancer/causes-prevention/risk/obesity/obesity-fact-sheet#q3

National Cancer Institute. "Tumor Grade: Questions and Answers." Available online at http://www.cancer.gov.

National Cancer Institute. *Laryngeal Cancer (PDQ) Treatment*. Washington, D.C.: Author. Available online at http://www.cancer.gov.

National Cancer Institute. *Radiation Therapy and You: A Guide to Self-Help During Cancer Treatment*. NIH Publication 01-2227. Bethesda, Md.: National Institutes of Health, 2001. Also available at http://www .cancer.gov.

National Cancer Institute. *Radiotherapy and You: Support for People with Cancer*. Available online at http://www .cancer.gov/cancertopics/radiation-therapy-and-you.

National Cancer Institute. *SEER Cancer Statistics Review, 1975-2004*. Bethesda, Md.: Author, 2006.

National Cancer Policy Forum, et al. (2014) Identifying and Addressing the Needs of Adolescents and Young Adults with Cancer: Workshop Summary 1st Edition. Washington, DC: National Academies Press.

National Commission for the Protection of Human Subjects of Biomedical and Behavioral Research. (1979). *The Belmont report. Ethical principles and guidelines for the protection of human subjects of research.* Washington, D.C: U.S. Department of Health and Human Services, Department of Health, Education, and Welfare.

National Institutes of Health (2009). Acupuncture from ancient practice to modern science. *NIH Medline Plus*, 4(1), 18. https://www.nlm.nih.gov/medlineplus/magazine/issues/winter09/articles/winter09pg18.html

National Institutes of Health. *Understanding Autoimmune Diseases*. NIH Publication 98-4273. Bethesda, Md.: Author, 1998.

_______. *What You Need to Know About Hodgkin's Disease*. Bethesda, Md.: National Institutes of Health, 1999.

_______ *What You Need to Know About Non-Hodgkin's Lymphoma*. Bethesda, Md.: National Institutes of Health, 1999.

_______. *Dry Mouth*. NIH Publication 99-3179. Bethesda, Md.: Author, 1999.

_______. *Disease-Specific Estimates of Direct and Indirect Costs of Illness and NIH Support*. Bethesda, Md.: Author, 2000.

_______. *Questions and Answers About Autoimmunity*. NIH Publication 02-4858. Bethesda, Md.: Author, 2002.

_______. *Understanding the Immune System: How It Works*. NIH Publication 03-5423. Bethesda, Md.: Author, 2003.

National Institutes of Health. "NIH Study Finds Avastin and Lucentis are Equally Effective in Treating Age-Related Macular Degeneration." (2011). Retrieved at: http://www.nih.gov/news-events/news-releases/nih-study-finds-avastin-lucentis-are-equally-effective-treating-age-related-macular-degeneration

National Research Council. *Carcinogens and Anticarcinogens in the Human Diet*. Washington, D.C.: National Academy Press, 1996.

_______. *Pesticides in the Diets of Infants and Children*. Washington, D.C.: National Academy Press, 1993.

National Science Foundation. *Overcoming the Past, Focusing on the Future*. Arlington, Va.: Author, 2003.

Neale, R. E., et al. "Basal Cell Carcinoma on the Trunk Is Associated with Excessive Sun Exposure." *Journal of the American Academy of Dermatology* 56, no. 3 (2007): 380-386.

Neff, B., et al. "The Molecular Biology of Vestibular Schwannomas: Dissecting the Pathogenic Process at the Molecular Level." *Otology and Neurotology* 27 (2006): 197-208.

Nemet, A. Y., P. Martin, R. Benger, et al. "Orbital Exenteration: A Fifteen-Year Study of Thirty-eight Cases." *Ophthalmic Plastic & Reconstructive Surgery* 23, no. 6 (November/December, 2007): 468-472.

Nessim, Susan. *Can Survive: Reclaiming Your Life After Cancer*. Boston: Houghton Mifflin, 2000.

Neumann, Hartmut P., A. Vortmeyer, et al. "Evidence of MEN-2 in the Original Description of Classic Pheochromocytoma." *New England Journal of Medicine* 357 (2007): 1311-1315.

Neumann, Hartmut P., B. Bausch, et al. "Germ-Line Mutations in Nonsyndromic Pheochromocytoma." *New England Journal of Medicine* 346 (2002): 1459-1466.

Neves, H. & Kwok, H. F. (2015). Recent advances in the field of anti-cancer immunotherapy. *BBA Clinical*, 3: 280–288. doi: 10.1016/j.bbacli.2015.04.001.

Neviani, P. & Fabbri, M. (2015). "Exosomic microRNAs in the tumor microenvironment." *Frontiers in Medicine* 2(47). doi: 10.3389/fmed.2015.00047.

New England Medical Center EPC. *Management of Cancer Symptoms: Pain, Depression, and Fatigue*. Rockville, Md.: U.S. Department of Health and Human Services, Public Health Service, Agency for Healthcare Research and Quality, 2002.

Nguyen, D. X., & Massague, J. (2007). Genetic determinants of cancer metastasis. *Nature Reviews (Genetics)*, 8: 341-352. http://www.ncbi.nlm.nih.gov/pubmed/17440531.

Niederhuber, J. E., Armitage, J., Doroshow, J., Kastan, M. & Tepper, J. (2013). *Abeloff's clinical oncology* (5th ed.). Philadelphia: Elsevier – Health Sciences Division.

Niida, H., & Nakanishi, M. (2006). DNA damage checkpoints in mammals. *Mutagenesis*, 21: 3-9.

Nikolakakos, Alexios P., ed. *Oral Cancer Research Advances*. New York: Nova Biomedical Books, 2007.

NIOSH Fast Facts: Protecting Yourself from Sun Exposure. The National Institute for Safety and Health. Retrieved from http://www.cdc.gov/niosh/docs/2010-116/

Nishikawa, H., & Sakaguchi, S. (2014). Regulatory T cells in cancer immunotherapy. *Current Opinions in Immunology*, 27: 1-7.

Nishimura, H., et al. "Proton-Beam Therapy for Olfactory Neuroblastoma." *International Journal of Radiation Oncology, Biology, Physics* 68, no. 3 (July 1, 2007): 758-762.

Nishino, M., et al. "The Thymus: A Comprehensive Review." *Radiographics* 26, no. 2 (March/April, 2006): 335-348.

Nissenkorn, A., & Ben-Zeev, B. (2015). Ataxia telangiectasia. *Handbook of Clinical Neurology,* 132: 199–214.

Nitta, R., Ning, G., Avilion, A. A., & Joseph, I. (2012). Inhibition of telomerase with imetelstat causes depletion of cancer stem cells. In M. A. Hayat (Eds.), *Stem cells and cancer stem cells: Therapeutic applications in disease and injury* (pp. 13-24). New York City, NY: Springer.

Noble, J. *Textbook of Primary Care Medicine*. 3rd ed. St. Louis: Mosby, 2001.

Northrop, Dorothy E., Stephen E. Cooper, and Kimberly Calder. *Health Insurance Resources: A Guide for People with Chronic Disease and Disability*. 2d ed. New York: Demos Medical, 2007.

Norton, A. J., J. Matthews, V. Pappa, et al. "Mantle Cell Lymphoma: Natural History Defined in a Serially Biopsied Population over a 20-Year Period." *Annals of Oncology* 6 (1995): 249-256.

NTP (National Toxicology Program). 2014. *Report on Carcinogens, Thirteenth Edition*. Research Triangle Park, NC: U.S. Department of Health and Human

Services, Public Health Service. http://ntp.niehs.nih.gov/pubhealth/roc/roc13/

Null, Gary. *Women's Health Solutions*. New York: Seven Stories Press, 2002.

Nuñez, Kevin R., ed. *Trends in Kidney Cancer Research*. New York: Nova Biomedical Books, 2006.

Nurse's Five-Minute Consult: Treatments. Philadelphia: Lippincott Williams & Wilkins, 2007.

Nursing 2008 Drug Handbook. Philadelphia: Lippincott Williams & Wilkins, 2008.

Nussey, S. S., and S. A. Whitehead. *Endocrinology: An Integrated Approach*. London: Taylor & Francis, 2001.

Nwodo, J.N, A. Ibezim, C.V. Simoben, & Ntie-Kang, F. (2015). Natural products from African medicinal plants, Part II: Alkaloids, terpenoids, and flavonoids. *Anticancer Agents and Medicinal Chemistry,* 16(1):108-127. Describes anti-cancer activity from plant-derived compounds from African flora.

Nygren, P. "The Pharmacist and Quality of Cancer Chemotherapy." *Acta Oncologica* 46, no. 6 (2007): 715-716.

O'Connell, T. X., et al. "Understanding and Interpreting Serum Protein Electrophoresis." *American Family Physician* 71, no. 1 (January 1, 2005): 105-112.

O'Connor, A., McNamara, D., & O'Moráin, C. A. (2013). Surveillance of gastric intestinal metaplasia for the prevention of gastric cancer. *Cochrane Database Systematic Reviews*, 9:CD009322. The authors performed a search of electronic databases to assess the utility and structure of surveillance programs for this condition and hand-searched for abstracts from relevant conferences. They found that there was lack of randomized data for this query. Given the ethical and acceptability for issues involved in randomizing surveillance, the authors recommended further non-randomized clinical studies focusing on surveillance protocols and on the role of *Helicobacter pylori* eradication that may be utilized as a more pragmatic means of preventing gastric cancer.

O'Connor, S. M., & Boneva, R. S. (2007). Infectious Etiologies of Childhood Leukemia: Plausibility and Challenges to Proof. *Environmental Health Perspectives,* 115(1): 146–150. http://doi.org/10.1289/ehp.9024

O'Donnell, M. R., Abboud, C. N., Altman, J., Appelbaum, F. R., Arber, D. A., Attar, E., … Gregory, K. M. (2012). Acute myeloid leukemia. *Journal of the National Comprehensive Cancer Network*, 10(8):984-1021. Comprehensive and well-written review of AML.

O'Donovan, Peter J., and Ellis G. R. Downes, eds. *Advances in Gynaecological Surgery*. San Francisco: GMM, 2002.

O'Dowd, G. J., et al. "The Gleason Score: A Significant Biologic Manifestation of Prostate Cancer Aggressiveness on Biopsy." *PCRI Insights* 4, no. 1 (January, 2001).

O'Keefe, Stephen J. D., et al. "Why Do African Americans Get More Colon Cancer than Native Africans?" *Journal of Nutrition* 137, no. 1 (January, 2003): 175-183.

O'Neill, Catherine E., ed. *New Developments in Bone Cancer Research*. New York: Nova Biomedical Books, 2006.

O'Reilly, Derek A., & Poston, Graeme J. (2007). Classification of colorectal liver metastases. *Advances in Gastrointestinal Cancer.* Retrieved February 26, 2016 from HighBeam Research: https://www.highbeam.com/doc/1G1-171137590.html

O'Sullivan, B., Brierley, J., D'Cruz, A., Fey, M., Pollock, R. E., Vermorken, J., & Huang, S. H. (Eds.). (2015). *Union for international cancer control manual of clinical oncology* (9th ed.). New Jersey: Wiley-Blackwell, 2015.

Oberdoerffer, P., & Sinclair, D. A. (2007). The role of nuclear architecture in genomic instability and ageing. *Nature Reviews Molecular Cell Biology*, 8, 692-702.

Offit, Paul A. *Vaccinated: One Man's Quest to Defeat the World's Deadliest Diseases*. New York: Collins, 2007.

Offit, Paul A., and Louis M. Bell. *Vaccines: What You Should Know*. New York: Wiley, 2003.

Ohgaki, H., and P. Kleihues. "Population-Based Studies on Incidence, Survival Rates, and Genetic Alterations in Astrocytic and Oligodendroglial Gliomas." *Journal of Neuropatholy and Experimental Neurology* 64, no. 6 (June, 2005): 479-489.

Ohta, S. "Contribution of Somatic Mutations in the Mitochondrial Genome to the Development of Cancer and Tolerance Against Anticancer Drugs." *Oncogene* 25 (2006): 4768-4776.

Okamura, M., Inagaki, T., Tanaka, T., & Sakai, J. (2010). Role of histone methylation and demethylation in adipogenesis and obesity. *Organogenesis,* 6(1): 24–32. http://www.ncbi.nlm.nih.gov/pmc/articles/PMC2861740/

Oktay, K. H., L. Beck, and J. D. Reinecke. *One Hundred Questions and Answers About Cancer and Fertility*. Sudbury, Mass.: Jones and Bartlett, 2008.

Oktay, Kutluk, H., Lindsay Nohr Beck, and Joyce Dillon Reinecke. *One Hundred Questions and Answers About Cancer and Fertility*. Sudbury, Mass.: Jones and Bartlett, 2008.

Old, L. J. "Immunotherapy for Cancer." *Scientific American* 275 (1996): 136-143.

Oleinika, K., Nibbs, R. J., Graham, G. J., & Fraser, A. R. (2013). Suppression, subversion and escape:The role of regulatory T cells in cancer progression. *Clinical and Experimental Immunology*, 171(1): 36-45.

Olsen, E. A., Rook, A. H., Zic, J., Kim, Y., Porcu, P., Querfeld, C., … Duvic M. (2011). Sézary syndrome: Immunopathogenesis, literature review of therapeutic options, and recommendations for therapy by the United States cutaneous lymphoma consortium (US-CLC). *Journal of the American Academy of Dermatology,* 64(2), 352-404.

Oncology Times. (2014). Reasons identified for link between Down syndrome and leukemia. *Oncology Times,* 36(10): 66-67.

Ondrus, D., et al. "Nonseminomatous Germ Cell Testicular Tumors Clinical Stage I: Differentiated Therapeutic Approach in Comparison with Therapeutic Approach Using Surveillance Strategy Only." *Neoplasma* 54, no. 5 (2007): 437-442.

Orentas, Rimas, James W. Hodge, and Bryon D. Johnson, eds. *Cancer Vaccines and Tumor Immunity*. Hoboken, N.J.: Wiley-Interscience, 2008.

Orin, Rhonda. *Making Them Pay: How to Get the Most from Health Insurance and Managed Care*. New York: St. Martin's Press, 2001.

Oritz, Lori M. *Facing the Mirror with Cancer: A Guide to Using Makeup to Make a Difference*. Chicago: Belle Press, 2004.

Osborn, Anne G. *Diagnostic Neuroradiology*. St. Louis: Mosby-Year Book, 1994.

Osborne, Helen. *Health Literacy from A to Z: Practical Ways to Communicate Your Health Message*. Sudbury, Mass.: Jones and Bartlett, 2005.

OSI Pharmaceuticals, LLC. (2015). Tarceva (erlotinib hydrochloride) prescribing information. Retrieved from http://www.gene.com/download/pdf/tarceva_prescribing.pdf

Osowski, M. J. "Spinal Cord Compression: An Obstructive Oncologic Emergency." *Topics in Advanced Practice Nursing eJournal* 2, no. 4 (2002).

Ostrosky-Zeichner, Luis, et al. "Deeply Invasive Candidiasis." *Infectious Disease Clinics of North America* 16 (2002): 821-835.

Ota, D. M. "What's New in General Surgery: Surgical Oncology." *Journal of the American College of Surgeons* 196, no. 6 (2003): 926-932.

Ott, Mary Jane. "Mind-Body Therapies for the Pediatric Oncology Patient: Matching the Right Therapy with the Right Patient." *Journal of Pediatric Oncology Nursing* 23, no. 5 (2006): 254-257.

Otto, S. E. *Oncology Nursing*. 4th ed. St. Louis: Elsevier, 2001.

Ou, Jing-hsuin James, & Yen, T. S. B. (2010). *Human oncogenic viruses*. Hackensack, NJ: World Scientific.

Owens, Annette F., and Mitchell S. Tepper, eds. *Sexual Health*. Westport, Conn.: Praeger, 2007.

Pagana, Kathleen Deska, and Timothy J. Pagana. *Mosby's Diagnostic and Laboratory Test Reference*. Philadelphia: Elsevier-Mosby, 2006.

Pagana, Kathleen Deska, and Timothy J. Pagana. *Mosby's Manual of Diagnostic and Laboratory Tests*. 3rd ed. St. Louis: Mosby Elsevier, 2006.

Pagé, Michel. *Tumor Targeting in Cancer Therapy*. Totowa, N.J.: Humana Press, 2004.

Pagliarulo, Michael A. (2012). *Introduction to Physical Therapy.* St. Louis: Elsevier Mosby.

Pai, G. S., et al. *Handbook of Chromosomal Syndromes*. Hoboken, N.J.: John Wiley & Sons, 2003.

Pal, S. K., and B. Mittal. "Fight Against Cancer in Countries with Limited Resources: The Post-genomic Era Scenario." *Asian Pacific Journal of Cancer Prevention* 5, no. 3 (July, 2004): 328-333.

Palmateer, Paige. "Interest Rises in Cancer Insurance." *Central New York Business Journal*, October 20, 2006.

Pals, S. D., and R. M. Wilkins. "Giant Cell Tumor of the Bone Treated by Curettage, Cementation, and Bone Grafting." *Orthopedics* 15 (1992): 703-708.

Panasci, Lawrence C., and Moulay A. Alaoui-Jamali, eds. *DNA Repair in Cancer Therapy*. Totowa, N.J.: Humana Press, 2004.

Panglossi, Harold V., ed. *Antioxidants: New Research*. New York: Nova Science, 2006.

Papaefthimiou, M., et al. "The Role of Liquid-Based Cytology Associated with Curettage in the Investigation of Endometrial Lesions from Postmenopausal Women." *Cytopathology* 16, no. 1 (February, 2005): 32-39.

Pappas, Alberto S., ed. *Pediatric Bone and Soft Tissue Sarcomas*. New York: Springer, 2006.

Pappas, Peter G., et al. "Guidelines for Treatment of Candidiasis." *Clinical Infectious Diseases* 38 (2004): 161-189.

Pappo, Alberto S., ed. *Pediatric Bone and Soft Tissue Sarcomas*. New York: Springer, 2005.

Parazzini, F., C. La Vecchia, L. Bocciolone, and S. Franceschi. "The Epidemiology of Endometrial Cancer." *Gynecologic Oncology* 41 (1991): 1-16.

Parbin, S., Kar, S., Shilpi, A., Sengupta, D., Deb, M., Rath, S. K., & Patra, S. K. (2013). Histone deacetylases: A saga of perturbed acetylation homeostasis in cancer. *Journal of Histochemistry & Cytochemistry,* 62(1): 11-33. Readable summary of the consequences of inhibiting HDACs in cancer cells.

Pardoll, D. M. "Therapeutic Vaccination for Cancer." *Clinical Immunology* 95, no. 1, pt. 2 (2000): S44-S62.

Pardoll, Drew. (2012). T cells take aim at cancer. *Proceedings of the National Academy of Sciences,* 99(25): 15840-15842.Retrieve at http://www.pnas.org/content/99/25/15840.full

Parikh, S.A., Kay, N.E., & Shanafelt, T. D. (2014). How we treat Richter syndrome. Blood, 123 (11), 1647-1657.

Parisi, S., et al. "Role of External Radiation Therapy in Urinary Cancers." *Annals of Oncology* 18 (2007): vi157-vi161.

Park, Alice. "The Cancer Test: Exposing a Growing Tumor's Secrets May Be as Simple as Drawing Blood." *Time*, June 25, 2007, 53.

Park, Stephen S. *Facial Plastic Surgery: The Essential Guide*. New York: Thieme, 2005.

Parker, James N. & Parker, Philip M. (Eds.). (2002). The official patient's sourcebook on adult acute myeloid leukemia: A revised and updated directory for the internet age. Icon Health Publications. A sourcebook for patients conducted independent internet-based research to complement their treatment, and provides information for patients to find information on topics related to acute myeloid leukemia.

Parker, James N., and Philip M. Parker, eds. *The Official Parent's Sourcebook of Ewing's Family of Tumors*. San Diego, Calif.: Icon Health, 2002.

Parker, James N., and Philip M. Parker, eds. *The Official Parent's Sourcebook on Retinoblastoma: Directory for the Internet Age*. San Diego, Calif.: Icon Health, 2005.

_______. *The Official Parent's Sourcebook on Wilms' Tumor: A Revised and Updated Directory for the Internet Age*. San Diego, Calif.: Icon Health, 2002.

Parker, James N., and Philip M. Parker, eds. *The Official Patient's Sourcebook on Chronic Lymphocytic Leukemia: A Revised and Updated Directory for the Internet Age*. San Diego, Calif.: Icon Health, 2002.

_______, eds. *The Official Patient's Sourcebook on Cushing's Syndrome: A Revised and Updated Directory for the Internet Age*. San Diego, Calif.: Icon Health, 2002.

_______, eds. *The Official Patient's Sourcebook on Testicular Cancer: A Revised and Updated Directory for the Internet Age*. San Diego, Calif.: Icon Health Publications, 2002.

_______, eds. *The Official Patient's Sourcebook on Adult Brain Tumors: A Revised and Updated Directory for the Internet Age*. San Diego, Calif.: Icon Health, 2002.

_______, eds. *The Official Patient's Sourcebook on Gestational Trophoblastic Tumors*. San Diego, Calif.: Icon Health, 2002.

_______, eds. *The Official Patient's Sourcebook on Adult Hodgkin's Disease: A Revised and Updated Directory for the Internet Age*. San Diego, Calif.: Icon Health, 2002.

_______. *The Official Patient's Sourcebook on Uterine Fibroids*. San Diego, Calif.: Icon Health, 2002.

_______. *The Official Patient's Sourcebook on Ovarian Epithelial Cancer*. San Diego, Calif.: Icon Health, 2002.

_______, eds. *The Official Patient's Sourcebook on Zollinger-Ellison Syndrome: A Revised and Updated Directory for the Internet Age*. San Diego, Calif.: Icon Health, 2002.

_______, eds. *The Official Patient's Sourcebook on Testicular Cancer: A Revised and Updated Directory for the Internet Age*. San Diego, Calif.: Icon Health, 2002.

_______. *The Official Patient's Sourcebook on Childhood Ependymoma: A Revised and Updated Directory for the Internet Age*. San Diego, Calif.: Icon Health, 2002.

_______, eds. *The Official Patient's Sourcebook on Hairy Cell Leukemia*. San Diego, Calif.: Icon Health, 2002.

_______, eds. *The Official Patient's Sourcebook on Barrett's Esophagus: A Revised and Updated Directory for the Internet Age*. San Diego, Calif.: Icon Health, 2004.

_______, eds. *The Official Patient's Sourcebook on Lip and Oral Cavity Cancer*. San Diego, Calif.: Icon Health, 2005.

Parker, R. G., N. A. Janjan, and M. T. Selch. *Radiation Oncology for Cure and Palliation*. New York: Springer, 2003.

Parker, Robert G. *Radiation Oncology for Cure and Palliation*. New York: Springer, 2003.

Parker, W. H., et al. "Elective Oophorectomy in the Gynecological Patient: When Is It Desirable?" *Current Opinion in Obstetrics and Gynecology* 19, no. 4 (August, 2007): 350-354.

Parker, W., E. Filion, D. Roberge, and C. R. Freeman. "Intensity-Modulated Radiotherapy for Craniospinal Irradiation: Target Volume Considerations, Dose Constraints, and Competing Risks." *International Journal of Radiation Oncology, Biology, Physics* 69, no. 1 (September 1, 2007): 251-257.

Parkman, Henry, and Robert S. Fisher, eds. *The Clinician's Guide to Acid/Peptic Disorders and Motility*

Disorders of the Gastrointestinal Tract. Thorofare, N.J.: SLACK, 2006.

Pascual Castroviejo, I. *Spinal Tumors in Children and Adolescents*. New York: Raven Press, 1990.

Pascuzzi, Robert M. "Myasthenia Gravis and Lambert-Eaton Syndrome." *Therapeutic Apheresis and Dialysis* 6, no. 1 (February, 2002): 57-68.

Pasic, Resad P., and Ronald Leon Levine. *A Practical Manual of Hysteroscopy and Endometrial Ablation Techniques: A Clinical Cookbook*. New York: Informa Healthcare, 2004.

Pasqualini, Jorge R., ed. *Breast Cancer: Prognosis, Treatment, and Prevention*. 2d ed. New York: Informa Healthcare, 2008.

Pass, Harvey I. *One Hundred Questions and Answers About Mesothelioma*. Sudbury, Mass.: Jones and Bartlett, 2004.

Pass, Harvey I., Nicholas J. Vogelzang, and Michele Carbone, eds. *Malignant Mesothelioma: Advances in Pathogenesis, Diagnosis, and Translational Therapies*. New York: Springer, 2005.

Pastwa, E., S. B. Somiari, M. Czyz, and R. I. Somiari. "Proteomics in Human Cancer Research." *Proteomics—Clinical Application* 1 (2007): 4-17.

Pasuawski, M., J. Zuomaniec, E. Ruci½ska, and W. Koutyk. "Synchronous Primary Esophageal and Gastric Cancers." *Annales Universitatis Mariae Curie-Skuodowska* 59, no. 1 (2004): 406-410.

Patel, K. N., and A. R. Shaha. "Poorly Differentiated and Anaplastic Thyroid Cancer." *Cancer Control* 13, no. 2 (2006): 119-128.

Patel, Uday, ed. *Carcinoma of the Kidney*. New York: Cambridge University Press, 2008.

Patti, Jay W., et al. "Radiofrequency Ablation for Cancer-Associated Pain." *The Journal of Pain* 3, no. 6 (2002): 471-473.

Pattou, François, & Proye, Charles. (2001). Endocrine tumors of the pancreas. In R. G. Holzheimer, & J. A. Mannick (Eds.), *Surgical treatment: Evidence-based and problem-oriented.* Munich: Zuckschwerdt. Retrieved from http://www.ncbi.nlm.nih.gov/books/NBK6889. An extended discussion of treatment strategies for endocrine tumors of the pancreas.

Pavlidis, N., and F. Peccatori. *Cancer and Pregnancy*. New York: Springer, 2007.

Pavlovich, C. P., Grubb, R. L., Hurley, K., Glenn, G. M., Toro, J., Schmidt, L. S., Linehan, W. M. (2005). Evaluation and management of renal tumors in the Birt-Hogg-Dubé syndrome. *American Journal of Surgical Pathology,* 173(5), 1482-1486.

Pazdur, R. (July 2, 2103). *FDA Approval for Cetuximab*. Retrieved from http://www.cancer.gov/about-cancer/treatment/drugs/fda-cetuximab

Pazdur, Richard, ed. *Medical Oncology: A Comprehensive Overview*. Huntington, N.Y.: PRR, 1995.

Pea, A., Hruban, R. H., & Wood, L. D. (2015). Genetics of pancreatic neuroendocrine Tumors: Implications for the Clinic." *Expert Review of Gastroenterology & Hepatology.* 9(11), 1-13. Advances in the genetics of pancreatic neuroendocrine tumors and the potential to use this information in diagnosis and treatment.

Peabody, T. D., et al. "Evaluation and Staging of Musculoskeletal Neoplasms." *The Journal of Bone and Joint Surgery: American Volume* 80, no. 8 (1998): 1204.

Pecorino, Lauren. (2012). Molecular biology of cancer (3rd ed.). New York: Oxford University Press.

Pectasides, D., and T. Economopoulos. "Fallopian Tube Carcinoma: A Review." *Oncologist* 11 (2006): 902-912.

Pectasides, D., D. Farmakis, and M. Pectasides. "The Management of Stage I Nonseminomatous Testicular Germ Cell Tumors." *Oncology* 71, nos. 3/4 (July 17, 2007): 151-158.

Pelengaris, Stella, & Khan, Michael. (Eds.). (2006). *The molecular biology of cancer.* Malden, Mass.: Blackwell.

Pelengaris, Stella, & Khan, Michael. (Eds.). (2013). *Molecular biology of cancer: A bridge from bench to bedside.* 2nd ed. Hoboken, NJ: Wiley-Blackwell.

Pelengaris, Stella, and Michael Khan, eds. *The Molecular Biology of Cancer*. Malden, Mass.: Blackwell, 2006.

Pennazio, M. "Capsule Endoscopy: Where Are We After Six Years of Clinical Use?" *Digestive and Liver Disease* 38, no. 12 (December, 2006): 867-878.

Pensiero, Laura, Michael Osborne, and Susan Oliviera. *The Strang Cancer Prevention Center Cookbook: A Complete Nutrition and Lifestyle Plan to Dramatically Lower Your Cancer Risk*. New York: McGraw-Hill, 2004.

Penson, D. F., M. S. Litwin, J. L. Gore, et al. "Quality of Life After Surgery, External Beam Irradiation, or Brachytherapy for Early Stage Prostate Cancer." *Urologic Oncology* 25, no. 5 (September/October, 2007): 442-443.

Penthoroudiaks, G., and Palvidis, N. "Management of Leptomeningeal Malignancy." *Expert Opinion on Pharmacotherapy* 6, no. 7 (June, 2005): 1115-1125.

Perantoni, Alan O. (1998). Carcinogenesis. In R. G. McKinnell, R. E. Parchment, A. O. Perantoni, G. B. Pierce, & I. Damjanov (Eds.), The biological basis of cancer (2nd ed.), (pp. 80-125). New York: Cambridge University Press.

Perazzoli, G., Prados, J., Ortiz, R. Caba, O., Cabeza, M.B., … Melguizo, C. (2015). Temozolomide resistance in Gliopastoma cell lines: Implication of MGMT, MMR, P-Glycoprdotein and CD 133 expression. *PLOS ONE,* 10(10). doi: 10.1371/journalpone.0140131.

Perboni, S., and A. Inui. "Anorexia in Cancer: Role of Feeding-Regulatory Peptides." *Philosophical Transactions of the Royal Society B: Biolocial Sciences* 361, no. 1471 (July 29, 2006): 1281-1289.

Pereira, Larissa S., ed. *Cancer Research Perspectives.* New York: Nova Science, 2008.

Perez, A., & Merli, G. J. (2013). Novel Anticoagulant Use for Venous Thromboembolism: A 2013 Update. *Current Treatment Options in Cardiovascular Medicine,* 15(2): 164-172.

Pérez-Peña, Richard. "A $100 Million Gift to Sloan-Kettering." *New York Times*, May 10, 2006, p. B3.

Perkins, G. L., et al. "Serum Tumor Markers." *American Family Physician* 68 (2003): 1075-1082.

Perkins, Kenneth A., Cynthia A. Conklin, and Michele D. Levine. *Cognitive-Behavioral Therapy for Smoking Cessation: A Practical Guidebook to the Most Effective Treatments.* New York: Routledge, 2008.

Perlman, S. L., Boder, E., Sedgewick, R. P. & Gatti, R. A. (2012). Ataxia–telangiectasia. *Handbook of Clinical Neurology,* 103: 307–332.

Perry, Angela, ed. *The American Medical Association Guide to Home Caregiving*. New York: J. Wiley & Sons, 2001.

Perry, Chris. (2013). What leaders can learn from Stand Up To Cancer's Latest Moonshot. *Forbes*. Retrieved from http://www.forbes.com/sites/chrisperry/2013/06/17/what-leaders-can-learn-from-stand-up-to-cancers-latest-moonshot

Perry, Michael C. (Ed.). (2012). *Perry's The Chemotherapy Source Book* (5th ed.). Philadelphia, PA: Wolters Kluwer Health/Lippincott Williams &; Wilkins. This book provides information on choosing chemotherapeutic agents, using combination chemotherapy, and toxicity of individual drugs. This book focuses on clinical use of chemotherapy.

Perry, Michael C., and James E. Wooldridge. *Companion Handbook to the Chemotherapy Source Book.* 2d ed. Philadelphia: Lippincott Williams & Wilkins, 2004.

Perry, Michael C., ed. *The Chemotherapy Source Book.* 4th ed. Philadelphia: Wolters Kluwer Health/Lippincott Williams & Wilkins, 2008.

Perry, Michael Clinton. (Ed.) (2008). *The Chemotherapy Source Book* (4th ed.). Philadelphia, PA: Wolters Kluwer Health.

Persson, I., et al. "Risk of Endometrial Cancer After Treatment with Oestrogens Alone or in Conjunction with Progestogens: Results of a Prospective Study." *British Medical Journal* 298, no. 6667 (January 21, 1989): 147-151.

Perth, Danial. (2013). *HPV and men*. Seattle, WA: Amazon Digital Services.

Peters, David, and Anne Woodham. *Encyclopedia of Natural Healing*. London: Dorling Kindersley, 2000.

Peters, W. A., N. B. Kuman, and G. W. Morley. "Carcinoma of the Vagina: Factors Influencing Treatment Outcome." *Cancer* 55 (1985): 892-897.

Petrek, J. A., P. I. Pressman, and R. A. Smith. "Lymphedema: Current Issues in Research and Management." *CA: A Cancer Journal for Clinicians* 50, no. 5 (September/October, 2000): 292-307.

Petricoin, E. F., et al. "Use of Proteomic Patterns in Serum to Identify Ovarian Cancer." *Lancet* 359 (2002): 572-577.

Petrou, I. M.D. (2012, April 1). Individualized melanoma chemoprevention may be possible in future. *Dermatology Times.* Retrieved from http://dermatologytimes.modernmedicine.com/dermatology-times/news/modernmedicine/modern-medicine-feature-articles/individualized-melanoma-chemo?page=full

Petruzelli, Guy, ed. *Practical Head and Neck Oncology*. San Diego: Plural, 2008.

Pfeiffer, David. "Social Security's Disability Insurance Program: A History." *Ragged Edge* 23, nos. 2/3 (2002).

Pfragner, Roswitha, and R. Ian Freshney, eds. *Culture of Human Cancer Cells*. Hoboken, N.J.: Wiley-Liss, 2004.

Pham, H. P., & Schwartz, J. (2015). How we approach a patient with symptoms of leukostasis requiring emergent leukocytapheresis. *Transfusion,* 55(10):2306-2311.

Phillips, Carmen. *Radiofrequency Ablation Making Inroads as Cancer Treatment*. Bethesda, Md.: National Cancer Institute, 2005. Also available online at http://www.cancer.gov.

Phillips, Theresa, Ph.D. (2008). The Role of Methylation in Gene Expression. *Nature Education,* 1(1), 116. Song, Chin-Xiao, and He, Chuan. (2012). Balance of DNA Methylation and Demethylation in Cancer Development. *Genome Biology*, 13: 173. http://www.genomebiology.com/2012/13/10/173

Physician's Desk Reference, 2008. 62d ed. Montvale, N.J.: Thomson Healthcare, 2007.

Phytoestrogen: Foods high in phytoestrogens and health benefits (2014, June 7). *Cholesterol and Fat Data Base.* Retrieved from http://www.dietaryfiberfood.com/phytoestrogen-hormones/phytoestrogen-food-sources.php

Piano, A., & Titorenko, V. I. (2015). The Intricate Interplay between Mechanisms Underlying Aging and Cancer. *Aging & Disease*, 6(1), 56-75. doi:10.14336/AD.2014.0209

Piasecki, J. H., and K. A. Gutowski. "Breast Reconstruction." *Clinical Obstetics and Gynecology* 49 (2006): 401-413.

Pickhardt, P. J. "The Natural History of Colorectal Polyps and Masses: Rediscovered Truths from the Barium Enema Era." *American Journal of Roentgenology* 188, no. 3 (March, 2007): 619-621.

Piekin, Steven R. *Gastrointestinal Health: The Proven Nutritional Program to Prevent, Cure, or Alleviate Irritable Bowel Syndrome (IBS), Ulcers, Gas, Constipation, Heartburn, and Many Other Digestive Disorders.* 3rd ed. Chino Hills, Calif.: Collins, 2005.

Pierson, D. J., S. K. Epstein, C. G. Durbin, Jr., et al. "Twentieth Annual New Horizons Symposium: Tracheostomy from A to Z." *Respiratory Care* 50 (2005): 473-549.

Ping Dou, Q. & Zonder, J. A. (2014*)*. Overview of proteasome inhibitor-based anti-cancer therapies: Perspective on bortezomib and second generation proteasome inhibitors versus future generation inhibitors of ubiquitin-proteasome system. *Current Cancer Drug Targets*, 14(6), 517-536.

Pingpank, Elizabeth. (2015). Takeda announces termination of alisertib phase 3 trial in relapsed or refractory peripheral T-cell lymphoma. Takeda remains committed to continuing the ongoing alisertib clinical development program. *Takeda News*, Retrieved from https://www.takeda.com/news/2015/20150513_6985.html

Pires, I. M., Ward, T. H., & Dive, C. (2010). Oxaliplatin responses in colorectal cancer cells are modulated by CHK2 kinase inhibitors. *British Journal of Pharmacology,* 159(6): 1326-1338.

Pisano, E. D., C. Gatsonis, E. Hendrick, et al. "Diagnostic Performance of Digital Versus Film Mammography for Breast-Cancer Screening." *New England Journal of Medicine* 353 (October 27, 2005): 1773-1783.

Pitot, Henry. *Fundamentals of Oncology*. 4th ed. New York: Marcel Dekker, 2002.

Pizzo, P. A., & Poplack, D. G. (Eds.). (2010). Principles and practice of pediatric oncology (6th ed.). Philadelphia, PA: Lippincott Williams & Wilkins.

Plotkin, Stanley A., Walter A. Orenstein, and Paul A. Offit, eds. *Vaccines*. 5th ed. Philadelphia: Saunders/Elsevier, 2008.

Pluschke, P. (Ed.). (204). Indoor air pollution. New York: Springer.

Pochapin, Mark B. *What Your Doctor May Not Tell You About Colorectal Cancer: New Tests, New Treatments, New Hope*. New York: Warner Books, 2004.

Podajcer, O. L., Lopez, M. V. &Mazzolini, G. (2007). Cytokine gene transfer for cancer therapy. *Cytokine and Growth Factor Reviews*, 18: 183-194. http://www.ncbi.nlm.nih.gov/pubmed/17320465

Podolsky, M. Lawrence. *Cures out of Chaos*. Newark, N.J.: Harwood Academic, 1997.

Poeppl, N., et al. "Does the Surface Structure of Implants Have an Impact on the Formation of a Capsular Contracture?" *Aesthetic Plastic Surgery* 31, no. 2 (March/April, 2007): 133-139.

Pohanish, Richard P. *Sittig's Handbook of Toxic and Hazardous Chemicals and Carcinogens*. 5th ed. Norwich, N.Y.: William Andrew, 2008.

Pollack, A. (2003, August 19). Theories vary on cancer vaccines. *The New York Times*. Retrieved from http://www.nytimes.com/2003/08/19/health/theories-vary-on-cancer-vaccines.html

Pollack, A. (2014, April 8). Sidestepping the biopsy with new tools to spot cancer. *New York Times*, pp. B1. http://www.nytimes.com/2014/04/08/business/cancer-analysis-tools-circumvent-biopsies.html?_r=0

Pollock, Raphael E., ed. *Surgical Oncology*. Boston: Kluwer Academic Press, 1997.

_______., ed. *Soft Tissue Sarcomas*. Lewiston, N.Y.: BC Decker, 2002.

Polovich, M., White, J. M., & Kelleher, L. O. (Eds.). (2005). *Chemotherapy and biotherapy guidelines* (2nd ed.). Pittsburgh, PA: Oncology Nursing Society.

Pomery, Chris. (2004). DNA and family history. Toronto, Ontario: Dundurn Press Limited.

Poole, Catherine M., and I. V. DuPont Guerry. *Melanoma: Prevention, Detection, and Treatment*. 2d ed. New Haven, Conn.: Yale University Press, 2005.

Poole, K., and K. Froggatt. "Loss of Weight and Loss of Appetite in Advanced Cancer: A Problem for the Patient, the Carer, or the Health Professional?" *Palliative Medicine* 16, no. 6 (November, 2002): 499-506.

Pope, C.A. III, Majid, E., & Dockery, D. W. (2009). Fine particle air pollution and life expectancy in the United States, *New England Journal of Medicine*, 360: 376-386.

Porta, M., et al. "Coffee Drinking: The Rationale for Treating It as a Potential Effect Modifier of Carcinogenic

Exposures." *European Journal of Epidemiology* 18, no. 4 (2003): 289-298.

Porter, Robert S., ed. *The Merck Manual of Women's and Men's Health*. 2d ed. New York: Simon & Schuster, 2006.

Post-menopausal hormone therapy after breast cancer. American Cancer Society. Retrieved from http://www.cancer.org/cancer/breastcancer/detailedguide/breast-cancer-after-post-menopausal-therapy

Potter, D. A., and J. S. Hanin. *What to Do When You Can't Get Pregnant: The Complete Guide to All the Technologies for Couples Facing Fertility Problems*. New York: Marlowe, 2005.

Pratt, William B., et al. *The Anticancer Drugs*. 2d ed. New York: Oxford University Press, 1994.

Predergast, G. C., & Jaffee, E. M. (2013). *Cancer immunotherapy* 2nd ed). Waltham, MA: Academic Press. This book discusses the role of the immune system in suppressing tumor development and provides basic and clinical cancer researchers with an overview of immunotherapy and chemotherapy in fight against cancer.

PREVENT Cancer Preclinical Drug Development Program (PREVENT). National Cancer Institute Division of Cancer Prevention. Retrieved from http://prevention.cancer.gov/major-programs/prevent-cancer-preclinical

Produce for Better Health Foundation. (2011). Fruits, vegetables, and health: A scientific overview. Retrieved from http://www.pbhfoundation.org/pdfs/about/res/pbh_res/PBH_Health_Benefit_Review.pdf.

Project Inform (1998). HIV Drug Book Revised. NY: Simon & Schuster.

Prosek, R., and L. Vreeland. "The Intelligibility of Time-Domain-Edited Esophageal Speech." *Journal of Speech, Language, and Hearing Research* 44, no. 3 (2001): 525-534.

Provides a meta analytic report (from research published between 2006 – 2011) on data regarding the effect of fruits and vegetables on health. Discusses the overall benefits of a diet rich in fruits and vegetables, and reviews data on the effects of fruits and vegetables on specific diseases and disorders, including cancer. Relays mixed results regarding the effect of fruit on the prevention and progression of different types of cancers.

Pucheril, D. & Sharma, S. (2011). The history and future of personalized medicine. *Managed Care Magazine*. Retrieved from: http://www.managedcaremag.com/content/history-and-future-personalized-medicine.

Pui, C-H, ed. *Childhood Leukemias*. 2d ed. New York: Cambridge University Press, 2006.

Putman, Charles E., and Carl E. Ravin. *Textbook of Diagnostic Imaging*. 2d ed. Philadelphia: W. B. Saunders, 1994.

Qasee, A., et al. "Screening Mammography for Women Forty to Forty-nine Years of Age: A Clinical Practice Guideline from the American College of Physicians." *Annals of Internal Medicine* 146, no. 7 (April 3, 2007): 511-515.

Querna, Elizabeth. "Breast Cancer Screening: What Is the Best Way to Find Out If You Have the Disease?" *U.S. News & World Report*, September 9, 2004.

Quillin, Patrick. *Beating Cancer with Nutrition*. 4th ed. Tulsa, Okla.: Nutrition Times Press, 2005.

Quinn, T., Ostrom, Q.T., Bauchet, L., Davis, F. G., Deltour, I., Fisher, J. L., ... Barnholtz-Sloan, J. S. (2014). The epidemiology of glioma in adults: a "state of the science" review. *Neuro-Oncology*, 16(7): 896-913.

Quint, Leslie E. "Imaging of Anterior Mediastinal Masses." *Cancer Imaging* 7 (2007): S56-S62.

Rabady, D. Z. "Pediatric Horner Syndrome: Etiologies and Roles of Imaging and Urine Studies to Detect Neuroblastoma and Other Responsible Mass Lesions." *American Journal of Ophthalmology* 144, no. 3 (September, 2007): 481-482.

Radbruch, Andreas, ed. *Flow Cytometry and Cell Sorting*. 2d ed. New York: Springer, 2000.

Raffle, P. B., et al., eds. *Hunter's Diseases of Occupations*. 8th ed. Boston: Arnold, 1994.

Raghavan, Derek. *Bladder Cancer: A Cleveland Clinic Guide—Information for Patients and Caregivers*. Cleveland: Cleveland Clinic Press, 2008.

Rai, K. R. & Jain, P. (2015). Chronic lymphocytic leukemia (CLL) — then and now. *American Journal of Hematology*, doi: 10.1002/ajh.24282.

Raj, P. Prithvi., ed. *Pain Medicine: A Comprehensive Review*. 2d ed. St. Louis: Mosby, 2003.

Raju, Tonse N. K. *The Nobel Chronicles: A Handbook of Nobel Prizes in Physiology or Medicine, 1901-2000*. Bloomington, Ind.: AuthorHouse, 2002.

Rakhimov, Artour. (2013). *Doctors Who Cure Cancer: Anticancer Biography and New Way of Life to Treat the Emperor of All Maladies*. Ontario: Artour Rakhimov.

Raloff, J. (2009). Desperately seeking moly. *Science News,* 176(7): 16-20.

Ramachandran, G. (2005). Occupational exposure assessment for air contaminants. New York: CRC Press.

Ramanakumar, A. V. "Need for Epidemiological Evidence from the Developing World to Know the

Cancer-Related Risk Factors." *Journal of Cancer Research and Therapeutics* 3 (2007): 29-33.

Randi, Giorgia, et al. "Marital Status and Cancer Risk in Italy." *Preventive Medicine* 38, no. 5 (May, 2004): 523-528.

Rando, Therese A. *How to Go on Living When Someone You Love Dies*. Lexington, Mass.: Bantam, 1991.

Rankin, Sally H., Karen Duffy Stallings, and Fran London. *Patient Education in Health and Illness*. 5th ed. Philadelphia: Lippincott Williams & Wilkins, 2005.

Rankin, Sheila C., ed. *Carcinoma of the Esophagus*. New York: Cambridge University Press, 2008.

Rankin, W., V. Grill, and T. Martin. "Parathyroid Hormone-Related Protein and Hypercalcemia." *Cancer* 80, no. 8 (1997): 1564-1571.

Ransohoff, D. F. (2003). Developing molecular biomarkers for cancer. *Science*, 299(5613): 1679-1680.

Rapaport, L. (2015,Sept.16). Cancer Remains Leading Cause of Death Among U.S. Hispanics. Reuters Health. Retrieved from http://www.reuters.com/article/us-health-hispanics-cancer-idUSKCN0RG2HG20150916

_______. (2016, Jan.4) Risk of heart damage follows some childhood cancer survivors. Reuters. Retrieved from http://mobile.reuters.com/article/idUSKBN0UI22O20160104?feedType=nl&feedName=healthNews

Rapp, Doris J. *Our Toxic World: A Wake Up Call*. New York: Environmental Medical Research Foundation, 2004.

Ravandi, F., and S. O'Brien. "Chronic Lymphoid Leukemias Other than Chronic Lymphocytic Leukemia: Diagnosis and Treatment." *Mayo Clinic Proceedings* 80, no. 12 (December, 2005): 1660-1674.

Rawls, George, Frank P. Lloyd, Jr., and Herbert Stern. *Managing Cancer: The African American's Guide to Prevention, Diagnosis, and Treatment*. Roscoe, Ill.: Hilton, 2001.

Raymond, Joan. "A Guide for Caregivers." *Newsweek*, June 18, 2007, 62-64.

Reang, P., M. Gupta, and K. Kohli. "Biological Response Modifiers in Cancer." *Medscape General Medicine* 14 (2006): 33.

Reber, Howard, ed. *Pancreatic Cancer: Pathogenesis, Diagnosis, and Treatment*. Totowa, N.J.: Humana Press, 1998.

Reed, James, Neil Shulman, and Charlene Shucker. *The Black Man's Guide to Good Health: Essential Advice for the Special Concerns of African-American Men*. New York: Berkley, 1994.

Reiber, A., K. Schramm, G. Helms, et al. "Breast-Conserving Surgery and Autogeneous Tissue Reconstruction in Patients with Breast Cancer: Efficacy of MRI of the Breast in the Detection of Recurrent Disease." *European Journal of Radiology* 13 (2003): 780-787.

Reichert, J. M., and V. E. Valge-Archer. "Development Trends for Monoclonal Antibody Cancer Therapeutics." *Nature Reviews Drug Discovery* 6 (2007): 349-356.

Reid, J. D., C. E. Parker, and C. H. Borchers. "Protein Arrays for Biomarker Discovery." *Current Opinion in Molecular Therapeutics* 9 (2006): 216-221.

Reid, M. D., Balci, S., Saka, B., & Adsay, N. V. (2014). Neuroendocrine tumors of the pancreas: Current concepts and controversies. *Endocrine Pathology,* 25(1), 65-79. A review of staging and prognostic indicators for islet cell tumors.

Rein, D., Breidenbach, M., & Curiel, D. T. (2006). Current developments in adenovirus-based cancer gene therapy. *Future Oncology,* 2(1), 137-143.

Rekate, Harold L. "Craniopharyngioma." *Journal of Neurosurgery (Pediatrics 4)* 103 (2005): 297-298.

Rendl, Michael. (Ed.). (2014). *Stem Cells in Development and Disease, Volume 107 (Current Topics in Developmental Biology*). Boston: Elsevier Academic Press.

Researchers reviewed data on almost 500,000 people enrolled in a longitudinal large scale study on cancer and nutrition in Europe. Results showed that eating a recommended (200g) of fruit per day decreased cancer risk slightly by 3% in females only, concluding a minimal benefit in terms of cancer prevention.

Reznek, Rodney, ed. *Cancer of the Ovary*. Cambridge, England: Cambridge University Press, 2007.

_______. *Cancer of the Ovary*. New York: Cambridge University Press, 2007.

Ricci, P. E. "Imaging of Adult Brain Tumors." *Neuroimaging Clinics of North America* 9 (1999): 651-669.

Rice, Jerry M. "The Carcinogenicity of Acrylamide." *Mutation Research/Genetic Toxicology and Environmental Mutagenesis* 580, nos. 1/2 (2005): 3-20.

Richards, R. I. "Fragile and Unstable Chromosomes in Cancer: Causes and Consequences." *Trends in Genetics* 17 (2001): 339-345.

Richardson, P. G., Mitsiades, C., Hideshima, T. & Anderson, K. C. (2006). Bortezomib: Proteasome inhibition as an effective anticancer therapy. *Annual Review of Medicine*, 57, 33-47.

Richon, V. M. (2006). Cancer biology: Mechanism of antitumour action of vorinostat (suberoylanilide hydroxamic acid), a novel histone deacetylase inhibitor.

British Journal of Cancer, 95: S2-S6. http://www.nature.com/bjc/journal/v95/n1s/full/6603463a.html

Ricks, Delthia. *Breast Cancer Basics and Beyond*. Alameda, Calif.: Hunter House Books, 2005.

Ridgway, E. B. "Skull Deformities." *Pediatric Clinics of North America* 5, no. 2 (2004): 359-387.

Riemenschneider, M. J., A. Perry, and G. Reifenberger. "Histological Classification and Molecular Genetics of Meningiomas." *Lancet Neurology* 5 (2006): 1045-1054.

Riess, H., A. Goerke, and H. Oettle, eds. *Pancreatic Cancer*. New York: Springer, 2008.

Rigel, Darrell S., et al., eds. *Cancer of the Skin*. Philadelphia: Elsevier, 2005.

Ringsrud, Karen Munson, and Jean Jorgenson Linne. *Urinalysis and Body Fluids: A Colortext and Atlas*. Philadelphia: Elsevier, 1994.

Risch, H. A. "Etiology of Pancreatic Cancer, with a Hypothesis Concerning the Role of N-Nitroso Compounds and Excess Gastric Acidity." *Journal of the National Cancer Institute* 95, no. 12 (July 2, 2003): 948-960.

Ritterbeck, Molly. Samantha Harris on beating cancer, staying fit and feeling happy. *Fitness Magazine*. Retrieved from http://www.fitnessmagazine.com/blogs/beauty-on-the-go/

Rizzo, Phillip A., and David G. Poplack, eds. *Principles and Practice of Pediatric Oncology*. Philadelphia: Lippincott Williams and Wilkins, 2002.

Robbins Pathologic Basis of Disease. 5th ed. Philadelphia: W. B. Saunders, 1994.

Robertson G. "Screening for Endometrial Cancer." *Medical Journal of Australia* 178, no. 12 (June 16, 2003): 657-659.

Robertson, E. S. (2005). *Epstein-Barr virus*. Portand, OR: Caister Academic Press.

Robertson, Erle. (Ed.). (2012). *Burkitt's Lymphoma* (Current Cancer Research) (2013th Edition). New York: Springer Science-Business Media.

Robertson, L. E., Pugh, W., O'Brien, S. O., Kantarjian, H., Hirsch-Ginsberg, C., Cork, A., … Keating, M. J. (1993). Richter's syndrome: A report on thirty-nine patients. *Journal of Clinical Oncology.* 11, 1985-1989.

Robins, H. Ian, et al. "Therapeutic Advances for Glioblastoma Multiforme: Current Status and Future Prospects." *Current Oncology Reports* 9, no. 1 (2007): 66-70.

Roche Group Media Relations. (2013, February 22). FDA approves Roche's Kadcyla (trastuzumab emtansine), the first antibody-drug conjugate for treating HER2-postiive metastatic breast cancer. *Roche Media Release*, Retrieved from http://www.roche.com/media/store/releases/med-cor-2013-02-22.htm

Roche Holding A.G. *The New York Times*. Retrieved from http://topics.nytimes.com/top/news/business/companies/roche-holding-ag/index.html

Rock, John A., and Howard W. Jones III, eds. *Te Linde's Operative Gynecology*. 9th ed. Philadelphia: Lippincott Williams & Wilkins, 2003.

Rodriguez, J., Keating, M. J., O'Brien, S., Champlin, R. E., & Khouri, I. F. (2000). Allogeneic haematopoietic transplantation for Richter's syndrome. *British Journal of Haematology,* 110, 897-899.

Rodriquez, Alejandro, and Wade J. Sexton. "Management of Locally Advanced Renal Cell Carcinoma." *Cancer Control: Journal of the Moffitt Cancer Center* 13 (July, 2006): 199-210.

Roh, Jong-Lyel, Jooryung Huh, and Cheolwon. Suh. "Primary Non-Hodgkin's Lymphomas of the Major Salivary Glands." *Journal of Surgical Oncology* 97, no. 1 (October 10, 2007): 35-39.

Rohatiner, Ama Z. S., Nancy L. Harris, Riccardo Dalla-Favera, and T. Andrew Lister. "Lymphoplasmacytic Lymphoma and Waldenström's Macroglobulinemia." In *Non-Hodgkin's Lymphomas*, edited by Peter Mauch et al. Philadelphia: Lippincott Williams & Wilkins, 2004.

Roila, F., S. Fatigoni, and G. Ciccarese. "Daily Challenges in Oncology Practice: What Do We Need to Know About Antiemetics?" *Annals of Oncology* 17, suppl. 10 (September, 2006): 90-94.

Rollandi, G. A., E. Biscaldi, and E. DeCicco. "Double Contrast Barium Enema: Technique, Indications, Results, and Limitations of a Conventional Imaging Methodology in the MDCT Virtual Endoscopy Era." *European Journal of Radiology* 61, no. 3 (March, 2007): 382-387.

Röllig, C., & Ehninger, G. (2015). How I treat hyperleukocytosis in acute myeloid leukemia. *Blood,* 125(21): 3246-3452.

Roncadin, C., Hitzler, J., Downie, A., Montour-Proulx, I., Alyman, C., Cairney, E., & Spiegler, B. J. (2015). Neuropsychological late effects of treatment for acute leukemia in children with Down syndrome. *Pediatric Blood Cancer,* 62: 854–858.

Rooney, R. J., et al. "Giant Cell Tumor of the Bone: A Surgical Approach." *International Orthopaedics* 17, no. 2 (1993): 87-92.

Ropeik, D., and G. M. Gray. *Risk: A Practical Guide for Deciding What's Really Safe and What's Dangerous in the World Around You*. Boston: Houghton Mifflin, 2002.

Rose, Noel R., and Ian R. Mackay. *The Autoimmune Diseases*. Amsterdam: Elsevier/Academic Press, 2006.

Rose, Susannah, and Richard Hara. *One Hundred Questions and Answers About Caregiving for Family or Friends with Cancer*. Sudbury, Mass.: Jones & Bartlett, 2004.

Rose, T., & Choi, J. (2015). Intravenous imaging contrast media complications: The basics that every clinician needs to know. *The American Journal of Medicine*, 128(9): 943-949.

Rosen, Paul Peter, and Syed A. Hoda. *Breast Pathology: Diagnosis by Needle Core Biopsy*. 2d ed. Philadelphia: Lippincott Williams & Wilkins, 2006.

Rosen, Winifred, & Weil, Andrew T. (2004). *From Chocolate to Morphine: Everything You Need to Know About Mind-Altering Drugs*. Rev. ed. Boston: Houghton Mifflin. Easy to read discussion about common every day drugs to a range of illicit substances and how they affect the body.

Rosenberg, S. M., & Partridge, A. H. (2013). Premature menopause in young breast cancer: Effects on quality of life and treatment interventions. *Journal of Thoracic Disease*, 5(1), 55–S61. doi: 10.3978/j.issn.2072-1439.2013.06.20.

Rosenberg, Steven A., ed. *Principles and Practice of the Biologic Therapy of Cancer*. 3rd ed. Philadelphia: Lippincott Williams & Wilkins, 2000.

Rosenberg, Tina. "What the World Needs Now Is DDT." *The New York Times*, May 23, 2004, p. 8.

Rosenblatt, Bob, and Carol Van Steenberg. *Handbook for Long-Distance Caregivers*. San Francisco: Family Caregiver Alliance of the National Center on Caregiving, 2003.

Rosenthal, D. I. "Radiologic Diagnosis of Bone Metastases." *Cancer* 80, suppl. 8 (1997): 1595-1607.

Rosenthal, M. Sara. *The Thyroid Sourcebook: Everything You Need to Know*. 3rd ed. Los Angeles: Lowell House, 1998.

Rosenthal, Sara M. *The Gynecological Sourcebook*. 4th ed. New York: McGraw-Hill Professional, 2003.

Roses, Daniel F. *Breast Cancer*. Philadelphia: Elsevier, 2005.

Rosman, A. S., and M. A. Korsten. "Meta-analysis Comparing CT Colonography, Air Contrast Barium Enema, and Colonoscopy." *American Journal of Medicine* 120, no. 3 (March, 2007): 203-210.

Ross, Joanna. *Occupational Therapy and Vocational Rehabilitation*. Hoboken, N.J.: John Wiley and Sons, 2007.

Ross, Walter S. *Crusade: The Official History of the American Cancer Society*. New York: Arbor House, 1987.

Rossi, A., C. Gandolfo, G. Morana, and P. Tortori-Donati. "Tumors of the Spine in Children." *Neuroimaging Clinics of North America* 17 (2007): 17-35.

Rossi, Carla. (2014). *The living end of cancer: One woman's faith-based journey through Non-Hodgkin lymphoma.* Seattle, WA: Amazon Digital Services LLC.

Roth, A. J. (2015). *Managing prostate cancer: A guide for living better.* New York: Oxford University Press.

Roth, Jack A., James D. Cox, and Waun Ki Hong, eds. *Lung Cancer*. 3rd ed. Malden, Mass.: Blackwell, 2008.

Rowley, R., M. Zorch, and D. B. Leeper. "Effect of Caffeine on Radiation-Induced Mitotic Delay: Delayed Expression of G2 Arrest." *Radiation Research* 97, no. 1 (January, 1984): 178-185.

Rubenstein, Joel H., Enns, Robert, Heidelbaugh, Joel, Barkun, Alan & the Clinical Guidelines Committee. (2015). American gastroenterological association institute guideline on the diagnosis and management of lynch syndrome. *Gastroenterology*, 149(3): 777–782. Guideline for clinicians who treat patients with Lynch Syndrome or HNPCC. It contains the official recommendations of the American Gastroenterological Association (AGA) Institute on the diagnosis and management of Lynch syndrome or HNPCC. This article is freely available at http://www.gastrojournal.org/article/S0016-5085%2815%2901031-8/abstract?referrer=http%3A%2F%2Fwww.ncbi.nlm.nih.gov%2Fpubmed%2F%3Fterm%3DRubenstein%252C%2BJoel%2BH.%252C%2BEnns%252C%2BRobert%252C

Rubin, A. D., and R. T. Sataloff. "Vocal Fold Paresis and Paralysis." *Otolaryngolic Clinic of North America* 40, no. 5 (October, 2007): 1109-1231.

Rubin, B. P., et al. "Gastrointestinal Stromal Tumor." *Lancet* 369 (2007): 1731-1741.

Rubin, Eva, and Jean F. Simpson. *Breast Specimen Radiography: Needle Localization and Radiographic Pathologic Correlation*. Philadelphia: Lippincott-Raven, 1998.

Rubin, H. "Cancer Cachexia: Its Correlations and Causes." *Proceedings of the National Academy of Sciences of the United States of America* 100, no. 9 (April 29, 2003): 5384-5389.

Ruddon, R. W. *Cancer Biology*. 4th ed. New York: Oxford University Press, 2007.

Ruddon, Raymond W. (2007). Cancer Biology (4th ed.). New York: Oxford University Press.

Ruddon, Raymond W. "Causes of Cancer." In *Cancer Biology*. 4th ed. New York: Oxford University Press, 2007.

Ruiz-Pesini, Eduardo, et al. "An Enhanced MITOMAP with a Global mtDNA Mutational Phylogeny." *Nucleic Acids Research* 35 (January 1, 2007): D823-D828.

Rumak, Carole M., S. R. Wilson, and J. W. Charboneau. *Diagnostic Ultrasound*. St. Louis: Mosby-Year Book, 1991.

Rumpf, T. P., & K. M. Hammitt. *The Sjögren's Syndrome Survival Guide*. Oakland, Calif.: New Harbinger, 2003.

Rushing, Lynda, and Nancy Joste. *Abnormal Pap Smears: What Every Woman Needs to Know*. Amherst, N.Y.: Prometheus Books, 2001.

Russell, B., Collins, A., Dowling, A., Dally, M., Gold, M., Murphy, M. Philip, J. (2016). Predicting distress among people who care for patients living longer with high-grade malignant glioma. *Support Care Cancer,* 24: 43-51. doi: 10.1007/s00520-015-2739-0.

Rustgi, A. K. "Hereditary Gastrointestinal Polyposis and Nonpolyposis Syndromes." *New England Journal of Medicine* 331 (1994): 1694.

Rustum, Youcef M., ed. *Fluoropyrimidines in Cancer Therapy*. Totowa, N.J.: Humana Press, 2003.

Ryan, C. J., Smith, M. R., de Bono, J. S., Molina, A., Logothetis, C. J. de Souza, P., Rathkopf, D. E. (2013). Abiraterone in metastatic prostate cancer without previous chemotherapy. *New England Journal of Medicine* 368(2): 138-148. http://dx.doi.org/10.1056/NEJMoa1209096

Ryan, C. J., Smith, M. R., Fizazi K., Saad, F., Mulders, P. F. A., Sternberg, C. N., ... Rathkopf, D. E. (2015). Abiraterone acetate plus prednisone versus placebo plus prednisone in chemotherapy-naive men with metastatic castration-resistant prostate cancer (COU-AA-302): Final overall survival analysis of a randomised, double-blind, placebo-controlled phase 3 study. *The Lancet Oncology* 16(2): 152-160. http://www.thelancet.com/journals/lanonc/article/PIIS1470-2045%2814%2971205-7/fulltext

Ryan, J. L., et al. "Mechanisms of Cancer-Related Fatigue." *The Oncologist* 12 (May, 2007): 22-34.

Rydzewski, R. M. (2008). *Real world drug discovery: A chemist's guide to biotech and pharmaceutical research*. Amsterdam: Elsevier.

Sabel, Michael S., Vernon K. Sondak, and Jeffrey J. Sussman, eds. *Surgical Foundations: Essentials of Surgical Oncology*. Philadelphia: Mosby Elsevier, 2007.

Saca-Hazboun, Hanan. "Empowering Patients with Knowledge: An Update on Trends in Patient Education." *ONS Connect* 22, no. 5 (May, 2007): 8-12.

Sadock, Benjamin James, & Sadock, Virginia Alcott. (2007). *Kaplan and Sadock's synopsis of psychiatry: Behavioral sciences clinical psychiatry* (10th ed.). Philadelphia: Wolter Kluwer/Lippincott Williams & Wilkins.

Sagar, Stephen M. *Restored Harmony: An Evidence Based Approach for Integrating Traditional Chinese Medicine into Complementary Cancer Care*. Hamilton, Ont.: Dreaming DragonFly Communications, 2001.

Sagi, M., Eilat, A., Ben Avi, L., Goldberg, Y., Bercovich, D., Hamburger, T., ... Lerer, I. (2011). Two BRCA1/2 founder mutations in Jews of Sephardic origin. *Familial Cancer,* 10(1): 59-63.

Sahakyan, K. R., Somers, V. K., Rodriguez-Escudero, J. P., Hodge, D. O., Carter, R. E., Sochor, O., . . . Lopez-Jimenez, F. (2015). Normal-Weight Central Obesity: Implications for Total and Cardiovascular Mortality. *Ann Intern Med,* 163(11), 827-835. doi:10.7326/m14-2525

Salamon, M. (2015). The truth behind three natural cancer "cures". Retrieved from https://www.mskcc.org/blog/truth-behind-three-natural-cures

Salmon, Charles G. *Adjuvant Therapy of Cancer*. Philadelphia: Lippincott Williams & Wilkins, 1993.

Sandborn, William J. (2014). Crohn's Disease evaluation and treatment: Clinical decision tool. *Gastroenterology,* 147(3), 702-705. This article conveys that the treatment of Crohn's Disease is in evolution and this clinical decision tool is designed to assist clinical providers in their identification, assessment and treatment of patients with Crohn's Disease. This article is available to the public and can be accessed free at http://www.gastrojournal.org/article/S0016-5085%2814%2900918-4/fulltext

Sandler, Martin P., R. Edward Coleman, and James A. Patton, eds. *Diagnostic Nuclear Medicine*. 4th ed. Philadelphia: Lippincott Williams & Wilkins, 2003.

Sanofi Clinical Trials. (n.d.) Retrieved January 11, 2016 from http://en.sanofi.com/rd/clinical_trials/clinical_trials.aspx

Sanofi Commitment. (n.d.) Retrieved January 11, 2016 from http://en.sanofi.com/our_company/our_commitment/our_commitment.aspx

Sanofi History. (n.d.) Retrieved January 11, 2016 from http://en.sanofi.com/our_company/history/history.aspx

Sanofi in the United States Homepage. (n.d.) Retrieved January 11, 2016 from http://www.sanofi.us/l/us/en/index.jsp

Sanofi Key Facts and Figures. (n.d.) Retrieved January 11, 2016 from http://en.sanofi.com/our_company/key_facts_and_figures/key_facts_and_figures.aspx

Sanofi Products. (n.d.) Retrieved January 11, 2016 from http://en.sanofi.com/products/products.aspx

Sansur, C. A., et al. "Spinal-Cord Neoplasms: Primary Tumours of the Bony Spine and Adjacent Soft Tissue." *The Lancet Oncology* 8 (2007): 137-147.

Saporito, B. (2013, May 20). Blood work. *Time Magazine*, 181(19). http://content.time.com/time/magazine/0,9263,7601130520,00.html

Sarg, M. J., and A. D. Gross. *The Cancer Dictionary*. 3rd ed. New York: Facts On File, 2006.

Sarwer, David B., and Thomas Pruzinsky, eds. *Psychological Aspects of Reconstructive and Cosmetic Plastic Surgery: Clinical, Empirical, and Ethical Perspectives*. Philadelphia: Lippincott Williams & Wilkins, 2006.

Saslow, D., et al. "American Cancer Society Guideline for Human Papillomavirus (HPV) Vaccine Use to Prevent Cervical Cancer and Its Precursors." *CA: A Cancer Journal for Clinicians* 57 (2007): 7-28.

Sass, Hans-Martin, Robert M. Veatch, and Ribito Kimura, eds. *Advance Directives and Surrogate Decision Making in Health Care: United States, Germany, and Japan*. Baltimore: Johns Hopkins University Press, 1998.

Sato, K., R. Shigenaga, S. Udea, et al. "Sentinel Lymph Node Biopsy for Breast Cancer." *Journal of Surgical Oncology* 96, no. 4 (September 15, 2007): 322-329.

Sawyer, Kathy. "Breast Cancer Drug Testing Will Continue: Potential of Tamoxifen Is Said to Outweigh Risks." *Washington Post*, May 12, 1994, p. A3.

Saygili, H. "Histopathologic Correlation of Dilatation and Curettage and Hysterectomy Specimens in Patients with Postmenopausal Bleeding." *European Journal of Gynaecological Oncology* 27, no. 2 (2006): 182-184.

Scarisbrick, J. J., Prince, H. M., Vermeer, M. H., Quaglino, P., Horwitz, S., Porcu, P., … Kim, Y. H. (2015). Cutaneous lymphoma international consortium study of outcome in advanced stages of mycosis fungoides and Sézary syndrome: Effect of specific prognostic markers on survival and development of a prognostic model. *Journal of Clinical Oncology,* 33(32), 3766-3773.

Scerri, E. (2013). *A tale of 7 elements*. New York: Oxford.

Schajowicz, F. *Tumors and Tumorlike Lesions of the Bone: Pathology, Radiology, and Treatment*. Berlin: Springer-Verlag, 1994.

Schally, A. V., and A. M. Comaru-Schally. "Hypothalamic and Other Peptide Hormones." In *Holland-Frei Cancer Medicine 7*, edited by D. W. Kufe et al. Hamilton, Ont.: BC Decker, 2006.

Scheuer, Peter J., and Jay H. Lefkowitch. *Liver Biopsy Interpretation*. 7th ed. Philadelphia: Elsevier Saunders, 2006.

Schiff, David, and Patrick Y. Wen, eds. *Cancer Neurology in Clinical Practice*. Totowa, N.J.: Humana Press, 2002.

Schindler, D., and H. Hoehn. *Fanconi Anemia: A Paradigmatic Disease for the Understanding of Cancer and Aging*. Basel, Switzerland: S. Karger, 2007.

Schlegel, W., et al., eds. *New Technologies in Radiation Oncology*. New York: Springer, 2006.

Schlehofer, B., et al. "Environmental Risk Factors for Sporadic Acoustic Neuroma." *European Journal of Cancer* 43 (2007): 1741-1747.

Schmeck, Jr. H.M. (1981). Study Links Coffee Use to Pancreas Cancer. *The New York Times*. http://www.nytimes.com/1981/03/12/us/study-links-coffee-use-to-pancreas-cancer.html

Schmeler, Kathleen, et al. "Prophylactic Surgery to Reduce the Risk of Gynecological Cancers in the Lynch Syndrome." *New England Journal of Medicine* 354 (January 19, 2006): 261-269.

Schmidt, C.W. (2006). Signs of the times: Biomarkers in perspective. *Environmental Health Perspectives,* 114(12): A700-A705. http://www.jstor.org/stable/4119581

Schoenberg, Mark P., et al. *The Guide to Living with Bladder Cancer*. Baltimore: Johns Hopkins University Press, 2000.

Schofield, Jill R., and William A. Robinson. *What You Really Need to Know About Moles and Melanoma*. Baltimore: Johns Hopkins University Press, 2000.

Scholz, Tim, et al. "Current Treatment of Malignant Pheochromocytoma." *Journal of Clinical Endocrinology and Metabolism* 92, no. 4 (2006): 1217-1225.

Schoonmaker, Michele, & William, Erin D. (2013). *Genetic testing: Scientific background and nondiscrimination legislation*. Columbus, OH: Bibliogov.

Schottenfeld, D., and J. F. Fraumeni, Jr., eds. *Cancer Epidemiology and Prevention*. New York: Oxford University Press, 2006.

Schover, Leslie R. *Sexuality and Fertility After Cancer*. New York: John Wiley & Sons, 1997.

Schrezenmeier, Hubert, and Andrea Bacigalupo, eds. *Aplastic Anemia: Pathophysiology and Treatment*. New York: Cambridge University Press, 2000.

Schrier, Robert W., ed. *Diseases of the Kidney and Urinary Tract.* 8th ed. Philadelphia: Wolters Kluwer Health/Lippincott Williams & Wilkins, 2007.

Schuchert, M. G., and J. D. Luketich. "Management of Barrett's Esophagus." *Oncology (Williston Park)* 21 (2007): 1382-1389.

Schulz, Volker, Hánsel, Rudolf, & Tyler, Varro E. (2001). *Rational phytotherapy*. New York, NY: Springer Science & Business Media.

Schuz, J., et al. "Cellular Telephone Use and Cancer Risk: Update of a Nationwide Danish Cohort." *Journal of the National Cancer Institute* 98 (2006): 1707-1713.

Schwamm, H. A., and C. L. Millward. *Histologic Differential Diagnosis of Skeletal Lesions*. New York: Igaku-Shoin, 1996.

Schwartz, Herbert S., ed. *Orthopaedic Knowledge Update: Musculoskeletal Tumors 2.* 2d ed. Rosemont, Ill.: American Academy of Orthopaedic Surgeons, 2007.

Schwartz, M., et al. "Strategies for the Management of Hepatocellular Carcinoma." *Nature Clinical Practice (Oncology)* 4 (2007): 424-432.

Schwartz, Seymour I. *Principles of Surgery*. New York: McGraw-Hill, 1984.

Schwarzbach, M., Y. Hormann, U. Hinz, et al. "Results of Limb-Sparing Surgery with Vascular Replacement for Soft Tissue Sarcoma in the Lower Extremity." *Journal of Vascular Surgery* 42, no. 1 (July, 2005): 88-97.

Scott, Andrew M., Wolchok, Jedd D., & Old, Lloyd J. (2012). Antibody therapy of cancer. *Nature Reviews Cancer* 12: 278-287. http://www.nature.com/nrc/journal/v12/n4/full/nrc3236.html

Scott, Kendall. (2015, February 13) How Cancer Taught Me to Cook. *Everyday Health* Retrieved from http://www.everydayhealth.com/columns/my-cancer-story/how-cancer-taught-me-cook/

Scott, Tamara. *Wilms' Tumor: A Handbook for Families.* Glenview, Ill.: Association of Pediatric Oncology Nurses, 2002.

Scott-Brown, Martin, Roy A. J. Spence, and Patrick G. Johnston, eds. *Emergencies in Oncology*. New York: Oxford University Press, 2007.

Scully, Crispian, et al. *Dermatology of the Lips*. Oxford, England: Isis Medical Media, 2000.

Segen, Joseph C., and Joseph Stauffer. *The Patient's Guide to Medical Tests*. New York: Facts On File, 1997.

Segnan, N., et al. "Randomized Trial of Different Screening Strategies for Colorectal Cancer: Patient Response and Detection Rates." *Journal of the National Cancer Institute* 97, no. 5 (2005): 347-357.

Seitz, H. K., and F. Stickel. "Molecular Mechanisms of Alcohol-Mediated Carcinogenesis." *Nature Reviews* 7 (2007): 599-612.

Seitz, H. K., B. Maurer, and F. Stickel. "Alcohol Consumption and Cancer of the Gastrointestinal Tract." *Digestive Diseases* 23 (2005): 297-303.

Semaan, N. "Integration of Complementary Disciplines into the Oncology Clinic. Part III, Herbal Medicine-Drug Interactions: The Role of the Pharmacist." *Current Problems in Cancer* 24, no. 4 (July/August, 2000): 213-222.

Sequist, L. V., et al. "Molecular Predictors of Response to Epidermal Growth Factor Receptor Antagonists in Non-Small-Cell Lung Cancer." *Journal of Clinical Oncology* 25 (2007): 587.

Serletti, J. M. "Breast Reconstruction with the TRAM Flap: Pedicled and Free." *Journal of Surgical Oncology* 94 (2006): 532-537.

Serraino, D., et al. "Risk of Cancer Following Immunosuppression in Organ Transplant Recipients and in HIV-Positive Individuals in Southern Europe." *European Journal of Cancer* 43, no. 14 (September, 2007): 2117-2123.

Sessler, J. L., & Miller, R. A. (2000). Texaphyrins: New drugs with diverse clinical applications in radiation and photodynamic therapy. *Biochemical Pharmacology,* 59: 733-739.

Sessler, J. L., Hemmi, G., Mody, T. D., Murai, T., Burrell, A., & Young, S. W. (1994). Texaphyrins: Synthesis and applications. *Accounts of Chemical Research,* 27: 43-50.

Sessler, J. L., Kral, V., Hoehner, M. C., Chin, O. A., & Davila, R. M. (1996). New texaphyrin-type expanded porphyrins. *Pure & Applied Chemistry,* 68: 1291-1295.

Shafer, William G., Maynard K. Hine, and Barnet M. Levy. *A Textbook of Oral Pathology*. 4th ed. Philadelphia: W. B. Saunders, 1983.

Shah, Manish A. Dx/Rx. Upper Gastrointestinal Malignancies: Cancers of the Stomach and Esophagus. Sudbury, Mass.: Jones and Bartlett, 2006.

Shah, N., & Dixon, D. S. (2009). New generation platinum agents for solid tumors. *Future Oncology*, 5(1): 33-42.

Shalauta, Saad R. "Barrett's Esophagus." *American Family Physician* 69, no. 9 (May 1, 2004): 2113-2118.

Shamin, Ahmad, and Sandra H. Kirk, eds. *Molecular Mechanisms of Fanconi Anemia*. New York: Springer, 2006.

Shankar, L. K., J. M. Hoffman, S. Bacharach, et al. "Consensus Recommendations for the Use of ^{18}F-FDG PET as an Indicator of Therapeutic Response in Patients in

National Cancer Institute Trials." *Journal of Nuclear Medicine* 47 (2006): 1059-1066.

Shannon, Joyce Brennfleck, ed. *Movement Disorders Sourcebook: Basic Consumer Health Information About* Neurological Movement Disorders. Detroit: Omnigraphics, 2003.

Shannon, Joyce Brennfleck, ed. *Death and Dying Sourcebook: Basic Consumer Health Information for the Layperson About End-of-Life Care and Related Ethical and Legal Issues.* 2d ed. Detroit: Omnigraphics, 2006.

Sharma, Prateek, and Richard E. Sampliner, eds. *Barrett's Esophagus and Esophageal Adenocarcinoma.* 2d ed. Malden, Mass.: Blackwell, 2006.

Sharma, R., et al. "Management of Chemotherapy-Induced Nausea, Vomiting, Oral Mucositis, and Diarrhea." *Lancet Oncology* 6 (2005): 93-102.

Sharma, Shikhar. (2012). *Epigenetic Inheritance of DNA Methylation Patterns: A DNMT3A and 3B Perspective.* Saarbrücken, Germany: LAP LAMBERT Academic Publishing.

Sharpe, Neil F., & Carter, R. F. (2006). *Genetic testing: Care, consent, and liability.* Hoboken, N.J.: Wiley-Liss. Kindle edition available.

Shehzad, K., et al. "Current Status of Minimal Access Surgery for Gastric Cancer." *Surgical Oncology* 16, no. 2 (June 6, 2007): 85-98.

Sheinfeld, Joel. *Testicular Cancer: An Issue of Urologic Clinics.* Philadelphia: Saunders, 2007.

Sheperd, J. T. *Inside the Mayo Clinic: A Memoir.* Afton, Minn.: Afton Historical Society Press, 2003.

Sherbert, Gajanan, and M. Lakshmi. *The Genetics of Cancer.* New York: Elsevier, 1997.

Sherman, M. E. "Theories of Endometrial Carcinogenesis: A Multidisciplinary Approach." *Modern Pathology* 13, no. 3 (March, 2000): 295-308.

Sherr, C. J. (2004). Principles of tumor suppression. *Cell,* 116, 235-246.Strano, S., Dell Orso, S., Di Agostino, S., Fontemaggi, G., Sacchi, A., & Blandino, G. (2007). Mutant p53: An oncogenic transcription factor. *Oncogene,* 26, 2212-2219.

Shi, Junwei, & Vakoc, Christopher R. (2014). "The mechanisms behind the therapeutic activity of BET bromodomain inhibition." *Molecular Cell* 54(5): 728-736.

Shields, Jerry A., and Carol L. Shields. *Intraocular Tumors: Atlas and Textbook,* 2d ed. Philadelphia: Lippincott Williams & Wilkins, 2008.

Shiloh, Y. (2006). The ATM-mediated DNA-damage response: Taking shape. *Trends in Biochemical Sciences,* 31: 402-410.

Shockney, Lille D. *Navigating Breast Cancer: A Guide for the Newly Diagnosed.* Sudbury, Mass.: Jones & Bartlett, 2006.

Shokat, Kevan M., (Ed.). (2014). *Methods in enzymology: Protein kinase inhibitors in research and medicine* (Vol. 548). Waltham, MA: Academic Press.

Shurr, Donald G., and John W. Michael. *Prosthetics and Orthotics.* Upper Saddle River, N.J.: Prentice Hall, 2001.

Siddiqui M. & Rajkumar S. V. (2012). The high cost of cancer drugs and what we can do about it. *Mayo Clinic Proceedings* 87(10):935-943.

Siegel, Bernie. *Love, Medicine, and Miracles.* New York: Harper & Row, 1986.

Siegel, C. A., et al. "Liver Biopsy 2005: When and How?" *Cleveland Clinic Journal of Medicine* 72, no. 3 (2005): 199-224.

"Silicone Gel-Filled Breast Implants Approved." *FDA Consumer* 41, no. 1 (January/February, 2007).

Silvera, S. A. N., and T. E. Rohan. "Trace Elements and Cancer Risk: A Review of the Epidemiologic Evidence." *Cancer Causes Control* 18 (2007): 7-27.

Silverman, Sol. *Oral Cancer.* Lewiston, N.Y.: BC Decker, 2003.

Simerville, Jeff A., William C. Maxted, and John J. Pahira. "Urinalysis: A Comprehensive Review." *American Family Physician,* March 15, 2005, 1153.

Simone, John. *The LCIS and DCIS Breast Cancer Fact Book.* Raleigh, N.C.: Three Pyramids Publishing, 2002.

Sinclair, Alison. "Genetics 101: Cytogenetics and FISH." *Canadian Medical Association Journal* 167 (2002): 373-374.

Singer, F. "Paget's Disease of the Bone." In *Endocrinology,* edited by L. J. DeGroot. Philadelphia: W. B. Saunders, 1995.

Singh, A. D., L. Bergman, and S. Seregard. "Uveal Melanoma: Epidemiologic Aspects." *Ophthalmology Clinics of North America* 18 (2005): 75-84.

Singh, Gurmit, and Shafaat A. Rabbani, eds. *Bone Metastasis.* Totowa, N.J.: Humana, 2005.

Singh, Siddharth & Loftus, Edward V. Jr. (2015). Crohn's disease: REACT to save the gut. The *Lancet,* 386(10006), 1800-1802. This article is a commentary on the most recent findings of the REACT Study that showed high quality evidence supporting the early treatment of Crohn's Disease in community gastroenterology practices using combined immunosuppression with an immunomodulator and antibody to TNF.

Sinha, D., Sarkar, N., Biswas, J., & Bishayee, A. (2016). Resveratrol for breast cancer prevention and therapy: Preclinical evidence and molecular mechanisms. *Seminars in Cancer Biology,* doi: 10.1016/j.semcancer.2015.11.00.

Sissell, Kara. "States, Retailers Push to Eliminate Phthalates from Toys." *Chemical Weekly* 170, no. 12 (April 14-21, 2008): 29.

________. "Study Links Phthalates and Infant Care Products." *Chemical Weekly* 170, no. 5 (February 11-18, 2008): 29.

Skandalakis, John E., Panajiotis N. Skandalakis, and Lee John Skandalakis. *Surgical Anatomy and Technique: A Pocket Manual*. 2d ed. New York: Springer, 2000.

Skeel, R. T. & Khlief, S. N. (2011). Handbook of cancer chemotherapy (8th ed.). Philadelphia: Lippincott Williams & Wilkins.

Skeel, Roland T. *Handbook of Cancer Chemotherapy*. 6th ed. Philadelphia: Lippincott Williams & Wilkins, 2003.

Skeel, Roland T. *Handbook of Cancer Chemotherapy*. 7th ed. Philadelphia: Lippincott Williams & Wilkins, 2007.

Skidmore-Roth, Linda. (2016). Mosby's 2016 nursing drugs reference. St. Louis: C. V. Mosby. This is the newest edition of a reference that has been valuable for over 30 years. More than 5,000 drugs are profiled, with an emphasis on patient safety.

Skilbeck, J., and S. Payne. "Emotional Support and the Role of Clinical Nurse Specialists in Palliative Care." *Journal of Advanced Nursing* 43, no. 2 (September, 2003): 521-530.

Skinner, H. B., ed. *Current Orthopedics: Diagnosis and Treatment*. 4th ed. New York: Lange Medical Books/McGraw-Hill, 2006.

Skinner, Harry B., ed. *Current Diagnosis and Treatment in Orthopedics*. 4th ed. New York: Lange Medical Books/McGraw-Hill, 2006.

Skloot, R. (Winter 2001). The marvels of telomerase. *Hopkins Medical News*. Retrieved from http://m.hopkinsmedicine.org/hmn/W01/top.html

Skloot, Rebecca. (2011). *The immortal life of Henrietta Lacks*. New York: Random House.

Slack, Jonathan. (2012). *Stem cells: A very short introduction*. New York, NY: Oxford University Press.

Slaga, Thomas J. "Fifty Years of the University of Texas M. D. Anderson Cancer Center and the Study of Carcinogenesis." *Molecular Carcinogenesis* 4, no. 6 (1991): 417-418.

Slamon, D., et al. "Use of Chemotherapy Plus a Monoclonal Antibody Against HER2 for Metastatic Breast Cancer That Overexpresses HER2." *New England Journal of Medicine* 344 (2001): 783-792.

Slap, Gail B. "Amenorrhea." In *The Gale Encyclopedia of Childhood and Adolescence*, edited by Jerome Kagan. Detroit: Gale, 1998.

Sloan, Frank A., and Hellen Gelband, eds. *Cancer Control Opportunities in Low- and Middle-Income Countries*. Washington, D.C.: National Academies Press, 2007.

Sloan, Sheila B., and John L. Dusseau. *Word Book in Pathology and Laboratory Medicine*. 2d ed. Philadelphia: Elsevier/Saunders, 1995.

Slotman, B. J., T. D. Solberg, and D. Verellen. *Extracranial Stereotactic Radiotherapy and Radiosurgery*. New York: Taylor and Francis, 2006.

Slovic, P. *The Perception of Risk*. London: Earthscan, 2000.

Smedby, K., Hjalgrim, H., Askling, J., Chang, E. T., Gregersen, H., Porwit-MacDonald, A., ... Adami, H-O. (2006). Autoimmune and chronic inflammatory disorders and risk of Non-Hodgkin lymphoma by subtype. *Journal of the National Cancer Institute,* 98, 51-60.

Smedley, Brian D., Adrienne Y. Steth, and Alan P. Nelson eds. *Unequal Treatment: Confronting Racial and Ethnic Disparities in Health Care*. Washington D.C.: National Academy Press, 2003.

Smeltzer, Suzanne C., et al., eds. *Brunner and Suddarth's Textbook of Medical-Surgical Nursing*. 11th ed. Philadelphia: Lippincott Williams & Wilkins, 2008.

Smith, Adam C., Sanaa Choufani, José C. Ferreira, and Rosanna Weksberg. "Growth Regulation, Imprinted Genes, and Chromosome 11p15.5." *Pediatric Research* 61, no. 5 (2007): 43R-47R.

Smith, E., S. Prues, and F. Ochme. "Environmental Degradation of Polyacrylamides: Effect of Artificial Environmental Conditions." *Ecotoxicology and Environmental Safety* 35 (1996): 121-135.

Smith, George F., and Timothy R. Toonen. "Primary Care of the Patient with Cancer." *American Family Physician* 75, no. 8 (April 15, 2007): 1207-1214.

Smith, K. B., & Pukall, C. F. (2009). An evidence-based review of yoga as a complementary intervention for patients with cancer. *Psycho-Oncology*, 18(5): 465-475.

Smith, S. M., O'Morain, C., & McNamara, D. (2014). Antimicrobial susceptibility testing for *Helicobacter pylori* in times of increasing antibiotic resistance. *World Journal of Gastroenterology,* 20(29), 9912–9921. http://www.ncbi.nlm.nih.gov/pmc/articles/PMC4123372. This article discusses the current treatment options for *Helicobacter pylori* infection in light of the recent challenges in eradication success rapid emergence of antibiotic resistant strains of *H. pylori.* Local surveillance of *Helicobacter pylori* antibiotic resistance by susceptibility testing is also discussed as a tool to inform clinicians in their choice of therapy for treating *Helicobacter pylori* infection.This article is available to the public and can be accessed free at the web link provided.

Smith, Terry L. *Breast Cancer: Current and Emerging Trends in Detection and Treatment*. New York: Rosen, 2006.

Smith, Tom. *Coping with Bowel Cancer*. London: Sheldon Press, 2006.

Smith, William, Keneth Adler, and Jo Brielyn. *Exercises for Cancer Wellness: Restoring Energy and Vitality While Fighting Fatigue.* Hobart, NY:Hatherleigh Press, 2016.

Snell, Clete. *Peddling Poison: The Tobacco Industry and Kids*. Westport, Conn.: Praeger, 2005.

Sobin, L. H. "TNM: Evolution and Relation to Other Prognostic Factors." *Seminars in Surgical Oncology* 21 (2003): 3-7.

Society of Urologic Oncology. "Advances in the Treatment of Genitourinary Cancer: Highlights from the Third Annual Meeting of the Society of Urologic Oncology, December 13-14, 2002, Washington, D.C." *Reviews in Urology* 5, no. 4 (Fall, 2003): 232-234.

_______. "Report from the Society of Urologic Oncology: Highlights from the Fourth Annual Meeting of the Society of Urologic Oncology, December 5-6, 2003, Bethesda, Md." *Reviews in Urology* 6, no. 4 (Fall, 2004): 193-199.

Soffritti, Morando, et al. "First Experimental Demonstration of the Multi-potential Carcinogenic Effects of Aspartame Administered in the Feed to Sprague-Dawley Rats." *Environmental Health Perspectives* 114, no. 3 (March, 2006): 379-385.

Sokoloff, M. H., G. F. Joyce, and M. Wise. "Urologic Diseases in America Project: Testis Cancer." *Journal of Urology* 177, no. (June, 2007): 2030-2041.

Sone, S., et al. "Long-Term Follow-up Study of a Population-Based 1996-1998 Mass Screening Programme for Lung Cancer Using Mobile Low-Dose Spiral Computed Tomography." *Lung Cancer*, August 3, 2007.

Sonis, Stephen T., Douglas E. Peterson, Deborah B. McGuire, and David A. Williams, eds. "Mucosal Injury in Cancer Patients: New Strategies for Research and Treatment." *Journal of the National Cancer Institute Monographs* 29 (2001): 1-54.

Sorscher, S. M. "Biological Therapy Update in Colorectal Cancer." *Expert Opinion on Biological Therapy* 7 (2007): 509-519.

Sosa, J. A., et al. "The Maturation of a Specialty: Workforce Projections for Endocrine Surgery." *Surgery* 142 (2007): 876-883.

Souhami, Robert, and Jeffrey Tobias. *Cancer and Its Management*. 5th Edition. Malden, Mass.: Blackwell, 2005.

Souhami, Robert, and Jeffrey Tobias. *Cancer and Its Management*. Malden, Mass.: Blackwell, 2005.

Souhami, Robert, et al., eds. *Oxford Textbook of Oncology*. 2d ed. New York: Oxford University Press, 2002.

Sparks, Martha E. *Cherish the Days: Inspiration and Insight for Long-Distance Caregivers*. Indianapolis, Ind.: Wesleyan, 2004.

Spear, S. L., and A. N. Mesbahi. "Implant-Based Reconstruction." *Clinics in Plastic Surgery* 34 (2007): 63-73.

Sperry, L. (2009). *Treatment of chronic medical conditions: Cognitive-behavioral therapy strategies and integrative treatment protocols.* Washington, D.C.: American Psychological Association.

Spiegel, Jeffrey H., and Scharukh Jalisi, eds. "Contemporary Diagnosis and Management of Head and Neck Cancer." *Otolaryngolic Clinics of North America* 30, no. 1 (2005).

Spiegel, *D.*, et al. "Effect of psychosocial treatment on survival of patients with metastatic breast cancer." *The Lancet* 2, no. 8668 (October, 1989): 888-891.

Spitz, M. R. "Epidemiology and Risk Factors for Head and Neck Cancer." *Seminars in Oncology* 31, no. 6 (2004): 726-733.

Spivak, J. L., et al. "Chronic Myeloproliferative Disorders." *Hematology/The Education Program of the American Society of Hematology* (2003): 200-224.

Sprod, L. K., Fernandez, I. D., Janelsins, M. C., Peppone, L. J., Atkins, J. N., Giguere, J., … Mustian, K. M. (2015). Effects of yoga on cancer-related fatigue and global side-effect burden in older cancer survivors. *Journal of Geriatric Oncology*, 6(1): 8-14.

St. Georgiev, Vassel. *Infectious Diseases in Immunocompromised Hosts*. Boca Raton, Fla.: CRC Press, 1998.

Stanberry, Lawrence. (2006). *Understanding herpes*. 2d ed. Jackson: University Press of Mississippi.

Stand Up To Cancer. (N.D.). Meet the SU2C Scientific Research Teams. Retrieved from http://www.standup2cancer.org/dream_teams/.

Staritz, M., et al., eds. *Side Effects of Cancer Chemotherapy on the Gastrointestinal Tract*. Boston: Kluwer Academic, 2003.

Stasney, C. Richard. *Atlas of Dynamic Laryngeal Pathology*. San Diego, Calif.: Singular, 1996.

Stavropoulos-Giokas C. & Papassavas, A. (2012). The role of HLA in cord blood transplantation. *Bone Marrow Research,* 2012, doi:10.1155/2012/485160.

Steen, Francis F. (1998). Landmarks in the history of genetics. Retrieved on February 15, 2016 from http://www.cogweb.ucla.edu/ep/dna-history.html. This document is a listing of landmarks in genetics.

Steen, R. Grant, and Joseph Mirro, eds. *Childhood Cancer: A Handbook from St. Jude Children's Research Hospital.* New York: Perseus, 2000.

Stefanick, M. L., et al. "Effects of Conjugated Equine Estrogens on Breast Cancer and Mammography Screening in Postmenopausal Women with Hysterectomy." *Journal of the American Medical Association* 295, no. 14 (2006): 1647-1657.

Stein, Kevin, et al. "The American Cancer Society's Studies of Cancer Survivors." *American Journal of Nursing* 106, no. 3 (March, 2006): 83-85.

Stein, R. (September, 2012). Scientists see upside and downside of sequencing their own genes. Retrieved from: http://www.npr.org/sections/health-shots/2012/09/19/160955379/scientists-see-upside-and-downside-of-sequencing-their-own-genes.

Sterman, Daniel, et al. *Thoracic Endoscopy: Advances in Interventional Pulmonology.* Malden, Mass.: Blackwell, 2006.

Stern, M., and R. Herrmann. "Overview of Monoclonal Antibodies in Cancer Therapy: Present and Promise." *Critical Reviews in Oncology/Hematology* 54, no. 1 (2005): 11-29.

Stern, Theodore A., and Mikkael A. Sekeres. *Facing Cancer: A Complete Guide for People with Cancer, Their Families, and Caregivers.* New York: McGraw-Hill, 2004.

Stevens, W. G., et al. "A Comparison of Five Hundred Prefilled Textured Saline Breast Implants Versus Five Hundred Standard Textured Saline Breast Implants: Is There a Difference in Deflation Rates?" *Plastic and Reconstruction Surgery* 117, no. 7 (June, 2006): 2175-2181.

Steward, W.P. & Brown, K. (2013, May 9). Cancer chemoprevention: A rapidly evolving field. British Journal of Cancer, 109: 1-7. Retrieved from http://www.nature.com/bjc/journal/v109/n1/full/bjc2013280a.html

Stewart, B. W., and P. Kleihues, eds. *World Cancer Report.* Geneva: World Health Organization, International Agency for Research on Cancer, 2003.

Stewart, Bernard W., and Paul Kleihues, eds. *World Cancer Report.* Lyon, France: IARC Press, 2003.

Stewart, K. A. (2014). How thalidomide works against cancer. *Science* 343(6168): 256-257.

Stidwill, Howard. *Exercise Therapy and the Cancer Patient: A Guide for Health Care Professionals and Their Patients.* Belgium, Wisc.: Champion Press, 2005.

Stine, Gerald. *AIDS Update: 2007.* New York: McGraw-Hill, 2007.

Stoller, David W. *Magnetic Resonance Imaging in Orthopedics and Sports Medicine.* Philadelphia: J. B. Lippincott, 1993.

Stoller, David W., et al. *Diagnostic Imaging: Orthopedics.* Salt Lake City, Utah: Amirsys, 2006.

Stolzenburg, J.-U., M. T. Gettman, and E. N. Liatsikis, eds. *Endoscopic Extraperitoneal Radical Prostatectomy: Laparoscopic and Robot-Assisted Surgery,* London: Springer, 2007.

Stowell, Cheri L., et al. "A Role for Sulfation-Desulfation in the Uptake of Bisphenol A into Breast Tumor Cells." *Chemistry and Biology* 13, no. 8 (2006): 891-897.

Strahm, B., and D. Malkin. "Hereditary Cancer Predisposition in Children: Genetic Basis and Clinical Implications." *International Journal of Cancer* 119, no. 9 (November 1, 2006): 2001-2006.

Strasfeld, L., & Chou, S. (2010). Antiviral drug resistance: Mechanisms and clinical implications. *Infectious Disease Clinics of North America* 24(2): 413-437.

Strashun, Arnold. (1992). Editorial: Adriamycin, Congestive Cardiomyopathy, and Metaiodobenzylguanidine. *The Journal of Nuclear Medicine* 33(2): 215-222. http://jnm.snmjournals.org/content/33/2/215.full.pdf

Strasinger, Susan King, and Marjorie Schaub Di Lorenzo. *Urinalysis and Body Fluids.* 5th ed. Philadelphia: F. A. Davis, 2008.

Straus, Joan Sutton. *A Legacy of Caring: The Society of Memorial Sloan-Kettering Cancer Center.* New York: The Society of Memorial Sloan-Kettering Cancer Center, 1996.

Strauss, James, and Ellen Strauss. *Viruses and Human Disease.* 2d ed. Burlington, Mass.: Elsevier Academic Press, 2008.

Strollo, Diane C., Melissa L. Rosado de Christenson, and James R. Jett. "Primary Mediastinal Tumors: Part 1, Tumors of the Anterior Mediastinum." *Chest* 112 (1997): 511-522.

_______. "Primary Mediastinal Tumors: Part 2, Tumors of the Middle and Posterior Mediastinum." *Chest* 112 (1997): 1344-1357.

Stroszczynski, E., ed. *Minimally Invasive Tumor Therapies.* New York: Springer, 2006.

Strother, D. R., et al. "Tumors of the Central Nervous System." In *Principles and Practice of Pediatric Oncology,* edited by P. A. Pizzo and D. G. Poplack. 4th ed. Philadelphia: Lippincott Williams & Wilkins, 2002.

Strum, Stephen, and Donna L. Pogliano. *A Primer on Prostate Cancer: The Empowered Patient's Guide*. Hollywood, Fla.: Life Extension Media, 2002.

Suda, Koichi, ed. *Pancreas: Pathological Practice and Research*. New York: Karger, 2007.

Sudarshan, Sunil, Peter A. Pinto, Len Neckers, and W. Marston Linehan. "Mechanisms of Disease: Hereditary Leiomyomatosis and Renal Cell Cancer—A Distinct Form of Hereditary Kidney Cancer." *Nature Clinical Practice—Urology* 4, no. 2 (February, 2007): 104-110.

Sugano, K., Tack, J., Kuipers, E. J., Graham, D. Y., El-Omar, E. M., Miura, S., … Kyoto Global Consensus Conference. (2015). Kyoto global consensus report on *Helicobacter pylori* gastritis. *Gut*, 264(9), 1353–1367. http://gut.bmj.com/content/64/9/1353.long. The article contains a global consensus developed for the first time on the: (1) classification of chronic gastritis and duodenitis, (2) clinical distinction of dyspepsia caused by *Helicobacter pylori* from functional dyspepsia, (3) appropriate diagnostic assessment of gastritis and (4) when, whom and how to treat *H. pylori* gastritis. This article is available to the public and can be accessed free at the web link provided.

Sugarbaker, Paul H. "New Standard of Care for Appendiceal Epithelial Neoplasms and Pseudomyxoma Peritonei Syndrome?" *Lancet Oncology* 7, no. 1 (January, 2006): 69-76.

Summers, D. S., M. D. Roger, P. L. Allan, and J. T. Murchison. "Accelerating the Transit Time of Barium Sulphate Suspensions in Small Bowel Examinations." *European Journal of Radiology* 62, no. 1 (April, 2007): 122-125.

Summers, N. *The Fundamentals of Case Management Practice: Skills for the Human Services*. 5th ed. Boston: Cengage Learning, 2016.

Summerton, Nicholas. *Diagnosing Cancer in Primary Care*. Abington, England: Radcliffe Medical, 1999.

Sun, C. L., et al. "Dietary Soy and Increased Risk of Bladder Cancer: The Singapore Chinese Health Study." *Cancer Epidemiology: Biomarkers and Prevention* 11, no. 12 (December, 2002): 1674-1677.

Sun, K.-X., Jiao, J.-W., Chen, S., Liu, B.-L., & Zhao, Y. (2015). MicroRNA-186 induces sensitivity of ovarian cancer cells to paclitaxel and cisplatin by targeting ABCB1. *Journal of Ovarian Research,* 8(80). doi: 10.1186/s13048-015-0207-6.

Surendran, A. "Studies Linking Breast Cancer to Deodorants Smell Rotten, Experts Say." *Nature Medicine* 10, no. 3 (2004): 216.

Surgical Care Made Incredibly Visual! Philadelphia: Lippincott Williams & Wilkins, 2006.

Surgical Care Made Incredibly Visual. Philadelphia: Lippincott Williams & Wilkins, 2007.

Suster, S. "Diagnosis of Thymoma." *Journal of Clinical Pathology* 59, no. 12 (December, 2006): 1238-1244.

Suster, S., and C. A. Moran. "Thymoma Classification: Current Status and Future Trends." *American Journal of Clinical Pathology* 125, no. 4 (April, 2006): 542-554.

Sutton, Amy, ed. *Cancer Sourcebook for Women*. 3rd ed. Detroit: Omnigraphics, 2006.

Swaminathan, D., & Swaminathan, V. (2015). Geriatric oncology: problems with under-treatment within this population. *Cancer Biology & Medicine*, 12(4), 275-283. doi:10.7497/j.issn.2095-3941.2015.0081

Swanson, Barbara M. *Careers in Health Care*. New York: McGraw Hill Professional, 2005.

Swartz, M. A., et al. "Incidence of Primary Urethral Carcinoma in the United States." *Urology* 68, no. 6 (2006): 1164.

Swerdlow, A. J., et al. "Fluorescent Lights, Ultraviolet Lamps, and Risk of Cutaneous Melanoma." *British Medical Journal* 297 (1988): 647-650.

Syngal, S., Brand, R. E., Church, J. M., Giardiello , F. M., Hampel, H. L., & Burt, R. W. (2015). American college of gastroenterology (ACG) clinical guideline: Genetic testing and management of hereditary gastrointestinal cancer syndromes. *American Journal of Gastroenterology*, 110(2): 223-262. Recommendations of the American College of Gastroenterology for the management of patients with hereditary gastrointestinal cancer syndromes. This article is freely available at http://www.ncbi.nlm.nih.gov/pmc/articles/PMC4695986/

Szeifert, G., et al. "The Role of the Gamma Knife in the Management of Cerebral Astrocytomas." *Progress in Neurological Surgery* 20 (2007): 150-163.

Tabor, Edward, (Ed.). (2006). *Viruses and liver cancer.* New York: Elsevier, 2006.

Takata, M., and T. Saida. "Early Cancers of the Skin: Clinical, Histopathological, and Molecular Characteristics." *International Journal of Clinical Oncology* 10 (2005): 391-397.

Talamonti, Mark S., and Sam G. Pappas, eds. *Liver-Directed Therapy for Primary and Metastatic Liver Tumors*. New York: Springer, 2001.

Talarico, L. D. (1998). Myeloproliferative disorders: A practical review. *Patient Care,* 30: 37-57.

Talpaz, Moshe, and Hagop M. Kantarjian, eds. *Medical Management of Chronic Myelogenous Leukemia*. New York: Dekker, 1998.

Tang, Y., & Dawn, D. (2015). *Mesenchymal Stem Cell Derived Exosomes: The Potential for Translational Nanomedicine*. Salt Lake City, UT: Academic Press.

Tannock, I. F., et al., eds. *The Basic Science of Oncology*. 4th ed. New York: McGraw Hill, 2005.

Tannock, Ian, et al. *The Basic Science of Oncology*. Columbus, Ohio: McGraw-Hill, 2005.

Tannock, Ian, et al. *The Basic Science of Oncology*. 5th ed. New York: McGraw-Hill, 2013.

Tao, K., Yin, Y., Shen, Q., Chen, Y., Li, R., Chang, W., … Zhang, P. (2016). Akt inhibitor MK-2206 enhances the effect of cisplatin in gastric cancer cells. *Biomedical Reports,* 4: 365-368. doi: 10.3892/br.2016.594.

Tao, Y., D. Lefkopoulos, D. Ibrahima, et al. "Comparison of Dose Contribution to Normal Pelvic Tissues Among Conventional, Conformal, and Intensity-Modulated Radiotherapy Techniques in Prostate Cancer." *Acta Oncologica*, September 28, 2007, 1-9.

Tareke, E., et al. "Analysis of Acrylamide, a Carcinogen Formed in Heated Foodstuffs." *Journal of Agriculture and Food Chemistry* 50, no. 17 (2002): 4998-5006.

Taso, C. J., Lin, H. S., Lin, W. L., Chen, S. M., Huang, W. T., & Chen, S. W. (2014). The effect of yoga exercise on improving depression, anxiety, and fatigue in women with breast cancer: a randomized controlled trial. *Journal of Nursing Research*, 22(3):155-164.

Taube, S. E., et al. "Cancer Diagnostics: Decision Criteria for Marker Utilization in the Clinic." *American Journal of Pharmacogenomics* 5 (2005): 357-364.

Taylor, M. Clare. *Evidence-Based Practice for Occupational Therapists*. Malden, Mass.: Blackwell, 2007.

Teeley, Peter, and Philip Bashe. *The Complete Cancer Survival Guide*. New York: Broadway Books, 2005.

_______. *Cancer Survival Guide*. Rev. ed. New York: Broadway Books, 2005.

_______. *The Complete Revised and Updated Cancer Survival Guide: The Most Comprehensive, Up-to-Date Guide for Patients and Their Families*. Rev. ed. New York: Broadway Books, 2005.

Tefferi, A. "The Forgotten Myeloproliferative Disorder: Myeloid Metaplasia." *Oncologist* 8, no. 3 (2003): 225-231.

_______., and D. G. Gilliland. "Oncogenes in Myeloproliferative Disorders." *Cell Cycle* 6, no. 5 (March 1, 2007): 550-566.

_______., Lasho, T. L., Begna, K. H., Patnaik, M. M., Zblewski, D. L., Finke, C. M., Pardanani, A. (2015). A Pilot Study of the Telomerase Inhibitor Imetelstat for Myelofibrosis. *New England Journal of Medicine*, 373(10): 908-919.

Tekes, Aylin, et al. "Dynamic MRI of Bladder Cancer: Evaluation of Staging Accuracy." *American Journal of Roentgenology* 184, no. 1 (January, 2005): 121-127.

Tenenbaum, D. J. "POPS in Polar Bears: Organochlorines Affect Bone Density." *Environmental Health Perspectives* 112, no. 17 (2004): A1011.

Ter-Ovanesyan, D. (2011). Exosomes: The little vesicles that could. *Boston Biotech Watch*, Retrieved from http://bostonbiotechwatch.com/2011/04/20/exosomes-the-little-vesicles-that-could.

Tezcan, G., Tunca, B., Ak, S., Cecener, G., & Egeli, U. (2016). Molecular approach to genetic and epigenetic pathogenesis of early-onset colorectal cancer. *World Journal of Gastrointestinal Oncology,* 8(1): 83-89.

Thaller, Seth R., and W. Scott McDonald. *Facial Trauma*. Miami: Informa Health Care, 2004.

The ABCs of the Initial Preventive Physical Examination (IPPE). Department of Health and Health and Human and Human Services Centers for Medicare and Medicaid. Retrieved from https://www.cms.gov/Outreach-and-Education/Medicare-Learning-Network-MLN/MLNProducts/downloads/mps_qri_ippe001a.pdf

The Annual Report to the Nation on the Status of Cancer, 1975-2011. National Cancer Institute. Retrieved from http://www.cancer.gov/research/progress/annual-report-nation

The D Dilemma. Skin Cancer Foundation. Retrieved from http://www.skincancer.org/healthy-lifestyle/vitamin-d/the-d-dilemma

The International Agency for Research on Cancer (2004). *Cruciferous Vegetables, Isothiocyanates and Indoles (IARC Handbooks of Cancer Prevention) 1st Edition.* Washington, DC: International Agency for Research on Cancer Press, WHO office.

"The Picture Problem: Mammography, Air Power, and the Limits of Looking." *The New Yorker*, December 13, 2004. http://www.gladwell.com/2004/2004_12_13_a_picture.html.

The Sanofi Foundation for North America. (n.d.) Retrieved January 11, 2016 from http://www.sanofi.us/l/us/en/layout.jsp?scat=2145DE58-C86E-4269-9E59-601ED265C686

Theroux, Nicole. *Ewing's Sarcoma Family of Tumors: A Handbook for Families*. Glenview, Ill.: Association of Pediatric Oncology Nurses, 1999.

Thiboldeaux, Kim, and Mitch Golant. *The Total Cancer Wellness Guide: Reclaiming Your Life After Diagnosis*. Dallas: BenBella Books, 2007.

Thinnes, C. C., England, K. S., Kawamura, A., Chowdhury, R., Schofield, C. J., & Hopkinson, R. J. (2014). Targeting histone lysine demethylases — Progress, challenges, and the future. *Biochimica et Biophysica*

Acta - Gene Regulatory Mechanisms, 1839(12): 1416–1432.

Thomas, J., and R. Keith. *Looking Forward: The Speech and Swallowing Guidebook for People with Cancer of the Larynx or Tongue*. New York: Thieme, 2005.

Thomas, Lewis. *The Fragile Species*. New York: Collier Books, 1992.

_______. *The Lives of a Cell: Notes of a Biology Watcher*. New York: Viking Press, 1974.

Thompson, Lester D. R., and Gretchen S. Folk. "Synovial Sarcoma (Disease Overview)." *Ear, Nose, and Throat Journal* 85 (2006): 418-419.

Thomsen, H., & Webb, J. (Eds.). (2014). *Contrast media: Safety issues and ESUR guidelines* (3rd ed.). Germany: Springer-Verlag Berlin Heidelberg.

Thornton, J. *Environmental Impacts of Polyvinyl Chloride* (PVC) Building Materials. Washington, D.C.: Healthy Building Network, 2002.

Thygerson, A., et al. *First Aid, CPR, and AED*. 5th ed. Sudbury, Mass.: American College of Emergency Physicians/Jones & Bartlett, 2006.

Tian, X., Shivapurkar, N., Zheng, W., Hwang, J.J., Pishvaian, M.J., Weiner, L.M., …He, A.R. (2016). Circulating microRHA profile predicts disease progression in patients receiving second-line treatment of lapatinib and capecitabine for metastatic pancreatic cancer. *Oncology Letters,* 11: 1645-1650. doi: 10.3891/ol.2016.4101.

Tisdale, James E., and Douglas A. Miller. *Drug-Induced Diseases: Prevention, Detection, and Management*. Bethesda, Md.: American Society of Health-System Pharmacists, 2005.

Tomatis, Lorenzo, & Huff, James. (2002). Evolution of research in cancer etiology. In William B. Coleman & Gregory T. Tsongalis (Eds.), The molecular basis of human cancer. Totowa, N.J.: Humana Press.

Tomatis, Lorenzo, and James Huff. "Evolution of Research in Cancer Etiology." In *The Molecular Basis of* Human Cancer, edited by William B. Coleman and Gregory T. Tsongalis. Totowa, N.J.: Humana Press, 2002.

Tomiyama, A. J., Hunger, J. M., Nguyen-Cuu, J., & Wells, C. (2016). Misclassification of cardiometabolic health when using body mass index categories in NHANES 2005-2012. *Int J Obes*. doi:10.1038/ijo.2016.17

Tomlinson, Deborah, and Nancy E. Kline, eds. *Pediatric Oncology Nursing: Advanced Clinical Handbook.* New York: Springer, 2005.

Tonato, M., ed. *Antiemetics in the Supportive Care of Cancer Patients*. New York: Springer, 1996.

Tonsgard, J. H. "Clinical Manifestations and Management of Neurofibromatosis Type 1." *Seminars in Pediatric Neurology* 13 (2006): 2-7.

Top 10 Green Companies in the World 2015. *Newsweek.* Retrieved from: http://www.newsweek.com/green-2015/top-10-green-companies-world-2015

Topham, N. J., & Hewitt, E. W. (2009). Natural Killer Cell Cytotoxicity: How Do They Pull the Trigger? *Immunology,* 128(1): 7-15.

Torosian, Michael H., ed. *Breast Cancer: A Guide to Detection and Multidisciplinary Therapy*. Totowa, N.J.: Humana Press, 2002.

Townsend, Courtney M., Jr., et al., eds. *Sabiston Textbook of Surgery*. 17th ed. Philadelphia: Elsevier Saunders, 2005.

Trafford, Abigail. "On the Streets of Philadelphia, Prescriptions for Progress." *Washington Post*, August 8, 2000, p. Z5.

Travis, W. D., et al. "Pulmonary Langerhans Cell Granulomatosis (Histiocytosis X): A Clinicopathologic Study of Forty-eight Cases." *American Journal of Surgical Pathology* 17 (1993): 971.

Treasure, T., et al. "Radical Surgery for Mesothelioma: The Epidemic Still to Peak and We Need More Research to Manage It." *British Medical Journal* 328 (2004): 237-238.

Trendowski, Matthew. (2015). Recent advances in the development of antineoplastic agents derived from natural products. Drugs, 75(17):1993-2016. A review journal article that covers recent advances in natural product based drug discovery and examines mechanisms of action and current clinical data.

Troch, M., et al. "Does MALT Lymphoma of the Lung Require Immediate Treatment? An Analysis of Eleven Untreated Cases with Long-Term Follow-Up." *Anticancer Research* 27, no. 5B (September/October, 2007): 3633-3637.

Trock, B. J., L. Hilakivi-Clarke, and R. Clarke. "Meta-analysis of Soy Intake and Breast Cancer Risk." *Journal of the National Cancer Institute* 98, no. 7 (April 5, 2006): 459-471.

Trondl, R., Heffeter, P., Kowol, C. R., Jakupec, M. A., Berger, W., & Keppler, B. K. (2014). NKP-1339, the first ruthenium-based anticancer drug on the edge to clinical application. *Chemical Science* 5: 2925-2932.

Tsao, S., Tsang, C.M., To, K., & Lo, K. (2015). The role of Epstein-Barr virus in epithelial malignancies. *Journal of Pathology*, 235, 323-333.

Tselis, A., &Jenson, H. B. (2006). Epstein-Barr virus. New York: Taylor & Francis.

Tsimberidou A. M., & Keating, M. J. (2005). Richter syndrome: Biology, incidence, and therapeutic strategies. *Cancer,* 103, 216-228.

Turk, Dennis C., and Caryn S. Feldman, eds. *Noninvasive Approaches to Pain Management in the Terminally Ill.* New York: Haworth, 1992.

Turkington, Carol A., and William LiPera, eds. *The Encyclopedia of Cancer.* New York: Facts on File, 2005.

Twombly, R. "Childhood Cancer Survivor Study Doubles to Examine Late Effects of New Treatments." *Journal of the National Cancer Institute* 99, no. 21 (November 7, 2007): 1574-1576.

Tyson, Leslie B., and Joanne Frankel Kelvin. *One Hundred Questions and Answers About Cancer Symptoms and Cancer Treatment Side Effects.* Sudbury, Mass.: Jones & Bartlett, 2005.

U.S. Department of Commerce. U.S. Census Bureau. *Profiles of General Demographic Characteristics: 2000 Census of Population and Housing.* Washington, D.C.: Author, 2001.

U.S. Department of Health and Human Services. *The Health Benefits of Smoking Cessation: A Report of the Surgeon General.* Washington, D.C.: Author, 1990.

U.S. Department of Health and Human Services. *United States Cancer Statistics: 1999-2002 Incidence and Mortality Web-Based Report.* Atlanta: Centers for Disease Control and Prevention and National Cancer Institute, 2005. Also available online at http://www.cdc.gov.

U.S. Department of Health and Human Services. *The Health Consequences of Involuntary Exposure to Tobacco Smoke: A Report of the Surgeon General.* Washington, D.C.: Author, 2006.

U.S. Department of Health and Human Services, National Institutes of Health, and the National Cancer Institute. *NCI International Portfolio: Addressing the Global Challenge of Cancer.* Bethesda, Md.: National Cancer Institute, 2006.

U.S. Department of Health and Human Services, National Institutes of Health (NIH).National Institute of Diabetes and Digestive and Kidney Diseases (NIDDK).The National Digestive Diseases Information Clearinghouse (NDDIC). (September, 2014). *Crohn's Disease.* NIH Publication No. 14–3410. Retrieved from http://www.niddk.nih.gov/health-information/health-topics/digestive-diseases/crohns-disease/Pages/facts.aspx. This is a government publication that provides basic information for patients regarding the identification, assessment, diagnosis and treatment of Crohn's Disease.

U.S. Department of Health and Human Services, Public Health Service, National Toxicology Program. *Eleventh Report on Carcinogens.* Research Triangle Park, N.C.: Author, 2005.

U.S. Environmental Protection Agency. Office of Research and Development. Office of Health and Environmental Assessment. *Health Assessment Document for 2,3,7,8-Tetrachlorodibenzo-p-dioxin (TCDD) and Related Compounds.* Washington, D.C.: Author, 1994.

_______. *The Effects of Great Lakes Contaminants on Human Health.* Report to U.S. Congress. EPA 95-R-95-107. Chicago: Author, 1995.

_______. *Toxicological Review of Beryllium and Compounds.* Washington, D.C.: Author, 1998.

_______. *Integrated Risk Information System (IRIS) on Beryllium.* Washington, D.C.: National Center for Environmental Assessment, Office of Research and Development, 1999.

U.S. Food and Drug Administration. *Guidance for Institutional Review Boards and Clinical Investigators: A Guide to Informed Consent.* Rockville, Md.: Author, 1998.

U.S. Occupational Safety and Health Administration. *Occupational Safety and Health Standards, Toxic and Hazardous Substances.* Code of Federal Regulations 29 CFR 1910.1000. Washington, D.C.: Author, 1998.

U.S. Preventive Services Task Force. "Genetic Risk Assessment and *BRCA* Mutation Testing for Breast and Ovarian Cancer Susceptibility: Recommendation Statement." *Annals of Internal Medicine* 143 (2005): 355-361.

Ulrich, Lawrence P. *The Patient Self-Determination Act: Meeting the Challenges in Patient Care.* Washington, D.C.: Georgetown University Press, 1999.

United Nations. (2015). Trends in Contraceptive Use Worldwide 2015. Retrieved from http://www.un.org/en/development/desa/population/publications/pdf/family/trendsContraceptiveUse2015Report.pdf.

United States Department of Health and Human Services, National Institutes of Health. *The NCI Strategic Plan for Leading the Nation to Eliminate the Suffering and Death Due to Cancer.* Washington, D.C.: National Cancer Institute, 2006.

United States Food and Drug Administration. (July 9, 2015). *Information on Cetuximab (marketed as Erbitux).* Retrieved from http://www.fda.gov/Drugs/DrugSafety/PostmarketDrugSafetyInformationforPatientsandProviders/ucm113714.htm

University of Rochester. (2011, June 17). Protein found that improves DNA repair under stress. *ScienceDaily.*

Retrieved February 10, 2016 from www.sciencedaily.com/releases/2011/06/110616142722.htm.

Update on genetic testing for heart disease. (2012), September 1. *Harvard Heart Letter*. http://www.health.harvard.edu/heart-health/update-on-genetic-testing-for-heart-disease

"Updated Guidelines: The Prevention and Treatment of Infection in Patients with an Absent or Dysfunctional Spleen." British Committee for Standards in Haematology. *BMJ*, June 2, 2001. Also available at http://www .bmj.com.

UpToDate. (2013). Patient information: Surgical procedures for breast cancer—Mastectomy and breast conserving therapy (Beyond the Basics). Retrieved from http://www.uptodate.com/contents/surgical-procedures-for-breast-cancer-mastectomy-and-breast-conserving-therapy-beyond-the-basics.

Uranus, S. *Current Spleen Surgery*. Munich: Zuckschwerdt, 1995.

Uronis, H. E., and J. C. Bendell. "Anal Cancer: An Overview." *Oncologist* 12, no. 5 (May, 2007): 524-534.

Utsunomiya, Joji, John J. Mulvihill, and Walter Weber, eds. *Familial Cancer and Prevention: Molecular Epidemiology, a New Strategy Toward Cancer Control.* New York: Wiley-Liss, 1999.

Uziel, G., and F. Taroni, eds. *Hereditary Leukoencephalop*athies and Demyelinating Neuropathies in Children. Eastleigh, England: John Libbey Eurotext Ltd, 2004.

Vadlamani, Lalit, et al. "Colorectal Cancer in Russian-Speaking Jewish Emigrés: Community-Based Screening." *American Journal of Gastroenterology* 96, no. 9 (2001): 2755-2760.

Valenzuela H. F., Fuller, T., Edwards, J., Finger, D., & Molgora, B. (2009). Cycloastragenol extends T cell proliferation by increasing telomerase activity. *Journal of Immunology* 182: 90.30.

Valle, R. F. "Development of Hysteroscopy: From a Dream to a Reality, and Its Linkage to the Present and Future." *Journal of Minimally Invasive Gynecology* 14, no. 4 (July/August, 2007): 407-418.

Van Deerlin V. & Reshef R. (2016). Chimerism testing in allogeneic hematopoietic stem cell transplantation. In Debra G.B. Leonard (Ed.), *Molecular Pathology in Clinical Practice* (pp. 823-848). New York, NY: Springer.

Van den Bent, M. J. "Advances in the Biology and Treatment of Oligodendrogliomas." *Current Opinion in Neurology* 17, no. 6 (December, 2004): 675-680.

Van Goethem, J. W., et al. "Spinal Tumors." *European Journal of Radiology* 50 (2004): 159-176.

van Kruijsdijk, R. C. M., van der Wall, E., & Visseren, F. L. J. (2009). Obesity and Cancer: The Role of Dysfunctional Adipose Tissue. *Cancer Epidemiology Biomarkers & Prevention,* 18(10), 2569-2578. doi:10.1158/1055-9965.EPI-09-0372

Van Lanshott, J. J., et al. "Hospital Volume and Hospital Mortality for Esophagectomy." *Cancer* 91 (2001): 1574.

Van Meir, E. G. "Turcot's Syndrome: Phenotype of Brain Tumors, Survival, and Mode of Inheritance." *International Journal of Cancer* 75 (1998): 162-164.

Van Vuuren, R. J., Visagie, M. H., Theron, A. E., & Joubert, A. M. (2015). Antimitotic drugs in the treatment of cancer. *Cancer chemotherapy and pharmacology,* 6(76): 1101-1112.

Vanderbilt University News. (2006, May 15). Vanderbilt-Ingram cancer center researchers find *Ginseng* may improve breast cancer outcomes. Retrieved from http://news.vanderbilt.edu/2006/03/vanderbilt-ingram-cancer-center-researchers-find-ginseng-may-improve-breast-cancer-outcomes-56874

Vanharanta S, & Massagué J. (2013). Origins of metastatic traits. *Cancer Cell*, 24(4):410-21. http://www.ncbi.nlm.nih.gov/pubmed/24135279

Vanneman, M., & Dranoff, G. (2012). Combining immunotherapy and targeted therapies in cancer treatment. *Nature Reviews Cancer*, 12(4): 237-251.

VanSonnenberg, Eric, William McMullen, and Luigi Solbiati. *Tumor Ablation: Principles and Practice*. New York: Springer, 2005.

Vardanyan, Ruben, & Hruby, Victor. (2006). Synthesis of essential drugs. Philadelphia: Elsevier. Provides descriptions of mechanism of action, implementation, and synthesis of medicinal drugs.

Varricchio, Claudette, et al., eds. *A Cancer Source Book for Nurses*. 8th ed. Sudbury, Mass.: Jones and Bartlett, 2004.

Vasen, H. F. A., Blanco, I., Aktan-Collan, K., Gopie, J. P., Alonso, A., Aretz, S., … the Mallorca Group. (2013). Revised guidelines for the clinical management of Lynch syndrome (HNPCC): Recommendations by a group of European experts. *Gut*, 62(6): 812-823. The Mallorca Group is a group of European experts who got together and developed this revised guidelines for the clinical management of Lynch syndrome (HNPCC). This article is freely available at http://gut.bmj.com/content/62/6/812.full

Vasilev, Steven A., ed. *Perioperative and Supportive Care in Gynelogic Oncology: Evidence-Based Management*. New York: Wiley-Liss, 2000.

Vázquez, G., and A. Pellón. "Polyurethane-Coated Silicone Gel Breast Implants Used for Eighteen Years." *Aesthetic Plastic Surgery* 31, no. 4 (July/August, 2007): 330-336.

Venkitaraman, A. R. "Cancer Susceptibility and the Functions of *BRCA1* and *BRCA2*: A Review." *Cell* 108, no. 2 (2002): 171-182.

Venn, A., D. Healy, and R. McLachlan. "Cancer Risk Associated with a Diagnosis of Infertility." *Best Practice and Research Clinical Obstetrics and Gynaecology* 17 (2003): 343-367.

Vermorken, J. B., et al. "Cisplatin, Fluorouracil, and Docetaxel in Unresectable Head and Neck Cancer." *New England Journal of Medicine* 357 (2007): 1695-1704.

Verona, Verne. (2001). *Nature's cancer fighting foods.* New York: Prentice Hall.

Verschuuren, J. J., et al. "Available Treatment Options for the Management of Lambert-Eaton Myasthenic Syndrome." *Expert Opinion on Pharmacotherapy* 7, no. 10 (July, 2006): 1323-1336.

Verweij, J., and Herbert M. Pinedo. *Targeting Treatment of Soft-Tissue Sarcomas*. Boston: Kluwer Academic, 2004.

Verweij, P. E., Chowdhary, A., Melchers, W. J. G., & Meis, J. F. (2016). Azole resistance in *Aspergillus fumigatus*: Can we retain the clinical use of mold-active antifungal azoles?" *Clinical Infectious Diseases,* 62(2): 362-368.

Veys, C. A. "ABC of Work Related Disorders: Occupational Cancer." *British Medical Journal* 313 (1996): 615-619.

Vij, D. F., and K. Mahesh, eds. *Medical Applications of Lasers*. Boston: Kluwer Academic, 2002.

Vinay, Kumar, Abul K. Abbas, and Nelson Fausto. *Robbins and Cotran Pathological Basis of Disease*. 7th ed. Philadelphia: Elsevier/Saunders, 2005.

Vincent, Angela, and Camilla Buckley. "Myasthenia Gravis and Other Antibody-Associated Neurological Diseases." In *The Autoimmune Diseases*, edited by Noel R. Rose and Ian R. Mackay. Boston: Elsevier/Academic Press, 2006.

Vliet, Elizabeth Lee. *It's My Ovaries, Stupid!* 2d ed. Tucson, Ariz.: Her Place Press, 2007.

Vogelstein, B., Sur, S. & Prives, C. (2010). p53: The most frequently altered gene in human cancers. *Nature Education,* 3(9): 6.

Vogelstein, Bert, and Kenneth Kinzler. The Genetic Basis of Human Cancer. New York: McGraw-Hill, 2002.

Vogelzang, N. J., Rusthoven, J. J., Symanowski, J., Denham, C., Kaukel, E., Ruffie, P., … Paoletti P. (2003). Phase III study of pemetrexed in combination with cisplatin versus cisplatin alone in patients with malignant pleural mesothelioma, *Journal of Clinical Oncology* 21(14): 2636-2644.

Vogt, P.K. (2012). Retroviral oncogenes: a historical primer. *Nature Reviews Cancer,* 12(9), 639-648. http://www.ncbi.nlm.nih.gov/pmc/articles/PMC3428493/

Voiland, Adam. "More Problems with Plastics: Like BPA, Chemicals Called Phthalates Raise Some Concern." *U.S. News & World Report*, May 19, 2008, p. 54.

Vom Saal, Frederick S., et al. "Chapel Hill Bisphenol A Expert Panel Consensus Statement: Integration of Mechanisms, Effects in Animals and Potential to Impact Human Health at Current Levels of Exposure." *Reproductive Toxicology* 24, no. 2 (2007): 131-138.

Vorburger, S., & Hunt, K. (2002). Adenoviral gene therapy. *The Oncologist*, 7(1), 46-59.

Waal, Isaac van der. *Diseases of the Salivary Glands Including Dry Mouth and Sjögren's Syndrome: Diagnosis and Treatment*. New York: Springer-Verlag, 1997.

Wahl, Richard L., ed. *Principles and Practice of Positron Emission Tomography*. Philadelphia: Lippincott Williams & Wilkins, 2002.

Wainrib, Barbara, et al. *Men, Women, and Prostate Cancer: A Medical and Psychological Guide for Women and the Men They Love*. Oakland, Calif.: New Harbinger, 2000.

Waisberg, M., P. Joseph, B. Hale, and D. Beyersmann. "Molecular and Cellular Mechanisms of Cadmium Carcinogenesis." *Toxicology* 192 (2003): 95-117.

Waldren, C. A., and I. Rasko. "Caffeine Enhancement of X-Ray Killing in Cultured Human and Rodent Cells." *Radiation Research* 73, no. 1 (January, 1978): 95-110.

Walko, C. M. and Lindley, C. (2005). Capecitabine: A review. *Clinical Therapeutics,* 27(1): 23–44. http://www.sciencedirect.com/science/article/pii/S0149291805000068

Wall, J.K. (2015, September 12). Lilly leaps into new frontier of cancer drugs. *Indianapolis Business Journal.* Retrieved from http://www.ibj.com/articles/54832-lilly-leaps-into-new-frontier-of-cancer-drugs

Wallace, D. J. (Ed.). (2004). *The new Sjögren's syndrome handbook* (3rd ed.). New York: Oxford University Press.

Wallach, Jacques. *Interpretation of Diagnostic Tests*. 8th ed. Philadelphia: Wolters Kluwer Health/Lippincott Williams & Wilkins, 2007.

Waller, A., and N. L. Caroline. *Handbook of Palliative Care in Cancer*. Boston: Butterworth-Heinemann, 2000.

Walsh, Mary. *Cushing's Syndrome, A Patient Guide: One Woman's Journey*. Rye, N.Y.: New Mill Press, 2001.

Walsh, P. C., & Farrar Worthington, J. (2013). Dr. *Patrick Walsh's guide to surviving prostate cancer.* New York: Grand Central Life & Style.

Walsh, Thomas J., & Andes, David R. (Eds.). (2015). Advances and new directions for echinocandins. Clinical Infectious Diseases, 61(suppl. 6): S601-S683.

Wang, J., Z. Lu, and J. L. Au. "Protection Against Chemotherapy-Induced Alopecia." *Pharmaceutical Research* 23, no. 11 (2006): 2505-2514.

Wang, K. K., et al. "American Gastroenterological Association Medical Position Statement: Role of the Gastroenterologist in the Management of Esophageal Carcinoma." *Gastroenterology* 128 (2005): 1468-1470.

Wang, L. L., et al. "Association Between Osteosarcoma and Deleterious Mutations in the *RECQ14* Gene in Rothmund-Thomson Syndrome." *Journal of the National Cancer Institute* 95, no. 9 (May 7, 2003): 669-674.

Wang, L., Ni, X., Covington, K. R., Yang, B. Y., Shiu, J., Zhang, X., Xi, L., … Duvic, M. (2015). Genomic profiling of Sézary syndrome identifies alterations of key T cell signaling and differentiation genes. *Nature Genetics,* 47(12), 1426-1434.

Wang, M., Qin, S., Zhang, T., Song. X., & Zhang, S. (2015). The effect of fruit and vegetable intake on the development of lung cancer: A meta analysis of 32 publications and 20,414 cases. *European Journal of Clinical Nutrition,* 69, 1184–1192.

Wang, X. Y., & Fisher, P. B. (Eds.). (2015). *Immunotherapy of cancer*, (Advances in Cancer Research), (Vol. 128). Waltham, MA: Academic Press, 2015. This book provides information on cancer research with expert reviews and is directed towards students and researchers.

Wang, X., et al. "Comparison of D&C and Hysterectomy Pathologic Findings in Endometrial Cancer Patients." *Archives of Gynecology and Obstetrics* 272, no. 2 (July, 2005): 136-141.

Wang, Y., et al. "Inhibition of the IGF-I Receptor for Treatment of Cancer: Kinase Inhibitors and Monoclonal Antibodies as Alternative Approaches." *Recent Results in Cancer Research* 172 (2007): 59-76.

Wang, Z. C., A. Buralmoh, J. D. Iglehart, and A. Richardson. "Genome-Wide Analysis for Loss of Heterozygosity in Primary and Recurrent Phyllodes Tumor and Fibroadenoma of Breast Using Single Nucleotide Polymorphism Arrays." *Breast Cancer Research and Treat*ment 97, no. 3 (2006): 301-309.

Wapner, Jessica. (2013). *The Philadelphia chromosome: A mutant gene and the quest to cure cancer at the genetic level.* New York: The Experiment.

Ward, E., et al. "Cancer Disparities by Race/Ethnicity and Socio-economic Status." *CA: A Cancer Journal for Clinicians* 54, no. 2 (2004): 78-93.

Ward, Elizabeth C., and Corina J. Van As-Brooks, eds. *Head and Neck Cancer: Treatment, Rehabilitation, and Outcomes*. San Diego, Calif.: Plural, 2006.

_______. *Head and Neck Cancer: Treatment, Rehabilitation, and Outcomes*. San Diego: Plural, 2007.

Watanabe, M., R. Tanaka, and N. Takeda. "Correlation of MRI and Clinical Features in Meningeal Carcinomatosis." *Neuroradiology* 35 (1993): 512-515.

Watanabe, N., Horikoshi, M., Yamada, M., Shimodera, S., Akechi, T., Miki, K. … Furukawa, T.A., (2015). Adding smartphone-based cognitive behavior therapy to pharmacotherapy for major depression (FLATT project): Study protocol for a randomized controlled trial. *BioMed Central,* 16(293). doi: 10.1186. s13063-015-0805-z.

Watson, Tim, ed. *Electrotherapy: Evidence-Based Practice*. 12th ed. New York: Churchill Livingstone, 2008.

Waye, Jerome D., Douglas K. Rex, and Christopher B. Williams, eds. *Colonoscopy: Principles and Practice*. Malden, Mass.: Blackwell, 2003.

Waynant, Ronald W. *Lasers in Medicine*. Boca Raton, Fla.: CRC Press, 2002.

Weaver, B. A. A., and D. W. Cleveland. "Does Aneuploidy Cause Cancer?" *Current Opinion in Cell Biology* 18 (2006): 658-667.

WebMD. (2014, July 14). *Resveratrol Supplements*. Retrieved from http://www.webmd.com/heart-disease/resveratrol-supplements

Wei, X., Yang, X., Han, Z., Qu, F., Shao, L., and Shi, Y. (2013). Mesenchymal stem cells: A new trend for cell therapy. *Acta Pharmacologia Sinica,* 34, 747 – 754.

Weinberg, R. A. *The Biology of Cancer*. New York: Garland Science, 2007.

_______. (2013). *The biology of cancer* (2nd ed.). New York: Garland Science.

_______. *The Biology of Cancer*. New York: Garland Science, Taylor & Francis, 2007.

Weinstein, S. L., and J. A. Buckwalter, eds. *Turek's Orthopaedics: Principles and Their Application*. Philadelphia: Lippincott Williams & Wilkins, 2005.

Weir, Robert F. *Abating Treatment with Critically Ill Patients: Ethical and Legal Limits to the Medical Prolongation of Life*. New York: Oxford University Press, 1989.

Weisbrot, Deborah M., and Alan B. Ettinger. *The Essential Patient Handbook: Getting the Health Care You Need—from Doctors Who Know*. New York: Demos Medical, 2004.

Weiss, G. "Acrylamide in Food: Uncharted Territory." *Science* 27 (2002): 297.

Weiss, Leonard. *Principles of Metastasis*. San Diego, Calif.: Academic Press, 1985.

Weiss, N. S. "Breast Cancer Mortality in Relation to Clinical Breast Examination and Breast Self-Evaluation." *Breast Journal* 9, suppl. 2 (May/June, 2003): S86-S89.

Weksberg, Rosanna, Cheryl Shuman, and Adam C. Smith. "Beckwith-Wiedemann Syndrome." *American Journal of Medical Genetics, Part C* 137C (2005): 12-23.

Welch, H. G. *Should I Be Tested for Cancer? Maybe Not and Here's Why*. Berkeley: University of California Press, 2004.

_______., L. M. Schwartz, and S. Woloshin. "Are Increasing Five-Year Survival Rates Evidence of Success Against Cancer?" *Journal of the American Medical Association* 283, no. 22 (June 14, 2000): 2975-2978.

Weldon, Glen, ed. *Dietary Options for Cancer Survivors: A Guide to Research on Foods, Food Substances, Herbals, and Dietary Regimens That May Influence Cancer*. Washington, D.C.: American Institute for Cancer Research, 2002.

Welte, K., Gabrilove, J., Bronchud, M. H., Platzer, E., & Morstyn, G. (1996). Filgrastim (r-metHuG-CSF): The first ten years. *Blood*, 88(6), 1907-1929.

Wen, P. Y., P. M. Black, and J. S. Loeffler. "Treatment of Metastatic Cancer." In *Cancer: Principles and Practice of Oncology*, edited by V. T. DeVita, Jr., S. Hellman, and S. A. Rosenberg. 6th ed. Philadelphia: Lippincott Williams & Wilkins, 2001.

Werth, James L., and Dean Blevins, eds. *Decision Making Near the End of Life: Issues, Development, and Future Directions*. New York: Brunner-Routledge, 2008.

Wesley, Merideth K., and Ingrid A. Sternbach, eds. *Smoking and Women's Health*. New York: Nova Science, 2008.

West, Alison C. & Johnstone, Ricky W. (2014). "New and emerging HDAC inhibitors for cancer treatment." *Journal of Clinical Investigation* 124(1): 30-39.

Westberg, Granger E. *Good Grief*. Minneapolis: Augsburg Fortress, 2006.

Westbrook, Catherine. *MRI in Practice*. 3rd ed. Malden, Mass.: Blackwell, 2005.

Wetherill, Y. B., et al. "Bisphenol A Facilitates Bypass of Androgen Ablation Therapy in Prostate Cancer." *Molecular Cancer Therapeutics* 5 (2006): 3181-3190.

Weycker, D., Li, X., Barron, R., Li, Y., Reiner, M., Kartashov, A., … & Garcia, J. (2015). Risk of chemotherapy-induced febrile neutropenia with early discontinuation of pegfilgrastim prophylaxis in US clinical practice. *Supportive Care in Cancer,* doi:10.1007/s00520-015-3039-4.

Weycker, D., Li, X., Figueredo, J., Barron, R., Tzivelekis, S. & Hagiwara, M. (2015). Risk of chemotherapy-induced febrile neutropenia in cancer patients receiving pegfilgrastim prophylaxis: Does timing of administration matter? *Supportive Care in Cancer,* doi:10.1007/s00520-015-3036-7.

What does Medicare cover for cancer? Medicare Matters. National Council on Aging. Retrieved from https://www.mymedicarematters.org/coverage/parts-a-b/conditions/?SID=569884b1e6002SID

What to Expect When Meeting with a Genetic Counselor. American Society of Clinical Oncology. Retrieved from http://www.cancer.net/navigating-cancer-care/cancer-basics/genetics/what-expect-when-meeting-genetic-counselor

Whiteside, T. L. (2012). What are regulatory T cells (Treg) regulating in cancer and why? *Seminars in Cancer Biology*, 22(4): 327-334.

Whittington, E. "Food for Thought: A Waste of Taste." *CURE* (Fall, 2006).

Wiederpass, E., et al. "Occurrence, Trends and Environment Etiology of Pancreatic Cancer." *Scandinavian Journal of Environmental Health* 24, no. 3 (June, 1998): 165-174.

Wiernik, Peter Harris, ed. *Neoplastic Diseases of the Blood*. 4th ed. New York: Cambridge University Press, 2003.

Wilander, Erik, Monalill Lundqvist, and Kjell Öberg. *Gastrointestinal Carcinoid Tumors*. New York: Fischer, 1989.

Wilcox, C. Mel, Miguel Muñoz-Navas, and Joseph J. Y. Sung. *Atlas of Clinical Gastrointestinal Endoscopy*. 2d ed. Philadelphia: Saunders Elsevier, 2007.

Wilcox, Ryan A. (2016). Cutaneous T-cell lymphoma: 2016 update on diagnosis, risk-stratification, and management. *American Journal of Hematology,* 91(1), 152-165.

Wilder, L. *The Mayo Clinic*. New York: Harcourt, Brace, 1942.

Wilkes, Gail M., and Terri B. Ades. *Patient Education Guide to Oncology Drugs*. 2d ed. Sudbury, Mass.: Jones and Bartlett, 2004.

Williams, Christopher Kwesi O., Olufunmilayo I. Olopade, and Carla I. Falkson, eds. *Breast Cancer in Women of African Descent*. London: Springer, 2006.

Williams, Nerys R. *Atlas of Occupational Health and Disease*. New York: Oxford University Press, 2004.

Williams, Simon J. *Medicine and the Body*. London: Sage Publications, 2003.

Wilson, A. Bennett, Jr. *A Primer on Limb Prosthetics*. Springfield, Ill.: Charles C Thomas, 1998.

Winawer, Sidney J., Moshe Shike, Philip Bashe, and Genell Subak-Sharpe. *Cancer Free: The Comprehensive Cancer Prevention Program.* New York: Fireside/Simon & Schuster, 1996.

Winchester, David J., et al. *Breast Cancer.* 2d ed. Hamilton, Ont.: BC Decker, 2006.

Winslow, R. (2015, October 8). Roche's MS Drug Reports Promising Results. *Wall Street Journal.* Retrieved from: http://www.wsj.com/articles/roche-reports-positive-late-stage-trial-results-for-ms-drug-1444325240

Winter, John C. *Tobacco Use by Native North Americans: Sacred Smoke, Silent Killer.* Norman: University of Oklahoma Press, 2000.

Wiseman, Sam M., et al. "Parathyroid Carcinoma: A Multicenter Review of Clinicopathologic Features and Treatment Outcomes." *Ear, Nose and Throat Journal* 83, no. 7 (July 1, 2004): 491-494.

Wisnia, Saul. *The Jimmy Fund of Dana-Farber Cancer Institute.* Charleston, S.C.: Arcadia, 2002.

Wittekind, C., et al. "TNM Residual Tumor Classification Revisited." *Cancer* 94 (2002): 2511-2516.

Wolbarst, Anthony Brinton. *Looking Within: How X-Ray, CT, MRI, Ultrasound, and Other Medical Images Are Created, and How They Help Physicians Save Lives.* Berkeley: University of California Press, 1999.

Wold, L. E., C. Adler, F. Sim, and K. Unni, eds. *Atlas of Orthopedic Pathology.* 2d ed. Philadelphia: Saunders, 2003.

Wold, W.S., & Toth, K. (2013). Adenovirus vectors for gene therapy. *Current Gene Therapy*, 13(6), 421-433.

Wong, S. T., et al. "Disparities in Colorectal Cancer Screening Rates Among Asian Americans and Non-Latino Whites." *Cancer* 104, no. 12 (2005): S2,940-S2,947.

Wood, B. J., et al. "Percutaneous Tumor Ablation with Radiofrequency." *Cancer* 94, no. 2 (2002): 443-451.

Wood, M. J. A. (2015). *Exosome Biology and Therapeutics.* Hoboken, New Jersey, Wiley-Blackwell.

Woodson, G. "Evolving Concepts of Laryngeal Paralysis." *The Journal of Laryngology and Otology* 122, no. 5 (May, 2008): 437-441.

Woodward, E. R., and E. R. Maher. "Von Hippel-Lindau Disease and Endocrine Tumour Susceptibility." *Endocrine Related Cancer* 32 (2006): 415-425.

Woodward, Kevin N. *Phthalate Esters: Toxicity and Metabolism.* Boca Raton, Fla.: CRC Press, 1988.

Worden, J. William. *Children and Grief: When a Parent Dies.* New York: Guilford Press, 1996.

Woznick, Leigh A., and Carol D. Goodheart. *Living with Childhood Cancer: A Practical Guide to Help Families Cope.* Washington, D.C.: APA Life Tools, 2002.

Wray, David, et al. eds. *Textbook of General and Oral Surgery.* New York: Churchill Livingstone, 2003.

Wright, Karen. "Testing Pesticides on Humans." *Discover* 3, no. 12 (December, 2003): 66-69.

Wright, Kenneth, et al. *Handbook of Pediatric Eye and Systemic Disease.* New York: Springer Science, 2006.

Wrightson, William R., ed. *Current Concepts in General Surgery: A Resident Review.* Georgetown, Tex.: Landes Bioscience, 2006.

Wu, A. H., D. Yang, and M. C. Pike. "A Meta-analysis of Soyfoods and Risk of Stomach Cancer: The Problem of Potential Confounders." *Cancer Epidemiology: Biomarkers and Prevention* 9, no. 10 (October, 2000): 1051-1058.

Wu, W. S. "The Signaling Mechanism of ROS in Tumor Progression." *Cancer Metastasis Reviews* 25 (2006): 695-705.

Wu, W., W. Hu, and J. J. Kavanagh. "Proteomics in Cancer Research." *International Journal of Gynecological Cancer* 12 (2002): 409-423.

Wyatt, A. J., G. D. Leonard, and D. L. Sachs. "Cutaneous Reactions to Chemotherapy and Their Management." *American Journal of Clinical Dermatology* 7, no. 1 (2006): 45-63.

Xavier, A. C., Edwards, H., Dombkowski, A. A., Balci, T. B., Berman, J. N., Dellaire, G., … Taub, J. W. (2011). A unique role of GATA1s in Down syndrome acute megakaryocytic leukemia biology and therapy. *PLoS ONE,* 6(11): e27486. doi:10.1371/journal.pone.0027486.

Xie, M., Jiang, Q. & Xie, Y. (2015). Comparison between decitabine and azacitidine for the treatment of myelodysplastic syndrome: A meta-analysis with 1392 participants. *Clinical Lymphoma, Myeloma & Leukemia,* 15(1):22-28.

Xu, H., Gong, Q., Vogl, F., Reiner, M. and Page, J. (2016). Risk factors for bone pain among patients with cancer receiving myelosuppressive chemotherapy and pegfilgrastim. *Supportive Care in Cancer,* doi:10.1007/s00520-015-2834-2.

Xu, J.-H., Hu, S.-L., Shen, G.-D., & Shen, G. (2016). Tumor suppressor genes and their underlying interactions in paclitaxel resistance in cancer therapy. *Cancer Cell International,* 16(13). doi: 10.1186/s12935-016-0290-9.

Yagi, H. & Kitagawa, Y. (2013). The role of mesenchymal stem cells in cancer development. *Frontiers in Genetics.* Retrieved from http://dx.doi.org/10.3389/fgene.2013.00261. Shah, K. (2014). *Mesenchymal Stem Cells in Cancer Therapy.* Cambridge, Mass: Academic Press.

Yamada, T., ed. *Textbook of Gastroenterology*. 4th ed. Philadelphia: Lippincott Williams & Wilkins, 2003.

Yamaguchi, Y. (Ed.). (2016). *Immunotherapy of cancer: An innovative treatment comes of age*. New York: Springer. A new book that summarizes present status and future for cancer immunotherapy.

Yan, L., and E. L. Spitznagel. "Meta-analysis of Soy Food and Risk of Prostate Cancer in Men." *International Journal of Cancer* 117, no. 4 (November 20, 2005): 667-669.

Yang, B.B., Savin, M.A., & Green, M. (2012). Prevention of chemotherapy-induced neutropenia with pegfilgrastim: Pharmakokinetics and patient outcomes. *Chemotherapy*, 58, 387-98.

Yap Y.S., Karapetis C., Lerose S., Iyer S., & Koczwara B. (2006). Reducing the risk of peripherally inserted central catheter line complications in the oncology setting. *European Journal of Cancer,* 15, 342-347.

Yarbro, C. H., M. H. Frogge, and M. Goodman. *Cancer Nursing: Principles and Practice*. 6th ed. Sudbury, Mass.: Jones and Bartlett, 2005.

Yarbro, C. H., M. H. Frogge, and M. Goodman. *Cancer Symptom Management*. 3rd ed. Sudbury, Mass.: Jones and Bartlett, 2005.

Yarbro, Connie H., Michelle Goodman, and Margaret H. Frogge, eds. *Cancer Symptom Management*. 3rd ed. Sudbury, Mass.: Jones and Bartlett, 2004.

Yarbro, Connie Henke, Margaret Hansen Frogge, and Michelle Goodman, eds. *Cancer Symptom Management*. Sudbury, Mass.: Jones and Bartlett, 2004.

Yavorkovsky, L. L., & Cook, P.(2001). Classifying chronic myelomonocytic leukemia. *Journal of Clinical Oncology,* 19: 3790-3792.

Yee, Judy. *Virtual Colonoscopy*. Philadelphia: Lippincott Williams & Wilkins, 2008.

Yirmiya, Raz, and Anna N. Taylor, eds. *Alcohol, Immunity, and Cancer*. Boca Raton, Fla.: CRC Press, 1993.

Yohay, K. "Neurofibromatosis Types 1 and 2." *The Neurologist* 12 (2006): 86-93.

Yoneda, T., and T. Hiraga. "Crosstalk Between Cancer Cells and Bone Microenvironment in Bone Metastasis." *Biochem Biophys Res Commun* 328, no. 3 (2005): 679-687.

Young, Carolyn, Cyndie Koopsen, and Daniel Farb. End of Life Care Issues Guidebook: *A Guide for Healthcare Providers and the Public on the Care of the Dying*. Los Angeles: University of Health Care, 2005.

Young, L. S., & Rickinson, A. B. Epstein-Barr virus: Forty years on. *Nature Reviews: Cancer*, 4(10), 757-768.

Your Guide to Medicare's Preventive Services. Centers for Medicare and Medicaid Services. Retrieved from https://www.medicare.gov/Pubs/pdf/10110.pdf

Ysunza, A., et al. "The Role of Laryngeal Electromyography in the Diagnosis of Vocal Fold Immobility in Children." *International Journal of Pediatric Otorhinolaryngology* 71, no. 6 (June, 2007): 949-958.

Yu L, Wang Y, Yao Y, Li W, Lai Q, Li J, Yang J. (2014). Eradication of growth of HER2-positive ovarian cancer with trastuzumab-DM1, an antibody-cytotoxic drug conjugate in mouse xenograft model. *International Journal of Gynecological Cancer,* 24(7): 1158-1164.

Yun, T. K. (2001). Brief introduction of *Panax ginseng* C.A. Meyer. *Journal of Korean Medical Science*, 16: S3-S5.

Yuspa, Stuart H., & Shields, Peter G. (2001). Etiology of cancer: Chemical factors. In Vincent T. DeVita, Jr., Theodore S. Lawrence, & Steven A. Rosenberg (Eds.), Cancer: Principles and practice of oncology (6th ed.), (pp 152-160). Philadelphia: Lippincott Williams & Wilkins. https://oncouasd.files.wordpress.com/2014/09/cancer-principles-and-practice-of-oncology-6e.pdf

_______, and Peter G. Shields. "Etiology of Cancer: Chemical Factors." In *Cancer: Principles and Practice of Oncology*, edited by Vincent T. DeVita, Jr., et al. 6th ed. Philadelphia: Lippincott Williams & Wilkins, 2001.

Zabalegui, A., S. Sanchez, P. D. Sanchez, and C. Juando. "Nursing and Cancer Support Groups." *Journal of Advanced Nursing* 51, no. 4 (2005): 369-381.

Zackheim, Herschel, ed. *Cutaneous T-cell Lymphoma: Mycosis Fungoides and Sézary Syndrome*. Boca Raton, Fla.: CRC Press, 2005.

Zafir-Lavie, I., Y. Michaeli, and Y. Reiter. "Novel Antibodies as Anticancer Agents." *Oncogene* 28 (2007): 3714-3733.

Zambetti, Gerald, (Ed.). (2005). Protein reviews: The p53 tumor suppressor pathway and cancer. New York: Springer.

Zeh, H. "Cancer of the Small Intestine." In *Cancer: Principles and Practice of Oncology*, edited by Vincent T. DeVita, Jr., Samuel Hellman, and Steven A. Rosenberg. 7th ed. Philadelphia: Lippincott Williams & Wilkins, 2005.

Zelman, K.M. (2008). The Buzz on Coffee. *WebMD*. http://www.webmd.com/diet/the-buzz-on-coffee

Zerwekh, Joyce V. *Nursing Care at the End of Life: Palliative Care for Patients and Families*. Philadelphia: F. A. Davis, 2006.

Zhang, L., et al. "Vascular Endothelial Growth Factor Overexpression by Soft-Tissue Sarcoma Cells: Implications for Tumor Growth, Metastasis, and Chemoresistance." *Cancer Research* 66 (2006): 8770-8778.

Zhang, Qunhao. "Complementary and Alternative Medicine in the United States." *Asia Pacific Biotech News* 8, no. 23 (December 1, 2004): 1274-1277.

Ziessman, Harvey A., Janis P. O'Malley, and James H. Thrall. *Nuclear Medicine: The Requisites*. 3rd ed. Philadelphia: Mosby Elsevier, 2006.

Zilberman, Daniel, and Henikoff, Steven. (2007). Genome-wide Analysis of DNA Methylation Patterns. *Development*, 3, 134, 3959-3965.

Zintzaras, E., M. Voulgarelis, and H. M. Moutsopoulos. (2005). The risk of lymphoma development in autoimmune diseases: A meta-analysis. *Archives of Internal Medicine,* 165, 2337-2344.

Zoler, Mitchel L., and Robert Finn. "Drug Update: Gastroesophageal Reflux Disease." *Family Practice News* 32, no. 9 (2002): 25.

Zonderman, Jon, & Shader, Laurel. (2006). *Birth control pills*. New York: Chelsea House.

Zuckerman, Eugenia, and Julie R. Ingelfinger. *Coping with Prednisone (and Other Cortisone-Related Medicines): It May Work Miracles, but How Do You Handle the Side Effects?* 2d ed. New York: St. Martin's Griffin, 2007.

Zuetenhorst, Johanna M., and Babs G. Taal. "Metastatic Carcinoid Tumors: A Clinical Review." *The Oncologist* 10, no. 2 (February, 2005): 123-131.

Zuzelo, Patti R. *Clinical Nurse Specialist Handbook*. Sudbury, Mass.: Jones and Bartlett, 2007.

▶ Index

A page number or range in boldface type indicates that an entire entry devoted to that topic appears in the set. Compounds are listed under their main root (hence, 4-Aminobiphenyl appears under "A").